Asthma, COPD, and Overlap:
A Case-Based Overview of Similarities and Differences

T0133689

Edited by
Jonathan A. Bernstein
Louis-Philippe Boulet
Michael E. Wechsler

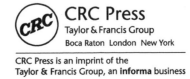

CRC Press
Taylor & Francis Group
Boca Raton London New York

CRC Press is an imprint of the
Taylor & Francis Group, an **informa** business

CRC Press
Taylor & Francis Group
6000 Broken Sound Parkway NW, Suite 300
Boca Raton, FL 33487-2742

© 2018 by Taylor & Francis Group, LLC
CRC Press is an imprint of Taylor & Francis Group, an Informa business

No claim to original U.S. Government works

Printed in Canada on acid-free paper

International Standard Book Number-13: 978-1-4987-5837-6 (Hardback)
978-1-4987-5841-3 (Paperback)

Visit the Taylor & Francis Web site at
http://www.taylorandfrancis.com

and the CRC Press Web site at
http://www.crcpress.com

Asthma, COPD, and Overlap

Dedication

Jonathan A. Bernstein: I would like to dedicate this book to my father, I. Leonard Bernstein, mother, Miriam, and wife, Lisa, who were always my strongest advocates professionally throughout my life. I am also blessed to have four great children, Alison, Joshua, Rebecca, and Caren, two awesome son-in-laws, Danny and Ronnie, and the cutest great grandson, Micah, who all inspire me to enjoy life each and every day.

Louis-Philippe Boulet: I would like to dedicate this book to my wife, Céline, who provided me her most appreciated support throughout my professional life, to my mother Suzanne, and to my wonderful daughters, Véronique and Geneviève, and granddaughters, Éliane and Sophie.

Michael E. Wechsler dedicates this book to his parents, Morris and Ann, and to his wife, Leora, each of whom has provided decades of love, support, and inspiration.

Contents

Preface

...on opening the cavity of the chest, the lungs did not collapse as they usually do when the air is admitted but remained distended, as if they had lost their power of contracting: the air cells on the surface of the trachea were somewhat inflamed.

James Wilson, December 15, 1784. Description of an autopsy finding on Dr. Samuel Johnson who had a history of being "troubled for several years with asthma" (Bailie M. *The Morbid Anatomy of Some of the Most Important Parts of the Human Body*, London: W Bulmer, 1803). Cited by Peter Warren *Canadian Respiratory Journal* 2009;16:14.

Since Hippocrates first used the term "asthma" more than 2000 years ago to describe episodic bouts of dyspnea, to the modern day recognition of the natural history of chronic obstructive pulmonary disease (COPD) detailed in the seminal work of Fletcher and colleagues in 1976 (*The Natural History of Chronic Bronchitis and Emphysema*, New York: Oxford University Press 1976), to the more recent debate about the definition and features of the asthma–COPD overlap, major progress has been made in gaining a better understanding of the characteristics and pathophysiology of obstructive airway diseases.

Unfortunately, asthma, COPD, and overlap are still responsible for an enormous human and socio-economic burden. Asthma is considered to affect more than 300 million individuals worldwide and COPD affects more than 210 million people, although it is still often under-diagnosed. The epidemiology of asthma–COPD overlap is still uncertain but a considerable number of patients who have asthma or COPD demonstrate evidence of this overlap. Allergy and smoking are two main causes of asthma and COPD, respectively; but various other genetic, developmental, and environmental factors have been identified as contributors to these illnesses.

There has been a recent debate about airways diseases taxonomy, as illustrated in the recent publication commissioned by *The Lancet* "After asthma: redefining airways diseases" in 2017. In this article, Pavord et al., suggested how important it is to "deconstruct" airway disease into its components before planning the treatment and focusing on traits that are identifiable and treatable. The recent development of imaging techniques, noninvasive airway inflammation assessment tools, and novel biomarkers can allow such phenotyping, or even better, endotyping of the disease, allowing for a more precise targeting of therapy.

However, in this rapidly changing environment of disease redefinition and progress in our understanding of diseases mechanisms, there is an important need to provide guidance to the clinician who may become confused with these new concepts and sophisticated assessment tools, which unfortunately are frequently not available in primary care settings. When we consider the current care gaps in the management of obstructive airway diseases such as insufficient preventive measures, insufficient use of pulmonary function testing to objectively assess airway obstruction and hyperresponsiveness, the lack of formal patient education on disease self-management and the persistent problem of poor adherence to therapy and follow-up, among other deficiencies, we realize that in many instances, proper care is not being provided, resulting in poor disease control and frequent unnecessary acute healthcare overuse.

We believe however that a good understanding of basic disease mechanisms, development of a practical multidisciplinary approach to patient assessment and treatment, with judicious selection of the most appropriate nonpharmacological and pharmacological therapies for patients with airways diseases could lead to a significant improvement in clinical outcomes, even for those patients presenting with severe disease.

In this book, we benefited from the expertise of world leaders in the field of asthma and COPD who have integrated the most recent evidence from cutting-edge research, into clinical management, using illustrative case examples, algorithms, tables, and figures to facilitate understanding of current concepts and recommendations. It thoroughly reviews similarities and differences between asthma, COPD and the overlap (previously called asthma–COPD overlap syndrome—ACO), regardless of whether one is inclined to accept or refute ACO as a diagnosis.

This book is intended to be a practical guide that will help clinicians distinguish and appreciate overlap nuances between obstructive airway diseases on a pathological and clinical basis, in order to develop appropriate management and treatment plans. We hope it will be useful to all those interested and/or involved in the care of patients with chronic obstructive airway diseases.

Jonathan A. Bernstein
Louis-Philippe Boulet
Michael E. Wechsler

Contributors

Mark H. Almond, MA, MRCP, PhD
Royal Brompton & Harefield NHS Trust
London, United Kingdom

Talya Alsaid-Habia, MA
Deparment of Psychology
University of Cincinnati
Cincinnati, Ohio

Kristina L. Bailey, MD
Department of Internal Medicine
Division of Pulmonary, Critical Care, Sleep & Allergy
University of Nebraska Medical Center
Omaha, Nebraska

Charles S. Barnes, PhD
Section of Allergy/Asthma/Immunology
Children's Mercy Kansas City
Kansas City, Missouri

Louis-Philippe Boulet, MD, FRCPC
Institut universitaire de cardiologie et de
   pneumologie de Québec (IUCPQ)
Université Laval
Québec, Canada

A. Bourdin, MD PhD
Department of Respiratory Diseases Montpellier
University Hospitals
Montpellier, France

Stephen Bujarski, MD
Section of Pulmonary and Critical Care Medicine
Baylor College of Medicine
Houston, Texas

Robert Busch, MD, MMSc
Channing Division of Network Medicine
Brigham and Women's Hospital and Harvard Medical
   School
Boston, Massachusetts

Thomas Casale, MD
Department of Internal Medicine
University of South Florida Morsani College of Medicine
Tampa, Florida

Pascal Chanez, MD PhD
Department of Respiratory Diseases
Aix-Marseille University
Marseille, France

Stephanie Christenson, MD, MAS
Department of Medicine
Division of Pulmonary Critical Care, Allergy and Sleep Medicine
University of California, San Francisco
San Francisco, California

Kian Fan Chung, MD, DSc, FRCP
Royal Brompton & Harefield NHS Trust
National Heart & Lung Institute
Imperial College London
London, United Kingdom

Gennaro D'Amato, MD, FAAAAI, FERS
Division of Respiratory and Allergic Diseases
Department of Respiratory Diseases
High Specialty A. Cardarelli Hospital
and
School of Specialization in Respiratory Diseases
University of Naples Federico II
Napoli, Italy

Maria D'Amato, MD
First Division of Pneumology
High Speciality Hospital "V. Monaldi"
and
University "Federico II" Medical School
Napoli, Italy

Angira Dasgupta, MD, MRCP (UK)
Department of Medicine
St. Joseph's Healthcare
and
McMaster University
Hamilton, Ontario, Canada

Max Feldman, MD
Department of Internal Medicine
University of South Florida Morsani College of Medicine
Tampa, Florida

Anne L. Fuhlbrigge, MDMS
Division of Pulmonary Sciences and Critical Care Medicine
University of Colorado School of Medicine
Aurora, Colorado

Arthur F. Gelb, MD
From the Pulmonary Division
Department of Medicine
Lakewood Regional Medical Center (LRMC)
Lakewood, California
and
Geffen School of Medicine at UCLA Medical Center
Los Angeles, California

Peter G. Gibson, MBBS, FRACP, FAPSR, FAAHMS
Centre of Excellence in Severe Asthma and Priority
    Research Centre for Healthy Lungs
University of Newcastle
Hunter Medical Research Institute
Newcastle, Australia

Krystelle Godbout, MD, FRCPC
Quebec Heart and Lung Institute
Laval University
Quebec, Canada

Qutayba Hamid, MD, PhD, MRCP (UK), FRCP (Canada), FRC Path. FRS
College of Medicine
University of Sharjah
Sharjah, United Arab Emirates

Nicola A. Hanania, MD, MS
Section of Pulmonary and Critical Care Medicine
Baylor College of Medicine
Houston, Texas

Craig P. Hersh, MD, MPH
Channing Division of Network Medicine
Brigham and Women's Hospital and Harvard Medical
    School
Boston, Massachusetts

Charles G. Irvin, PhD, FERS
Vermont Lung Center
Department of Medicine
University of Vermont
Burlington, Vermont

Adrienne L. Johnson, PhD
Department of Psychology
University of Cincinnati
Cincinnati, Ohio

David A. Kaminsky, MD
Vermont Lung Center
Department of Medicine
University of Vermont
Burlington, Vermont

Robert Ledford, MD
Department of Internal Medicine
University of South Florida Morsani College of
    Medicine
Tampa, Florida

Mark L. Levy, MBChB (Pret) FRCGP
Kenton Bridge Medical Centre
Harrow, United Kingdom

Bassam Mahboub, MBBS, FRCPC
College of Medicine
University of Sharjah
Sharjah, United Arab Emirates

Lisa A. Maier, MD, MSPH
Division of Environmental and Occupational Health
    Sciences
Department of Medicine
National Jewish Health
and
Department of Medicine, School of Medicine
Environmental and Occupational Health Department
Colorado School of Public Health
University of Colorado
Denver, Colorado

François Maltais, MD, FRCPC
Institut universitaire de cardiologie et de
    pneumologie de Québec (IUCPQ)
Université Laval
Québec, Canada

Christine F. McDonald, MBBS, PhD
Department of Respiratory & Sleep Medicine
Institute for Breathing & Sleep
Austin Hospital
University of Melbourne
Victoria, Australia

Vanessa M. McDonald, DipHlthScien (Nurs), BNurs, PhD
Centre of Excellence in Severe Asthma and Priority
    Research Centre for Healthy Lungs
University of Newcastle
Hunter Medical Research Institute
Newcastle, Australia

Alison C. McLeish, PhD
Department of Psychological and Brain Sciences
University of Louisville
Louisville, Kentucky

Antonio Molino, MD
First Division of Pneumology
High Speciality Hospital "V. Monaldi"
and
University "Federico II" Medical School
Napoli, Italy

Jay A. Nadel, MD
Departments of Medicine, Physiology
Radiology, and Cardiovascular Research Institute
University of California
San Francisco, California

Parameswaran Nair, MD, PhD, FRCP, FRCPC
Department of Medicine
St. Joseph's Healthcare
and
McMaster University
Hamilton, Ontario, Canada

Amber J. Oberle, MD
Division of Pulmonary
Allergy & Critical Care Medicine
Duke University School of Medicine
Durham, North Carolina

Karin A. Pacheco, MD, MSPH
Division of Environmental and Occupational Health
    Sciences
Department of Medicine
National Jewish Health
and
Environmental and Occupational Health Department
Colorado School of Public Health
University of Colorado
Denver, Colorado

Laurie Pahus, PharmD
Department of Respiratory Diseases
Aix-Marseille University
Marseille, France

Alain Palot, MD
Department of Respiratory Diseases
Aix-Marseille University
Marseille, France

Ralph J. Panos, MD
Department of Medicine
Division of Pulmonary, Critical Care, and Sleep Medicine
Cincinnati Veteran Affairs Medical Center
University of Cincinnati College of Medicine
Cincinnati, Ohio

Amit Parulekar, MD, MS
Section of Pulmonary and Critical Care Medicine
Baylor College of Medicine
Houston, Texas

Rakhee K. Ramakrishnan, MSc
College of Medicine
University of Sharjah
Sharjah, United Arab Emirates

Brian H. Rowe, MD, MSc, CCFP(EM), FCCP, FCAHS
Institute of Circulatory and Respiratory Health (ICRH)
Canadian Institutes of Health Research (CIHR)
and
Department of Emergency Medicine
University of Alberta
Edmonton, Alberta, Canada

Svien A. Senne, MD
Department of Internal Medicine
Division of Pulmonary, Critical Care, Sleep & Allergy
University of Nebraska Medical Center
Omaha, Nebraska

Don D. Sin, MD, MPH
Centre for Heart Lung Innovation
St. Paul's Hospital & Department of Medicine (Division of
    Respiratory Medicine)
University of British Columbia (UBC) Vancouver
    British Columbia, Canada

Neil C. Thomson, MD, FRCP, FERS
Institute of Infection, Immunity & Inflammation
University of Glasgow
Glasgow, United Kingdom

Diane Tissier-Ducamp, MD
Department of Respiratory Diseases
Aix-Marseille University
Marseille, France

Céline Tummino, MD
Department of Respiratory Diseases
Aix-Marseille University
Marseille, France

Cristina Villa-Roel, MD, MSc, PhD
Department of Emergency Medicine
University of Alberta
Edmonton, Alberta, Canada

Carolina Vitale, MD
First Division of Pneumology
High Speciality Hospital "V. Monaldi"
and
University "Federico II" Medical School
Napoli, Italy

Definitions of asthma and COPD and overlap

KRYSTELLE GODBOUT, VANESSA M. MCDONALD, AND PETER G. GIBSON

1.1 INTRODUCTION

Asthma and chronic obstructive pulmonary disease (COPD) are the two most prevalent chronic respiratory diseases and are therefore frequently encountered by clinicians. Although considered distinct diseases, overlap in the features of these two conditions is increasingly recognized, making straightforward distinction more challenging. Clinicians who manage patients with overlapping features of asthma and COPD struggle with a lack of evidence to guide them in obtaining a diagnosis and selecting a therapy. Recent guidelines have attempted to address this problem.[1-3] The criteria proposed by these latest guidelines and how they perform when applied to real-world patients are addressed in this chapter.

1.2 ASTHMA AND COPD

Asthma and COPD have been recognized and described for several centuries. The definitions have however dramatically evolved since the 1990s as our knowledge of the diseases increased. The most significant change probably lies in the recognition of chronic airway inflammation as a crucial feature in the pathophysiology of both diseases and its further measurement in clinical practice.

Several definitions arising from respiratory societies now exist for both asthma and COPD, but none is clearly superior to another. Definitions from the strategy documents of the Global Initiative for Asthma (GINA) and the Global Initiative for Chronic Obstructive Lung Disease (GOLD) are shown below.

Definition of asthma

Asthma is a heterogeneous disease, usually characterized by chronic airway inflammation. It is defined by the history of respiratory symptoms such as wheeze, shortness of breath, chest tightness and cough that vary over time and in intensity, together with variable airflow limitation.[4]

Definition of COPD

COPD, a common preventable and treatable disease, is characterized by persistent airflow limitation that is usually progressive and associated with an enhanced chronic inflammatory response in the airway and the lung to noxious particles or gases. Exacerbations and comorbidities contribute to the overall severity in individual patients.[5]

The terms chronic bronchitis and emphysema were previously included in the definition of COPD[6] but were abandoned in the first GOLD strategy documents in 2001 to be regarded as phenotypes of COPD. However, they also exist as independent disorders when they are identified without the presence of the fixed airflow limitation necessary for the diagnosis of COPD (Figure 1.1). Emphysema is diagnosed on pathology or radiology and is characterized by an abnormal permanent enlargement of the airspaces

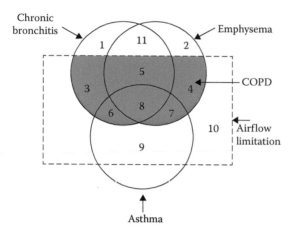

Figure 1.1 Nonproportional Venn diagram of COPD showing subsets of patients with chronic bronchitis, emphysema, and asthma produced by the American Thoracic Society.[6] The subsets comprising COPD are shaded. Subset areas are not proportional to actual relative subset sizes. Asthma is by definition associated with reversible airflow obstruction, although in variant asthma special maneuvers may be necessary to make the obstruction evident. Patients with asthma whose airflow obstruction is completely reversible (subset 9) are not considered to have COPD. Because in many cases it is virtually impossible to differentiate patients with asthma whose airflow obstruction does not remit completely from persons with chronic bronchitis and emphysema who have partially reversible airflow obstruction with airway hyperreactivity, patients with unremitting asthma are classified as having COPD (subsets 6, 7, and 8). Chronic bronchitis and emphysema with airflow obstruction usually occur together (subset 5), and some patients may have asthma associated with these two disorders (subset 8). Individuals with asthma exposed to chronic irritation, as from cigarette smoke, may develop chronic productive cough, a feature of chronic bronchitis (subset 6). Such patients are often referred to in the United States as having asthmatic bronchitis or the asthmatic form of COPD. Persons with chronic bronchitis and/or emphysema without airflow obstruction (subsets 1, 2, and 11) are not classified as having COPD. Patients with airway obstruction due to diseases with known etiology or specific pathology, such as cystic fibrosis or obliterative bronchiolitis (subset 10), are not included in this definition.

(Reprinted with permission of the American Thoracic Society. Copyright ©2016 American Thoracic Society. From Standards for the diagnosis and care of patients with chronic obstructive pulmonary disease. *Am J Respir Crit Care Med* 152(5), S77–121, 1995.)

distal to the terminal bronchioles.[6] Chronic bronchitis on the other hand is a clinical diagnosis identified by the presence of cough and sputum production for at least 3 months per year during two consecutive years.[6]

1.2.1 TRADITIONAL METHOD FOR DEFINITION AND DIAGNOSIS

As the exact mechanisms leading to the development of asthma and COPD remain unknown, their definitions are syndromic, stressing the typical characteristics seen in each disease. These features, summarized in Table 1.1, also serve to distinguish between the two disorders in clinical practice.

However, the reality is that asthma and COPD are heterogeneous diseases and few patients display all features. For example, asthmatics may not demonstrate the typical eosinophilic airway inflammation or airway hyperresponsiveness (AHR) seen in asthma.[2] Furthermore, no feature is specific for only one disease, and there is considerable overlap between the two diseases. Therefore, relying on these nonspecific characteristics for diagnosis may lead to diagnostic inaccuracies (Table 1.2).

1.2.2 DIAGNOSTIC CRITERIA FOR ASTHMA AND COPD

Despite their overlapping features, clinical-practice guidelines have developed criteria to help distinguish between asthma and COPD. Many respiratory societies have published their own criteria but they usually involve the same phenotypic characteristics. For asthma, its definition consists of the association of compatible symptoms and variable airflow limitation (Table 1.3). The diagnosis of COPD on the other hand only requires the demonstration of chronic airflow limitation, although it is suspected on clinical grounds by chronic respiratory symptoms, history of exposure to a risk factor, and family history of COPD. GOLD strategy recommend the use of a fixed post-bronchodilator (BD) forced expiratory volume in one second/ forced vital capacity (FEV_1/FVC) ratio lower than 0.7 for a diagnosis of COPD.[5]

1.3 OVERLAP OF ASTHMA AND COPD: A NEW ENTITY?

As mentioned above, asthma and COPD share several phenotypic features and are frequently difficult to differentiate in clinical practice, although traditionally considered as distinct entities in guidelines. Coexistence of the two obstructive diseases has been recognized for decades as illustrated in the Venn diagram from the 1995 American Thoracic Society (ATS) COPD guidelines (Figure 1.1). However, this topic received little attention until recently, when the scientific community took interest in phenotyping of asthma and COPD. Since then, the subject has been extensively reviewed,[7–10] and most studies on obstructive diseases now

Table 1.1 Clinical and physiological characteristics of asthma, COPD, and ACO

Features	Asthma	COPD	ACO
Airway inflammation	Predominantly eosinophilic	Predominantly neutrophilic	Eosinophilic and/or neutrophilic[11,12]
Symptoms	Circadian variability	Constant with day to day variation	More wheezing and dyspnea than asthma or COPD[13]
	Triggered by a variety of stimuli	Exertional	Conflicting data about cough and phlegm[13]
Past history	Allergies	Exposure to noxious particles or gases	Smoking common[9] and necessary for diagnosis in some studies[12,14–17]
	Family history of asthma and atopy	Family history of COPD	Atopy more common than in COPD[7,10,14]
Lung function and AHR	Variable airflow limitation	Chronic airflow limitation	Chronic airflow limitation similar to COPD[9]
	Hyperresponsiveness		Significant BDR in less than half[7,14,18,19]
			AHR very common and more severe than in asthma[20]
Exacerbation and comorbidities	Exacerbations occur	Comorbidities and exacerbations contribute to impairment	Exacerbations more frequent and severe than in asthma and COPD[9,13]
		Systemic inflammation	Systemic inflammation[21,22]
			Comorbidities usually present[7,13]

Note: AHR, airway hyperresponsiveness; BDR, bronchodilator reversibility.

recognize the overlap as a specific phenotype of asthma and COPD. Their overlap is also increasingly considered as a separate entity and the term asthma-COPD overlap (ACO) has been widely adopted to describe it.

1.3.1 RELEVANCE OF IDENTIFYING AND DEFINING ACO

We may question the importance of recognizing ACO independently from asthma and COPD in clinical practice. First, the literature has shown that the overlap between asthma and COPD is common, affecting 20% of patients with obstructive airway disease and 2% of the general population.[7] Clinical findings regarding ACO are then relevant for a large proportion of patients identified with airflow limitation. Furthermore, studies have consistently shown that ACO is associated with a greater morbidity and worse prognosis compared with asthma or COPD alone, emphasizing an increased need to recognize and treat these patients earlier in the course of disease to improve their clinical outcomes. Finally, the response to treatment in this large subgroup of obstructive airway disease is unknown, as they have been excluded from large randomized-control trials in asthma and COPD. The potential benefits and harms of medication, particularly long-actingβ-2-agonists (LABA) and inhaled corticosteroids (ICS), could be different from other obstructive airway diseases.

1.3.2 DEFINITIONS ARISING FROM STUDIES

Currently, one major problem with ACO lies in the absence of a widely accepted definition. The concept is that ACO is the coexistence of both asthma and COPD in the same patient. Evidence of irreversible airflow limitation, which is the key diagnostic criterion of COPD, seems to be well accepted. Apart from clinical feature, no other characteristic has been widely accepted for its inclusion in the definition of ACO. Consequently, definitions used for ACO vary among studies, although they usually fall in one of three classification schemes illustrated in Figure 1.2.[8]

In addition to these criteria, some studies also require a significant smoking history or evidence of emphysema for the diagnosis of ACO. As a result, there is considerable heterogeneity in the studied populations, making any results difficult to generalize and apply to clinical practice.

1.3.3 SELECTING CHARACTERISTICS FOR DEFINING ACO

To better describe and define ACO, its clinical and physiological features have been studied, often plotting them against those of asthma and COPD alone to highlight differences. Table 1.1 displays a summary of the findings.

Table 1.2 Issues with using the typical clinical and physiological features to differentiate between asthma and COPD

Features	Problems in differentiating asthma and COPD
Airway inflammation	Heterogeneity in inflammation occurs in both diseases
	Eosinophilic COPD and neutrophilic asthma frequently encountered[11,23]
Age of onset	Asthma can start anytime in life
	e.g., late onset non allergic asthma, occupational asthma
Symptoms	May be specific to the underlying pathophysiological component rather than the diagnosis
	e.g., mucus hypersecretion (chronic bronchitis) can occur in asthma
Atopy	Association with atopy is weak in adult-onset asthma[24,25]
	Atopy occurs in around 20% of COPD[26,27]
Smoking	25%–45% of COPD patients are never smokers[28]
Lung function and AHR	A subgroup of asthmatics develop chronic airflow limitation, particularly in severe, long standing asthma[29]
	BDR and AHR are common in COPD[30]
Disease course	Some asthmatics experience a steep rate of decline in FEV_1 despite treatment[31]
	High proportion of COPD show stable lung function[32]

Note: AHR, airway hyperresponsiveness; BDR, bronchodilator response.

Table 1.3 Diagnostic criteria for asthma from GINA[4]

Criteria for asthma diagnosis

Variable respiratory symptoms
Wheezing
Shortness of breath
Chest tightness
Cough

Airflow limitation
Reduced FEV_1/FVC (< 0.75–0.8 in adults) at least once

Excessive variability in lung function
Positive bronchodilator reversibility test
Excessive variability in PEF
Increase in lung function with treatment
Positive exercise challenge test
Positive bronchial challenge test
Excessive variation in lung function between visits

Note: PEF, peak expiratory flow.

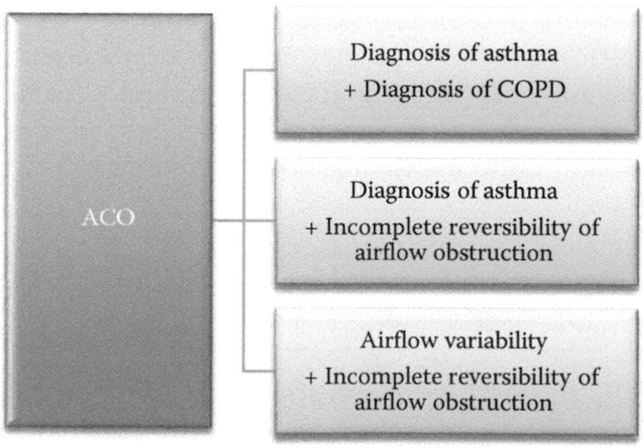

Figure 1.2 ACO definitions used in studies.

Needless to say, the clinical characteristics of the studied ACO populations are influenced by the definition used for its identification and the population it is derived from (i.e, asthma with features of COPD or COPD with features of asthma).[7] Nevertheless, the phenotypic characteristics of patients with ACO include features of both, with the exception of exacerbations, which tend to be more frequent and severe in ACO populations.

An alternate way of defining ACO is to select phenotypic features that can predict the different risk, quality of life, and treatment response seen in ACO. Bronchodilator reversibility (BDR) has proven ineffective in detecting asthma in patients with COPD.[1] It is also is not reproducible, not related to other asthma features,[33] and does not predict ICS responsiveness in this population.[34] However, ICS responsiveness was predicted by a high sputum eosinophil count, which also proved to be a useful marker to detect COPD patients with asthma.[17] Fraction of exhaled nitric oxide (FeNO) failed to demonstrate the same results.[35] As for chronic airflow limitation, it was shown to be predictive of an enhanced response to long-acting muscarinic antagonists (LAMA) in patients with asthma.[36,37] Given these results, it may be concluded that sputum eosinophilia and fixed airflow limitation are useful criteria for defining ACO in a way BDR and FeNO are not.

1.3.4 DEFINITIONS AND CRITERIA ARISING FROM GUIDELINES

Despite the lack of high quality evidence, some respiratory societies have proposed criteria to diagnose ACO in clinical practice guidelines. In 2012 the respiratory community in Spain was the first to publish a consensus statement specifically on the subject of the asthma-COPD overlap phenotype in COPD.[1] Diagnostic criteria for ACO were developed by selecting statements that reached a level of agreement of more than 70% among COPD experts in the country (Table 1.4). These Spanish criteria were also adopted by the Finnish Respiratory Society in their latest COPD guidelines, in which ACO was given special attention.[38] However, they added "typical PEF" (peak expiratory flow) as a minor criterion.

GINA and GOLD since joined forces in 2014 in order to release a consensus document for patients presenting with chronic airway disease, including ACO as a specific entity.[2] The strategy documents include a descriptive definition of ACO:

ACO definition from GINA/GOLD consensus document

Asthma-COPD overlap (ACO) is characterized by persistent airflow limitation with several features usually associated with asthma and several features usually associated with COPD. ACO is therefore identified in clinical practice by the features that it shares with both asthma and COPD.

A specific definition for ACO cannot be developed until more evidence is available about its clinical phenotypes and underlying mechanisms.[2]

Table 1.4 Diagnostic criteria for asthma-COPD overlap from the Spanish consensus Statement and the Czech Pneumological and Phthisiological Society

Spanish	Czech
DEFINITE DIAGNOSIS OF COPD	
Not specified	$FEV_1/FVC < LLN$
MAJOR CRITERIA	
Very positive bronchodilator test ($\uparrow FEV_1 \geq 15\%$ and ≥ 400 mL)	Very positive bronchodilator test ($\uparrow FEV_1 \geq 15\%$ and ≥ 400 mL)
Eosinophilia in sputum (threshold not specified)	Sputum eosinophils $\geq 3\%$ and/or FENO ≥ 45–50 ppb
Personal history of asthma before the age of 40	Personal history of asthma
	Positive bronchial challenge test
MINOR CRITERIA	
Positive bronchodilator test ($\uparrow FEV_1 \geq 12\%$ and ≥ 200 mL)	Positive bronchodilator test ($\uparrow FEV_1 \geq 12\%$ and ≥ 200 mL)
High total IgE	High total IgE
Personal history of atopy	Personal history of atopy

Note: ACO is confirmed by the presence of 2 major criteria or 1 major plus 2 minor criteria in addition to a COPD diagnosis. FeNO, fraction of exhaled nitric oxide; IgE, Immunoglobulin E; LLN, lower limit of normal values.

Because the GINA/GOLD task force was unable to clearly identify criteria for the diagnosis of ACO, they developed a syndromic approach to be applied after an initial evaluation confirming the presence of chronic airway disease. The method involves a comparison of classical clinical features of asthma and COPD present in the same patient (Table 1.5). Three or more features of one disease provides a high likelihood of the correct diagnosis and if there are a similar number of asthma and COPD features, then the overlap of asthma-COPD overlap can be considered. Spirometry is recommended afterward to confirm the diagnosis of obstructive disease. The result of this test serves as support for the diagnosis made with the syndromic approach, as no spirometric finding is specific for either disease.

The Czech COPD guidelines of 2013 also included an asthma-COPD phenotype diagnosed with the criteria presented in Table 1.4.[3] These criteria are similar to those of the Spanish consensus statement, with the addition of AHR and FeNO as features for diagnosis.

The current guidelines do not identify pathognomonic criteria for ACO, but rather list features that increase the probability of diagnosis of asthma, COPD, or ACO. There are similarities between most of these guidelines, which suggest some consensus between international bodies on how to diagnose ACO.

1.4 CLINICAL VIGNETTES

The utility of the guidelines for the diagnosis of ACO can best be assessed by their application to real-life clinical vignettes. We present four clinical scenarios of patients with obstructive airway diseases referred to a specialist clinic. These clinical vignettes are real world and illustrate difficulties or issues encountered when attempting to classify airway diseases.

CLINICAL VIGNETTE 1.1: A MALE PATIENT WITH ASTHMA AND A SIGNIFICANT SMOKING HISTORY

A 53-year-old male with a diagnosis of atopic asthma since age two presents to clinic as a result of worsening symptoms. In the last 3 years, he noticed an increase in his exertional dyspnea and is now bothered by a daily production of white phlegm. A short-acting β-agonist (SABA) provides only minimal symptom relief.

He is a former cigarette smoker with a history of 18 pack years, and he currently smokes marijuana twice weekly. He is prescribed a combination ICS/LABA, LAMA, and SABA for asthma; a nasal corticosteroid spray for allergic rhinitis; and a proton pump inhibitor for gastroesophageal reflux.

Atopy was previously confirmed by positive skin prick tests and an elevated total Immunoglobulin E (IgE) (234 kU/L). Centrilobular emphysema was found on a former CT-scan but the current chest X-ray is normal. His spirometry shows severe obstruction without improvement post-BD (post-BD FEV$_1$ 1.06 L [32%] and FEV$_1$/FVC [33%]). Sputum induction was performed, which provoked a 53% fall in FEV$_1$ after 2.5 minutes on hypertonic saline, confirming AHR. The sputum cell counts were normal (2.75% eosinophils and 47% neutrophils) suggesting a paucigranulocytic inflammatory phenotype. A FeNO was normal at 11.8 ppb.

CLINICAL VIGNETTE 1.2: A FEMALE WITH LONG-STANDING ASTHMA AND CHRONIC AIRFLOW LIMITATION

A 70-year-old woman presents to the clinic following an increase in her respiratory symptoms over the last 5 years. She is now severely dyspneic and has a chronic cough productive of white phlegm. The symptoms are worse at night, and they increase with cold air and dust exposure.

She was diagnosed with asthma at age 5 and has been treated for this condition ever since. She is currently on a combination ICS/LABA, LAMA, SABA, and a daily macrolide antibiotic, azithromycin. She has never smoked nor did she have significant passive smoke exposure as a child.

She has symptoms of allergic rhinitis with positive skin prick tests to house dust mite and elevated total IgE (334 kU/L). Her spirometry demonstrates moderate airflow obstruction without significant improvement post-BD (post-BD FEV$_1$ 1.10 L [53%] and FEV$_1$/FVC [48%]). A hypertonic saline challenge was positive. Sputum eosinophils were increased (4.5%) and a FeNO was increased (68 ppb) consistent with eosinophilic airway inflammation.

CLINICAL VIGNETTE 1.3: A FEMALE COPD PATIENT WITH EOSINOPHILIC INFLAMMATION

A 62-year-old female is referred for a new onset of cough, wheezing and shortness of breath following a hospitalization for pneumonia, 2 months ago. The symptoms are worse early in the morning and often wake her up at night.

One year ago, she was found to have abnormal lung function during a preoperative assessment for a knee replacement (spirometry unavailable). She was put on a LAMA and SABA despite being asymptomatic at the time. Subsequently she stopped smoking but her history was significant for 77 pack years. She has no personal history of asthma, atopy, or previous respiratory difficulties.

Her current spirometry demonstrated a severe obstructive defect (pre-BD FEV$_1$ 1.01 L [48%] and FEV$_1$/FVC [60%]) with a significant increase in her FEV$_1$ of 300 mL or 29% post-BD (post-BD FEV$_1$ 1.31 L [61%] and FEV$_1$/FVC [66%]). Her DLCO is low at 71%. Sputum induction provoked a 17% drop in FEV$_1$ after 1.5 minutes on hypertonic saline, consistent with AHR. The sputum analysis revealed an eosinophilic bronchitis with 35% eosinophils. Her blood eosinophils were also elevated at 1000/microL but her FeNO was normal at 13 ppb.

CLINICAL VIGNETTE 1.4: AN OLDER FEMALE WITH VARIABLE AIRFLOW LIMITATION

A 72-year-old female presents with intermittent breathlessness without other respiratory symptoms. She reports no diurnal variation in her symptoms but they are more severe in spring and triggered by smoke exposure.

She was diagnosed with asthma at age 60 based on a spirometry, which demonstrated a 29% increase in FEV$_1$ post-BD (pre-BD FEV$_1$ 1.64 L [64%] and FEV$_1$/FVC [33%]; post-BD FEV$_1$ 2.11 L [82%] and FEV$_1$/FVC [63%]). She is currently treated with a combination ICS/LABA and SABA. She has no history of smoking or passive smoke exposure.

Her current spirometry shows a normal FEV$_1$ (2.22 L [91%]) with a FEV$_1$/FVC ratio of 67% (only post-BD spirometry available). She is nonatopic (skin prick tests negative and total IgE 27 kU/L). She was unable to produce sputum for analysis, but her FeNO was 26 ppb.

1.5 APPLYING DEFINITIONS TO CLINICAL VIGNETTES AND RELATED ISSUES

The diagnostic criteria of asthma, COPD, and ACO presented were applied to the clinical vignettes. Results are shown in Table 1.6.

Despite some clear differences, all clinical vignettes were classified as having both asthma and COPD by the respective GINA and GOLD strategy documents. This is because the definitions of airway diseases were developed to have a high sensitivity, at the expense of their specificity. Patients fitted under one definition consequently form a heterogeneous population, with diverse clinical characteristics, prognosis, and

Table 1.5 Syndromic diagnosis of airway diseases according to GINA/GOLD

Feature	More likely to be asthma if several of	More likely to be COPD if several of
Age of onset	• Onset before age 20 years	• Onset after age 40 years
Pattern of respiratory symptoms	• Variation in symptoms over minutes, hours, or days • Symptoms worse during the night or early morning • Symptoms triggered by exercise, emotions including laughter, dust, or exposure to allergens	• Persistence of symptoms despite treatment • Good and bad days but always daily symptoms and exertional dyspnea • Chronic cough and sputum preceded onset of dyspnea, unrelated to triggers
Lung function	• Record of variable airflow limitation (spirometry, peak flow)	• Record of persistent airflow limitation (post-bronchodilator $FEV_1/FVC < 0.7$)
Lung function between symptoms	• Lung function normal between symptoms	• Lung function abnormal between symptoms
Past history or family history	• Previous doctor diagnosis of asthma • Family history of asthma, and other allergic conditions (allergic rhinitis or eczema)	• Previous doctor diagnosis of COPD, chronic bronchitis or emphysema • Heavy exposure to a risk factor: tobacco smoke, biomass fuels
Time course	• No worsening of symptoms over time. Symptoms vary either seasonally, or from year to year • May improve spontaneously or have an immediate response to BD or to ICS over weeks	• Symptoms slowly worsening over time (progressive course over years) • Rapid-acting bronchodilator treatment provides only limited relief
Chest X-ray	• Normal	• Severe hyperinflation

Source: Data from Global Initiative for Asthma (GINA) and Global Initiative for Chronic Obstructive Lung Disease (GOLD). "Diagnosis of Diseases of Chronic Airflow Limitation: Asthma, COPD and Asthma-COPD Overlap (ACO)" 2015. Available at *http://www.ginasthma.org/*. With permission.

Table 1.6 Diagnostic criteria applied to clinical vignettes

	Asthma Dx GINA	COPD Dx GOLD	ACO Dx		
			Spanish	GINA/GOLD	Czech
Clinical vignette 1.1	POSITIVE	POSITIVE	1–2 majors,[a] 2 minors	5 asthma	2 majors, 2 minors
			POSITIVE	7 COPD (COPD)	POSITIVE
Clinical vignette 1.2	POSITIVE	POSITIVE	2 majors, 2 minors	6 asthma	3 majors, 3 minors
			POSITIVE	5 COPD (ASTHMA)	POSITIVE
Clinical vignette 1.3	POSITIVE	POSITIVE	1 major, 1 minor	4 asthma	2 majors, 1 minor
			NEGATIVE (COPD)	6 COPD (COPD)	POSITIVE
Clinical vignette 1.4	POSITIVE	POSITIVE	1 major, 1 minor	6 asthma	2 majors and 1 minor but no definite diagnosis of COPD[b]
			NEGATIVE (COPD)	3 COPD (ASTHMA)	NEGATIVE (ASTHMA)

Note: Criteria for asthma, COPD and ACO were applied to the clinical vignettes. When the criteria for ACO were not met, the diagnosis (asthma or CPOD) was given in parenthesis.

[a] The Spanish consensus statement does not specify their sputum eosinophilia threshold, which varies between 2% and 3% according to references. We could therefore not determine whether 2.75% was a positive criterion.

[b] The Czech guidelines require an $FEV_1/FVC < LLN$ (lower limit of normal) to diagnose COPD.

treatment responses. This lack of specificity earned asthma and COPD the designation "umbrella terms." ACO is no different, usually including three separate phenotypes: COPD with features of asthma (Clinical vignette 1.3), asthma with current or past history of smoking (Clinical vignette 1.1), and long-standing asthma with partially reversible airflow limitation (Clinical vignette 1.2). The suitability of reclassifying these various phenotypes with likely different underlying pathophysiology under a single definition is unclear. In particular, the inclusion of the group with long-standing asthma and no history of smoking or exposure to noxious particles has been debated. Although it is generally accepted as an ACO phenotype, some still prefer the use of a distinctive denomination, such as irreversible asthma or asthma with chronic obstruction.[39]

However, if all the above clinical vignettes had a diagnosis of both asthma and COPD, none of them were categorized as having ACO with all the definitions (Table 1.6). This shows that diagnosing ACO is more complex than the mere demonstration of concurrent variable airflow limitation (in keeping with GINA diagnosis of asthma) and fixed airflow limitation (GOLD diagnosis of COPD), a definition frequently used for ACO in recent studies. Other features of asthma (patterns of symptoms, inflammation, associated conditions, risk factors) must be considered to establish a real overlap diagnosis. This is largely explained by the lack of specificity of variable airflow limitation in the COPD population (Table 1.2), where it does not necessarily represent an asthmatic phenotype.[33]

There has also been disagreement between the different set of criteria for ACO (Table 1.6), illustrating the imprecision in the current ACO definition and the resulting inconsistency in the existing diagnostic sets.

In the case of the GINA/GOLD syndromic approach, no case achieved a diagnosis of ACO (considered when there is an equal number of asthma and COPD characteristics) even though all the cases had three or more features of asthma and COPD, making both diagnoses likely. This finding highlights the principal weakness of the GINA/GOLD approach: the equal weight given to each feature in predicting the diagnosis of asthma and COPD. Yet, COPD is principally associated with age and smoking,[40] and eczema and familial asthma are strongest predictors for asthma.[41] The GINA/GOLD approach however has the advantage of requiring no specialized testing. With the two other sets of diagnostic criteria (Spanish and Czech), long-standing asthmatics with chronic airflow limitation achieved more stability in their diagnoses (Clinical vignettes 1.1 and 1.2) than those presenting with late onset of symptoms (Clinical vignettes 1.3 and 1.4), once again highlighting the complexity in defining the asthmatic phenotype in the COPD population.

Making the diagnosis of chronic airflow limitation lies in the demonstration of a low FEV_1/FVC ratio. However, this ratio falls with age, making the distinction between normality and obstruction more difficult in older patients. Using a fixed FEV_1/FVC ratio as advised by GOLD strategy documents has been linked to over diagnosis in healthy older adults,[42,43]

but also under diagnosis in the young adult population.[44] To avoid these diagnostic inaccuracies, some respiratory societies, like the ATS and ERS advise using the lower limit of normal threshold (fifth centile of a normal population) as diagnostic of airflow limitation.[45] However, there is currently no literature supporting the superiority of this method that can also lead to underdiagnosis.[46] Clinical vignette 1.4 illustrated how this area of uncertainty may affect the diagnosis of airway disease. In this clinical vignette, the post-BD FEV_1/FVC of 67% is above the lower limit of normal values (LLN) (66% in that case) but below 70%. The patient was thus classified as having COPD by the GOLD criteria but not by the Czech guidelines that use the LLN threshold. Missing the COPD diagnostic criteria, she could not be classified as having ACO despite filling the other Czech criteria (Table 1.6).

1.6 ASTHMA, COPD, OR ACO, DOES IT MATTER?

We have presented how airway diseases are currently classified, the imprecision in their definitions, and the sometimes difficult task of making a specific diagnosis. Given the limitations, one question is to be asked: Does making the distinction matter?

The purpose of accurately categorizing patients with airway disease is to select the appropriate treatment, predict the evolution, and define a group for research. However, the heterogeneity and complexity of the populations selected with the current definitions make these objectives difficult to achieve. The emergence of ACO as a unique clinical entity aimed to address these issues. However, ACO is still poorly defined and is likely as heterogeneous as asthma and COPD diagnoses alone. Therefore, existing classifications only partially resolves issues pertaining to the ACO definition.

A revised taxonomy of obstructive airway disease is needed, although the best classification method is still subject to debate. One widespread approach consists in further dividing asthma and COPD in clusters with shared biological mechanisms, whether confirmed or hypothesized. This approach using phenotypes and endotypes will be further discussed in Chapter 12.

Another strategy recently put forward is to consider airway diseases as a continuum with possible shared biological mechanisms, therefore abandoning the labels of asthma, COPD, and ACO. This approach, far from new, was first advanced more than 50 years ago in what would later become the Dutch hypothesis. Based on the hypothesis that asthma and COPD share common origins with expression modulated by endogenous (age and sex) and exogenous (environmental) factors, Orie and colleagues recommended a broader vision of airway diseases, unhampered by the diagnostic labels of asthma and COPD.[47] They suggested the use of a single generic term (chronic nonspecific lung disease) for airway diseases with further characterization using predetermined phenotypic features. The concept was recently modernized by the present authors[22,48,49] and later by Agusti et al., who suggested a label-free definition of airway disease based on the identification of "treatable traits."[50] This approach was put forward to facilitate personalized medicine in which the choice of therapy is guided by the presence of specific characteristics and biomarkers rather than the underlying airway diagnostic. Agusti proposed to define airway disease by these targets for intervention that he named treatable traits. These so-called traits can be a manifestation of the airway disease itself or represent a comorbidity, risk factor, or behavioral problem, contributing to the airway disease. Although this concept is appealing, it is still largely hypothetical. Evidence exists for some treatable traits (e.g., sputum eosinophils predict a response to corticosteroids independently of the underlying diagnosis, whether asthma or COPD) but further research is needed before implementing this approach.

1.7 CONCLUSIONS

Asthma and COPD are currently defined as composites of typical clinical and physiological features. However, none of the defining characteristics are restricted to one condition, leading to considerable heterogeneity in the asthmatic and COPD populations as well as a significant overlap between the two entities. The recognition and recent interest in these overlapping features led to the creation of the overlap syndrome, frequently referred to as ACO. Although the acknowledgment of this important subgroup of obstructive diseases is mostly accepted, ACO is still ill-defined. The criteria required for its diagnosis are still subject to debate, and that further limits its research and use in clinical practice. Then again, given the imprecision in the current classification of obstructive airway disease and the emergence of individualized medicine, a new taxonomy is inevitable. Interesting suggestions have been presented as to what form this will take and over what time period will it be adopted, but only future research will be able to adequately address these questions.

REFERENCES

1. Soler-Cataluña JJ, Cosío B, Izquierdo JL et al. Consensus document on the overlap Phenotype COPD–Asthma in COPD. *Arch Bronconeumol.* 2012;48(9):331–337.
2. Diagnosis of Diseases of Chronic Airflow Limitation: Asthma, COPD and Asthma-COPD Overlap Syndrome (ACO): Global Initiative for Asthma (GINA) and Global Initiative for Chronic Obstructive Lung Disease (GOLD); 2015. Available at http://www.ginasthma.org/.
3. Koblizek V, Chlumsky J, Zindr V et al. Chronic obstructive pulmonary disease: Official diagnosis and treatment guidelines of the Czech Pneumological and Phthisiological society; a novel phenotypic approach to COPD with patient-oriented care. *Biomed Pap Med Fac Univ Palacky Olomouc Czech Repub.* 2013;157(2):189–201.
4. Global Strategy for Asthma Management and Prevention: Global Initiative for Asthma (GINA); 2015. Available at http://www.ginasthma.org/.
5. Global Strategy for the Diagnosis, Management and Prevention of COPD: Global Initiative for Chronic Obstructive Lung Disease (GOLD); 2016. Available at http://www.goldcopd.org/.
6. Standards for the diagnosis and care of patients with chronic obstructive pulmonary disease. *Am J Respir Crit Care Med.* 1995;152(5 Pt 2):S77–121.
7. Gibson PG and McDonald VM. Asthma-COPD overlap 2015: Now we are six. *Thorax.* 2015;70(7):683–691.
8. Wurst KE, Kelly-Reif K, Bushnell GA et al. Understanding asthma-chronic obstructive pulmonary disease overlap syndrome. *Respir Med.* 2016;110:1–11.
9. Alshabanat A, Zafari Z, Albanyan O et al. Asthma and COPD overlap syndrome (ACO): A systematic review and meta analysis. *PLoS ONE.* 2015;10(9);1–15.
10. Gibson PG and Simpson JL. The overlap syndrome of asthma and COPD: What are its features and how important is it? *Thorax.* 2009;64(8):728–735.
11. D'silva L, Hassan N, Wang HY et al. Heterogeneity of bronchitis in airway diseases in tertiary care clinical practice. *Can Respir J.* 2011;18(3):144–148.
12. Iwamoto H, Gao J, Koskela J et al. Differences in plasma and sputum biomarkers between COPD and COPD-asthma overlap. *Eur Respir J.* 2014;43(2):421–429.
13. Nielsen M, Bårnes CB, and Ulrik CS. Clinical characteristics of the asthma-COPD overlap syndrome-a systematic review. *Int J Chron Obstruct Pulmon Dis.* 2015;10:1443–1454.
14. Hardin M, Silverman EK, Barr RG et al. The clinical features of the overlap between COPD and asthma. *Respir Res.* 2011;12(1):127.
15. Izquierdo-Alonso JL, Rodriguez-Gonzálezmoro JM, De Lucas-Ramos P et al. Prevalence and characteristics of three clinical phenotypes of chronic obstructive pulmonary disease (COPD). *Respir Med.* 2013;107(5):724–731.
16. Kauppi P, Kupiainen H, Lindqvist A et al. Overlap syndrome of asthma and COPD predicts low quality of life. *J Asthma.* 2011;48(3):279–285.
17. Kitaguchi Y, Komatsu Y, Fujimoto K et al. Sputum eosinophilia can predict responsiveness to inhaled corticosteroid treatment in patients with overlap syndrome of COPD and asthma. *Int J Chron Obstruct Pulmon Dis.* 2012;7:283–289.
18. Hardin M, Cho M, McDonald ML et al. The clinical and genetic features of COPD-asthma overlap syndrome. *Eur Respir J.* 2014;44(2):341–350.

19. Miravitlles M, Soler-Cataluña JJ et al. Treatment of COPD by clinical phenotypes: Putting old evidence into clinical practice. *Eur Respir J.* 2013;41(6):1252–1256.

20. Lee HY, Kang JY, Yoon HK et al. Clinical characteristics of asthma combined with COPD feature. *Yonsei Med J.* 2014;55(4):980–986.

21. Fu JJ, Gibson PG, Simpson JL et al. Longitudinal changes in clinical outcomes in older patients with asthma, COPD and asthma-COPD overlap syndrome. *Respiration.* 2014;87(1):63–74.

22. McDonald VM, Simpson JL, Higgins I et al. Multidimensional assessment of older people with asthma and COPD: Clinical management and health status. *Age Ageing.* 2011;40(1):42–49.

23. Simpson JL, Scott R, Boyle MJ et al. Inflammatory subtypes in asthma: Assessment and identification using induced sputum. *Respirology.* 2006;11(1):54–61.

24. Antó JM, Sunyer J, Basagaña X et al. Risk factors of new-onset asthma in adults: A population-based international cohort study. *Allergy.* 2010;65(8):1021–1030.

25. Jamrozik E, Knuiman MW, James A et al. Risk factors for adult-onset asthma: A 14-year longitudinal study. *Respirology.* 2009;14(6):814–821.

26. Jamieson DB, Matsui EC, Belli A et al. Effects of allergic phenotype on respiratory symptoms and exacerbations in patients with chronic obstructive pulmonary disease. *Am J Respir Crit Care Med.* 2013;188(2):187–192.

27. Fattahi F, ten Hacken NHT, Löfdahl CG et al. Atopy is a risk factor for respiratory symptoms in COPD patients: Results from the EUROSCOP study. *Respir Res.* 2013;14(1):10.

28. Salvi SS and Barnes PJ. Chronic obstructive pulmonary disease in non-smokers. *Lancet.* 2009;374(9691):733–743.

29. Lee JH, Haselkorn T, Borish L et al. Risk factors associated with persistent airflow limitation in severe or difficult-to-treat asthma: Insights from the TENOR study. *Chest.* 2007;132(6): 1882–1889.

30. Tashkin DP., Celli B, Decramer M et al. Bronchodilator responsiveness in patients with COPD. *Eur Respir J.* 2008;31(4):742–750.

31. Ulrik CS and Backer V. Nonreversible airflow obstruction in life-long nonsmokers with moderate to severe asthma. *Eur Respir J.* 1999;14(4):892–896.

32. Casanova C, De Torres JP, Aguirre-Jaíme A et al. The progression of chronic obstructive pulmonary disease is heterogeneous: The experience of the BODE cohort. *Am J Respir Crit Care Med.* 2011;184(9):1015–1021.

33. Albert P, Agusti A, Edwards L et al. Bronchodilator responsiveness as a phenotypic characteristic of established chronic obstructive pulmonary disease. *Thorax.* 2012;67(8):701–708.

34. Fingleton J, Travers J, Williams M et al. Treatment responsiveness of phenotypes of symptomatic airways obstruction in adults. *J Allergy Clin Immunol.* 2015;136(3):601–609.

35. Dummer JF, Epton MJ, Cowan JO et al. Predicting corticosteroid response in chronic obstructive pulmonary disease using exhaled nitric oxide. *Am J Respir Crit Care Med.* 2009;180(9):846–852.

36. Peters SP, Bleecker ER, Kunselman SJ et al. Predictors of response to tiotropium versus salmeterol in asthmatic adults. *J Allergy Clin Immunol.* 2013;132(5):1068–1074.

37. Lee LA, Yang S, Kerwin E et al. The effect of fluticasone furoate/umeclidinium in adult patients with asthma: A randomized, dose-ranging study. *Respir Med.* 2015;109(1):54–62.

38. Kankaanranta H, Harju T, Kilpeläinen M et al. Diagnosis and pharmacotherapy of stable chronic obstructive pulmonary disease: The finnish guidelines. *Basic Clin Pharmacol Toxicol.* 2015;116(4):291–307.

39. Lange P. Persistent airway obstruction in asthma. *Am J Respir Crit Care Med.* 2013;187(1):1–2.

40. Price DB, Tinkelman DG, Nordyke RJ et al. Scoring system and clinical application of COPD diagnostic questionnaires. *Chest.* 2006;129(6):1531–1539.

41. Castro-Rodríguez JA, Holberg CJ, Wright AL et al. A clinical index to define risk of asthma in young children with recurrent wheezing. *Am J Respir Crit Care Med.* 2000;162(4 Pt I): 1403–1406.

42. Hardie JA, Buist AS, Vollmer WM et al. Risk of over-diagnosis of COPD in asymptomatic elderly never-smokers. *Eur Respir J.* 2002;20(5):1117–1122.

43. Sorino C, Battaglia S, Scichilone N et al. Diagnosis of airway obstruction in the elderly: Contribution of the SARA study. *Int J Chron Obstruct Pulmon Dis.* 2012;7:389–395.

44. Cerveri I, Corsico AG, Accordini S et al. Underestimation of airflow obstruction among young adults using $FEV_1/FVC < 70\%$ as a fixed cut-off: A longitudinal evaluation of clinical and functional outcomes. *Thorax.* 2008;63(12):1040–1045.

45. Pellegrino R, Viegi G, Brusasco V et al. Interpretative strategies for lung function tests. *Eur Respir J.* 2005;26(5):948–968.

46. Mohamed Hoesein FAA, Zanen P, and Lammers JWJ. Lower limit of normal or $FEV_1/FVC < 0.70$ in diagnosing COPD: An evidence-based review. *Respir Med.* 2011;105(6):907–915.

47. Postma DS, Weiss ST, Van Den Berge M et al. Revisiting the Dutch hypothesis. *J Allergy Clin Immunol.* 2015;136(3):521–529.

48. Gibson PG, McDonald VM, and Marks GB. Asthma in older adults. *The Lancet.* 2010;376(9743):803–813.

49. McDonald VM, Higgins I, and Gibson PG. Managing older patients with coexistent asthma and chronic obstructive pulmonary disease: Diagnostic and therapeutic challenges. *Drugs Aging.* 2013;30(1):1–17.

50. Agusti A, Bel E, Thomas M et al. Treatable traits: Toward precision medicine of chronic airway diseases. *Eur Respir J.* 2016;47(2):410–419.

Epidemiology of asthma, COPD, and asthma-COPD overlap

ANNE L. FUHLBRIGGE

2.1 INTRODUCTION

CLINICAL VIGNETTE 2.1

A 52-year-old woman presents to discuss her chronic obstructive pulmonary disease (COPD) and specifically the problem she is having with exacerbations and the amount of time she has missed work. She is a heavy smoker, and has been diagnosed with COPD by prior physicians. However, she also has a history of childhood asthma and allergic rhinitis. Recent spirometry is consistent with obstructive lung disease (OLD) although she had some reversibility (250 mL and 20%) with a post-bronchodilator forced expiratory volume in 1 second (FEV_1) of 60% predicted.

CLINICAL VIGNETTE 2.2

A 46-year-old woman presents for evaluation of symptoms of increasing shortness of breath and recurrent episodes of "bronchitis." She is a nonsmoker but her father smoked. She immigrated to the United States approximately 10 years ago, and while growing up, she frequently helped her mother in preparing meals in a two-room house with an open fire for cooking and heating. She reports frequent respiratory infections as a child and young adult. She has never been diagnosed with asthma but has two siblings who have asthma.

OLD is a group of respiratory disorders characterized by airway obstruction, and is a leading cause of morbidity and mortality worldwide. The most common examples of OLD are asthma and COPD. However, many patients present with overlapping features of both asthma and COPD. In 2015, the Global Initiative for Asthma (GINA)[1] and the Global Initiative for Chronic Obstructive Lung Disease (GOLD)[2] issued a joint document describing this phenotype and identifying it as a distinct clinical entity, asthma-COPD overlap syndrome (ACOS, more recently named ACO) (Figure 2.1).

All three disorders (asthma, COPD, and ACO) present with similar clinical features (dyspnea, coughing, wheezing, and expectoration) and share pathophysiologic mechanisms such as airway limitation and underlying airway inflammation. Some experts have cautioned against labeling ACO as a unique disease entity because studies addressing this patient population are limited.[3] Historically, clinical trials have consistently excluded these patients: patients with COPD excluded from asthma clinical trials and patients with a history of asthma excluded from COPD clinical trials. As the focus on characterizing this population increases, reliable data on the epidemiology of the disease and its relationship to asthma and COPD will improve.

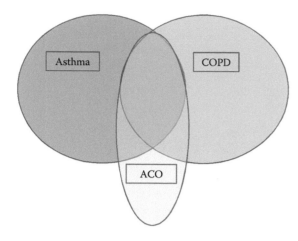

Figure 2.1 Venn diagram illustrating the overlapping nature of asthma, COPD, and asthma-COPD overlap.

2.2 ASTHMA

Asthma is a disease of reversible airflow obstruction, bronchial hyperresponsiveness, and underlying airway inflammation.[4] Wheezing in young children is a common, but heterogeneous condition. Its presence in children under 6 years is frequently a benign condition reflecting smaller airways that improves or resolves as the child grows.[5]

2.2.1 RISK FACTORS

A family history of asthma is a strong risk factor for persistence of wheeze and persistence of wheezing into adolescence is associated with a high rate of persistence of wheeze into adulthood and development of asthma. Identical twins are more likely to both be asthmatic compared with nonidentical twins, suggesting a genetic component.[6] Yet, in approximately half of the identical twins with one asthmatic twin, both twins do not have asthma, indicating the importance of complex gene–environment interactions and/or nongenetic factors.

A second factor important in the development of asthma is atopy, with sensitization and exposure to airborne allergens (e.g., house-dust mites). The increasing prevalence of asthma worldwide has been associated with a parallel increase in atopic sensitization and other allergic disorders such as eczema and rhinitis. Weinmayr et al. observed that the prevalence rates of asthma symptoms and atopic sensitization in children are linked, yet, the prevalence rates vary widely between countries, and the link between atopic sensitization and asthma symptoms may be modified by other factors such as economic development.[7] Economic development and urbanization have a direct impact on a child's living conditions and health status; with the rate of asthma increasing as communities adopt western lifestyles.[8] Analyzing data from the World Health Survey performed in 64 countries, Sembajwe and colleagues observed a bimodal distribution of asthma symptoms. Interestingly, the highest distribution of asthma symptoms was found in high- and low-income countries whereas middle-income countries

had the lowest prevalence.[9] This U-shape pattern may represent competing effects of multiple factors on asthma risk that are unique to high-income and low-income countries. Within the United States, significant effort has been focused on the "inner-city asthma epidemic" and trying to understand which factors present in poor urban environments are associated with a high asthma prevalence and morbidity. However, the independent effects of race/ethnicity, poverty, and area of residence are debated. Some analyses have observed that a large proportion of the racial/ethnic differences in the prevalence of asthma are explained by factors related to income, area of residence, and level of education.[10] In contrast, other studies suggest the differences in asthma prevalence are largely explained by demographic factors and not by living in an urban neighborhood[11]; the prevalence of current asthma is higher in inner-city versus non–inner-city areas, but this difference is not significant after adjusting for race/ethnicity, region, age, and sex. In adjusted models, black race, Puerto Rican ethnicity, and lower household income are independent risk factors for current asthma, but not residence in poor or urban areas. Several other factors may contribute to the risk of developing asthma, including changes in diet; physical activity and obesity; infectious disease and microbial exposures, including viral respiratory infections (respiratory syncytial virus [RSV] and rhinovirus); increased exposure to antibiotics; environmental factors (exposure to indoor irritants including tobacco smoke); psychosocial stressors including violence; occupational exposures; and the effects of industrial and motor vehicle pollution.[12] Finally, gender affects the risk of asthma in an age-dependent manner, but the complex biological mechanisms that cause these sex-associated differences is not yet fully understood.

2.2.2 PREVALENCE

The prevalence of asthma continues to rise. In the United States, the 2010 National Health Interview Survey (NHIS) sample estimated that one in 12 people (8%) of the population had asthma, compared with 1 in 14 (7%) in 2001. The NHIS data also demonstrate that race and ethnicity play a role. The asthma prevalence among white persons (7.2%) is intermediate between the prevalence seen in black persons (11.2%) and that seen among Asian (5.2%) and Hispanic persons (6.5%). Among Hispanics, Puerto Ricans (16.1%) are more likely to have asthma compared with Mexican persons (5.4%). In addition, the overall prevalence rate in females is greater than in males. However, age modifies the effect of gender on asthma prevalence. Among adults 18 years and older, females are more likely than males to have asthma. However, the pattern is reversed among children. The current asthma prevalence is higher among male children aged 0–4 years (7.7%) and aged 5–14 years (12.4%), compared with female children in the same age group (4.7% and 8.8%, respectively) (Figure 2.2).[13]

Asthma prevalence also varies by geography, but whether this variation is a result of environmental exposures or related to sociodemographic features of the population within a given geographic area remains uncertain. The International Study of Asthma and Allergies in Childhood (ISAAC) compared

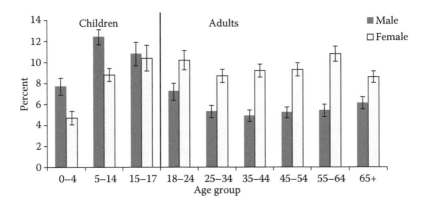

Figure 2.2 Asthma Prevalence by age and gender: The prevalence of asthma in the United States is plotted by age groups (age 0–4 to 65+ yrs.), stratified by gender. The National Surveillance of Asthma: United States, 2001–2010.

(Taken from CDC, Center for Disease Control and Prevention. *National Surveillance of Asthma: United States, 2001–2010.* Center for Disease Control and Prevention and National Center for Health Statistics, Editors. Hyattsville, MD: U.S. Department of Health and Human Services; November 2012.)

the prevalence of disease, between two age groups (13–14 and 6–7 years old), across a wide array of countries. ISAAC Phase One reported marked variations in the prevalence of asthma symptoms, with up to fifteen-fold differences between countries. The major differences between populations were thought to be due to environmental factors.[14] A follow-up evaluation using the same methodology in 2009 showed continued wide variations in the symptom prevalence of childhood asthma worldwide, with up to a 13-fold difference between countries among 6–7-year-old age group and 9-fold difference in the 13–14-year-old age group based on questionnaire data.[15] In addition, the authors confirmed prior reports of an association between asthma prevalence and economic development, with asthma symptoms being more prevalent in affluent countries. However, despite a lower prevalence of asthma, persons in less affluent countries reported more severe disease.

2.2.3 MORBIDITY AND MORTALITY

Asthma is a leading cause of activity limitation and is the primary cause for days lost from school in children. In 2008 the condition accounted for an estimated 14.4 million lost school days in children as well as 14.2 million lost work days in adults.[16] Rates of hospital admissions demonstrate a U-shaped distribution with highest rates among children under 15 years old and older adults over the age of 65. The association between other factors such as race/ethnicity, region, sex, and asthma morbidity are similar to those reported for asthma prevalence.[11] Additional factors, such as chronic rhinitis and gastroesophageal reflux disease (GERD), are known to worsen asthma severity and systemic processes including cardiovascular disease, obesity, and depression which have also been associated with an increase in asthma morbidity.[17] Importantly, asthma in older adults (persons over the age of 65) is associated with different risk factors, including an increased number of comorbid conditions, which influence the presentation, diagnosis, and management. As discussed, the differentiation between

asthma and COPD in this age group can be difficult due to substantial overlap in disease presentation and symptoms. Routine collection of data on hospital discharges is almost entirely restricted to high-income countries, limiting the value of admission rates for surveillance of the burden of asthma on a global scale.

Asthma deaths are rare among children and increase with age. The Global Burden of Disease Study (GBD) Study reported that age-standardized death rates from asthma fell by about one-third between 1990 and 2010. This improvement was seen across all ages and in both males and females.[18] Within the United States, the number of deaths due to asthma is also decreasing. The death rate in 2009 was approximately 27% lower than the number of deaths seen in 1999, with the age-adjusted death rate for females being approximately 50% greater than the rate seen in males and 75% higher among blacks compared with whites. Black women had the highest age-adjusted mortality rate due to asthma.[19] Age-adjusted death rates in Hispanics are lower than non-Hispanic blacks, but higher than non-Hispanic whites, with Puerto Ricans demonstrating higher age-adjusted death rates than all other Hispanic subgroups and non-Hispanic whites and blacks.[20]

2.3 COPD

COPD is "a common preventable and treatable disease characterized by persistent airflow limitation that is usually progressive and associated with an enhanced chronic inflammatory response in the airways and the lung to noxious particles or gases."[2] Traditionally, COPD is subdivided into the two phenotypes: chronic bronchitis and emphysema. However, based on a better understanding of the multiple influences (environmental, clinical, biological, and genetic), which lead to differences in outcome and/or management, there is recent support for defining additional phenotypes within the umbrella term of COPD.[21–23]

2.3.1 RISK FACTORS

The most important risk factor for developing COPD is tobacco exposure, which results in an accelerated FEV_1 decline with age. Smoking duration and pack years are directly associated with the diagnosis of COPD, after controlling for current smoking behavior.[24] Yet, not all smokers develop COPD, which in a subset of smokers is likely based on genetic risk factors, making them less "susceptible" to the damaging effects of smoking tobacco. Similarly, not all patients that develop COPD have significant smoking exposure, therefore, implicating occupational and other exposures in the development of COPD.[25] The American Thoracic Society (ATS) estimates that approximately 15% of COPD cases in the general population is attributable to occupational sources[26] supported by a meta-analysis of population-based studies that demonstrated an association between the presence of obstructive disease and self-reported occupational exposure to vapor-gas, dust, or fumes.[27] Looking globally, Ryu and colleagues conducted a meta-analysis of epidemiological studies investigating the relationship between COPD and occupational exposure to vapors, gases, dusts, or fumes (VGDF). In a random effects model meta-analysis, the pooled OR for exposure to VGDF was 1.43 for COPD (95% CI: 1.19–1.73) compared with no exposure to VGDF.[28]

Outside of the workplace, environmental exposures and respiratory infections are also associated with the development of COPD.[25] Furthermore, air pollution may influence the development of COPD and associated morbidity. Air pollution can affect lung development in childhood,[29] and exposure over several days to elevated levels of air pollution has been clearly shown to exacerbate preexisting COPD, resulting in increased morbidity and mortality.[30] Gender also influences the prevalence and morbidity associated with COPD. There is evidence for sex-specific susceptibility to environmental exposures with nonsmokers who develop COPD more likely to be women.[31] In addition, women with COPD are more likely to have a chronic bronchitis phenotype, potentially related to sex-specific environmental exposures. These include higher exposure risk to indoor air pollutants, such as biomass fuel fumes used for cooking and heating in low-income countries and differences in types of occupational exposures, such as cleaning agents, which are more commonly used by females compared to males in higher-income countries.[32] Finally, genetic factors are very important in the developing lung and even more so are "gene by environment" interactions, which are thought to play a pivotal role in susceptibility to environmental exposures and disease development. In addition, several other genes have been implicated in COPD susceptibility.[33] For example, alpha-1 antitrypsin deficiency is the best described known genetic risk factor for susceptibility to develop COPD.

In addition to the accelerated decline in lung function associated with environmental exposures, impaired lung growth in childhood is another pathophysiologic mechanism related to the development of COPD. Normal individuals achieve maximum lung growth in young adulthood followed by a plateau and then a slow decline with age (Figure 2.3). Prospective cohorts have demonstrated that factors, such as asthma, may lead to a pattern of reduced lung growth early in life leading to lower maximally attained lung volumes in young adulthood and subsequent increased risk for developing COPD later in life.[34-36] The combination of low maximally attained lung volume in young adulthood and environmental exposures are additive and potentially synergistic to further increasing the risk of developing COPD.

2.3.2 PREVALENCE

Accurate ascertainment of the true prevalence of COPD has been difficult. Recent estimates suggest more that 15 million people in the United States[37] and more that 210 million people worldwide[38] have COPD, but the prevalence of COPD varies by diagnostic criteria used. The GOLD and the Burden of Obstructive Lung Disease (BOLD) both recommend spirometry as the gold standard for diagnosing COPD, as estimates of COPD prevalence

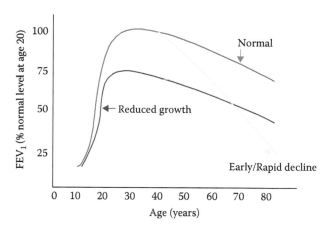

Figure 2.3 Longitudinal lung function growth and decline curves. Lung function growth and decline curves during the first three decades of life are shown. Lung function, as the percentage of the maximum forced expiratory volume in 1 second (FEV_1) in a person without lung disease is plotted by age. (a) the normal pattern of lung function growth and decline is characterized by an increase during childhood/adolescence, a plateau in early adulthood, and a gradual decline into old age (blue line). Abnormal growth and decline curves include (b) reduced growth (red line), (c) normal growth with an early/rapid decline (yellow line). A person can develop COPD from either the reduced growth curve or an early/rapid decline curve.

(Adapted from Speizer, F. E. and Tager, I. B., *Epidemiol Rev.*, 1, 124–142, 1979; McGeachie, M. J., Yates, K. P., Zhou, X. et al., *N Engl J Med.*, 374, 1842–1852, 2016.)

based on spirometry double the estimates derived from self-reported information. Further variability is related to differences in the quality of measurement, use of pre- versus post-bronchodilator values and inconsistency in the values for defining obstruction present in the literature.[39,40] Rycroft and colleagues, who published a review of all litera- ture reviews between 2000 and 2010, noted estimates for COPD prevalence varied from 0.2% (Japan) to 37% (United States) and that the higher estimates were based on GOLD spirometry criteria to define COPD.[41]

COPD has traditionally been a disease of men. However, in the United States, the prevalence of COPD in women has surpassed the prevalence in men. Although recent estimates from NHIS (2009 and 1998), demonstrate that prevalence of COPD appears to have stabilized, the prevalence remains higher in women than in men.[42] The rapid increase in the prevalence, morbidity, and mortality of COPD in women over the last three decades has largely been attributed to the increase in tobacco abuse among women. However, there is evidence that care providers continue to harbor a gender bias, leading to underdiagno- sis and/or delayed diagnosis of COPD in women, which may impact their morbidity.[32]

The prevalence of COPD is also known to vary by other demographic factors. Puerto Rican and non-Hispanic white adults have a higher prevalence of disease compared to non-Hispanic blacks and Mexican American adults, while adults with family income below the poverty level have a higher prevalence of disease across all racial and ethnic groups but with a similar relative distribution by race/ethnicity.[42] Prevalence also varies by urban/rural sta- tus and region within the United States.[43-45] Worldwide, the prevalence of COPD has not stabilized. In developing countries, where exposure to smoke from coal and bio- mass fossil fuels used in heating and cooking is common, a continued increase in the prevalence of COPD has been demonstrated.[46]

2.3.3 MORBIDITY AND MORTALITY

Within the United States, the overall age-adjusted death rate for COPD stabilized between 1999 and 2010, how- ever, there was a decline in the death rates for persons aged 55–64 years and 65–74 years that was offset by an increase in adults aged 45–54 years and American Indian/Alaska natives.[45] In contrast, the progress in primary prevention seen in the United States is not reported globally. The World Health Organization (WHO) reports that, globally, the morbidity and mortality associated with COPD continue to increase. COPD is now the fourth-leading cause of death and by 2030 is expected to rise to the third-leading cause of death. In 2005 almost 90% of these deaths occurred in low- to middle-income countries. Independent of geography, there is increased understanding that COPD is a systemic inflammatory disease as COPD patients report a higher prevalence of comorbid conditions, which significantly

impact diagnosis, management, and associated morbidity. In addition, the presence of multiple comorbidities has a cumulative effect on mortality.[47]

2.4 ACO

Asthma and COPD overlap (ACO) is used to describe patients with an overlapping phenotype where asthma patients exhibit COPD features/symptoms and/or COPD patients exhibit asthma features/symptoms. However, there is currently no consensus definition for this entity, which limits our ability to capture the prevalence of this complex disease accurately. Similar to asthma and COPD, ACO includes several phenotypes where risk factors, clinical pre- sentation, and response to treatment may vary.

2.4.1 RISK FACTORS

ACO shares risk factors and clinical characteristics with asthma alone, but among young adults, people with ACO were noted to have an earlier age of asthma onset and more frequent hospitalizations.[48] ACO may arise from severe, early onset asthma that develops a component of fixed air- flow obstruction. This is consistent with recent data pub- lished from the longitudinal cohort of children enrolled in the Childhood Asthma Management Program (CAMP) fol- lowed until young adulthood.[35] Childhood impairment of lung function was a significant predictor of abnormal lon- gitudinal patterns of lung-function growth and decline. In the CAMP population, 11% of the cohort met the GOLD spirometry criteria for COPD, and these individuals were more likely to have a reduced pattern of lung growth. Others have reported similar findings. Silva et al. observed that physician-diagnosed asthma was significantly associ- ated with an increased risk for chronic bronchitis, emphy- sema, and COPD,[49] while Tagiyeva et al. found that wheezy bronchitis and asthma are associated with an increased risk for COPD and reduced lung function (Tagiyeva et al. 2016). Similarly, Tai and colleagues reported that children with severe asthma are at increased risk for developing COPD.[50] Shritcliffe et al. found that among a random population sample aged 25–75 years, childhood asthma emerged as the strongest predictor for GOLD-defined COPD.[51] In their analysis, diagnosis of childhood asthma was associated with an increased risk for developing COPD that equated a 22-year increase in age or a 62-pack-year smoking exposure.

2.4.2 PREVALENCE

The prevalence of ACO varies based on the population studied: general population sample vs. smokers vs. individuals with known OLD. Population-based surveys from the United States suggest a prevalence of 3.1%.[52] The prevalence of ACO in gen- eral population samples globally is similar. In an Italian general

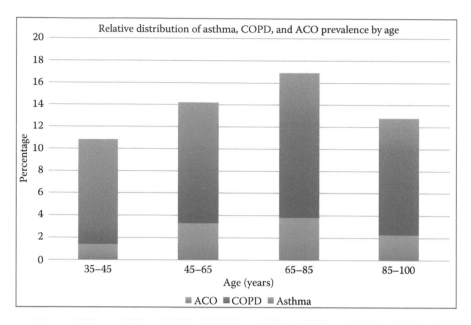

Figure 2.4 Relative Prevalence of Asthma, COPD and Asthma-COPD Overlap across different age groups.
(Adapted from Kumbhare, S., Pleasants, R., Ohar, J. A. et al., *Ann Am Thorac Soc.*, 13, 803–810, 2016.)

population sample, De Marco reported estimates of 1.6%, 2.1%, and 4.5%, for people age 20–44 years versus 45–64 years versus 65–84 years, respectively,[53] whereas Chung and colleagues observed that 2.3% of the South Korean population met criteria for ACO, based on the National Health and Nutrition Examination Survey.[54] Among high-risk populations, smokers or subjects with known OLD, the prevalence of ACO is much higher with estimates ranging between 12% and 55%, depending on the population being studied, the definition of ACO being used, and how that information is being gathered (e.g., self-report, medical records, or prospective/retrospective review).[55]

Kumbhare and colleagues analyzed the 2012 Behavioral Risk Factor Surveillance System (BRFSS) to examine the relative distribution of asthma, COPD, and ACO within the United States. Overall, the prevalence of ACO was lower than the prevalence of either asthma or COPD alone. However, the relative distribution of each diagnosis changes with age. For people between the ages of 35 and 45 years, the relative prevalence of asthma is greater than the prevalence of either COPD or ACO. However, between the ages of 45 and 85 years, the prevalence of COPD and ACO increase while the prevalence of asthma decreases. After age 85, the absolute prevalence of all three conditions declines but the relative prevalence of COPD remains higher than that of either asthma or ACO (Figure 2.4).[52]

As expected, the prevalence of ACO varies with smoking status. Patients with ACO report rates of current or former cigarette smoking that are intermediate between rates reported for patients with COPD alone and persons with asthma. However, the prevalence of current or former tobacco use is reported to be only slightly lower among persons with ACO compared to persons with COPD alone. Among asthma patients who smoke, the degree of smoking is a significant predictor of ACO.[56] In addition, other

demographic factors play a role in the relative distribution between the three diagnoses. ACO is more prevalent in women, people of a nonwhite race, lower-income populations, and those with a lower education level relative to persons diagnosed with asthma or COPD. Finally, ACO populations have a greater prevalence of obese and morbidly obese subjects.[52]

2.4.3 MORBIDITY AND MORTALITY

Patients with ACO reflect an associated morbidity of disease greater than that reported for either asthma or COPD alone. Retrospective analyses suggest an increase in resource utilization and costs compared to asthma or COPD alone.[57] Additional cross-sectional data suggests patientswith ACO have more respiratory-related exacerbations and hospitalizations.[53] Other reports suggests ACO had a significant impact on physical performance and affects health-related quality of life (HRQL), the latter[58] which has been reported to be worse for persons with ACO compared to those with asthma or COPD alone.[59] Consistent with this observation is preliminary data published in abstract form only, which suggests an increased mortality in persons with ACO compared with either asthma or COPD alone. This is in contrast to longitudinal data from subjects over a 15 year period, which demonstrated that the mortality rate of ACO was similar to patients with COPD, although higher than that of patients with asthma or controls. In addition, ACO patients have an increase in comorbid conditions. Kumbhare and colleagues reported that ACO patients had a higher prevalence of comorbidities compared with asthma or COPD patients alone, and this relationship persisted despite controlling for age, sex, race, marital status, income, employment, body mass index, and smoking status.[52] Some authors have suggested the increase in morbidity associated with ACO is secondary to health impairment of the comorbid conditions.[54]

2.5 CONCLUDING REMARKS

OLD (asthma, COPD, and ACO) is a leading cause of morbidity and mortality worldwide. As our knowledge of the clinical phenotypes and underlying mechanisms within asthma, COPD, and asthma-COPD overlap improves, the epidemiology will continue to evolve. A "diagnostic label-free" (i.e., COPD vs. asthma vs. ACO) approach has been recommended in some publications,[60] and others propose focusing on the unique phenotypes that have therapeutic and/or prognostic implications.[61,62] Regardless, a consensus approach to diagnosis of ACO is essential for generating meaningful and consistent worldwide epidemiologic information about this condition.

REFERENCES

1. Global Strategy for Asthma Management and Prevention: GINA Global Initiative for Asthma; 2016. Available at http://ginasthma.org/gina-reports/.
2. GOLD. *Global Initiative for Chronic Obstructive Lung Disease, Global Strategy for the Diagnosis, Management, and Prevention of Chronic Obstructive Pulmonary Disease.* 2016. Available at http://gold-copd.org/.
3. Postma DS and Rabe KF. The Asthma–COPD overlap syndrome. *N Engl J Med.* 2015;373:1241–1249.
4. NAEPP. Expert panel report 3: Guidelines for the diagnosis and management of asthma; 2007. Available at https://www.nhlbi.nih.gov/health-pro/resources/lung/naci/asthma-info/naepp.htm
5. Martinez FD, Wright AL, Taussig LM et al. Asthma and Wheezing in the first six years of life. *N Engl J Med.* January 19, 1995;332:133–138.
6. Moffatt MF, Gut IG, Demenais F et al. A large-scale, consortium-based genome wide association study of asthma. *N Engl J Med.* 2010;363:1211–1221.
7. Weinmayr G, Weiland SK, Bjorksten B et al. Atopic sensitization and the international variation of asthma symptom prevalence in children. *Am J Respir Care Med.* 2007;176:565–574.
8. Weinberg E. Urbanization and childhood asthma: An African perspective. *J Allergy Clin Immunol.* 2000;105:224–231.
9. Sembajwe G, Cifuentes M, Tak SW et al. National income, self-reported wheezing and asthma diagnosis from the World Health Survey. *Eur Respir J.* 2010;35:279–286.
10. Litonjua AA, Carey VJ, Weiss ST et al. Race, socio-economic factors, and area of residence are associated With Asthma prevalence. *Pediatr Pulmonol.* December 1999;28(6):394–401.
11. Keet CA, McCormack MC, Pollack CE et al. Neighborhood poverty, urban resident, race/ethnicity and asthma: Rethinking the inner city asthma epidemic. *J Allergy Clin Immunol.* March 3, 2015;135:655–662.
12. Wright R. Exploring biopsychosocial influences on asthma expression in both the family and community context. *Am J Respir Crit Care Med.* January 15, 2008;177:129–130.
13. CDC, Center for Disease Control and Prevention. *National Surveillance of Asthma: United States, 2001–2010.* Center for Disease Control and Prevention and National Center for Health Statistics, Editors. Hyattsville, MD: U.S. Department of Health and Human Services; November 2012. https://www.cdc.gov/nchs/data/series/sr_03/sr03_035.pdf
14. ISAAC. Worldwide variations in the prevalence of asthma symptoms: The International Study of Asthma and Allergies in Childhood (ISAAC). *Eur Respir J.* August 1998;12(2):315–335.
15. Lai CKW, Beasley R, Crane J et al. Global variation in the prevalence and severity of asthma symptoms: Phase three of the International Study of Asthma and Allergies in Childhood (ISAAC). *Thorax.* June 2009;64:476–483.
16. CDC, Center for Disease Control And Prevention. *Asthma Facts.* D.o.H.a.H. Services, Editor. National Asthma Control Program Grantees; July 2013. https://www.cdc.gov/asthma/pdfs/asthma_facts_program_grantees.pdf
17. Boulet LP and Boulay ME. Asthma-related comorbidities. *Exp Rev Resp Med.* June 2011;5:377–393.
18. Benziger CP, Roth GA, and Moran AE. The Global burden of disease study and the preventable burden of NCD. *Glob Heart.* 2016;11(4):393–397.
19. Akinbami LJ, Moorman JE, Bailey C et al. Trends in asthma prevalence, health care use, and mortality in the United States, 2001–2010. *NCHS Data Brief.* 2012;94:1–8.
20. Homa D, Mannino DM, and Lara M. Asthma mortality in U.S. Hispanics of Mexican, Puerto Rican, and Cuban heritage, 1990-1995. *Am J Respir Crit Care Med.* Feb 2000;161:504–509.
21. Vestbo J. COPD: Definition and phenotypes. *Clin Chest Med.* 2014;35:1–6.
22. Miravitlles M, Calle M, and Soler-Cataluña J. Clinical phenotypes of COPD: Identification, definition and implications for guidelines. *Arch Bronconeumol.* 2012;48(3):86–98.
23. Miravitlles M, Soler-Cataluna JJ, Calle M et al. Treatment of COPD by clinical phenotypes: Putting old evidence into clinical practice. *Eur Respir J.* 2013;41:1252–1256.

24. Liu Y, Pleasants RA, Croft JB et al. Smoking duration, respiratory symptoms, and COPD in adults aged ≥45 years with a smoking history. *Int J Chron Obstruct Pulmon Dis.* 2015;10:1409–1416.

25. Walter R, Gottlieb DJ, and O'Connor GT. Environmental and genetic risk factors and gene-environment interactions in the pathogenesis of chronic obstructive lung disease. *Environ Health Perspect.* August 2000;108:733–742.

26. Balmes J, Becklake M, Blanc P et al. American thoracic society statement: Occupational contribution to the burden of airway disease. *Am J Respir Crit Care Med.* March 2003;167:787–797.

27. Alif SM, Dharmage S. Bowatte G et al. Occupational exposure and risk of chronic obstructive pulmonary disease: A systematic review and meta-analysis. *Expert Rev Respir Med.* Aug 2016;10(8):861–872.

28. Ryu JY, Sunwoo YE, Lee SY et al. Chronic obstructive pulmonary disease (COPD) and vapors, gases, dusts or fumes (VGDF): A meta-analysis. *COPD J Chronic Obstruct Pulm Dis.* 2015;12:374–380.

29. Schikowski T, Mills IC, Anderson HR et al. Ambient air pollution: A cause of COPD? *Eur Respir J.* January 2014;43:250–263.

30. Sint T, Donohue JF, and Ghio AJ. Ambient air pollution particles and the acute exacerbation of chronic obstructive pulmonary disease. *Inhal Toxicol.* January 2008;20:25–29.

31. Kennedy SM, Chambers R, Du W et al. Environmental and occupational exposures: Do they affect chronic obstructive pulmonary disease differently in women and men? *Proc Am Thorac Soc.* 2007;4(8):692–694.

32. Aryal S, Diaz-Guzman E, and Mannino. Influence of sex on chronic obstructive pulmonary disease risk and treatment outcomes. *Int J Chron Obstruct Pulmon Dis.* October 14, 2014;9:1145–1154.

33. Berndt A, Leme AS, and Shapiro SD. Emerging genetics of COPD. *EMBO Mol Med.* November 2012;4(11):1144–1155.

34. Speizer FE and Tager IB. Epidemiology of chronic mucus hypersecretion and obstructive airways disease. *Epidemiol Rev.* 1979;1:124–142.

35. McGeachie MJ, Yates KP, Zhou X et al. Patterns of growth and decline in Lung function in persistent childhood Asthma. *N Engl J Med.* May 12, 2016;374:1842–1852.

36. Lange P, Celli B, Agusti A et al. Lung-function trajectories leading to chronic obstructive pulmonary disease. *N Engl J Med.* July 9, 2015;373:111–122.

37. CDC, Center for Disease Control and Prevention. Chronic pulmonary obstructive disease among adults—United States, 2011. *MMWR Morb Mortal Wkly Rep.* 2012;61(46):938–942.

38. Bousquet J, Kiley J, Bateman ED et al. Prioritised research agenda for prevention and control of chronic respiratory diseases. *Eur Respir J.* 2010;36(5):995–1001.

39. Mannino DM, Homa DM, Akinbami LJ et al. Chronic obstructive pulmonary disease surveillance—United States, 1971–2000. *MMWR Surveill Summ.* 2002;51(6):1–16.

40. Celli BR, Halbert RJ, Isonaka S et al. Population impact of different definitions of airway obstruction. *Eur Respir J.* 2003;22(2):268–273.

41. Rycroft CE, Heyes A, Lanza L et al. Epidemiology of chronic obstructive pulmonary disease: A literature review. *Int J Chron Obstruct Pulmon Dis.* 2012;7:457–494.

42. Akinbami LJ and Liu X. Chronic obstructive pulmonary disease among adults aged 18 and over in the united states, 1998–2009. *NCHS Data Brief.* 2011;63:1–8.

43. Halbert RJ, Natoli JL, Gano A et al. Global burden of COPD: Systematic review and meta-analysis. *Eur Respir J.* 2006;28(3):523–532.

44. Buist AS, McBurnie MA, Vollmer WM et al. International variation in the prevalence of COPD (the BOLD Study): A population-based prevalence study. *Lancet.* September 1, 2007;370(9589):741–750.

45. Ford ES, Croft JB, Mannino DM et al. COPD surveillance-United States, 1999-2011. *Chest.* 2013;144(1):284–305.

46. Hu G, Zhou Y, Tian J et al., Risk of COPD from exposure to biomass smoke: A metaanalysis. *Chest.* 2010;138(1):20–31.

47. Miller J, Edwards LD, Agustí A et al. Comorbidity, systemic inflammation and outcomes in the ECLIPSE cohort. *Respir Med.* 2013;107(9):1376–1384.

48. Tagiyeva N, Devereux G, Fielding S et al. Outcomes of childhood Asthma and Wheezy bronchitis. A 50-year cohort study. *Am J Resp Crit Care Med.* 2016;193(1):23–30.

49. Silva GE, Sherrill DL, Guerra S et al. Asthma as a risk factor for COPD in a longitudinal study. *Chest.* 2004;126:59–65.

50. Tai A, Tran H, Roberts M et al. The association between childhood asthma and adult chronic obstructive pulmonary disease. *Thorax.* 2014;69(9):805–810.

51. Shirtcliffe P, Marsh S, Travers J et al. Childhood asthma and GOLD-defined chronic obstructive pulmonary disease. *Int Med J.* 2012;42(1):83–88.

52. Kumbhare S, Pleasants R, Ohar JA et al. Characteristics and prevalence of Asthma/Chronic obstructive pulmonary disease overlap in the United States. *Ann Am Thorac Soc.* 2016;13(6):803–810.

53. de Marco R, Pesce G, Marcon A et al. The coexistence of asthma and chronic obstructive pulmonary disease (COPD): Prevalence and risk factors in young, middle-aged and elderly people from the general population. *PLOS ONE.* 2013;8(5):e62985.

54. Chung JW, Kong KA, Lee JH et al. Characteristics and self-rated health of overlap syndrome. *Int J COPD.* 2014;9:795–804.

55. Ding B and Enstone A. Asthma and chronic obstructive pulmonary disease overlap syndrome (ACOS): Structured literature review and physician insights. *Expert Rev Respir Med.* 2016;10(3):363–371.

56. Kiljander T, Helin T, Venho K et al. Prevalence of asthma–COPD overlap syndrome among primary care asthmatics with a smoking history: A cross-sectional study. *NPJ Prim Care Respir Med.* 2015;25:15047.

57. Shaya FT, Dongyi D, Akazawa MO et al. Burden of concomitant asthma and COPD in a Medicaid population. *Chest.* 2008;134(1):14–19.

58. Sorino C, Pedone P, and Scichilone N. Fifteen-year mortality of patients with asthma–COPD overlap syndrome. *Eur J Int Med.* 2016;34:72–77.

59. Kauppi P, Kupiainen H, Lindqvist A et al. Overlap syndrome of asthma and COPD predicts low quality of life. *J Asthma.* 2011;48(3):279–285.

60. Agusti A, Bel E, Thomas M et al. Treatable traits: Toward precision medicine of chronic airway diseases. *Eur Respir J.* 2016;47:410–419.

61. Turner AM, Tamasi L, Schleich F et al. Clinically relevant subgroups in COPD and asthma. *Eur Respir Rev.* 2015;24(136):283–98.

62. Barnes P. Therapeutic approaches to asthma–chronic obstructive pulmonary disease overlap syndromes. *J Allergy Clin Immunol.* 2015;136:531–545.

The genetics of asthma, COPD, and the asthma-COPD overlap

ROBERT BUSCH AND CRAIG P. HERSH

3.1 CLINICAL VIGNETTE

CLINICAL VIGNETTE 3.1

A 10-year old, otherwise healthy male is brought to your office by his mother for wheezing over the last month. The wheezing is episodic and occurs during vigorous exercise, or exposure to cigarette smoke or dusty rooms. The boy describes that his "breathing feels tight," and is accompanied by nonproductive coughing. The patient's mother and father are lifelong nonsmokers, and there are no sources of indoor air pollutants in the home, such as kerosene heaters, wood-burning stoves, or fireplaces.

The patient's mother and father received "health-related genetic risk assessments" through an online commercial genotyping service prior to changes in the regulation of those services in 2013. The mother self-identifies as African American, while her husband self-identifies as Caucasian of central European descent. The patient's mother has no relevant family history of lung disease, while the patient's father has a strong family history of emphysema and liver disease. The patient's paternal grandfather smoked cigarettes and was identified as having alpha-1 antitrypsin deficiency (AATD) after presenting with severe emphysema at an early age. The patient's father was told after a blood test that he was a "carrier" of the gene for AATD by his doctor, and he saw this on his commercial genetic risk report as well.

The patient's mother is concerned because both of their commercial genetic risk assessments stated that they had greater-than-average risk for both asthma and chronic obstructive pulmonary disease (COPD), and she asks what effect this may have on her child's health. The mother also wants to know whether her son has asthma, COPD, or both.

3.2 CLINICAL VIGNETTE: MANAGEMENT

CLINICAL VIGNETTE 3.2

Based on the clinical presentation, this child likely has asthma as a cause of his wheezing. A thorough history and physical should focus on wheeze triggers, family history, associated atopic and allergic comorbidities, and identifying potential alternative sources of wheezing. Additional testing, such as spirometry and allergy testing, may be indicated. If asthma is diagnosed, symptom severity will help guide therapy with bronchodilators, inhaled corticosteroids, and additional medications as per current guidelines. It is unlikely that the patient has COPD at age 10. However, he and his family members should be advised about the dangers of tobacco smoking as a risk factor for COPD and other diseases, as he may be exposed to the opportunity to smoke in his teenage years or earlier.

But how does the genetic data play into decision-making with this child? While Food and Drug Administration (FDA) regulations have changed the way commercially available health-related genetic data is reported to consumers, patients and their family members may still have received these data previously, potentially with little or no guidance in interpretation. Most commercially-available genetic data of this sort prior to 2013 were not approved by the United States FDA,[1,2] and not performed in a lab compliant with the Clinical Laboratory Improvement Amendments (CLIA) standards set forth by the United States government, and should not be used for clinical interpretation. The patient's father reports a family history of AATD along with knowledge of carrier status through medical testing by his physician, although it is unclear which mutations in the *SERPINA1* gene responsible for AATD might be present. The Z-allele and S-allele are the most common pathogenic mutations among populations of European genetic ancestry.[3,4]

In this case, a thorough family history should be obtained focusing on emphysema, COPD, and liver disease, in addition to asthma, allergies, and atopy, to guide clinical decision-making regarding the child's risk for AATD. If it is determined that the patient's risk of inheriting AAT alleles is significant, the family should be referred to an expert in AATD or a genetic counselor to discuss diagnostic testing and counseling regarding the risk for the potential future fathering of children.[5] If the patient has even one copy of the *SERPINA1* Z-allele (MZ genotype), studies have shown that his risk for emphysema, COPD, and liver disease are higher than control populations.[6,7] Intravenous augmentation therapy is indicated in patients with severe AATD (most commonly due to ZZ genotype) and reduced forced expiratory volume in 1 second (FEV_1).[8]

Currently, there is no clinically available genetic test to distinguish between asthma, COPD, or asthma-COPD overlap (ACO). However, genetic research has made great strides in determining genetic risk factors that may contribute to the pathogenesis of these complex diseases, and has helped reveal pathways for potential treatment and for further study.

3.3 BACKGROUND

ACO has been recognized as a distinct entity by both the Global Initiative for Chronic Obstructive Lung Disease (GOLD) and the Global Initiative for Asthma (GINA),[9] the leading international organizations on obstructive lung diseases. While the GOLD/GINA guidelines of 2014 acknowledge the burden and importance of this syndrome, they also make mention of the different underlying mechanisms and phenotypes that make up the spectrum of ACO disease, the uncertainty associated with definitively diagnosing ACO, and the lack of novel therapeutic options for this disease entity. The guidelines include a call for further research into this evolving area of obstructive lung disease, and genetic research has the potential to play a key role in further defining both the diagnosis and management of ACO.

Genetic investigation has already greatly influenced our knowledge of asthma and COPD. This chapter will summarize the principles of genome-wide association studies (GWAS), discuss genetic variants implicated in asthma and COPD, and then summarize the challenges and limitations of current genetic studies in ACO.

3.4 GENETIC RESEARCH METHODOLOGY

3.4.1 HUMAN GENETIC VARIATION

When discussing genetic studies, certain biological principles are important to review. The approximately three billion base pairs that make up the human DNA sequence are organized in 23 pairs of chromosomes: 22 autosomes and a pair of sex chromosomes. While the vast majority (greater than 99.9%) of human DNA is identical between any two individuals, certain areas of the genome are polymorphic due to distant mutation and recombination events. At any area of variation in the human genome, differences in DNA sequence—known as genetic variants—can consist of changes affecting only one base pair position or larger changes involving multiple nucleotide positions. Simple one-base changes are known as single nucleotide polymorphisms (SNPs). Small insertions or deletions encompassing tens to hundreds of base pairs are commonly referred to as "indels." In addition, larger structural changes such as translocations or copy number variants (CNV) can be sources of variation in the genome encompassing hundreds to millions of base pairs.

Humans are diploid organisms, and they inherit one haploid copy of the genome from each parent. This inheritance leads to both a maternal allele and a paternal allele at each locus within the genome. The specific pattern of alleles passed on to offspring by one parent makes up a haplotype, while the information obtained from the combination of both alleles is referred to as the genotype. Characteristic patterns of polymorphisms may develop in different populations due to natural selection, population drift, founder effects, and other forces. Most variation in the human genome is found outside of protein-coding regions. Polymorphisms in protein-coding regions (exons) can change the translated protein sequence (nonsynonymous variant), or the protein can remain unchanged (synonymous variant).

Heritable diseases can be passed to offspring through multiple patterns of inheritance. Broadly, genetic diseases can be classified as Mendelian or non-Mendelian (complex). Classic Mendelian diseases such as sickle cell anemia are caused by highly penetrant rare variants that result in an amino acid change in the translated protein. This aberrant amino acid causes a structural change in the protein that changes its activity, and the resultant defective protein is the pathologic cause of the disease phenotype in homozygotes. In contrast, the genetic contribution to complex diseases such as asthma and COPD is thought to occur through regulatory variation at multiple genetic loci rather than direct changes in protein structure. While each regulatory variant contributes only a small risk of disease individually, the combined burden of multiple risk variants at different genetic loci may exceed a threshold after which the disease phenotype is displayed.

3.4.2 COMPLEX DISEASES: GENES AND ENVIRONMENT

While this chapter is primarily focused on the relationship of genetic variation to disease, the complex interaction of multiple genetic variants and environmental exposures contribute to both COPD and asthma. Environmental factors such as cigarette smoke, dusts, and allergens may modulate genetic effects on lung disease through gene-by-environment interactions, epigenetic mechanisms, or direct inflammatory effects mediated by the immune system.

3.4.3 HISTORY OF GENETIC STUDIES

Genetic research methodology evolved drastically over the last few decades, leading to major changes in how we understand complex respiratory disease. Twin-study methodologies yielded information on the heritability of COPD and asthma as early as the 1970s, and twin studies continue to be a powerful tool for both genetic and epigenetic investigation using modern techniques. In the 1980s and 1990s, familial linkage studies helped locate genetic risk factors on the megabase scale.[10] In the 1990s and early 2000s, investigation of candidate genes led to many new disease associations for individual genes. Most recently, the application of genome-wide genotyping approaches as well as whole genome sequencing has led to an explosion of new genetic data in the realms of asthma and COPD.[11]

3.4.4 GWAS METHODOLOGY

GWAS rely on a simple, yet powerful, methodology. In a typical case-control GWAS, subjects are ascertained on a trait of interest (e.g., smokers with COPD, individuals with an asthma diagnosis), and their genetic information is compared to controls (e.g., smokers without COPD, individuals who do not have asthma). Family- or pedigree-based GWAS are alternative study designs that recruit affected probands (e.g., child with atopic asthma) and their family members who may or may not be affected by the disease. Genotyping is performed at millions of SNPs for each subject. Each directly genotyped SNP is representative of a block of polymorphisms in linkage disequilibrium, meaning that the genotypes of all SNPs in the block are correlated with the genotyped SNP (tag SNP). The patterns of linkage disequilibrium between SNPs allow statistical imputation of the values of the unmeasured SNPs, enabling the investigator to gain reliable genome-wide genetic information while only testing a subset of all the polymorphisms in the genome.

For each SNP, statistical testing is performed to determine whether a disproportionately large number of a particular allele is found in those subjects with the phenotypic trait (risk allele) or without the phenotypic trait (protective allele). Because millions of individual SNPs are tested at once for association with the phenotype, rigorous correction for multiple testing is required to avoid false positives; statistical significance is generally only declared when the p-value for association between a particular SNP and the phenotypic trait is less than 5×10^{-8}. Because of this stringent cutoff, one of the major limitations of GWAS is recruiting enough subjects to achieve the necessary statistical power.

When a statistically significant association between a genetic variant and a phenotype is discovered, it indicates one of two possibilities. In rare situations, the measured SNP itself is directly responsible for the association; however, the association is more commonly driven by another causal variant that is in linkage disequilibrium with the measured SNP. Once the causal variant is identified, additional investigation and validation are required to establish a biologically plausible mechanism relating the causal variant to the disease process.

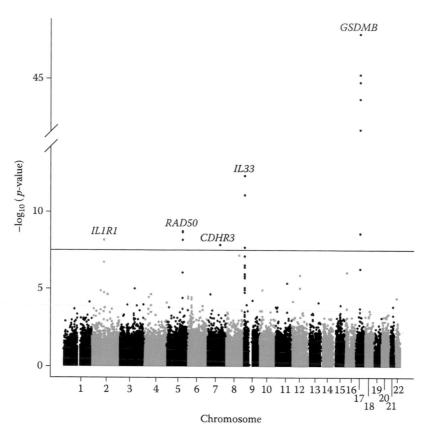

Figure 3.1 Manhattan Plot. The plot displays association results from a GWAS meta-analysis of asthma by Bønnelykke K. et al., *Nat. Genet.*, 46, 51–55, 2014. Coordinates on the *x*-axis represent the SNP's chromosomal position, while the *y*-axis coordinates indicate the negative base-10 logarithm of the *p*-value for association with early childhood asthma with severe exacerbations. SNPs that surpassed or approached the genome-wide significance threshold (horizontal line) are labeled with the gene name of the locus. Used with permission.

GWAS results are often presented using two characteristic figures. First, the Manhattan Plot (Figure 3.1) displays results for every SNP investigated in the GWAS plotted by chromosome on the *x*-axis, along with the negative base-10 logarithm of the *p*-value for association on the *y*-axis. In this figure, a point higher on the *y*-axis indicates greater statistical evidence for a region's association with the phenotype, and the genome-wide significance threshold is often noted on the *y*-axis. The second type of plot is a Local Association Plot (Figure 3.2), also called a LocusZoom plot,[12] which examines SNPs within a smaller region of the genome in more detail. Similar to the Manhattan Plot, SNPs in the Local Association Plot are organized by base-pair position on the *x*-axis and negative base-10 logarithm of the *p*-value on the *y*-axis. This plot also contains additional information about the position of nearby genes, and color codes the plotted points to convey information about the linkage disequilibrium values between SNPs within the locus.

3.4.5 GWAS ADVANTAGES AND DISADVANTAGES

GWAS has many advantages over previous genetic study designs. GWAS is considered an unbiased or "hypothesis-free" study design, because analysis is not influenced by prior information about the function of any particular gene. New disease associations may be found at any position in the genome without any prior knowledge related to the locus. Since a person's DNA sequence is established at conception, genetic variation is not confounded by environmental exposures or unmeasured variables. Once genetic information is obtained for a group of subjects, those data could be used to examine multiple different related phenotypes, as long as care is taken to account for the method of ascertainment.

Disadvantages of GWAS methodology include the large sample size requirements for adequate power to discover associations and the aforementioned need for additional studies to find and validate the specific causal variant. Additionally, sampling from a nonhomogeneous population can lead to spurious association results driven by population stratification, in which both the disease frequency and a particular allele frequency cluster within a subgroup that is not representative of the larger population. On the other hand, genetic association results found in one cohort may not be applicable to members of a separate cohort with different genetic ancestry (such as different racial groups), so GWAS cohorts must be diverse in order for the results to be generalizable. Overall, this has led to a strategy of larger studies that recruit subjects from multiple genetic ancestry groups, while analysis strategies require that each genetic ancestry group be analyzed separately to control for

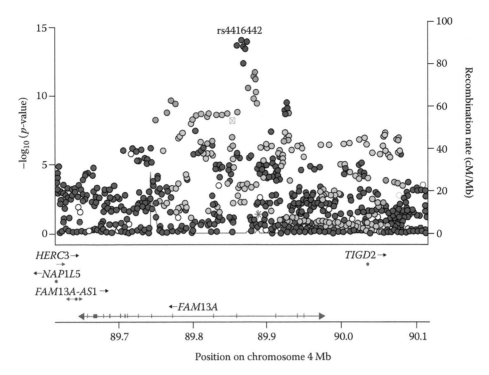

Figure 3.2 Local Association Plot. The plot shows association results of the chromosome 4q22.1 region from a GWAS meta-analysis of COPD by Cho MH et al., *Lancet Respir. Med.*, 2, 214–225, 2014. Coordinates on the x-axis represent the SNP's base-pair position, the y-axis encodes the negative base-10 logarithm of the p-value for association with COPD, and the color of the plotted point indicates the linkage disequilibrium (LD, measured by r^2 value) within the locus. Known gene transcripts within the region are noted on the x-axis. Used with permission.

population stratification. The end result of this strategy is a requirement for even larger study samples. While genotyping costs have dropped significantly over the last decade, the cost of obtaining thorough phenotype data on patients has remained relatively constant. Because of all of these factors, careful planning and study design is required to conduct a GWAS, and an understanding of these limitations is required to appropriately interpret the results.

3.4.6 GWAS IN ASTHMA, COPD, AND ACO

Numerous GWAS have been previously performed for asthma and COPD (and related phenotypes), yielding many novel associations (Tables 3.1 and 3.2). These associations have led to a better understanding of the genetic basis of obstructive lung diseases, and genetic associations identified in asthma and COPD may play a role in our understanding of ACO as well. Conversely, genetic studies of ACO as a phenotype have been limited by multiple factors: a lack of accurate disease definitions for case-control studies, few ACO-related biomarkers (such as characteristic biochemical assays, imaging findings, or pulmonary function testing findings), and lower sample size due in part to the fact that many ACO studies are subgroups of larger investigations of either asthma or COPD. However, GWAS may be a promising methodology to investigate ACO. Genetic studies may help influence characterization

of ACO subtypes related to disease mechanisms, may lead to more accurate identification of subjects at risk of ACO and to more accurate diagnosis of ACO, and may potentially identify novel therapeutic targets.

3.5 GENETIC INVESTIGATIONS OF ASTHMA

3.5.1 ASTHMA PHENOTYPES

Asthma is largely a clinical diagnosis (as defined by GINA guidelines[15]) that relies on characteristic symptomatology, associated comorbidities, such as atopy, family history, and physical exam findings. Laboratory testing such as methacholine challenge testing, circulating eosinophil counts, IgE levels, and exhaled nitric oxide levels are supportive of the diagnosis, but have not been fully integrated as diagnostic tools into clinical practice guidelines. Asthma severity is also defined primarily by clinical presentation and symptoms, although spirometry also is included in current guidelines. While heterogeneity in subphenotypes such as atopic and nonatopic asthma is apparent, unambiguous definitions of these specific phenotypes for the purposes of genetic studies have been elusive. Most asthma studies have relied on a doctor's diagnosis of asthma as the primary phenotype, while a subset of investigations has further classified subjects as atopic or nonatopic.

Table 3.1 Genome-wide significant associations with asthma phenotypes

Chromosome region	Genes	Phenotype
1q23.1	PYHIN1	Asthma, among subjects of African descent[23]
1q31.3	DENND1B	Asthma[32]
2q12.1	IL1RL1/IL18R1	Asthma[21]
3q27.3	RTP2	Asthma, among subjects of Latino descent[23]
5q22.1	TSLP	Asthma[23]
5q31.1	RAD50/IL13	Asthma[21]
6p21.32	HLA-DQ/HLA-DR	Asthma[21]
9p24.1	IL33	Asthma[21]
15q22.33	SMAD3	Asthma[23]
17q21	ZPBP2/ORMDL3/GSDMB/IKFZ3	Asthma, childhood onset[16]
22q12.3	IL2RB	Asthma[23]

Table 3.2 Genome-wide significant associations with COPD and related phenotypes

Chromosome region	Genes	Phenotype
4p15.2	DHX15	Upper to lower lobe emphysema ratio among Chinese[72]
4q22.1	FAM13A	COPD[60]
4q24	NPNT	COPD[56]
4q31	HHIP	COPD[50]
6p21.32	HLA-DQB1/HLA-DQA2	COPD[56]
6p21.32	PPT2/AGER	Quantitative emphysema[72]
11q22.3	MMP12	Severe COPD[14]
12q23.1	SNRPF/CCDC38	Quantitative emphysema[72]
14q22.33	RIN3	COPD[14]
15q25	CHRNA3/CHRNA5/IREB2	COPD[50]
17q21	TGFB2	Severe COPD[14]
17q21.31	KANSL1	COPD[56]
17q25.1	TSEN4	COPD in never smokers[56]
17q25.2	MGAT5B	Upper to lower lobe emphysema ratio among Chinese[72]
19p13.2	MAN2B1	Upper to lower lobe emphysema ratio among Hispanics[72]
19q13	RAB4B/EGLN2/CYP2A6	COPD[52]

3.5.2 ZPBP2/ORMDL3/GSDMB/IKFZ3

One of the earliest GWAS examining asthma and asthma-related phenotypes met with success despite relatively small discovery populations. This study by Moffatt et al.,[16] representing the GABRIEL consortium, compared 994 patients with asthma with 1243 nonasthmatics, using both family-based and case-control panels of subjects. After genotyping and association analysis, a group of SNPs in linkage disequilibrium with each other at the 17q21 locus was found to be significantly associated with asthma. Further conditional analysis with a focus on the 17q21 region identified three SNPs that showed statistically independent effects within the linkage disequilibrium block. The top SNP, rs7216389, yielded an odds ratio of 1.45 for association with asthma (p-value 9×10^{-11}). In two replication populations, the 17q21 region consistently showed statistical significance and comparable effect sizes to the discovery analysis. This entire block of SNPs was in close proximity to the Zona Pellucida

Binding Protein 2 (ZPBP2), Gasdermin B (GSDMB), IKAROS family zinc finger 3 (IKZF3), and Orosomucoid-like 3 (ORMDL3) genes.

Once the potential risk alleles in the 17q21 region were identified, additional gene expression assays were performed to identify genes with increased or decreased levels of expression associated with these genetic variants (expression quantitative trait loci or eQTLs). The asthma risk variant at the rs7216389 SNP was associated with higher levels of ORMDL3 gene expression and was shown to account for 29.5% of the variance in expression of the ORMDL3 gene.[16] A subsequent study by Verlaan et al. quantifying allelic expression differences at the 17q21 locus provided a more detailed map of regulatory variation at this region and showed that the asthma-associated SNPs within 17q21 exerted regulatory effects on ZPBP2, GSDMB, and ORMDL3 through chromatin remodeling effects.[17] When taken together with the GWAS data, these additional results support the hypothesis that causal variants in the 17q21 region exerts their effect on asthma risk through differences in gene expression of both the *ORMDL3* and *GSDMB* genes. Both *ORMDL3* and *GSDMB* are biologically plausible effectors of asthma pathogenesis. Yeast homologs of the *ORMDL3* gene product are involved in sphingolipid regulation and metabolism,[18] and dysregulation of homologous sphingolipids pathways in human airways have been shown to contribute to airway inflammation in asthma.[19] *GSDMB* is involved in maintaining the differentiation state of epithelial cells,[20] and it is highly expressed in both CD4 and CD8 T-cells, which could have implications for airway immune response.[17]

The 17q21 locus has been robustly replicated in subsequent GWAS. In a follow-up study conducted by the GABRIEL Consortium,[21] the 17q21 locus showed a significant association with childhood onset asthma. In a separate large candidate gene study performed by the EVE consortium,[22] and in a later GWAS meta-analysis by the same group[23] including multiple asthma study populations, the 17q21 locus association was replicated in subjects of European, Latino, and African ancestry in the discovery phase. Notably, while some SNPs within the 17q21 region showed association in each ethnic and racial group, the African-descent replication populations in the candidate gene study did not corroborate the *ORMDL3* association at rs7216389, although other genotyped SNPs in the area did show a significant association. It has been hypothesized that this result may reflect the limited ability of genotyping platforms to accurately assess the more diverse common variation within populations of African descent.[22] Additional studies further confirmed and refined the 17q21 locus asthma association[24-26] with additional associations to childhood age of onset,[21,27,28] greater asthma severity,[27] more frequent exacerbations,[29,30] and an interaction with smoking.[31]

3.5.3 DENND1B

Sleiman et al. performed an asthma GWAS meta-analysis utilizing several cohorts of children of both European and African ancestry.[32] The discovery phase of this study focused on 793 subjects with persistent asthma treated with inhaled glucocorticoid therapy and 1988 matched controls, all of whom were North Americans of European ancestry. This investigation revealed several SNPs within a locus at 1q31.3 that were statistically significantly associated with asthma, and these associations were replicated in cohorts of European children (917 adults and children with asthma, 1546 children and adults without asthma) and North American children of African ancestry (1667 children with asthma, 2045 children without asthma). The DENN/MADD containing domain 1B (*DENND1B*) gene in this locus is a plausible asthma candidate, as its gene product is a protein found in natural killer cells, memory T-cells, and dendritic cells that interact with tumor-necrosis-factor alpha receptor type-1[33] to modulate inflammatory signaling cascades.[34]

3.5.4 IL33 AND IL1RL1 REGIONS

In 2010, Moffatt et al.[21] published the GABRIEL Consortium's expanded investigation of genetic variants associated with asthma including 10,365 subjects with asthma as well as 16,110 controls in an ancestry-matched case-control GWAS meta-analysis. This study found statistically significant associations between atopic asthma and genetic variants in five additional loci. Two of these regions were the chromosome 9p24.1 locus flanking Interleukin (*IL*)*33* and the chromosome 2q12.1 locus near *IL1RL1/IL18R1*. While both of these loci had previously been implicated in asthma in a study of eosinophil count in an Icelandic population,[35] the association at 9p24.1 was affirmed as genome-wide significant in the Moffatt study.

IL-33, the protein product of the *IL33* gene, is a member of the IL-1-like cytokine family that interacts with the IL1RL1 receptor[36] to activate human eosinophils and regulate eosinophil-mediated inflammation,[37] like that seen in asthma. In addition, IL33 has been detected in airway epithelial cells, and increased expression of *IL33* has been documented in the airway smooth muscle cells of subjects with severe asthma.[38] IL-33 has also been shown to regulate Th2-mediated inflammation by activating members of the nuclear factor kappa B (NF-κB) and mitogen-activated protein (MAP) kinase pathways. Thus the causal variants within these asthma-associated loci are hypothesized to exert their action through modulating eosinophilic inflammation and Th2 immune response pathways in the lung.

Subsequent studies have replicated the genome-wide significant signal at the chromosome 2q12.1 locus[23] containing *IL1RL1*, and genetic variants in the 2q12.1 locus flanking *IL33* also approached genome-wide significance in the same study.

3.5.5 TSLP

In their 2011 GWAS of the EVE consortium cohorts, Torgerson et al.[23] provided genome-wide validation of an association with thymic stromal lymphopoietin (*TSLP*), which had been noted in the candidate gene era.[39] The asthma-associated SNP on chromosome 5q22.1 was near the *TSLP* gene, and increased expression of *TSLP* had previously been shown to correlate with disease severity in asthmatic airways[40] by Ying and colleagues. Further work also linked increased expression of *TSLP* with increased expression of Th2 cytokines and selective infiltration of CD4(+)/CCR4(+) T-cells in biopsy specimens from asthmatic airways.[40] Subsequent genetic association studies replicated the 5q22.1 association with other asthma phenotypes,[41] including asthma with hay fever.[42] Additional study led to the design of a monoclonal antibody against the TSLP protein that prevented receptor interaction. A double-blind, randomized, placebo-controlled, proof-of-concept study showed that subjects treated with the monoclonal antibody showed decreased levels of allergen-induced bronchoconstriction and decreased markers of systemic inflammation at multiple timepoints when compared to placebo,[43] and the antibody is now undergoing additional clinical trials.

3.5.6 ADDITIONAL ASTHMA LOCI: HLA-DQ, SMAD3, IL13, IL2RB, RTP2

Many additional loci have been implicated in asthma through GWAS. While not all have been robustly replicated to date, they remain as potential objectives for further studies. In their expanded GABRIEL Consortium study,[21] Moffatt et al. discovered associations with genetic variants near the HLA-DQ region (chromosome 6p21.32). The HLA-DQ locus was again associated with asthma in a GWAS by Li et al.[44] albeit not at a genome-wide significance level. The GABRIEL group also found genome-wide significant asthma associations for loci near SMAD3 (chromosome 15q22.33) and a locus near IL2RB (chromosome 22q12.3).[21] A locus near *IL13* (chromosome 5q31.1) had approached genome-wide significant association with asthma,[44] and achieved genome-wide significance level in fixed effect meta-analysis in the GABRIEL study, but not in the random effects model. While it did not reach significance in meta-analysis of all racial subgroups, PYHIN1 (chromosome 1q23.1) showed genome-wide significant association in individuals identifying as African American and African Caribbean. Evidence of further ancestry-specific associations is supported by loci near PYHIN1 (chromosome 1)[23] and C11orf71 (chromosome 11),[23] which approached genome-wide significance in populations of African descent. Similarly, the chromosome 3q27.3 locus near RTP2 was associated with asthma among Latino subjects in the initial phase of the EVE study,[23] but not in replication. Association studies that identify distinct phenotypic subpopulations have also provided additional insight into classification of asthma within narrower target populations, such as the GWAS of early childhood asthma with severe exacerbations by Bønnelykke et al.[13] (Figure 3.1). Additional loci such as PDE4D (chromosome 5q12)[45] and RORA (chromosome 15q22)[21] approached genome-wide significance in previous studies and may still overcome this stringent threshold if larger samples sizes are examined.

3.5.7 CANDIDATE GENE ASSOCIATIONS

While GWAS has discovered multiple genes associated with asthma and asthma-related phenotypes, prior methodologies such as linkage studies and candidate gene analyses have led to important genetic associations that may represent viable targets for further study and pharmacologic intervention. Notable genes include disintegrin and metallopeptidase domain 33 (*ADAM33*) on chromosome 20p13,[46] dipeptidyl peptidase X (*DPP10*)[47] in the same region of chromosome 2q14 containing IL-1, and filaggrin[48] (*FLG*) on chromosome 1q21.3. Mechanistic roles have been implicated for these genes in phenotypes such as asthma, asthma progression, and atopic dermatitis with asthma. Despite the

evidence presented through these additional studies, these regions have not been identified as significant in GWAS to date.

3.6 GENETIC INVESTIGATIONS OF COPD

3.6.1 COPD PHENOTYPES

COPD is a chronic, progressive disease characterized by airflow obstruction. Both genetic and environmental risk factors such as cigarette smoking play a role in susceptibility to COPD. However, even early classifications of COPD patients recognized that multiple subtypes exist, defined by phenotypic features such as chronic bronchitis, emphysema, and the frequency of exacerbations. This disease heterogeneity led to a multitude of COPD-related phenotypes used in genetic association studies, each of which may relate to different aspects of disease pathogenesis. Most larger GWAS investigations of COPD have reported associations to COPD defined by the GOLD spirometric criteria,[49] defined by the ratio of FEV_1 to forced vital capacity (FVC) less than 0.7; severity grade is subsequently defined by FEV_1. Many genetic studies have focused on moderate, severe, or very severe disease ($FEV_1 < 80\%$ predicted, corresponding to GOLD spirometric stages 2–4). In contrast to genetic studies of asthma, in which the majority of subjects have limited tobacco smoke exposure, COPD GWAS have generally focused on smokers with and without COPD.

3.6.2 CHRNA3/CHRNA5/IREB2

One of the first GWAS to report genome-wide significant associations with COPD was conducted by Pillai et al.[50] in 2009, which discovered genome-wide significant associations at the chromosome 15q25 region, near a complex cluster of genes including iron-responsive-element binding protein 2 (*IREB2*), nicotinic cholinergic receptors alpha3 (*CHRNA3*), and alpha5 (*CHRNA5*). The discovery phase of this GWAS used the GenKOLS Norwegian case-control study population, with replication in the International COPD Genetics Network (ICGN) family-based study and a case-control population composed of cases from the National Emphysema Treatment Trial (NETT) and controls from the Normative Aging Study (NAS). SNPs within this complex region have consistently shown association with COPD in multiple subsequent studies of COPD,[14,51,52] emphysema,[53] smoking,[54] and lung function.[55,56]

3.6.3 HHIP

In an article by Wilk et al.[57] and a companion article by Pillai et al.[50] in 2009, the hedgehog-interacting protein (*HHIP*) locus on chromosome 4q31 was significantly associated with lung function (as measured by FEV_1) and reached near-genome-wide significance in the COPD association analysis (p-value 1.47×10^{-7}). Further work by Zhou et al.[58] demonstrated that lung tissue samples from subjects with COPD showed long-range regulation of HHIP mRNA expression and protein levels through differential binding of the Sp3 transcription factor in an upstream enhancer region of HHIP; this same region contained previously COPD-associated GWAS variants that were responsible for the differential binding of Sp3. Subsequent studies linked lower levels of HHIP to emphysema susceptibility in mice[59] as well as changes in extracellular matrix and cell proliferation in murine lung tissue, further supporting the mechanistic link of COPD-associated variants in *HHIP*. This locus has been robustly replicated in multiple subsequent GWAS of COPD,[14,52] emphysema,[53] and lung function.[56]

3.6.4 FAM13A

An additional COPD-associated locus was discovered on chromosome 4q22.1 (Figure 3.2) by Cho et al.[60] in a GWAS meta-analysis including the GenKols cohort, the NETT/NAS cohort, and subjects from Evaluating COPD Longitudinally to Identify Predictive Surrogate Endpoints (ECLIPSE). Replication confirmed the finding in a subset of the Genetic Epidemiology of COPD study (COPDGene), ICGN, and the Boston Early-Onset COPD Study. Significantly associated SNPs centered on the *FAM13A* gene, and this locus has been replicated in additional studies.[14]

3.6.5 RAB4B/EGLN2/CYP2A6

Further reinforcing the genetic connection between COPD and smoking-related behaviors, a study by Cho et al.[52] in 2012 identified a genome-wide significant association with COPD at the 19q13 locus near the genes member-RAS Oncogene Family (*RAB4B*), Egl-9 family hypoxia-Inducible Factor 2 (*EGLN2*), and cytochrome P450 2A6 (*CYP2A6*). While the *RAB4B/EGLN2/CYP2A6* locus had previously been implicated in GWAS of smoking-related behaviors,[54,61] the direct pathogenic links between this locus, smoking, and COPD have not been fully investigated.

3.6.6 MMP12, RIN3, AND TGFB2

In a large GWAS meta-analysis including the COPDGene, ECLIPSE, NETT/NAS, GenKOLS, and ICGN cohorts including 6633 COPD cases and 5704 controls, Cho et al.[14] showed a significant association with moderate-to-severe COPD (GOLD stage 2–4) at one novel locus as well as confirming previously discovered associations with COPD. The first locus was near the matrix metalloproteinase-12 (*MMP12*) locus on chromosome 11q22.3. Hautamaki and colleagues previously showed that MMP12-deficient mice did not develop emphysema in response to cigarette smoking.[62] This proteolytic enzyme has also been associated with FEV_1, COPD risk, and time of COPD onset in previous candidate gene studies in humans.[63] Polymorphisms in the *MMP12* gene promoter were

also previously associated with decreased promoter activity and decreased binding of activator protein-1 (AP-1),[64] while decreased binding of AP-1 was associated with decreased expression of *MMP12*.[65] This body of evidence supports the role of *MMP12* in COPD through dysregulated proteolytic activity on extracellular matrix proteins in the lung, although precisely defining its role has remained a challenge.

Two additional loci stood out in the Cho et al. meta-analysis[14] when testing for association with more severe COPD. The ras and rab interactor 3 (*RIN3*) locus at chromosome 14q32 and the transforming growth factor beta-2 (*TGFB2*) at chromosome 1q41 both approached genome-wide significance for association with severe COPD (GOLD stage 3–4).

3.6.7 AGER/PPT2 AND EMPHYSEMA-ASSOCIATED LOCI

Associations between lung function (FEV_1 and FEV_1/FVC) and SNPs within the *AGER* gene on chromosome 6p21 were discovered in a large population-based GWAS[66] and subsequent meta-analysis[67] in 2010. Additional work by Wu et al.[68] and Cheng et al.[69] showed that systemic soluble receptor for advanced glycation end products (sRAGE) protein levels were increased in COPD, and that the sRAGE protein was a biomarker of emphysema in COPD patients. In addition, Cheng et al. demonstrated that the rs2070600 SNP in the *AGER* locus was associated with circulating sRAGE levels. While the rs2070600 SNP has shown promise in GWAS of COPD,[70,71] additional SNPs in the *AGER/PPT2* region reached genome-wide significance in the Multi-Ethnic Study of Athersclerosis (MESA) GWAS meta-analysis of quantitative emphysema[72] and in an emphysema GWAS meta-analysis[53] including subjects from COPDGene, ECLIPSE, GenKOLS, and others. Despite the current lack of robust genome-wide associations of variants in the *AGER* gene with COPD susceptibility, associations with both lung function and emphysema phenotypes make this gene locus a promising candidate for future studies of COPD.

The MESA meta-analysis discovered an additional association with quantitative emphysema at the 12q23.1 locus near *SNRPF/CCDC38*. Examination of upper-to-lower lobe ratio of emphysema distribution yielded additional associations within specific racial and ethnic groups as well.

3.6.8 ALPHA-1 ANTITRYPSIN DEFICIENCY AND SERPINA1

AATD was first discovered in 1963 by Laurell and Eriksson[73] using protein electrophoresis. Severe AATD has long been recognized as a genetic cause of emphysema[74] among smokers, and the link between rare polymorphisms in the *SERPINA1* gene (Z and S alleles) and protein dysfunction of AAT has been well-described at a molecular level.[3] While lung disease in AATD follows an autosomal recessive inheritance pattern, additional genetic and environmental factors modify emphysema risk among those with polymorphisms in AAT.[75]

Due to statistical issues and study design, a genome-wide significant association between known risk alleles in the *SERPINA1* gene and either COPD or emphysema has been elusive. The Z and S alleles are rare variants in North American and European populations (Z-allele frequency: 0.014–0.049; S-allele frequency: 0.056–0.14),[4] and many GWAS have removed rare variants from analysis due to methodological problems with quality control and statistical power. In addition, most GWAS of COPD and emphysema have specifically excluded subjects with AATD. However, several studies have shown that heterozygote carriers may be at increased risk of airflow obstruction,[6,7] and the genetic signal of this increased risk may still be present in population studies of lung function and case-control studies of COPD. Further supporting the increased risk associated with Z-allele heterozygosity, variants in linkage disequilibrium with the Z allele in the *RIN3* locus were associated with emphysema in a GWAS meta-analysis by Cho et al.[53] This association was attenuated by conditioning upon the Z allele, further supporting the involvement of *SERPINA1*. Cho et al. concluded that these tagging SNPs may be capturing a signal related to pathogenic variants in *SERPINA1*, but further investigation is needed to definitively identify the causal variants in this association region.

3.6.9 THE UNITED KINGDOM BIOBANK

The UK Biobank Lung Exome Variant Evaluation (UK BiLEVE) study[56] published a well-powered GWAS of lung function. They also investigated the relationships of their novel genome-wide significant lung function loci to COPD. They discovered that the *NPNT* (chromosome 4q24), *HLA-DQB1/HLA-DQA2* (chromosome 6p21.32, rs9274600), and *KANSL1* (chromosome 17q21.31) loci achieved genome-wide significant association with COPD (GOLD stage 2–4) in a meta-analysis of never- and heavy-smoking case-control datasets. Additionally, the *TSEN4* locus (chromosome 17q25.1) showed significant association with COPD among never smokers. Thus these genes may represent links between the genetic architecture of lung function and COPD.

3.6.10 FUTURE STUDIES

As of the writing of this chapter, large, well-powered GWAS meta-analyses from groups such as the International COPD Genetics Consortium[76] and the UK BiLEVE group[77] are underway. The sample sizes of these studies are significantly larger than previous investigations, and they will likely reveal multiple new associations with lung function and COPD that may lead to treatment targets and further mechanistic insight. Additionally, whole genome sequencing projects like the Trans-Omics for Precision Medicine (TOPMed) initiative offer new opportunities for pinpointing causal variants and investigating rare variants in COPD and asthma.

3.7 GENETIC INVESTIGATIONS OF ASTHMA-COPD OVERLAP

Variants hypothesized to identify promising genes for further study in ACO come from many sources: variants associated with ACO, variants associated with both asthma and COPD in a meta-analysis strategy, and variants associated with phenotypes shared between COPD and asthma (e.g., lung function, pharmacologic response to bronchodilators, inflammatory pathways). In each experimental design, robust replication among ACO populations will contribute to the veracity of the findings. Each of these techniques may identify associations with different genetic aspects of ACO and provide different insights into similarities between asthma, COPD, and ACO.

ACO has only recently been formally recognized through international guidelines, and accordingly there are fewer genetic studies that have directly investigated this syndrome. A GWAS by Hardin et al.[78] was the first study to investigate genetic variation in subjects with ACO in the COPDGene cohort. This study compared subjects with COPD that also carried a physician's diagnosis of asthma ($n = 450$) to subjects with COPD alone ($n = 3120$). The investigation found several suggestive associations (Figure 3.3), but none reached genome-wide significance levels. Suggestive associations included the *CSMD1* (chromosome 8p23.2), *SOX5* (chromosome 12p12.1), and *RMST* (chromosome 12q23.1) loci among non-Hispanic whites. The *CSMD1* gene has previously been associated with emphysema,[79] while the *SOX5* gene has previously been associated with COPD and lung development.[80] The analysis of African Americans revealed suggestive associations at the *PKD1L1* (chromosome 7p12.3), *ATP11A* (chromosome 13q34), and *REEP3* loci (chromosome 10q21.3), though the p-values were not genome-wide significant. Meta-analysis of the two racial groups revealed suggestive associations in a cluster of SNPs near the *GPR65* locus on chromosome 14q31.3, as well as two variants in the *CYP11B2* locus on chromosome 8q24.3. Similar to the experience in other complex disease GWAS, this study was likely underpowered due to a relatively small sample size.

In an alternative study design, Smolonska and colleagues utilized an asthma case-control study and a separate COPD study in a GWAS meta-analysis to identify common genetic variants that affected both conditions.[81] Results of this meta-analysis revealed one genome-wide significant association with obstructive lung disease and two loci with suggestive associations at sub-genome-wide significance levels. The G-protein subunit gamma 5 pseudogene 5 (*GNG5P5*) locus was associated with obstructive lung disease at genome-wide significance in meta-analysis (chromosome 13q14.2). The two additional sub-genome-wide significant loci were

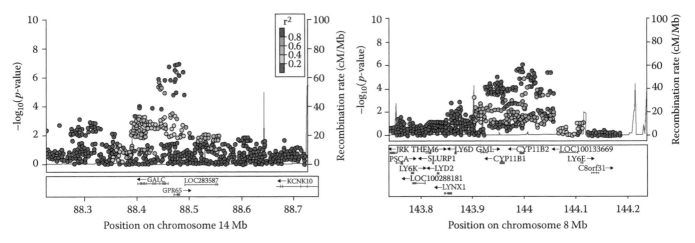

Figure 3.3 Top association results of the chromosome 14q31.3 region (left) and 8q24.3 region (right) from a GWAS of ACO by Hardin M et al., *Eur. Respir. J.*, 44, 341–350, 2014 presented as local association plots. Used with permission.

of interest due to their connection to inflammatory pathways. The first of these loci (chromosome 2p24.3) is a complex region containing multiple genes, pseudogenes, and long noncoding RNA, as well as the DEAD-box polypeptide 1 (*DDX1*) gene approximately 139 kb away. The second locus (chromosome 5q23.1) contains the COMM domain containing 10 (*COMMD10*) protein. Both the *DDX1* and *COMMD10* genes play a regulatory role in the NF-κB pathway; DDX1 acts as a coactivator of NF-κB transcription by interacting with the subunits of NF-κB directly, while COMMD10 interacts with other members of the COMM domain containing proteins to inhibit NF-κB pathway activation. While this study did not directly investigate ACO, it highlighted a method to increase statistical power by investigating genetic variation shared between both diseases.

GWAS and meta-analyses of phenotypes related to both asthma and COPD provide interesting candidate genes for future ACO investigations, particularly in the studies of lung function. Decreased lung function is a unifying feature between asthma, COPD, and ACO. It stands to reason that genes related to lung function might also be involved in ACO. Population-based investigations of lung function have benefitted from large sample sizes as well as robust and objective phenotyping through spirometry. Multiple genome-wide significant loci have been identified related to measure of lung function such as FEV_1,[56,66,67,82,83] FVC,[83,84] and the ratio of FEV_1 to FVC (Tables 3.3 through 3.5).[67,82,83,85]

3.8 CHALLENGES FOR FUTURE GENETIC STUDIES OF ACO

The most prominent challenge in studying ACO through GWAS methodologies is the lack of statistical power due to small sample sizes. While larger studies of ACO may be necessary to identify genome-wide significant associations, other methodological concerns must also be addressed. First, there may be a fundamental difference on the genetic level between subtypes of ACO patients. For example, a

hypothetical ACO patient might be characterized by severe persistent asthma since childhood that leads to chronic progressive airflow obstruction over time, atopic symptoms and triggers, frequent exacerbations, and minimal or no emphysema or other COPD-related phenotypes. A second ACO patient may have had a diagnosis of intermittent asthma during childhood, smoked tobacco throughout their adult life, and experience the onset in middle age of manifestations of COPD such as persistent obstruction and emphysema along with some degree of reversible airflow obstruction and some asthma-like features. Currently, it is unclear whether these two patients share common genetic pathways. Most investigations of ACO to date have used subjects from studies of COPD. Fewer data exist in the group of subjects with long-standing asthma with fixed airflow obstruction in the absence of tobacco smoke exposure.

Second, while the GINA/GOLD guidelines give muchneeded credibility to the diagnosis of ACO, unambiguous objective diagnostic criteria are needed to clearly define ACO for genetic studies. While the diagnosis of COPD by spirometry is well-established, asthma phenotyping for large-scale genetic studies has largely relied on various combinations of a physician's clinical diagnosis, asthma-related medication use, and symptoms. Efforts to further classify asthma subjects into atopic and nonatopic subgroups have also differed by study. Additional supportive diagnostic tests such as exhaled nitric oxide and biomarkers related to atopy might help to further refine phenotyping and decrease noise in the genetic signal. Gene expression signatures related to Th2 inflammatory profiles have been hypothesized to define relevant subphenotypes of asthma by Woodruff et al.,[86] and similar efforts related to other disease characteristics could refine our classifications of asthma, COPD, and ACO. Christenson and colleagues examined a Th2 gene expression signature in asthma and COPD cohorts in order to determine associations with clinical features of COPD.[87] This study did not reveal associations between Th2 gene expression signatures and subjects diagnosed with the ACO. However, this Th2 gene expression signature did correlate

Table 3.3 GWAS associations with forced expiratory volume in one second (FEV$_1$)

Chromosome region	Genes	Phenotype
1p12	SPAG17/TBX15	Low vs. high FEV$_1$[56]
1q21.3	MCL1/ENSA	FEV$_1$[83]
2q22.1	DARS/CSCR4	Low vs. high FEV$_1$[56]
2q35	TNS1	FEV$_1$[66]
3p14.3	SLMAP	Low vs. high FEV$_1$[56]
3q25.32	RSRC1	Low vs. high FEV$_1$ in heavy smokers[56]
3q26.2	MECOM/EVI1	FEV$_1$[82]
4q24	GSTCD/INTS12/NPNT	FEV$_1$[67]
4q24	TET2	Low vs. high FEV$_1$ in never smokers[56]
4q24	NPNT	Low vs. high FEV$_1$ in never smokers[56]
5q32	HTR4	FEV$_1$[66]
6p21.32	HLA-DQB1/HLADQA2	Low vs. high FEV$_1$ in never smokers[56]
6p22.1	ZKSCAN3	FEV$_1$[82]
10p13	CDC123	FEV$_1$[82]
10q22.3	C10orf11	FEV$_1$[82]
12p11.22	TBX3	FEV$_1$[83]
12p11.22	CCDC91	Low vs. high FEV$_1$ in never smokers[56]
12q24.21	RBM19/TBX5	Low vs. high FEV$_1$ in heavy smokers[56]
14q32.12	TRIP11	FEV$_1$[83]
14q32.12	RIN3	FEV$_1$[83]
17q21.31	KANSL1	Low vs. high FEV$_1$ in never smokers[56]
17q24.3	KCNJ2	FEV$_1$-by-smoking interaction term[85]
17q25.1	TSEN54	Low vs. high FEV$_1$ in never smokers[56]
20p12.3	FERMT1/BMP2	Low vs. high FEV$_1$[56]
22q11.21	MICAL3	Low vs. high FEV$_1$[56]
22q12.1	MIAT/MN1	FEV$_1$[83]

Table 3.4 GWAS associations with forced vital capacity (FVC)

Chromosome region	Genes	Phenotype
2p16.1	EFEMP1	FVC[84]
2q21.3	TMEM163	FVC[84]
3q25.32	AK097794	FVC[83]
6p24.3	BMP6	FVC[84]
9q34.3	LHX3	FVC[83]
11p11.2	HSD17B12	FVC[84]
11p11.2	PRDM11	FVC[84]
12p11.22	PTHLH/CCDC91	FVC[83]
16q23.1	WWOX	FVC[84]
17q24.3	KCNJ2	FVC[84]

with clinical features among subjects with COPD such as lower lung function, bronchodilator response, peripheral blood eosinophilia, and improvement in hyperinflation in response to corticosteroid therapy.

Third, current genetic studies of ACO have not been able to adequately represent groups that show health disparities related to asthma and COPD. Women and African Americans have higher rates of ACO than other groups; however, these have represented only a small portion of most investigations in the field. While the GWAS of Hardin

and colleagues[78] did include women and African Americans with ACO, a larger stratified analysis would be necessary to better define genetic associations that could contribute to these disparities.

3.9 OPPORTUNITIES FOR FUTURE ACO STUDIES

Current genetic investigations of ACO are largely limited by power. Large-scale meta-analyses have attempted to address these limitations in complex diseases such as COPD and asthma, and similar strategies using well-phenotyped subjects may increase power in studies of ACO. Additionally, large-scale genotyping efforts connected to extensive medical records such as the UK Biobank may allow investigators to choose sampling populations with adequate statistical power.

Evolving genetic technologies as well as evolving methods in epigenetics, gene expression, proteomics, and network medicine are revolutionizing the investigation of obstructive lung diseases. Whole genome sequencing projects are refining our ability to examine rare variants and their effects on complex disease. Efforts like the TOPMed project sponsored by the National Institutes

Table 3.5 GWAS associations with FEV$_1$/FVC ratio

Chromosome region	Genes	Phenotype
1p36.13	MFAP2	FEV$_1$/FVC[82]
1q41	TGFB2-LYPLAL1	FEV$_1$/FVC[82]
1q41	LYPLAL1/RNUSF-1	FEV$_1$/FVC[83]
2p24.2	KCNS3/NT55C1B	FEV$_1$/FVC[83]
2q36.3	PID1	FEV$_1$/FVC[67]
2q36.3	DNER	FEV$_1$/FVC-by-smoking interaction term[85]
2q37.3	HDAC4-FLJ43879	FEV$_1$/FVC[82]
3p24.2	RARB	FEV$_1$/FVC[82]
4q22.1	FAM13A	FEV$_1$/FVC[67]
4q24	NPNT	FEV$_1$/FVC[83]
4q31.21	HHIP	FEV$_1$/FVC[67]
5q15	SPATA9-RHOBTB3	FEV$_1$/FVC[82]
5q32	HTR4	FEV$_1$/FVC[67]
5q33.3	ADAM19	FEV$_1$/FVC[67]
6p21.32	AGER/PPT2	FEV$_1$/FVC[67]
6p21.32	HLA-DQB1	FEV$_1$/FVC-by-smoking interaction term[85]
6p21.33	NCR3-AIF1	FEV$_1$/FVC[82]
6q21	ARMC2	FEV$_1$/FVC[82]
6q24.1	GPR126/LOC153910	FEV$_1$/FVC[67]
6q24.2	GPR126/LOC153910	FEV$_1$/FVC[83]
9q22.32	PTCH1	FEV$_1$/FVC[67]
9q33.1	ASTN2	FEV$_1$/FVC[83]
10p13	CDC123	FEV$_1$/FVC[82]
12q13.3	LRP1	FEV$_1$/FVC[82]
12q23.1	CCDC38	FEV$_1$/FVC[82]
15q23	THSD4	FEV$_1$/FVC[66]
16p13.13	EMP2/TEKT5	FEV$_1$/FVC[83]
16q21	MMP15	FEV$_1$/FVC[82]
16q23.1	CFDP1	FEV$_1$/FVC[82]
19q13.2	LTBP4	FEV$_1$/FVC[83]
21q22.11	KCNE2-LINC00310/C21 or f82	FEV$_1$/FVC[82]
Xp22.2	AP1S2/GRPR	FEV$_1$/FVC[83]

of Health are creating a wealth of genomic data consisting of more than 60,000 complete human genomes that can be leveraged to investigate asthma, COPD, and ACO. Epigenetic studies of differential DNA methylation, transcription-factor binding, and histone modification are providing information about transcriptional regulation that may affect disease pathways. RNA sequencing allows for the quantification of gene expression in multiple tissue types. Reviews of these findings in these fields and integrative analyses of these complementary technologies are discussed elsewhere.[88,89]

3.10 CONCLUSIONS

GWAS have yielded valuable insights into the pathogenesis of COPD and asthma. While larger studies are needed to completely define the genetic architecture responsible for COPD,

asthma, and ACO, substantial progress has been made. Promising candidate genes for ACO include those derived from studies of COPD, asthma, and lung function. While current guidelines rely on clinical diagnosis, further study may allow us to contribute to the accurate definition of ACO through genetic risk markers. Ultimately, understanding of the genetic mechanisms contributing to ACO may lead to novel therapeutic targets for this disease, as well as personalized strategies for treatment.

3.11 ACKNOWLEDGMENTS

The authors thank Dr. Edwin K. Silverman and Dr. Jessica Lasky-Su for their helpful comments.

Funded by U.S. National Institutes of Health grants P01HL105339, R01HL094635, R01HL125583, R01HL130512, and T32HL007427.

REFERENCES

1. The FDA and me. *Nature*. 2013;504:7–8.
2. Yim SH and Chung YJ. Reflections on the US FDA's warning on direct-to-consumer genetic testing. *Genomics Inform*. 2014;12:151–155.
3. Carrell RW, Jeppsson JO, Laurell CB et al. Structure and variation of human alpha 1-antitrypsin. *Nature*. 1982;298:329–334.
4. de Serres FJ and Blanco I. Prevalence of alpha1-antitrypsin deficiency alleles PI*S and PI*Z worldwide and effective screening for each of the five phenotypic classes PI*MS, PI*MZ, PI*SS, PI*SZ, and PI*ZZ: A comprehensive review. *Ther Adv Respir Dis*. 2012;6:277–295.
5. American Thoracic Society/European Respiratory Society statement: Standards for the diagnosis and management of individuals with alpha-1 antitrypsin deficiency. *Am J Respir Crit Care Med*. 2003;168:818–900.
6. Sorheim IC, Bakke P, Gulsvik A et al. alpha(1)-Antitrypsin protease inhibitor MZ heterozygosity is associated with airflow obstruction in two large cohorts. *Chest*. 2010;138:1125–1132.
7. Silverman EK. Risk of lung disease in PI MZ Heterozygotes. Current status and future research directions. *Ann Am Thorac Soc*. 2016;13 Suppl 4:S341–345.
8. Sandhaus RA, Turino G, Brantly ML et al. The diagnosis and management of Alpha-1 antitrypsin deficiency in the adult. *Chronic Obstr Pulm Dis (Miami)*. 2016;3:668–682.
9. Global IfAGIfCOLDGG. Asthma, COPD, and Asthma-COPD Overlap Syndrome; 2015. Available at http://goldcopd.org/asthma-copd-asthma-copd-overlap-syndrome/.
10. Marsh DG, Neely JD, Breazeale DR et al. Linkage analysis of IL4 and other chromosome 5q31.1 markers and total serum immunoglobulin E concentrations. *Science*. 1994;264:1152–1156.
11. Center DM, Schwartz DA, Solway J et al. Genomic medicine and lung diseases. *Am J Respir Crit Care Med*. 2012;186:280–285.
12. Pruim RJ, Welch RP, Sanna S et al. LocusZoom: Regional visualization of genome-wide association scan results. *Bioinformatics*. 2010;26:2336–2337.
13. Bønnelykke K, Sleiman P, Nielsen K et al. A genome-wide association study identifies CDHR3 as a susceptibility locus for early childhood asthma with severe exacerbations. *Nat Genet*. 2014;46:51–55.
14. Cho MH, McDonald ML, Zhou X et al. Risk loci for chronic obstructive pulmonary disease: A genome-wide association study and meta-analysis. *Lancet Respir Med*. 2014;2:214–225.
15. Global IfAG. Global Strategy for Asthma Management and Prevention; 2016. Available at www.ginasthma.org.
16. Moffatt MF, Kabesch M, Liang L et al. Genetic variants regulating ORMDL3 expression contribute to the risk of childhood asthma. *Nature*. 2007;448:470–473.
17. Verlaan DJ, Berlivet S, Hunninghake GM et al. Allele-specific chromatin remodeling in the ZPBP2/GSDMB/ORMDL3 locus associated with the risk of asthma and autoimmune disease. *Am J Hum Genet*. 2009;85:377–393.
18. Breslow DK, Collins SR, Bodenmiller B et al. Orm family proteins mediate sphingolipid homeostasis. *Nature*. 2010;463:1048–1053.
19. Nixon GF. Sphingolipids in inflammation: Pathological implications and potential therapeutic targets. *Br J Pharmacol*. 2009;158:982–993.
20. Carl-McGrath S, Schneider-Stock R, Ebert M et al. Differential expression and localisation of gasdermin-like (GSDML), a novel member of the cancer-associated GSDMDC protein family, in neoplastic and non-neoplastic gastric, hepatic, and colon tissues. *Pathology*. 2008;40:13–24.
21. Moffatt MF, Gut IG, Demenais F et al. A large-scale, consortium-based genomewide association study of asthma. *N Engl J Med*. 2010;363:1211–1221.
22. Galanter J, Choudhry S, Eng C et al. ORMDL3 gene is associated with asthma in three ethnically diverse populations. *Am J Respir Crit Care Med*. 2008;177:1194–1200.
23. Torgerson DG, Ampleford EJ, Chiu GY et al. Meta-analysis of genome-wide association studies of asthma in ethnically diverse North American populations. *Nat Genet*. 2011;43:887–892.
24. Leung TF, Sy HY, Ng MC et al. Asthma and atopy are associated with chromosome 17q21 markers in Chinese children. *Allergy*. 2009;64:621–628.
25. Madore AM, Tremblay K, Hudson TJ et al. Replication of an association between 17q21 SNPs and asthma in a French-Canadian familial collection. *Hum Genet*. 2008;123:93–95.
26. Sleiman PM, Annaiah K, Imielinski M et al. ORMDL3 variants associated with asthma susceptibility in North Americans of European ancestry. *J Allergy Clin Immunol*. 2008;122:1225–1227.
27. Halapi E, Gudbjartsson DF, Jonsdottir GM et al. A sequence variant on 17q21 is associated with age at onset and severity of asthma. *Eur J Hum Genet*. 2010;18:902–908.
28. Wu H, Romieu I, Sienra-Monge JJ et al. Genetic variation in ORM1-like 3 (ORMDL3) and gasdermin-like (GSDML) and childhood asthma. *Allergy*. 2009;64:629–635.
29. Bisgaard H, Bonnelykke K, Sleiman PM et al. Chromosome 17q21 gene variants are associated with asthma and exacerbations but not atopy in early childhood. *Am J Respir Crit Care Med*. 2009;179:179–185.

30. Tavendale R, Macgregor DF, Mukhopadhyay S et al. A polymorphism controlling ORMDL3 expression is associated with asthma that is poorly controlled by current medications. *J Allergy Clin Immunol.* 2008;121:860–863.

31. Flory JH, Sleiman PM, Christie JD et al. 17q12–21 variants interact with smoke exposure as a risk factor for pediatric asthma but are equally associated with early-onset versus late-onset asthma in North Americans of European ancestry. *J Allergy Clin Immunol.* 2009;124:605–607.

32. Sleiman PM, Flory J, Imielinski M et al. Variants of DENND1B associated with asthma in children. *N Engl J Med.* 2010;362:36–44.

33. Del Villar K and Miller CA. Down-regulation of DENN/MADD, a TNF receptor binding protein, correlates with neuronal cell death in Alzheimer's disease brain and hippocampal neurons. *Proc Natl Acad Sci USA.* 2004;101:4210–4215.

34. Willinger T, Freeman T, Hasegawa H et al. Molecular signatures distinguish human central memory from effector memory CD8 T cell subsets. *J Immunol.* 2005;175:5895–5903.

35. Gudbjartsson DF, Bjornsdottir US, Halapi E et al. Sequence variants affecting eosinophil numbers associate with asthma and myocardial infarction. *Nat Genet.* 2009;41:342–347.

36. Schmitz J, Owyang A, Oldham E et al. IL-33, an interleukin-1-like cytokine that signals via the IL-1 receptor-related protein ST2 and induces T helper type 2-associated cytokines. *Immunity.* 2005;23:479–490.

37. Cherry WB, Yoon J, Bartemes KR et al. A novel IL-1 family cytokine, IL-33, potently activates human eosinophils. *J Allergy Clin Immunol.* 2008;121:1484–1490.

38. Prefontaine D, Lajoie-Kadoch S, Foley S et al. Increased expression of IL-33 in severe asthma: Evidence of expression by airway smooth muscle cells. *J Immunol.* 2009;183:5094–5103.

39. He JQ, Hallstrand TS, Knight D et al. A thymic stromal lymphopoietin gene variant is associated with asthma and airway hyperresponsiveness. *J Allergy Clin Immunol.* 2009;124:222–229.

40. Ying S, O'Connor B, Ratoff J et al. Thymic stromal lymphopoietin expression is increased in asthmatic airways and correlates with expression of Th2-attracting chemokines and disease severity. *J Immunol.* 2005;174:8183–8190.

41. Harada M, Hirota T, Jodo AI et al. Thymic stromal lymphopoietin gene promoter polymorphisms are associated with susceptibility to bronchial asthma. *Am J Respir Cell Mol Biol.* 2011;44:787–793.

42. Ferreira MA, Matheson MC, Tang CS et al. Genome-wide association analysis identifies 11 risk variants associated with the asthma with hay fever phenotype. *J Allergy Clin Immunol.* 2014;133:1564–1571.

43. Gauvreau GM, O'Byrne PM, Boulet LP et al. Effects of an anti-TSLP antibody on allergen-induced asthmatic responses. *N Engl J Med.* 2014;370:2102–2110.

44. Li X, Howard TD, Zheng SL et al. Genome-wide association study of asthma identifies RAD50-IL13 and HLA-DR/DQ regions. *J Allergy Clin Immunol.* 2010;125:328–35 e11.

45. Himes BE, Hunninghake GM, Baurley JW et al. Genome-wide association analysis identifies PDE4D as an asthma-susceptibility gene. *Am J Hum Genet.* 2009;84:581–593.

46. Van Eerdewegh P, Little RD, Dupuis J et al. Association of the ADAM33 gene with asthma and bronchial hyperresponsiveness. *Nature.* 2002;418:426–430.

47. Allen M, Heinzmann A, Noguchi E et al. Positional cloning of a novel gene influencing asthma from chromosome 2q14. *Nat Genet.* 2003;35:258–263.

48. Palmer CN, Irvine AD, Terron-Kwiatkowski A et al. Common loss-of-function variants of the epidermal barrier protein filaggrin are a major predisposing factor for atopic dermatitis. *Nat Genet.* 2006;38:441–446.

49. Global IfCOLDG. Global Strategy for the Diagnosis, Management and Prevention of COPD 2016; 2016. Available at http://goldcopd.org.

50. Pillai SG, Ge D, Zhu G et al. A genome-wide association study in chronic obstructive pulmonary disease (COPD): Identification of two major susceptibility loci. *PLoS Genet.* 2009;5:e1000421.

51. DeMeo DL, Mariani T, Bhattacharya S et al. Integration of genomic and genetic approaches implicates IREB2 as a COPD susceptibility gene. *Am J Hum Genet.* 2009;85:493–502.

52. Cho MH, Castaldi PJ, Wan ES et al. A genome-wide association study of COPD identifies a susceptibility locus on chromosome 19q13. *Hum Mol Genet.* 2012;21:947–957.

53. Cho MH, Castaldi PJ, Hersh CP et al. A Genome-Wide association study of emphysema and airway quantitative imaging phenotypes. *Am J Respir Crit Care Med.* 2015;192:559–569.

54. Tobacco and Genetics Consortium. Genome-wide meta-analyses identify multiple loci associated with smoking behavior. *Nat Genet.* 2010;42:441–447.

55. Wilk JB, Shrine NR, Loehr LR et al. Genome-wide association studies identify CHRNA5/3 and HTR4 in the development of airflow obstruction. *Am J Respir Crit Care Med.* 2012;186:622–632.

56. Wain LV, Shrine N, Miller S et al. Novel insights into the genetics of smoking behaviour, lung function, and chronic obstructive pulmonary disease (UK BiLEVE): A genetic association study in UK Biobank. *Lancet Respir Med.* 2015;3:769–781.

57. Wilk JB, Chen TH, Gottlieb DJ et al. A genome-wide association study of pulmonary function measures in the framingham heart study. *PLoS Genet.* 2009;5:e1000429.

58. Zhou X, Baron RM, Hardin M et al. Identification of a chronic obstructive pulmonary disease genetic determinant that regulates HHIP. *Hum Mol Genet*. 2012;21:1325–1335.

59. Lao T, Jiang Z, Yun J et al. Hhip haploinsufficiency sensitizes mice to age-related emphysema. *Proc Natl Acad Sci U S A*. 2016;113:E4681–4687.

60. Cho MH, Boutaoui N, Klanderman BJ et al. Variants in FAM13A are associated with chronic obstructive pulmonary disease. *Nat Genet*. 2010;42:200–202.

61. Thorgeirsson TE, Gudbjartsson DF, Surakka I et al. Sequence variants at CHRNB3-CHRNA6 and CYP2A6 affect smoking behavior. *Nat Genet*. 2010;42:448–453.

62. Hautamaki RD, Kobayashi DK, Senior RM et al. Requirement for macrophage elastase for cigarette smoke-induced emphysema in mice. *Science*. 1997;277:2002–2004.

63. Hunninghake GM, Cho MH, Tesfaigzi Y et al. MMP12, lung function, and COPD in high-risk populations. *N Engl J Med*. 2009;361:2599–2608.

64. Jormsjo S, Ye S, Moritz J et al. Allele-specific regulation of matrix metalloproteinase-12 gene activity is associated with coronary artery luminal dimensions in diabetic patients with manifest coronary artery disease. *Circ Res*. 2000;86:998–1003.

65. Wu L, Tanimoto A, Murata Y et al. Matrix metalloproteinase-12 gene expression in human vascular smooth muscle cells. *Genes Cells*. 2003;8:225–234.

66. Repapi E, Sayers I, Wain LV et al. Genome-wide association study identifies five loci associated with lung function. *Nat Genet*. 2010;42:36–44.

67. Hancock DB, Eijgelsheim M, Wilk JB et al. Meta-analyses of genome-wide association studies identify multiple loci associated with pulmonary function. *Nat Genet*. 2010;42:45–52.

68. Wu L, Ma L, Nicholson LF, and Black PN. Advanced glycation end products and its receptor (RAGE) are increased in patients with COPD. *Respir Med*. 2011;105:329–336.

69. Cheng DT, Kim DK, Cockayne DA et al. Systemic soluble receptor for advanced glycation endproducts is a biomarker of emphysema and associated with AGER genetic variants in patients with chronic obstructive pulmonary disease. *Am J Respir Crit Care Med*. 2013;188:948–957.

70. Soler Artigas M, Wain LV, Repapi E et al. Effect of five genetic variants associated with lung function on the risk of chronic obstructive lung disease, and their joint effects on lung function. *Am J Respir Crit Care Med*. 2011;184:786–795.

71. Castaldi PJ, Cho MH, Litonjua AA et al. The association of genome-wide significant spirometric loci with chronic obstructive pulmonary disease susceptibility. *Am J Respir Cell Mol Biol*. 2011;45:1147–1153.

72. Manichaikul A, Hoffman EA, Smolonska J et al. Genome-wide study of percent emphysema on computed tomography in the general population. The Multi-Ethnic study of atherosclerosis lung/SNP health association resource study. *Am J Respir Crit Care Med*. 2014;189:408–418.

73. Laurell CB and Eriksson S. The electrophoretic alpha1-globulin pattern of serum in alpha1-antitrypsin deficiency. 1963. *Copd*. 2013;10 Suppl 1:3–8.

74. Gross P, Babyak MA, Tolker E et al. Enzymatically produced pulmonary emphysema; A preliminary report. *J Occup Med*. 1964;6:481–484.

75. DeMeo DL and Silverman EK. Alpha1-antitrypsin deficiency. 2: Genetic aspects of alpha(1)-antitrypsin deficiency: Phenotypes and genetic modifiers of emphysema risk. *Thorax*. 2004;59:259–264.

76. Hobbs BD, de Jong K, Lamontagne M et al. Genetic loci associated with chronic obstructive pulmonary disease overlap with loci for lung function and pulmonary fibrosis. *Nat Genet*. 2017;49:426–432.

77. Wain LV, Shrine N, Artigas MS et al. Genome-wide association analyses for lung function and chronic obstructive pulmonary disease identify new loci and potential druggable targets. *Nat Genet*. 2017;49:416–425.

78. Hardin M, Cho M, McDonald ML et al. The clinical and genetic features of COPD-asthma overlap syndrome. *Eur Respir J*. 2014;44:341–350.

79. Kong X, Cho MH, Anderson W et al. Genome-wide association study identifies BICD1 as a susceptibility gene for emphysema. *Am J Respir Crit Care Med*. 2011;183:43–49.

80. Hersh CP, Silverman EK, Gascon J et al. SOX5 is a candidate gene for chronic obstructive pulmonary disease susceptibility and is necessary for lung development. *Am J Respir Crit Care Med*. 2011;183:1482–1489.

81. Smolonska J, Koppelman GH, Wijmenga C et al. Common genes underlying asthma and COPD? Genome-wide analysis on the Dutch hypothesis. *Eur Respir J*. 2014;44:860–872.

82. Soler Artigas M, Loth DW, Wain LV et al. Genome-wide association and large-scale follow up identifies 16 new loci influencing lung function. *Nat Genet*. 2011;43:1082–1090.

83. Soler Artigas M, Wain LV, Miller S et al. Sixteen new lung function signals identified through 1000 genomes project reference panel imputation. *Nat Commun*. 2015;6:8658.

84. Loth DW, Soler Artigas M, Gharib SA et al. Genome-wide association analysis identifies six new loci associated with forced vital capacity. *Nat Genet*. 2014;46:669–677.

85. Hancock DB, Soler Artigas M, Gharib SA et al. Genome-wide joint meta-analysis of SNP and SNP-by-smoking interaction identifies novel loci for pulmonary function. *PLoS Genet*. 2012;8:e1003098.

86. Woodruff PG, Modrek B, Choy DF et al. T-helper type 2-driven inflammation defines major subphenotypes of asthma. *Am J Respir Crit Care Med.* 2009;180:388–395.

87. Christenson SA, Steiling K, van den Berge M et al. Asthma-COPD overlap. Clinical relevance of genomic signatures of type 2 inflammation in chronic obstructive pulmonary disease. *Am J Respir Crit Care Med.* 2015;191:758–766.

88. Hobbs BD and Hersh CP. Integrative genomics of chronic obstructive pulmonary disease. *Biochem Biophys Res Commun.* 2014;452:276–286.

89. Sharma S, Chhabra D, Kho AT et al. The genomic origins of asthma. *Thorax.* 2014;69:481–487.

Asthma-chronic obstructive pulmonary disease overlap: A distinct pathophysiological and clinical entity

RAKHEE K. RAMAKRISHNAN, BASSAM MAHBOUB, AND QUTAYBA HAMID

CLINICAL VIGNETTE 4.1

A 49-year-old male presents to the clinic with a case of dyspnea upon exertion. He also complains of post-viral cough that "goes all the way down to his chest" and which requires an antibiotic. He is prescribed steroid tablets once or twice for one week.

His past medical history revealed seasonal hay fever with occasional wheeze and cough, sometimes after playing football, for which he used to take salbutamol for relief. He started smoking at the age of 23 and currently smokes one pack a day. His past medical history is otherwise unremarkable.

On physical examination, he showed mild decrease in air entry on both sides with end expiratory wheeze. Spirometry reported a FEV_1 of 62% predicted and FVC of 70% predicted, which was irreversible with bronchodilators indicating persistent airflow obstruction. His allergy profiles were normal.

4.1 INTRODUCTION

Asthma and chronic obstructive pulmonary disease (COPD) are two of the most common obstructive airway diseases. The amount of individuals affected by asthma is continually on the rise, with over 300 million asthmatics worldwide and roughly 250,000 asthma-associated deaths.[1] Certain risk factors including environmental factors (such as allergen exposure, air pollution, occupational exposure, respiratory infections) and genetic predisposition (such as atopy, family history of asthma, airway hyperresponsiveness and low

lung function) have been held responsible for the dramatic rise in the occurrence of this disease.[2,3] The global burden of COPD is estimated at 384 million individuals affected by COPD and a rising mortality rate.[4] Tobacco smoke constitutes the primary risk factor for the development of COPD[5] and unsurprisingly, most COPD patients are either former, passively exposed, or active smokers.[6]

Furthermore, some patients demonstrate phenotypic characteristics of both asthma as well as COPD.[7] In some instances, a history of asthma with features of eosinophilic T helper type 2 (Th2) inflammation associated with increased blood immunoglobulin E (IgE), peripheral eosino-phil levels and airway hyperresponsiveness (AHR) may precede the development of COPD in cigarette smokers.[7] The Global Initiative for Asthma (GINA) and the Global Initiative for Chronic Obstructive Lung Disease (GOLD) committees together termed this mixed phenotype asthma-COPD overlap (ACO) in order to highlight the therapeutic and diagnostic challenges that are frequently encountered by physicians who manage these patients.[8]

Presently, ACO is a poorly characterized disease but it is more prevalent than previously realized after applying the proposed characteristics of this condition to patients with a diagnosis of asthma or COPD. However, there remains no universally accepted case definition of ACO. The prevalence of ACO is estimated to include one-half of asthma and one-third of COPD cases.[9] ACO appears to be more prevalent in the elderly, women, former and current smokers.[10] A longitudinal study in young European adults reported that the ACO subjects were associated with early-onset asthma, fixed airflow obstruction and highest hospitalization rates and therefore, ACO seemed to represent a severe form of asthma.[11] Asthma and COPD emerge as two distinct entities in the early or mild stage of the disease, which may eventually converge in the same patient later in life as their disease becomes more severe. Thus, the increasing prevalence of asthma and COPD likely increases the probability of overlap with increasing age. Patients with long-standing asthma, who are also former or current smokers, are particularly more susceptible to ACO. Some potential risk factors for ACO include smoking, increasing age, frequent respiratory exacerbations and AHR.

Patients demonstrating features of both asthma and COPD are frequently observed in clinical settings. A recent study highlighted the applicability of ACO characteristics to a patient prediagnosed with asthma.[12] The 64-year-old current smoker with a medical history of childhood asthma presented with deteriorating clinical symptoms. The patient displayed clinical features such as increased blood eosinophil count (429/μL) and total IgE levels (1089 U/mL), positive skin prick tests and increased post-bronchodilator forced expiratory volume in 1 second (FEV$_1$), which are suggestive of asthma. However, the patient being a heavy smoker also exhibited clinical features such as persistent clinical symptoms and airflow limitation post therapy with long-acting β_2-agonist (LABA)/inhaled corticosteroids (ICS)/long-acting muscarinic antagonist (LAMA), which are suggestive of COPD. Despite regular therapy with LABA/ICS/LAMA, the post-bronchodilator FEV$_1$ continued to decrease indicating a rapid decline in lung function. Another recent case report illustrated the case of a 77-year-old ex-smoker COPD patient who resumed smoking.[13] The patient demonstrated marked eosinophilia which constituted 61.5% of the total peripheral white blood cells. The patient further showed low FEV$_1$ along with emphysematous changes and diffuse bilateral pulmonary infiltrates in the lung. Treatment with prednisolone remarkably improved his peripheral blood eosinophil count and the abnormal shadows on his chest X-ray film. Prednisolone in combination with bronchodilators led to better management of his clinical symptoms and this case was categorized as elderly ACO.

Asthma and COPD share common symptoms such as cough, increased sputum production, and shortness of breath further confounding the ability of physicians to correctly diagnose these diseases.[14] At the same time, they also differ from each other with respect to their disease progression, pathogenesis, prognosis, and treatment options.[15] It is essential to differentiate asthma cases from COPD cases to advise the correct treatment regimen. However, early diagnosis and deciding on proper treatment present a challenge to even some experienced specialists and primary care physicians.[16] Therefore, it is important to follow a systematic guideline-based approach to appropriately diagnose and treat these lung diseases. Against this background, the current chapter investigates the pathophysiology of asthma, COPD, and ACO, to improve their early detection and to help distinguish one from the other. The information presented in this chapter may be used to improve the guidelines for pharmacological treatment options for these diseases.

4.2 ASTHMA AND COPD – SIMILARITIES AND DIFFERENCES

Asthma and COPD possess similarities in some of their clinical features. For instance, airflow limitation, and symptoms, including cough, sputum, wheezing, and dyspnea, are shared by both conditions. Chronic inflammation is common to both diseases and is associated with cellular and structural changes leading to airway remodeling and airway wall thickening, which constricts the airways and initiates airflow restriction.[17–19] However, they exhibit distinct pathophysiological features. Although airway inflammation is common to both, asthma is predominantly eosinophilic while COPD is predominantly neutrophilic. Eosinophils, mast cells, T lymphocytes and CD4+ cells are predominantly involved in asthma and neutrophils, macrophages, T lymphocytes and CD8+ cells are predominantly involved in COPD (Figure 4.1). Neutrophil infiltration into the airway wall is also commonly observed in the severe forms of both diseases. Moreover, while asthma displays a Th2 cytokine bias, COPD is biased toward Th1 cytokines and cytotoxic T cells.[20,21] Smooth muscle thickening in mainly observed in the large airways in severe asthma and are more common in the small airways in COPD.[22] Expiratory airflow limitation also demonstrates subtle differences between the two conditions. Airflow limitation is mostly episodic in asthma with complete or near complete reversibility observed during treatment or periods of stability.[20] In contrast, the airflow limitation is more persistent and often progressive in COPD.[21] Although reversibility of airway obstruction with treatment is a characteristic of early asthma, the reversibility gradually reduces and can even disappear with the progression of the disease. More severe cases of asthma may present with limited reversibility and additionally, patients with COPD also frequently exhibit reversibility of airway obstruction.[23,24] Thus broadly, while asthma is characterized by reversible airflow obstruction and COPD by largely irreversible airflow obstruction, a considerable number of asthma patients do exhibit persistent obstruction and substantial COPD patients do present with

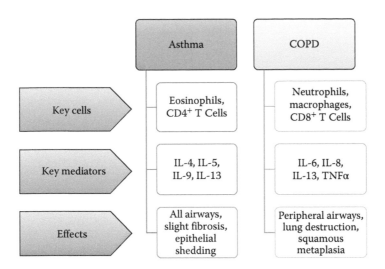

Figure 4.1 Inflammatory components and their role in asthma and COPD. The figure compares the key inflammatory cells and mediators involved in asthma and COPD, and their effects on the pathogenesis of asthma and COPD.

reversible obstruction.[25] The airways also undergo structural changes that result in airway remodeling in both diseases. The narrowing of the airway lumen due to inflammatory cells and mucus hypersecretion, secondary to proliferation of mucus-producing goblet cells, resulting in thickening of the airway mucosa layer and bronchial wall are characteristically seen in both asthma and COPD.[19] However, the obliteration and fibrosis of alveolar attachments is unique to COPD.[26]

Furthermore, asthma and COPD also tend to differ in their clinical presentation. Asthma usually develops during the early childhood years, then proceeds to a remission phase in the adolescent or young adulthood years and may reappear during middle age. However, in adult-onset asthma, the patients typically start exhibiting symptoms in their 40s or 50s.[27] Long-term exposure to biomass fuel or cigarette smoke is the key risk factor responsible for the manifestation of COPD.[28,29] Patients with a long smoking history pose a conundrum to physicians due to the difficulty in distinguishing between asthma and COPD as the patient may have features of both diseases.[6] Additionally, aging is another major risk factor for COPD, with COPD being rare before the age of 30 and its occurrence increasing exponentially beyond the age of 40. Whereas asthma is a disease that can continue into old age, the life expectancy in COPD patients is considerably reduced. It must be highlighted that although common phenotypic and clinical characteristics are observed in asthma and COPD, they constitute distinct diseases with different origins.[30] Moreover, there does not exist a curative treatment for either asthma or COPD.

Thus, in general, asthma is a Th2 cytokine-driven disease, which is more frequently associated with atopy that develops in the early childhood, showing signs of reversible airflow obstruction with an episodic course, and a favorable prognosis with good response to anti-inflammatory and/or bronchodilator therapeutics. In contrast, COPD is typically observed in cigarette smokers, develops in mid-to-later life, with signs of partly reversible or irreversible airflow obstruction and/or smoking-induced emphysema and chronic bronchitis, which

contribute to an accelerated decline in lung function and premature death. It is essential to understand the pathophysiologies of asthma and COPD in depth in order to improve our understanding of ACO. Furthermore, studying ACO may provide mechanistic insights into the development of COPD.

4.3 PATHOPHYSIOLOGY OF ASTHMA

Asthma is a chronic immunologically-mediated lung disease associated with defects in the normal airway repair mechanisms, resulting in airway inflammation and remodeling, which together contribute to most of the clinical manifestation of the disease. Asthma is thus, typically characterized by inflammation and remodeling of the airways, including both the smaller and larger airways, with episodic airway obstruction as well as AHR, resulting in intermittent clinical symptoms of coughing, wheezing, chest tightness, and breathlessness.[31] As shown in Figure 4.2a, histological airway sections from asthma patients typically show chronic infiltration of inflammatory cells along with thickening of sub-epithelial reticular basement membrane and smooth muscle layers.

4.3.1 ATOPY

Atopy denotes the genetic predisposition to develop an intensified allergic immune response to commonly encountered allergens such as inhaled and food allergens. Atopy is a significant risk factor for asthma development and a considerable proportion of asthma patients are atopic. Nevertheless, not all individuals with atopy are asthmatics and not all asthma patients exhibit increased allergic response. The pathogenesis of asthma is invariably associated with dysregulated immune responses, involving increased eosinophil infiltration into lungs, increased serum IgE levels, excessive release of inflammatory mediators from mast cells, airway inflammation and a skewed Th1/Th2 response.[32] Blood eosinophilia is a widely accepted marker of atopy. Asthma patients demonstrate increased sensitivity of the airways to a

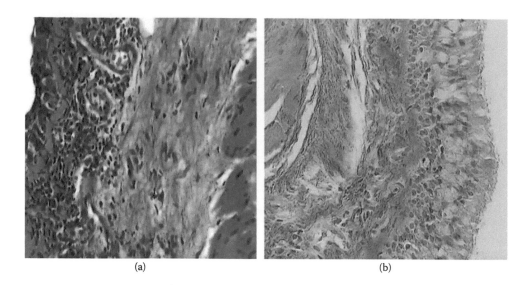

(a)
(b)

Figure 4.2 Histological illustration of asthma and COPD sections. (a) Asthma airway section showing thickening of the sub-epithelial layer with chronic inflammatory infiltrate and a thickened layer of smooth muscle cells. (b) COPD airway section showing transitional epithelium, thickening of the basement membrane, and sub-epithelial fibrosis.

variety of specific and non-specific stimuli, including allergens and chemical stimulants. For instance, in individuals genetically predisposed to atopy, repeated exposures to environmental allergens elicits an increased Th2 cytokine response that promotes specific IgE responses, however non-atopic patients may have similar immunologic Th2 cytokine responses without eliciting specific IgE responses.

4.3.2 AIRWAY HYPERRESPONSIVENESS

AHR refers to the heightened bronchoconstrictor response to inhaled specific stimuli (such as allergens) or non-specific stimuli (such as dry and cold air). AHR is a hallmark of asthma and often serves as a risk factor for disease development. The distal airways in particular are highly sensitive to stimuli, such as cigarette smoke, perfumes, cold air, and other non-specific stimuli.[2,17] Various factors can contribute to hyperresponsiveness; the most notable of which are epithelial shedding, enhanced neurogenic activity, enhanced smooth muscle mass and reactivity, greater airway wall thickness, reduced airway diameter, airway inflammation, enhanced (peri)bronchial vascularity and loss of elastic recoil.[33] For instance, epithelial shedding promotes AHR through sensory nerve exposure leading to reflex neural effects on the airways, loss of enzymes responsible for degrading the inflammatory mediators, and loss of barrier function allowing allergen penetration.[34] In asthma patients, the underlying eosinophilic inflammation,[35] airway smooth muscle alterations,[36] small airway dysfunction[37] and altered glucocorticoid response[38] are important predictors of the degree of hyperresponsiveness.

4.3.3 AIRWAY REMODELING

Some of the major structural and pathological traits of asthma include increased mass of airway smooth muscles due to migration, hyperplasia or hypertrophy, epithelial shedding,

mucus gland hyperplasia resulting in mucus hypersecretion, and infiltration of inflammatory cells into the bronchial wall resulting in chronic inflammation; all of which contributes to airway remodeling and subsequent sub-epithelial fibrosis due to abnormal repair mechanisms.[39] These changes are more pronounced in poorly controlled or untreated asthma which leads to reversible or irreversible structural changes in the cells and tissues along the respiratory tract.[40] The structural remodeling of the airways is the major contributor to the long-term narrowing of airways in asthma and to the progression of major asthma symptoms, such as sputum, cough, and shortness of breath, also common to COPD.[19] Bronchospasm, referring to the sharp contractions experienced by the bronchial smooth muscles, also contributes to airway narrowing. Moreover, the airway capillaries may dilate and leak. As a consequence of this microvascular leakage, edema, impaired mucociliary clearance and increased airway secretion are observed, which may further add to the narrowing and hyperresponsivenes of the airways.[34] In addition, asthmatic airways are often obstructed by hypersecretion of mucus, and associated irreversible structural airway remodeling.[26] Uncontrolled asthma is associated with proliferation of mucus-secreting goblet cells in the airways causing the mucus glands to expand with hypersecretion of mucus that can occlude the airways due to the development of viscid mucus plugs.[41] Asthma is also characterized by damage to the epithelial cells lining the airways causing them to peel away. Sub-epithelial changes may also occur, such as collagen deposition, primarily collagen type I, type III and type V, in the sub-epithelial layer contributing to sub-epithelial reticular basement thickening and sub-epithelial fibrosis.[40]

4.3.4 AIRWAY INFLAMMATION

Inflammation is another important contributing factor in the pathogenesis of asthma. In asthma, inflammatory cells, particularly eosinophils and T cells, are recruited into the central airways, distal lung,[42,43] and lung parenchyma.[44] Abundant concentration of Th2 cytokines, such as IL-4, IL-5, IL-9 and IL-13, as well as chemokines, such as eotaxin and RANTES, can also be observed in these sites[43,45] (Figure 4.1). The eosinophil infiltration and mast cell activation frequently observed in asthma are driven by the activation of Th2 cells. In addition to the classical Th2 pathways, pathways involving GATA-3, IL-33, type 2 innate lymphoid cells and CRTH2 receptors have been reported to play a significant role in eosinophil recruitment.[46] IgE-mediated bronchi hypersensitivity to aeroallergens such as pollen, fungal spores, dust mites, and dander, is a characteristic feature in 50% of asthma patients, and it is often associated with increased mucus secretion. While allergen-induced airway inflammation is predominantly eosinophilic, eosinophils also play a prominent role in non-allergic asthma.

Asthma affects the entire length of the respiratory tract, including the trachea, bronchi and bronchioles. In addition to the central airways, inflammation and remodeling of the airways are observed in the small airways as well as the lung parenchyma.[47] However, in asthma, lung parenchymal changes are usually rare and are more often associated with acute exacerbations or the severe form of the disease.[48]

Thus, asthma is a heterogeneous disease with many different clinical phenotypes arising from the complex interplay between the various environmental factors and susceptibility genes.[49] Although individually-tailored therapeutic options are available to manage most of the clinical manifestations of asthma, this chronic disease still remains incurable.[1]

4.4 PATHOPHYSIOLOGY OF COPD

Tobacco smoke is the main risk factor responsible for the development of COPD.[5] Whereas biomass smoke predominantly induces airway remodeling and less emphysema, cigarette smoke exposure contributes to airway remodeling and centrilobular emphysema.[50] Hereditary predisposition makes individuals with alpha-1-protease inhibitor deficiency more susceptible to developing COPD at an earlier age.[3] Alpha-1-antitrypsin deficiency results in unobstructed proteolytic injury to the alveolar capillary membrane and this differs from a mutation in the protein sequence of alpha-1-protease inhibitor which primarily triggers increased lung inflammation.[5,6] This deficiency leads to accelerated airway remodeling, less conspicuous than the events triggered by cigarette smoke such as panlobular emphysema.[51]

Inflammation and remodeling of the large and small airways in particular are the sentinel pathological characteristics of COPD that result in the destruction of the respiratory bronchioles and distal lung parenchyma leading to emphysematous lung changes.[52] In addition to the structural changes in the small conducting airways, emphysema promotes airflow limitation and is an independent contributor toward airflow obstruction in COPD.[53] Emphysematous lesions together with its chronic inflammatory infiltrates cause dilatation and destruction of the lung parenchymal tissue reducing the elastic recoiling capacity of the lung to drive out air and thereby, resulting in decreased maximum expiratory airflow.[52] Patients with COPD who experience recurrent lung infections have further accelerated damage to their lung tissue. Comorbidities, including depression, diabetes, hypertension, osteoporosis, lung cancer, or coronary artery disease, which dramatically worsen symptoms and impair the quality of life, are frequently observed in the later stages of COPD.

4.4.1 AIRWAY HYPERRESPONSIVENESS

Although a characteristic of asthma, AHR has emerged as a risk factor for disease development in COPD as well.[54] A recent study has correlated the degree of bronchial hyperresponsiveness in COPD to residual volume which is associated with small airway dysfunction.[55] Furthermore, the pattern of airway inflammation characteristically observed in COPD patients, with elevated neutrophil, lymphocyte, and macrophage counts in bronchial biopsy and sputum samples[55] and elevated eosinophil and CD8 lymphocyte counts in peripheral lung tissues,[56] also contribute to bronchial hyperresponsiveness. AHR in COPD is considered however to be largely due to airway caliber, as opposed to inflammatory bronchoconstriction as is the case in asthma.[56]

4.4.2 AIRWAY OBSTRUCTION

Patients with COPD suffer from persistent and often progressive airflow limitation with concomitant chronic inflammation of the airways and lungs. Pathologically, small airway abnormalities and parenchymal destruction are two different but often co-existing features. Pathological changes in the small conducting airways result in airflow limitation due to narrowing and destruction of the airway lumen as well as to active airway constriction that contribute to increased airway resistance. In contrast, pathological changes in the lung parenchyma result in airflow limitation due to the reduction in the elastic recoil of the lung because of damage to the parenchyma, in addition to reduction in the elastic load on the airways because of damage to the alveolar walls directly attached to the airways (alveolar attachments). Thus, COPD involves structural and pathological alterations to the airways, the lung parenchyma, and the lung vasculature,[57] which correlate with the clinical disease presentation and the observed alterations in lung function tests. Thickening of the smooth muscle layer in the peripheral airways in COPD patients can be correlated to the degree of airflow limitation, with increased area of smooth muscles contributing to more severe airway obstruction and lower FEV_1.[58] The increased smooth muscle mass contributes to airway wall thickening, via hyperplasia and hypertrophy of the smooth muscle cells, possibly in response to the activity of growth factors, cytokines, and inflammatory mediators.

4.4.3 CIGARETTE SMOKE-INDUCED DAMAGE

Cigarette smoke induces pathological changes in the small airways in smokers even in the absence of airflow limitation.[59]

An inflammatory response in the peripheral airways is one of the earliest histologic abnormality observed in smokers, suggesting early pathological changes in the peripheral airways of smokers may develop before the occurrence of COPD.[60] Cigarette smoking damages the lung epithelium resulting in the release of endogenous damage-associated molecular pattern (DAMP) molecules. The receptor for advanced glycation end-products (RAGE) and high-mobility group box 1 (HMGB1) are elevated in smokers' lungs and may interact with toll-like receptors and activate an innate immune response.[61] Several pathological lesions in the peripheral airways of smokers with COPD, such as inflammatory cell infiltrate, squamous cell and goblet cell hyperplasia and metaplasia, mucus gland hypertrophy, increased smooth muscle cell hyperplasia and hypertrophy, and fibrosis, all contribute to airway lumen narrowing and loss of tethering function of the lung parenchyma, thereby reducing expiratory airflow in COPD.[57] Cigarette smoking-induced damage to the airway epithelium leads to goblet cell and squamous cell metaplasia and mucosal ulcers.[59] The peripheral airway epithelium of COPD smokers is enriched with mucus-secreting goblet cells and their increased numbers can be correlated to the degree of lung function decline, as measured by the FEV_1/forced vital capacity (FVC) ratio.[62] The functional consequence of goblet cell metaplasia is the development of airway obstruction through excess mucus secretion. Occlusion of the airway lumen by inflammatory exudates or mucus plugs is a common observation in COPD smokers.[63]

4.4.4 INFLAMMATION AND REMODELING

The establishment of COPD in smokers is associated with a parallel increase in the inflammatory response and structural abnormalities in the airways and lung parenchyma.[58,64] Inflammation in COPD is not confined to the lungs as elevated levels of inflammatory mediators are observed in the blood, which may worsen comorbidities, including depression, metabolic syndrome, heart failure, ischemic heart disease, renal disease, and anemia.[65]

Various inflammatory cell subtypes infiltrate the peripheral airways, central airways and lung parenchyma in smokers with COPD (Figure 4.1). The characteristic pattern of inflammation in COPD involves increased neutrophil and macrophage infiltration which is driven by Th1, Th17 and CD8+ T cells, and the lack of mast cell activation generally accounts for the irreversibility. An increased number of macrophages and lymphocytes, in particular CD8+ T and B lymphocytes, are detected in smokers who develop COPD.[58,63] Inflammation can contribute to mild airflow limitation and functional bronchial constriction by the release of inflammatory mediators acting directly on the bronchiolar smooth muscles.[57] On the other hand, chronic inflammation also results in fibrosis of the airways and increase in smooth muscle mass, either directly by inflammation or indirectly by chronically increasing

muscle tone.[57] These changes increase the airway wall thickness and promotes narrowing of the airways and airflow limitation. Furthermore, the inflammation of the airways induces obliteration of the alveolar attachments and reduces the tethering function of the lung parenchyma, causing deformation and narrowing of the airway walls.[66]

Fibrosis is an important aspect of airway and alveolar wall remodeling in COPD. Human lung fibroblasts are subjected to oxidative stress due to cigarette smoking, resulting in the initiation of repair mechanisms and collagen deposition.[67] Fibrotic remodeling may also involve an interaction between inflammatory cells and fibroblasts. Mast cells, with profibrotic and prorepair properties, are increasingly observed in the airways of COPD patients, especially in those having centrilobular emphysema.[68] In addition to an increase in smooth muscle mass and inflammatory mediators, fibrosis also significantly contributes to increasing the thickness of the airway wall and inducing changes in its mechanical characteristics (Figure 4.2b). The pathological changes of the small airways in COPD is followed by a repair process, culminating in fibrosis and airway wall thickening.[69]

Thus, inflammation, smooth muscle hypertrophy and fibrosis lead to thickening of the airway wall and may initiate the detachment of the airways from the lung parenchyma, further stimulating airway closure.

4.5 PATHOPHYSIOLOGY OF ACO

Asthma and COPD overlap (ACO) represents a subset of asthma and COPD patients that demonstrate overlapping characteristics in their immune responses (Figure 4.3). ACO cannot be constrained to a clinical phenotype, as COPD subgroups or endotypes may show similar biological characteristics to asthma. For instance, the drivers of airway inflammation in asthma are superficially quite different from those in COPD. While airway inflammation is driven by eosinophilic and Th2 pathways in asthma, neutrophils play a predominant role in COPD. However, increasing data suggests this demarcation of the two diseases to be oversimplified. Nevertheless, mounting evidence suggests eosinophilic and Th2 type inflammation, a hallmark of asthma, is also involved to some extent in COPD.

4.5.1 AIRWAY INFLAMMATION

Eosinophils are a commonly used biomarker to measure treatment response to therapeutics in asthma. Eosinophils are becoming increasing relevant in COPD as 30%–40% of COPD patients exhibit elevated eosinophil count in both their sputum as well as peripheral blood.[70] Small randomized controlled trials (RCTs) have demonstrated that treatment with systemic and ICS induce slight improvements in FEV_1 and symptom scores in COPD patients.[71–73] Additionally, therapeutic intervention to minimize sputum

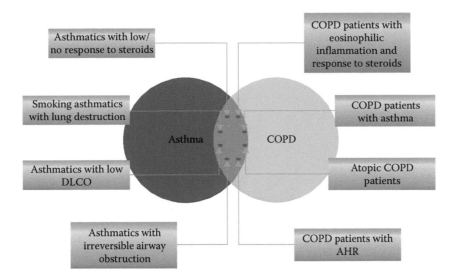

Figure 4.3 Characterization of ACO patients. ACO represents a subset of asthma and COPD patients that demonstrate overlapping characteristics in their immune responses. DLCO, diffusing capacity of the lung for carbon monoxide; COPD, chronic obstructive pulmonary disease; AHR, airway hyperresponsiveness.

eosinophil counts in COPD is associated with a decline in severe exacerbations.[74] Furthermore, two large parallel RCTs have demonstrated that supplementing LABA with ICS leads to improved exacerbation rates in COPD patients with elevated blood eosinophil counts.[75] These findings taken together suggest that elevated eosinophil counts are observed in a subgroup of COPD patients and are associated with their response to therapeutics. Furthermore, an abundant neutrophil population has been reported in the airways of many asthmatics, in particular older asthmatics exhibiting moderate to severe symptoms.

The Th2 bias in asthma may no longer be unique to asthma due to the display of asthmatic biosignature in COPD airways. The type 2-associated inflammation is less thoroughly studied in COPD and this may be due to the difficulty in directly assessing the Th2 cytokine levels, such as IL-4, IL-5 and IL-13, in biospecimens. A transcriptomics study demonstrated the enrichment of genes implicated in the Th2 inflammatory pathway, comprising the "asthma" genomic signature, in the COPD airways when compared to healthy controls and smokers without COPD.[76] More importantly in this study, the COPD patients who displayed a Th2 gene expression profile were found to have tissue and peripheral eosinophilia, improved bronchodilator reversibility and a more favorable response to ICS compared with COPD patients without the Th2 biosignature. These COPD patients with their airway-enriched Th2 biosignature may be speculated to represent ACO, although additional studies are essential to validate this speculation. Thus, in addition to eosinophilic inflammation, a type 2-proinflammatory pathway may play a role in the pathophysiology of COPD in a subset of patients. Although less defined in asthma, systemic inflammation with elevated levels of TNF-α, IL-6, surfactant protein A, C-reactive protein, and reduced plasma levels of soluble RAGE is a common observation in ACO resembling the systemic inflammatory profile of COPD.[77]

Ghebre et al. employed cluster analysis to distinguish between asthma and COPD.[78] Three distinct biological clusters were identified based on sputum cytokine profiling: asthma predominant with eosinophilic and high type 2 cytokines, asthma and COPD overlap with neutrophilia, and COPD predominant with mixed eosinophilia and neutrophilia. This study demonstrated the largest overlap among study participants with a predominance of non-eosinophilic or type 2 inflammation, and helped establish ACO on a biological level. Thus, considerable overlap exists between asthma and COPD and this overlap may be much broader than eosinophilic and type 2 inflammation, and may involve the inflammatory mediators from both diseases (Figure 4.4).

4.5.2 AIRWAY OBSTRUCTION

ACO patients are also characterized by incompletely reversible airway obstruction with increased airflow variability.[79] Due to the lack of clinical trials investigating ACO, the majority of our understanding about the disease stems from studies on patients having features of both asthma and COPD (Figure 4.3). These include patients with asthma who are smokers, asthmatics who develop incompletely reversible airflow obstruction and COPD patients who are non-smokers. Asthma patients who smoke resemble COPD and have less likelihood of developing an eosinophilic inflammation[80] and more likelihood of increased airway neutrophilia.[81] Incomplete reversible airflow obstruction is observed in some patients with long-term asthma.[82] Furthermore, asthmatic patients with incomplete reversibility of airflow obstruction exhibited increased airway neutrophils.[83] In a study with older adults (>55 years) having stable asthma and/or COPD, 65% of the participants exhibited an overlap with an intermediate rate of atopy (64%).[79] Patients with overlap syndrome also had the highest sputum neutrophil and total cell population. The data from

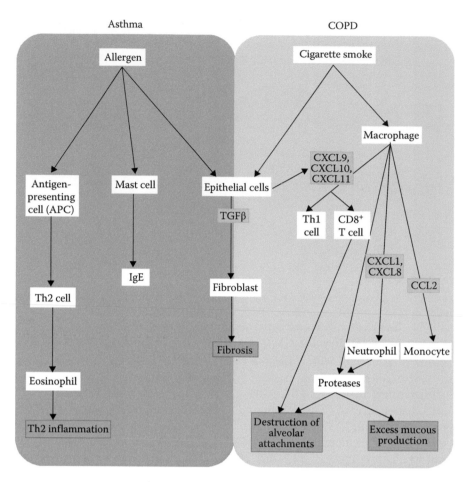

Figure 4.4 Inflammatory pathways involved in ACO. The figure depicts the characteristic inflammatory pathways involved in asthma and COPD and an overlap of these pathways is observed in ACO.

this study implicates ACO to be more common in the older population and to resemble COPD in terms of the pattern of airway inflammation with increased neutrophil infiltration.

4.5.3 AIRWAY REMODELING

The overlap syndrome is also characterized by increased airway remodeling with high-resolution computed tomography (HR-CT) showing increased bronchial wall thickening.[84] Although both asthma and COPD show features such as goblet cell hyperplasia and thickening of the airway epithelium, which contribute to airway remodeling, these features are more pronounced in asthma than in COPD.[85]

Even among smokers, patients with ACO demonstrate more airway disease and less emphysema. Upon phenotyping ACO versus pure COPD patients, patients with ACO displayed greater airway wall thickness, less emphysema, and more frequent and severe respiratory exacerbations than COPD patients.[86] In another study using inspiratory and expiratory CT images, ACO patients were found to have less gas trapping and less emphysema burden post-bronchodilators compared to pure COPD.[87] Although genome-wide association studies have implied a weak genetic component in ACO, genetic analysis of ACO revealed significant hits in GPR65, SOX5, and CSMD1 genes.[86] These cumulative results suggest

a link between ACO and the molecular drivers of asthma, and cigarette smoke appears to amplify these drivers.

4.6 CONCLUSIONS

Asthma is typically characterized by pathological changes that affect both the small and large airways. Airway inflammation in asthma is predominantly eosinophilic involving Th2 lymphocyte- and Th2 cytokine-driven pattern of inflammation. Airway obstruction runs an episodic course in asthma and is usually completely reversible. Spasms of the thickened smooth muscle layer, increased airway mucus secretion and heightened inflammatory infiltrates contribute to this airway obstruction. In contrast, COPD targets the small airways in particular and patients with COPD often exhibit co-existing conditions of chronic bronchitis with airways infiltrated by inflammatory cells, and emphysema with inflammatory infiltrates around areas of alveolar tissue breakdown. Airway inflammation in COPD is predominantly neutrophilic involving cytotoxic CD8+ T lymphocytes. The persistent airway obstruction in COPD is usually irreversible and is a consequence of a combination of factors, including constriction of the smooth muscle layer, excess airway mucus and loss of elastic recoil resulting in closure of the airways.

The ACO phenotype may be characterized by neutrophilic, type 2 and eosinophilic immune responses. An attempt to list the proposed characteristic features of ACO derived from current understanding of its pathology is seen in Table 4.1. However, the best possible way to characterize the ACO subset in order to attain maximum therapeutic benefit remains an enigma. The GINA and the GOLD committees in collaboration have released the 2015 Asthma, COPD, and ACO document, which provides guidelines for the identification of ACO patients and treatment regimens to be followed. The majority of the studies on ACO are cross-sectional and lack randomized controlled therapeutic intervention. Also, biomarker studies suggest that clinical characteristics alone cannot be used to identify the patients most likely to respond to directed therapies, such as ICS. Therapeutic approaches to ACO must focus on novel therapeutics in addition to the current arsenal of oral corticosteroids, ICS, LABA, LAMA and omalizumab. ACO-relevant inflammatory pathways and the proteolytic cascade responsible for lung tissue breakdown may serve as putative targets for these therapies with the objective to prevent irreversible structural changes.

No large scale therapeutic trials currently exist on ACO patients. Generally, ACO patients are at an increased risk of respiratory exacerbations, and present with more symptoms (cough and dyspnea) and worse health status than patients with either pure asthma or pure COPD. ACO patients are heavily burdened by their symptoms and poor quality of life and there exists an increased risk of hospitalizations in this subset of patients. Furthermore, they experience rapid deterioration in their lung function when compared to pure asthma or pure COPD patients, and are at the highest risk of COPD-related mortality. Even with the great burden and poor prognosis associated with ACO patients, literature-based evidence is scarce to guide therapeutic decisions in these patients. Although there is an increasing belief that ICS would be effective in providing a better response in ACO patients, there is a striking scarcity of data to support this belief. Nonetheless, until more reliable research data are made available, the rational first line therapy for ACO patients includes a combination of ICS and LABA.

Thus, the significant burden of this disease on patients necessitates high quality therapeutic clinical trials to be conducted in order to determine optimal management approaches for ACO patients. There also exists an urgent need to characterize easily accessible and inexpensive biomarkers so as to correctly identify ACO patients and guide therapeutic decisions. Further studies are inevitable to understand the underlying mechanisms of ACO that

Table 4.1 Pathological characteristics of asthma, COPD, and ACO. ACO is a poorly characterized disease at present and is defined by the features it shares with both asthma and COPD.

Feature	Asthma	COPD	ACO
Airway involvement	Central and peripheral airways	Peripheral airways	Central and peripheral airways
Airway inflammation	Predominantly eosinophilic with Th2 pattern	Predominantly neutrophilic with Th1 pattern	Predominantly neutrophilic with eosinophilic and Th2 pattern
Inflammatory infiltrate	Eosinophils, mast cells, T lymphocytes and CD4+ cells	Neutrophils, macrophages, T lymphocytes and CD8+ cells	Eosinophils, neutrophils, and T lymphocytes
Atopy	High	Low	Intermediate
Airway hyperresponsiveness	Common	Rare	Intermediate
Airflow limitation/Airway obstruction	Episodic and mostly reversible	Persistent and mostly irreversible	Fixed and incompletely reversible
Airway wall remodeling	Epithelial shedding, early sub-epithelial reticular basement membrane thickening, sub-epithelial fibrosis, goblet cell and mucus gland hypertrophy and hyperplasia, airway smooth muscle hypertrophy and hyperplasia (large airways), vascular congestion, edema	Airway smooth muscle hypertrophy and hyperplasia (small airways), squamous and goblet cell metaplasia, goblet cell and mucus gland hypertrophy and hyperplasia, airway wall fibrosis, loss of alveolar attachments	Mucosal edema, epithelial damage, basement membrane thickening, smooth muscle hypertrophy and hyperplasia, goblet cell hyperplasia, mucus hypersecretion
Alveolar wall destruction	Absent	Present with alveolar wall fibrosis	Present

should aid in the identification of novel therapeutic targets and the development of improved treatment and management strategies for ACO patients.

REFERENCES

1. Cukic V, Lovre V, Dragisic D et al. Asthma and chronic obstructive pulmonary disease (COPD) - differences and similarities. *Materia Socio-Medica.* 2012;24(2):100–105.

2. Bleecker ER. Similarities and differences in asthma and COPD. The Dutch hypothesis. *Chest.* 2004;126(Suppl. 2):93S–95S; discussion 159S–161S.

3. Kaneko Y, Yatagai Y, Yamada H et al. The search for common pathways underlying asthma and COPD. *Int J Chron Obstruct Pulmon Dis.* 2013;8:65–78.

4. Adeloye D, Chua S, Lee C et al. Global and regional estimates of COPD prevalence: Systematic review and meta-analysis. *J Glob Health.* 2015;5(2):020415.

5. Sutherland ER and Martin RJ. Airway inflammation in chronic obstructive pulmonary disease: Comparisons with asthma. *J Allergy Clin Immunol.* 2003;112(5):819–827; quiz 28.

6. Kardos P, Brutsche M, Buhl R et al. Combination of asthma and COPD: More frequent as considered to be? *Pneumologie (Stuttgart, Germany).* 2006;60(6):366–372.

7. Gibson PG and McDonald VM. Asthma-COPD overlap 2015: Now we are six. *Thorax.* 2015;70(7):683–691.

8. GINA/GOLD Joint Report. Asthma, COPD and Asthma-COPD overlap syndrome (ACOS) 2015. Available at http://ginasthma.org/asthma-copd-and-asthma-copd-overlap-syndrome-acos/. Accessed February 15, 2017.

9. Kitaguchi Y, Komatsu Y, Fujimoto K et al. Sputum eosinophilia can predict responsiveness to inhaled corticosteroid treatment in patients with overlap syndrome of COPD and asthma. *Int J Chron Obstruct Pulmon Dis.* 2012;7:283–289.

10. de Marco R, Pesce G, Marcon A et al. The coexistence of asthma and chronic obstructive pulmonary disease (COPD): Prevalence and risk factors in young, middle-aged and elderly people from the general population. *PLOS ONE.* 2013;8(5):e629–685.

11. de Marco R, Marcon A, Rossi A et al. Asthma, COPD and overlap syndrome: A longitudinal study in young European adults. *Eur Respir J.* 2015;46(3):671–679.

12. Lee H, Tho NV, Nakano Y et al. A diagnostic approach and natural course of a patient with asthma–COPD overlap syndrome. *Respirol Case Rep.* 2015;3(4):119–121.

13. Suzuki H, Yoshida K, and Teramoto S. A case of acute respiratory failure in an elderly patient with elderly asthma-COPD overlap syndrome (ACOS) is differentiated from acute eosinophilic pneumonia. *Nihon Ronen Igakkai Zasshi Japan J Geriatr.* 2015;52(3):278–284.

14. Carolan BJ and Sutherland ER. Clinical phenotypes of chronic obstructive pulmonary disease and asthma: Recent advances. *J Alle Clin immunol.* 2013;131(3):627–34; quiz 35.

15. Chang J and Mosenifar Z. Differentiating COPD from asthma in clinical practice. *J Intensive Care Med.* 2007;22(5):300–309.

16. Rothe T. COPD and Asthma: Same same but different. *Praxis.* 2012;101(4):233–237.

17. Miglino N, Roth M, Tamm M et al. Asthma and COPD—The C/EBP Connection. *Open Respir Med J.* 2012;6:1–13.

18. Nakawah MO, Hawkins C, and Barbandi F. Asthma, chronic obstructive pulmonary disease (COPD), and the overlap syndrome. *JABFM.* 2013;26(4):470–477.

19. Gorska K, Krenke R, Kosciuch J et al. Relationship between airway inflammation and remodeling in patients with asthma and chronic obstructive pulmonary disease. *Eur J Med Res.* 2009;14(Suppl. 4):90–96.

20. Reddel HK, Bateman ED, Becker A et al. A summary of the new GINA strategy: A roadmap to asthma control. *Eur Respir J.* 2015;46(3):622–639.

21. Vestbo J, Hurd SS, Agusti AG et al. Global strategy for the diagnosis, management, and prevention of chronic obstructive pulmonary disease: GOLD executive summary. *Am J Respir Crit Care Med.* 2013;187(4):347–365.

22. Skold CM. Remodeling in asthma and COPD–differences and similarities. *Clin Respir J.* 2010;4(Suppl. 1):20–27.

23. Postma DS, Reddel HK, ten Hacken NH et al. Asthma and chronic obstructive pulmonary disease: Similarities and differences. *Clin Chest Med.* 2014;35(1):143–156.

24. Bleecker ER, Emmett A, Crater G et al. Lung function and symptom improvement with fluticasone propionate/salmeterol and ipratropium bromide/albuterol in COPD: Response by beta-agonist reversibility. *Pulm Pharmacol Ther.* 2008;21(4):682–688.

25. Donohue JF. Therapeutic responses in asthma and COPD. *Bronchodilators. Chest.* 2004;126(Suppl. 2): 125S–37S; discussion 59S–61S.

26. Aoshiba K and Nagai A. Differences in airway remodeling between asthma and chronic obstructive pulmonary disease. *Clin Rev Alle Immunol.* 2004;27(1):35–43.

27. Gibson PG, McDonald VM, and Marks GB. Asthma in older adults. *Lancet (London, England).* 2010;376(9743):803–813.

28. Barnes PJ, Burney PG, Silverman EK et al. Chronic obstructive pulmonary disease. *Nat Rev Dis Primers.* 2015;1:150–176.

29. Po JY, FitzGerald JM, and Carlsten C. Respiratory disease associated with solid biomass fuel exposure in rural women and children: Systematic review and meta-analysis. *Thorax.* 2011;66(3):232–239.

30. Vermeire PA and Pride NB. A "splitting" look at chronic nonspecific lung disease (CNSLD): Common features but diverse pathogenesis. *Eur Respir J.* 1991;4(4):490–496.

31. Levy ML, Fletcher M, Price DB et al. International Primary Care Respiratory Group (IPCRG) Guidelines: Diagnosis of respiratory diseases in primary care. *Prim Care Respir J:J Gen Pract Ai Group.* 2006;15(1):20–34.

32. Toskala E and Kennedy DW. Asthma risk factors. *Int Forum Alle Rhinol.* 2015;5(Suppl. 1):S11–16.

33. Postma DS and Kerstjens HA. Characteristics of airway hyperresponsiveness in asthma and chronic obstructive pulmonary disease. *Am J Respir Crit Care Med.* 1998;158(5 Pt 3):S187–192.

34. Barnes PJ. Pathophysiology of asthma. *Bri J Clin Pharmacol.* 1996;42(1):3–10.

35. Wardlaw AJ, Dunnette S, Gleich GJ et al. Eosinophils and mast cells in bronchoalveolar lavage in subjects with mild asthma. Relationship to bronchial hyperre-activity. *Am Rev Respir Dis.* 1988;137(1):62–69.

36. Gunst SJ and Panettieri RA, Jr. Point: Alterations in airway smooth muscle phenotype do/do not cause airway hyperresponsiveness in asthma. *J Appl Physiol* (Bethesda, MD: 1985). 2012;113(5):837–839.

37. Brown RH, Pearse DB, Pyrgos G et al. The structural basis of airways hyperresponsiveness in asthma. *J Appl Physiol* (Bethesda, MD: 1985). 2006;101(1):30–39.

38. Prosperini G, Rajakulasingam K, Cacciola RR et al. Changes in sputum counts and airway hyperre-sponsiveness after budesonide: Monitoring anti-inflammatory response on the basis of surrogate markers of airway inflammation. *J Alle Clin Immunol.* 2002;110(6):855–861.

39. Dunnill MS. The pathology of asthma, with special reference to changes in the bronchial mucosa. *J Clin Pathol.* 1960;13:27–33.

40. Rees J. *Asthma in Adults.* US: Wiley-Blackwell; 2010. Available at http://med.utq.edu.iq/images/books/ABC%20Of%20Astham%202010.pdf. Accessed February 15, 2017.

41. Ward JPT, Ward J, and Leach RM. *The Respiratory System at a Glance.* 3th Edition. US: Wiley-Blackwell; 2010.

42. Hamid Q, Song Y, Kotsimbos TC et al. Inflammation of small airways in asthma. *J Alle Clin Immunol.* 1997;100(1):44–51.

43. Minshall EM, Hodd JC, and Hamid QA. Cytokine mRNA expression in asthma is not restricted to the large airways. *J Alle Clin Immunol.* 1998; 101(3):386–390.

44. Kraft M, Djukanovic R, Wilson S et al. Alveolar tissue inflammation in asthma. *Am J Respir Crit Care Med.* 1996;154(5):1505–1510.

45. Taha RA, Minshall EM, Miotto D et al. Eotaxin and monocyte chemotactic protein-4 mRNA expression in small airways of asthmatic and nonasthmatic individu-als. *J Alle Clinl Immunol.* 1999;103(3):476–483.

46. Postma DS and Rabe KF. The Asthma-COPD overlap syndrome. *New Eng J Med.* 2015;373(13):1241–1249.

47. Hamid Q. Pathogenesis of small airways in asthma. *Respir; Int Rev Thorac Dis.* 2012;84(1):4–11.

48. Gelb AF, Yamamoto A, Verbeken EK et al. Unraveling the pathophysiology of the asthma-COPD overlap syndrome: Unsuspected mild centrilobular emphysema is responsible for loss of lung elastic recoil in never smokers with asthma with persistent expiratory airflow limitation. *Chest.* 2015;148(2):313–320.

49. Murphy DM and O'Byrne PM. Recent advances in the pathophysiology of asthma. *Chest.* 2010;137(6):1417–1426.

50. Camp PG, Ramirez-Venegas A, Sansores RH et al. COPD phenotypes in biomass smoke- versus tobacco smoke-exposed Mexican women. *Eur Respir J.* 2014;43(3):725–734.

51. McDonough JE, Yuan R, Suzuki M et al. Small-airway obstruction and emphysema in chronic obstructive pulmonary disease. *New Eng J Med.* 2011;365(17):1567–1575.

52. Hogg JC. Pathophysiology of airflow limitation in chronic obstructive pulmonary disease. *Lancet (London, England).* 2004;364(9435):709–721.

53. Patel BD, Coxson HO, Pillai SG et al. Airway wall thickening and emphysema show indepen-dent familial aggregation in chronic obstructive pulmonary disease. *Am J Respir Crit Care Med.* 2008;178(5):500–505.

54. Rijcken B, Schouten JP, Xu X et al. Airway hyperre-sponsiveness to histamine associated with acceler-ated decline in FEV_1. *Am J Respir Crit Care Med.* 1995;151(5):1377–1382.

55. van den Berge M, Vonk JM, Gosman M et al. Clinical and inflammatory determinants of bron-chial hyperresponsiveness in COPD. *Eur Respir J.* 2012;40(5):1098–1105.

56. Lancas T, Kasahara DI, Gross JL et al. Cholinergic hyperresponsiveness of peripheral lung parenchyma in chronic obstructive pulmonary disease. *Respir; Int Rev Thorac Dis.* 2011;82(2):177–184.

57. Baraldo S, Turato G, and Saetta M. Pathophysiology of the small airways in chronic obstructive pulmonary disease. *Respir; Int Rev Thorac Dis.* 2012;84(2):89–97.

58. Saetta M, Di Stefano A, Turato G et al. CD8+ T-lymphocytes in peripheral airways of smokers with chronic obstructive pulmonary disease. *Am J Respir Crit Care Med.* 1998;157(3 Pt 1):822–826.

59. Cosio MG, Saetta M, and Agusti A. Immunologic aspects of chronic obstructive pulmonary disease. *New Eng J Med.* 2009;360(23):2445–2454.

60. Niewoehner DE, Kleinerman J, and Rice DB. Pathologic changes in the peripheral airways of young cigarette smokers. *N Engl J Med.* 1974;291(15):755–758.

61. Ferhani N, Letuve S, Kozhich A et al. Expression of high-mobility group box 1 and of receptor for advanced glycation end products in chronic obstructive pulmonary disease. *Am J Respir Crit Care Med.* 2010;181(9):917–927.

62. Saetta M, Turato G, Baraldo S et al. Goblet cell hyperplasia and epithelial inflammation in peripheral airways of smokers with both symptoms of chronic bronchitis and chronic airflow limitation. *Am J Respir Crit Care Med.* 2000;161(3 Pt 1):1016–1021.

63. Hogg JC, Chu F, Utokaparch S et al. The nature of small-airway obstruction in chronic obstructive pulmonary disease. *N Engl J Med.* 2004;350(26):2645–2653.

64. Turato G, Zuin R, and Saetta M. Pathogenesis and pathology of COPD. *Respir; In Re Thorac Dis.* 2001;68(2):117–128.

65. van Eeden SF and Sin DD. Chronic obstructive pulmonary disease: A chronic systemic inflammatory disease. *Respir; Int Rev Thorac Dis.* 2008;75(2):224–238.

66. Saetta M, Ghezzo H, Kim WD et al. Loss of alveolar attachments in smokers. A morphometric correlate of lung function impairment. *Am Rev Respir Dis.* 1985;132(4):894–900.

67. Carnevali S, Luppi F, D'Arca D et al. Clusterin decreases oxidative stress in lung fibroblasts exposed to cigarette smoke. *Am J Respir Crit Care Med.* 2006;174(4):393–399.

68. Ballarin A, Bazzan E, Zenteno RH et al. Mast cell infiltration discriminates between histopathological phenotypes of chronic obstructive pulmonary disease. *Am J Respir Crit Care Med.* 2012;186(3):233–239.

69. Deveci F, Murat A, Turgut T et al. Airway wall thickness in patients with COPD and healthy current smokers and healthy non-smokers: Assessment with high resolution computed tomographic scanning. *Respir; Int Rev Thorac Dis.* 2004;71(6):602–610.

70. Singh D, Kolsum U, Brightling CE et al. Eosinophilic inflammation in COPD: Prevalence and clinical characteristics. *Eur Respir J.* 2014;44(6):1697–700.

71. Brightling CE, Monteiro W, Ward R et al. Sputum eosinophilia and short-term response to prednisolone in chronic obstructive pulmonary disease: A randomised controlled trial. *Lancet (London, England).* 2000;356(9240):1480–1485.

72. Brightling CE, McKenna S, Hargadon B et al. Sputum eosinophilia and the short term response to inhaled mometasone in chronic obstructive pulmonary disease. *Thorax.* 2005;60(3):193–198.

73. Leigh R, Pizzichini MM, Morris MM et al. Stable COPD: Predicting benefit from high-dose inhaled corticosteroid treatment. *Eur Respir Jl.* 2006;27(5):964–971.

74. Siva R, Green RH, Brightling CE et al. Eosinophilic airway inflammation and exacerbations of COPD: A randomised controlled trial. *Eur Respir J.* 2007;29(5):906–913.

75. Pascoe S, Locantore N, Dransfield MT et al. Blood eosinophil counts, exacerbations, and response to the addition of inhaled fluticasone furoate to vilanterol in patients with chronic obstructive pulmonary disease: A secondary analysis of data from two parallel randomised controlled trials. *Lancet Respir Med.* 2015;3(6):435–442.

76. Christenson SA, Steiling K, van den Berge M et al. Asthma-COPD overlap. Clinical relevance of genomic signatures of type 2 inflammation in chronic obstructive pulmonary disease. *Am J Respir Crit Care Med.* 2015;191(7):758–766.

77. Fu JJ, McDonald VM, Gibson PG et al. Systemic inflammation in older adults with asthma-COPD overlap syndrome. *Alle, Asthma Immunol Res.* 2014;6(4):316–324.

78. Ghebre MA, Bafadhel M, Desai D et al. Biological clustering supports both "Dutch" and "British" hypotheses of asthma and chronic obstructive pulmonary disease. *J Alle Clin Immunol.* 2015;135(1):63–72.

79. Gibson PG and Simpson JL. The overlap syndrome of asthma and COPD: What are its features and how important is it? *Thorax.* 2009;64(8):728–735.

80. Chalmers GW, MacLeod KJ, Thomson L et al. Smoking and airway inflammation in patients with mild asthma. *Chest.* 2001;120(6):1917–1922.

81. Boulet LP, Lemiere C, Archambault F et al. Smoking and asthma: Clinical and radiologic features, lung function, and airway inflammation. *Chest.* 2006;129(3):661–668.

82. Backman KS, Greenberger PA, and Patterson R. Airways obstruction in patients with long-term asthma consistent with 'irreversible asthma'. *Chest.* 1997;112(5):1234–1240.

83. Shaw DE, Berry MA, Hargadon B et al. Association between neutrophilic airway inflammation and airflow limitation in adults with asthma. *Chest.* 2007;132(6):1871–1875.

84. Bumbacea D, Campbell D, Nguyen L et al. Parameters associated with persistent airflow obstruction in chronic severe asthma. *Eur Respir J.* 2004;24(1):122–128.

85. Bosken CH, Wiggs BR, Pare PD et al. Small airway dimensions in smokers with obstruction to airflow. *Am Rev Respir Dis.* 1990;142(3):563–570.

86. Hardin M, Cho M, McDonald ML et al. The clinical and genetic features of COPD-asthma overlap syndrome. *Eur Respir J.* 2014;44(2):341–350.

87. Gao Y, Zhai X, Li K, Zhang H et al. Asthma COPD overlap syndrome on CT densitometry: A distinct phenotype from COPD. *Copd.* 2016;13(4):471–476.

Pathophysiology of asthma, COPD, and the overlap

CHARLES G. IRVIN AND DAVID A. KAMINSKY

CLINICAL VIGNETTE 5.1

A 65-year-old woman presents with history of lifelong asthma and allergies for evaluation of increased respiratory symptoms. She has never smoked. She is allergic to dogs, but owns multiple dogs and is active in dog shows throughout the region. Her medications include: fluticasone/salmeterol 250 mcg/50 mcg, one inhalation, once daily; montelukast, 10 mg daily; and tiotropium, one inhalation, once daily. She has been on omalizumab for the past 5 years in an attempt to reduce asthma exacerbations and because of documented elevated IgE. This treatment regime has resulted in improved asthma control.

A physical exam reveals an elderly, obese woman (BMI = 40 kg/m². Lungs have soft, expiratory wheezes throughout with good air movement. Heart sounds are normal. There is no jugular venous distension or peripheral edema.

Pulmonary function tests (PFTs) (absolute, [% predicted])
Total lung capacity (TLC) = 3.85 (L) (89)
Functional residual capacity (FRC) = 2.53(L) (104)
Residual volume (RV) = 2.29(L) (124)
Forced vital capacity (FVC) = 1.49(L) (57)
Forced expiratory volume in 1 second (FEV$_1$) = 0.74 (L) (37)
FEV$_1$/FVC = 0.49 (lower limit of normal [LLN] = 0.66)
No bronchodilator response
sGaw (L/cmH$_2$0*s) = 0.10 (reduced)
Diffusing capacity of the lungs for carbon monoxide (DLCO) (ml/min/mmHg) = 17.34 (105)
DLCO/VA (ml/min/mmHg/L) = 5.47 (105)
VA (L) = 3.17 (73)

Impression: This is the case of an older, allergic asthmatic with fixed airflow limitation, gas trapping, elevated airway resistance (as seen by reduced sGaw), and normal DLCO. Despite a lack of response to bronchodilator, she shows improvement in symptoms from bronchodilators, suggesting a likely beneficial effect on reducing gas trapping or airway resistance not detected by spirometry.

CLINICAL VIGNETTE 5.2

A 23-year-old female presents with asthma since childhood for further evaluation. She is a current 2-pack-per-day smoker for the past 8 years. Previous allergy evaluation reveals that she was nonatopic. Her medications include budesonide/formoterol 160 mcg/4.5 mcg, two inhalations, twice daily, and montelukast, 10 mg, once daily. Despite this treatment regime, she continues to experience respiratory symptoms. As a result, she continues to use albuterol rescue medication 4–6 times per day.

A physical exam shows an obese woman (BMI = 35 kg/m²). Lung auscultation reveals diffuse inspiratory and expiratory wheezes. Heart sounds are normal but mildly tachycardic. There is no jugular venous distention and no peripheral edema.

PFTs (absolute, [% predicted])
FVC (L) = 4.14 (105)
FEV_1 (L) = 2.86 (84)
FEV_1/FVC = 0.69 (LLN = 0.76)
No bronchodilator response

Impression: This is a young, obese asthmatic who is a smoker with fixed airflow limitation. The negative BDR and low FEV_1/FVC suggests ACO, which may be due to asthma in the setting of persistent smoking. Alternatively, the patient may have a suboptimal response to or adherence with asthma therapy. Obesity may be complicating her clinical condition.

CLINICAL VIGNETTE 5.3

A 27-year-old female who has a history of being born prematurely and has a diagnosis of bronchopulmonary dysplasia and is experiencing increased dyspnea with exercise. She has evidence of mild emphysema on chest CT. She is allergic only to dust mites, and reports frequent bouts of wheezing and shortness of breath as a child. There is no history of smoking. She is being treated with beclomethasone HFA 40 mcg, two inhalations, twice daily, and has been prescribed albuterol as a rescue medication. She has no daily or nocturnal symptoms other than symptoms consistent with mild exercise-induced bronchospasm.

A physical exam shows a thin, young woman with clear lungs on auscultation and normal heart exam.

PFTs (absolute [% predicted])
FVC = 3.29(L) (98)
FEV_1= 2.20 (L) (76)
FEV_1/FVC = 0.67 (LLN = 0.75)
No bronchodilator response

Impression: This patient likely has congenital emphysema with fixed airway obstruction as a consequence of her bronchopulmonary dysplasia. A DLCO determination would be helpful to assess the degree to which the emphysema component is contributing to her airflow limitation.

CLINICAL VIGNETTE 5.4

A 53-year-old male with 40 pack-year history of smoking (quit 3 years prior) presents with stable dyspnea on exercise and productive occasional cough. He has multiple environmental allergies. Previous blood counts reveal elevated peripheral eosinophils (> 200 HPF) on at least one occasion. Current medications include fluticasone/salmeterol HFA 115 mcg/21 mcg, two inhalations, twice daily; tiotropium, one inhalation, once daily; and albuterol for rescue.

A physical exam shows an obese male (BMI = 30 kg/m²) with clear lungs on auscultation. Heart sounds are normal, and there is no jugular venous distension or peripheral edema.

PFTs (absolute, [% predicted])
TLC = 7.13 (L) (102), no change after bronchodilator
FRC = 4.28 (L) (119), no change after bronchodilator
RV = 3.57 (L) (169), 10% fall after bronchodilator
FVC = 3.19 (L) (63), 11% increase after bronchodilator
FEV_1 = 1.54 (L) (40), 7% increase after bronchodilator
FEV_1/FVC = 0.48 (LLN = 0.67)
sGaw (L/cmH$_2$0*s) = 0.06 (reduced), improves to 0.07 after bronchodilator

Impression: This is an example of a COPD patient with allergies, occasional eosinophilia, with fixed airflow limitation. Obtaining a DLCO and retesting for BDR on another occasion when allergy symptoms are reduced might help clarify whether this patient has ACO.

CLINICAL VIGNETTE 5.5

A 54-year-old female with 20 pack-year history of smoking presents with complaints of dyspnea on exertion, nocturnal wheezing, and periodic shortness of breath. Medications include fluticasone/salmeterol 250 mcg/50 mcg, one inhalation, twice daily; tiotropium, once daily, and albuterol as needed.

Physical examination reveals a healthy-appearing woman (BMI = 22 kg/m²) with diminished breath sounds throughout, but with no audible wheeze or rhonchi. Her heart sounds are normal, without evidence of a murmur, and there is no jugular venous distension or peripheral edema.

PFTs (absolute, [% predicted])
TLC = 4.02 (L) (93)
FRC = 2.64 (L) (110)
RV = 2.47(L) (152)
FVC = 1.53(L) (53), 14% increase after bronchodilator
FEV_1 = 1.07 (L) (47), 22% increase after bronchodilator
FEV_1/FVC = 0.70 (LLN = 0.69)
sGaw (L/cmH$_2$0*s) = 0.17 (within normal limits)
DLCO (ml/min/mmHg) = 9.76 (43)
DLCO/VA (ml/min/mmHg/L) = 3.03 (58)
VA (L) = 3.22 (74)

Impression: This case represents a COPD patient with emphysema and a significant bronchodilator response. It is a case of ACO with many clinical features of asthma and a BDR but with a preserved FEV_1/FVC ratio that at first seems to be more consistent with asthma. The sGaw being within normal limits in the face of a low FEV_1/FVC suggests peripheral disease. However, the DLCO is much more consistent with a COPD/emphysema diagnosis.

5.1 INTRODUCTION

Patients with asthma and Chronic obstructive pulmonary disease (COPD) are frequently visitors to pulmonary and primary care clinics given the high prevalence and incidences of both disorders. Some asthma patients smoke and some COPD patients are atopic, whereas others were born premature and all have lungs that age. In addition to these groups, there are other clusters of presenting features. Accordingly, patients will present with overlapping features of both asthma and COPD, thus confusing both diagnosis and best treatment to initiate for each of these phenotypes and the prognosis in terms of lung function. Further complicating the situation, patients presenting with overlapping features in the clinic often lack definitive pathophysiologic findings, and, therefore, diagnosis and treatment is based primarily on clinical presentation and augmented with limited laboratory results. It is important to stress that the pathophysiology of these two disorders can be very obscure in many cases, and solely relying on symptoms may lead to initial treatment missteps. Thus, understanding the pathophysiology of these common pulmonary disorders is critical for diagnosis as well as understanding the mechanisms targeted by treatment regimens and the functional impact of treatment.

As emphasized by the Global Initiative for Asthma (GINA)[1] and Global Initiative for Chronic Obstructive Lung Disease (GOLD),[2] lung dysfunction, most often assessed by spirometry, is a key feature of both disorders and provides objective evidence of functional impairment and serves as a basis for prognosis. When assessing the phenotypes of asthma[3] or COPD,[4] physiology, as measured by lung function tests, often plays a pivotal role in the diagnosis and assessment. This chapter will initially summarize the physiological features of asthma and COPD and then apply these concepts to those patients who have a less-clear presentation or overlap. We would suggest that similar to how a patient with mixed restriction/obstruction is evaluated, considering both ends of the spectrum of asthma and COPD helps illuminate the middle ground. This chapter will also discuss the physiology behind the common lung function tests used because, in unclear cases, appreciating what a test measures can be helpful in considering a particular patient's results.

5.2 ASTHMA

Asthma is a syndrome best characterized by objective measures of lung function.[5] The relationships between the inflammatory process and immune/cellular dysfunction have been reviewed before,[6] but the essence of the pathophysiologic presentation is that an asthmatic patient should at some point exhibit periodic bronchospasm, airway hyperresponsiveness (AHR), and with time, often exhibits a progressive loss of lung function. However, patients with mild disease frequently have lung function within normal limits.

Bronchospasm, as well as more permanent airway narrowing and/or obstruction, are most commonly assessed by spirometry, a mainstay of diagnostic assessment. Bronchodilator responsiveness (BDR) is an essential part of any assessment of a patient with lung disease (i.e., RV and TLC). It is important to understand that spirometry is a nonspecific measure that can be influenced by any number of factors, such as airway narrowing, changes in the lung volumes (as TLC and RV define the vital capacity), and muscular effort (which determines achieving maximal TLC) (Figure 5.1). All of these parameters can be impaired in patients with asthma or COPD. A common misconception is that a low FEV_1 in 1 second is solely the result of airway narrowing. In fact the fall in FEV_1 is largely the result of the fall in FVC due to a rise in RV, which is reflected by the tight correlation of FVC and FEV_1 in asthma.[7,8] As asthmatics often display a positive bronchodilator response,[5] this raises the issue of exactly how bronchodilation improves FEV_1 since it is hard to conceptualize how relaxation of airway smooth muscle would result in a fall in RV. Those patients who manifest a decrease in RV after bronchodilator are termed volume responders,[9] whereas those who respond with changes in FEV_1 or the FEV_1/FVC are referred to as flow responders. Patients who exhibit a volume response (fall in FCV) are likely to be obese, have more severe symptoms, and require oral steroid therapy.[10,11]

Obstructive lung diseases, such as chronic bronchitis, emphysema, and asthma, all result in increases in lung volume.[5] Changes in lung volume, especially a rise in TLC, serve to mitigate falls in FEV_1, by keeping pace with the rise

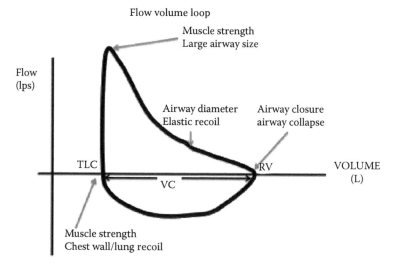

Flow volume loop

Figure 5.1 A stylized flow volume loop where flow in liters per second is plotted on the y axis and volume in liters on the x-axis. To perform the maximal flow volume maneuver, the patient inhales maximally to total lung capacity (TLC). That point is based on maximal muscle effort, overcoming elastic recoil of both the lung and the thorax. The patient then exhales maximally. The peak flow is effort dependent and is influenced by the caliber of larger airways. Soon after the peak flow, flow becomes effort independent and is largely a function of the driving pressure (elastic recoil), airway closure/compression (important in some patients), and peripheral airway narrowing. The volume exhaled finally reaches the other extreme, residual volume (RV). Residual volume is also determined by muscle strength (to overcome chest wall and lung recoil) and, in particular, airway closure. The FEV_1 is the volume exhaled in 1 second and is influenced by all these factors making it a multifaceted outcome measure. In asthmatics, it is largely influenced by the size of the vital capacity that in turn is determined by the factors that influence TLC and RV. In patients with airway remodeling/loss of recoil, bronchospasm will cause flow at any given time to fall even farther, manifested as a fall in the FEV_1/FVC ratio. Hence, a low FEV_1 is impossible to interpret in terms of pathophysiology without further information, but like a robust questionnaire that assesses many factors, it still performs well.

in RV, resulting in a preserved VC. However, overdistension of the thorax is associated with increased symptoms as seen in COPD.[9]

Maximal expiratory airflow is also determined by the driving pressure or static elastic recoil.[12,13] Elastic recoil in asthma patients is often reported as being within normal limits, but several studies dating from the 1960s[12–14] have reported that some asthma patients exhibit reduced recoil and can experience a rapid fall in driving pressure.[14] A fall in elastic recoil would explain falls in maximal airflow. While these decreases in elastic recoil are significant, they usually are not as profound, especially at high lung volumes (TLC), as the fall in recoil observed in patients with emphysema.[5] Lastly, in the few clinical studies of elastic recoil in normal subjects, some normal individuals have intrinsically low elastic recoil,[12] but how this impacts acquisition of a low and/or unresponsive FEV_1 is unknown.

AHR was at one time considered to be the sine qua non for asthma. AHR is an exaggerated response to a specific (allergen, etc.) or nonspecific trigger (cold, exercise, etc.) that normally would not trigger or worsen asthma and explains much of the variation in asthma symptoms.[10] However, several studies have shown that AHR is not a stable phenotype as it is responsive to treatment and exhibits substantial variability, which is especially dependent on exposure to antigenic and/or irritant triggers.[15–17] Clinical studies that target AHR as a clinical endpoint have demonstrated that this approach is more effective than traditional methods for assessing asthma improvement.[10] One interesting phenomenon is that not all asthmatics are hyperresponsive to all bronchial challenge modalities (e.g., direct versus indirect modalities), suggesting AHR can be used for more detailed phenotyping.[16,18]

Periodicity of airflow limitation and symptoms are defining asthma characteristics and represent the periodic/effervescent nature of the disease. Patients demonstrate marked variability in lung function (e.g., peak flow) that can fluctuate hour-to-hour, day to night, based on triggers and by season, making diagnosis and investigations of the mechanisms difficult. Further complicating the problem, patients can have little or no detectable functional abnormalities between bouts of asthma.[19,20] There is no consensus as to how best to measure periodicity of airflow limitation.[18–21] Whether overlap patients exhibit this degree of variability has not been studied.

5.3 CHRONIC OBSTRUCTIVE PULMONARY DISEASE

Chronic obstructive pulmonary disease (COPD) has many similarities to asthma but also a number of marked differences.[5] The current definition of COPD most used is the one based on the GOLD statement.[2] Like asthma, inflammatory processes are implicated in COPD. It is known that these inflammatory processes, similar to those occurring in the asthmatic lung, are complex, so it should come as no surprise that the clinical expression of COPD is also

heterogeneous.[2,4] Expiratory airflow limitation, measured as FEV_1 or FEV_1/FVC, forms a central part of the assessment and diagnosis of the COPD patient.[2,4]

Similar to asthma, a fall in FEV_1 in the COPD patient is not pathognomonic for any specific physiological alterations. Although related to the rise in RV and FRC, the relationship is not as interrelated,[22] as there is a fall in FEV_1/FVC. The fall in FEV_1 in the COPD patient reflects airway obstruction, especially in the case of bronchitis, where there is a loss of lung volume and dynamic closure of airways as the transmural pressure increases during expiration.[23,24] Pathologically there is a loss of parenchymal structure adjacent to the airway and the loss of tethering connections of the adjacent parenchyma that are broken during the destruction of small airway tracts,[25] leading to the formation of centrilobular bullae and emphysema.

Like asthma, the pathologic process of COPD begins in the small airways (< 2 mm in diameter). For example, patients with mild COPD and asymptomatic smokers demonstrate airway flow inhomogeneity[26–28] much the same as an asthmatic. Indeed peripheral resistance in both patients with mild forms of asthma[29] and COPD[30] is 4- to 10-fold higher than normal, and involves larger and larger airways as the disease progresses. More recently an intriguing report[31] has identified COPD patients with significant symptoms and exacerbation but preserved FVC. These patients have lower FEV_1/FVC and CT evidence of airways disease, as well as limited exercise capacity; as such, they resemble mild asthma patients between asthma attacks.

The loss of airflow during progression of COPD is a mixed process of airway occlusion, loss of communicating volume, air trapping, and loss of static elastic recoil.[30] Without careful, detailed lung function assessments that include placement of an esophageal balloon, which is beyond the capabilities of all but a few laboratories, the exact nature of the loss of lung function is largely a surmise.[32]

AHR is also observed in patients with COPD, is more common in women, and is predictive of declines in FEV_1, disease-specific mortality, and all-cause mortality.[33–35] The mode of testing for AHR is important, as the type of provocation (e.g., direct versus indirect) used to assess hyperresponsiveness will result in an outcome that is not the same in all patients. Bronchodilator responsiveness is generally less or about the same in patients with asthma.[2] However, several studies have shown bronchodilator responses in COPD patients[36] that, like asthma, fluctuate with time.[37]

One defining characteristic of the pathophysiology of the COPD patient, and, in particular, the emphysema patient, is the prevalence of low diffusing capacity of the lung for carbon monoxide (DLCO). Patients with mild asthma or bronchitis have a DLCO that is within normal limits, whereas patients with emphysema show a decline in DLCO[5,38] that correlates to emphysemous structural changes as assessed by pathology or CT scans. Asthma patients, on the other hand, will sometimes exhibit a rise in DLCO related to disease severity. Hence, the general changes in lung function in asthma and COPD are quite similar with the general exception of DLCO (Table 5.1).

Table 5.1 Physiologic features of asthma, COPD, and ACO (overlap)

Physiologic assessment	Asthma	COPD	ACO
Airflow limitation	± Yes	Yes	Yes
Thick wall CT	±	+	++
BDR	+	±	+
AHR	++	+	++
Exercise-induced AHR	+	−	?
Hyperinflation	+	+	?
Loss of elastic recoil	Sometimes	Yes	?
DLCO	Normal or ↑	↓	?

Note: Thick wall CT: airway wall thickness by CT; AHR, airway hyperresponsiveness; BDR, bronchodilator responsiveness; DLCO, diffusion capacity of the lung.

In a majority of cases, a battery of lung function tests, that include spirometry with flow volume loops, lung volumes, DLCO, bronchodilator responsiveness, and bronchial challenge tests, coupled with a careful history, results in a clear picture of the disease process and its severity. The difficulty occurs when features of asthma and COPD coexist.

5.4 PHYSIOLOGICAL FEATURES OF ASTHMA-COPD OVERLAP PATIENTS

It is important to emphasize that there is no universally accepted definition, criteria, or even terminology for describing patients with an asthma-COPD overlap presentation (see Chapter 1). For the purposes of this section and given the heterogeneity of overlap patients, we will consider the potential pathophysiology of four groups as germane examples of ACO: (1) patients with asthma who smoke; (2) patients with COPD with a bronchodilator response and/or atopy; (3) patients who had asthma as children; and (4) older patients with asthma. We will only consider the structure-function relationship as the genetic and molecular mechanisms are considered in Chapter 3. The major limitation to any discussion of ACO is the paucity of studies investigating ACO patients that contain lung function measurements that extend beyond spirometry, that is the FEV_1 and FVC.

Low lung function (low FEV_1): As previously reviewed,[39,40] the FEV_1 of patients who are either asthmatics or asthmatics with COPD features show a remarkable consistency of spirometric impairment, ranging from 60% to 66% predicted, and most report a long duration of asthma or asthma-like features. It is well appreciated that poorly controlled and poorly treated asthma leads to fixed airflow limitation.[41,42] The most common assumption is that chronic uncontrolled asthma leads to airway remodeling that is the root cause

for the permanent decreases of FEV_1.[6] As previously discussed,[43] IL-6 is an inflammatory cytokine commonly encountered in overlap patients. We have reported that the loss of central airway function as measured by FEV_1/FVC is related to IL-6 presence known to drive TGFβ release and fibrosis.[44,45] IL-6 is a plausible inflammatory mediator of interest because it is implicated in multiple settings of epithelial injury.[45] Alternatively, the loss or persistent loss of elastic recoil, especially if coupled with airway fibrosis, would contribute to the significant loss of FEV_1 in this group in some, in an as of yet, undefined synergistic fashion.

Bronchodilator reversibility (BDR): Many authors state that COPD is characterized by a lack of response to bronchodilators; although this is not true, the changes are often small and usually are less than 100 mL even with combined therapies.[46,47] The situation is complicated by the fact that there is little consensus on the best approach to determine broncho-reversibility.[20] Moreover, there is little consensus on the minimal clinically important difference (MCID) for FEV_1, which range from 75 mL[47] to 200 mL.[20] The most frequently used criteria used for BDR are 12% and 200 mL, but it must be recognized that this standard was a compromise between 10% and 15%.[48] Moreover, it is known that BDR is not helpful in distinguishing asthma from COPD nor is BDR even reproducible in patients with COPD.[46] If BDR were to be a useful biomarker for ACO, then it may be necessary to set the BDR threshold higher than current standards. Nevertheless, BDR remains a central feature of the patient with ACO.

AHR: When measured, AHR is a common feature of the patient with ACO, which should come as no surprise given that AHR is reported in patients with either asthma or COPD. As there are many mechanisms that cause AHR,[10] those involved in ACO may be driven by mechanisms that cause AHR in either asthma or COPD or something completely different. It is not known whether the patient with ACO will have a positive response to all forms of bronchial challenge. Only one study investigating ACO patients taken from an asthma cohort reported this group to be hyperresponsive to both mannitol and methacholine.[49] Mannitol might not be positive in an ACO group that is derived from a COPD cohort, but when measured, several studies with ACO patients show AHR to methacholine.[49,50] Moreover, in a study by De Marco et al.,[50] ACO patients were the most responsive to methacholine, but further investigation seems warranted.

Other measures of lung function: There is very little known about the alterations in lung volume in ACO patients with the exception of one report[51] that curiously did not show these ACO patients to be hyperinflated. A frequently useful test in the case of ACO is the DLCO that is usually reduced in emphysema, unchanged in bronchitis, and unchanged or elevated in asthma[38]; however, two studies in patients with ACO report that DLCO was not different.[52,53] Although the forced oscillation technique has been shown to differentiate between patients with asthma and COPD,[54] another report did not show a difference.[51] Given the poor quality of life in patients with overlap,[55] and the importance of differentiating ACO versus asthma or COPD, further characterization and detailed physiological investigation seems warranted.

5.5 OTHER MECHANISMS OF FIXED AIRFLOW LIMITATION

Two other groups that are often identified with ACO are patients with fixed airflow limitation who reported asthma in early life and older patients. Children with severe asthma in early life often have reduced lung function in adulthood that does not respond to bronchodilators. Indeed early life asthma leads to a profound increase in the odds[35] for COPD.[56] Early onset asthma also leads to accelerated declines in lung function, which in time would manifest as ACO as the patient would be expected to present with fixed airflow limitation.[57] If the lung function of a person fails to reach its structural developmental maximal then it is difficult to envision a therapeutic option (a ceiling effect).

At the other end of the spectrum lies the insidious fall in lung function with age. Lung function declines with age but it does so in a variable fashion.[58] Moreover, in a patient with an overlay of disease such as asthma or especially COPD, there is an acceleration of this fall with age.[59–61] Surprisingly little is known about the variable effects of aging on the lung in the context of disease other than the resultant fixed loss of FEV_1 that fails to respond to treatment.[62] Interestingly, most studies report that ACO patients are older.

5.6 CONCLUSIONS

The pathophysiology of ACO patients is frequently characterized by a reduced FEV_1 that fails to respond adequately to an acute treatment with short-acting bronchodilator agents. However, other patients with ACO do exhibit a significant BDR. In this chapter, we have developed the concept that FEV_1 is a complex parameter that assesses the intersection of at least three synergistic processes of obstruction: loss of elastic recoil, loss of lung volume, and fixed narrowing of airways due to structural changes (Figure 5.2). At least one study[50] shows that ACO patients have a much reduced FEV_1 compared to patients with either COPD or asthma alone. Airway-wall thickening probably best explains this finding, as several studies show that ACO patients have evidence of thickened airways on CT scans.[53,63] Furthermore, ACO patients frequently exhibit significant AHR. However, since there is a relative paucity of carefully conducted detailed assessments of ACO patients, a clear picture of the pathophysiology and pathogenesis is missing. Moreover, given the profound underutilization of lung function in general and simple spirometry in particular,[64,65] this situation is unlikely to improve. Until this situation changes our diagnosis and understanding of the pathogenesis of ACO will remain incomplete.

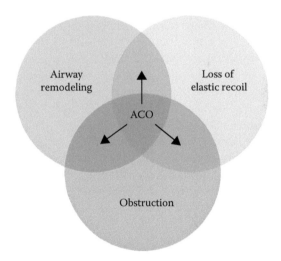

Figure 5.2 A schematic Venn diagram to help appreciate the primary factors that influence the low FEV_1 observed in patients with overlapping airway disease: static elastic recoil such as seen in some asthmatics, patients with emphysema, or the elderly; airway remodeling, such as is observed in younger patients with previously untreated airway asthma or patients with occupational airway injury; and obstruction caused by secretions and mucus, such as in bronchitis or acute-status asthma. Patients with more than one derangement (as represented by the overlapping areas) would be expected to have larger declines in FEV_1. Moreover, those with structural abnormalities would be predicted not to reverse totally with therapy.

REFERENCES

1. Global Initiative for Asthma (GINA). Global Strategy for Asthma Management and Prevention; 2015. Available at http://www.ginaasthma.org/.

2. Global Initiative for Chronic Obstructive Lung Disease (GOLD). Global Strategy for the Diagnosis, Management, and Prevention of COPD; 2016. Available at http://www.goldcopd.org/.

3. Moore WC, Meyers DA, Wenzel SE et al. Identification of asthma phenotypes using cluster analysis in the severe asthma research program. *Am J Respir Crit Care Med.* 2010;181(4):315–323.

4. Han MK, Agusti A, Calverley PM et al. Chronic obstructive pulmonary disease phenotypes: The future of COPD. *Am J Respir Crit Care Med.* 2010;182(5):598–604.

5. Irvin CG. Pulmonary physiology. In PJ Barnes, JM Drazen, SI Rennard et al., eds. *Asthma and COPD.* 2nd ed. Boston, MA: Elsevier Academic Press.

6. Bosse Y, Riesenfeld EP, Pare PD et al. It's not all smooth muscle: Non-smooth-muscle elements in control of resistance to airflow. *Annu Rev Physiol.* 2010;72:437–462. PMID: 20148684.

7. Brown RH, Pearse DB, Pyrgos G et al. The structural basis of airways hyperresponsiveness in asthma. *J Appl Physiol (1985).* 2006;101(1):30–39.

8. Irvin CG. Lessons from structure-function in asthma: Myths and truths about what we teach. Invited editorial. *J Appl Physiol.* 2006;101:7–9.

9. Pare PD, Lawson LM, and Brooks LA. Patterns of response to inhaled bronchodilators in asthmatics. *Am Rev Respir Dis.* 1983;127(6):680–685.

10. Chapman DG and Irvin CG. Mechanisms of airway hyper-responsiveness in asthma: The past, present and yet to come. *Clin Exp Allergy: J Br Soc Allergy Clin Immunol.* 2015;45(4):706–719.

11. Gibbons WJ, Sharma A, Lougheed D et al. Detection of excessive bronchoconstriction in asthma. *Am J Respir Crit Care Med.* 1996;153(2):582–589.

12. Woolcock AJ, Vincent NJ, and Macklem PT. Frequency dependence of compliance as a test for obstruction in the small airways. *J Clin Invest.* 1969;48(6):1097–1106.

13. McCarthy DS and Sigurdson M. Lung elastic recoil and reduced airflow in clinically stable asthma. *Thorax.* 1980;35(4):298–302.

14. Mansell A, Dubrawsky C, Levison H et al. Lung mechanics in antigen-induced asthma. *J Appl Physiol.* 1974;37(3):297–301.

15. Cartier A, Thomson NC, Frith PA et al. Allergen-induced increase in bronchial responsiveness to histamine: Relationship to the late asthmatic response and change in airway caliber. *J Allergy Clin Immunol.* 1982;70(3):170–177.

16. Sumino K, Sugar EA, Irvin CG et al. Variability of methacholine bronchoprovocation and the effect of inhaled corticosteroids in mild asthma. *Ann Allergy Asthma Immunol.* 2014;112(4):354–360. e351.

17. Sumino K, Sugar EA, Irvin CG et al. Methacholine challenge test: Diagnostic characteristics in asthmatic patients receiving controller medications. *J Allergy Clin Immunol.* 2012;130(1):69–75. e66.

18. Irvin CG. Asthma: Bronchial challenge. UpToDate in Pulm Disease and Critica Care. Available at https://www.uptodate.com/contents /bronchoprovocation-testing.

19. Reddel HK. Peak flow monitoring in clinical practice and clinical asthma trials. *Curr Opin Pulm Med.* 2006;12(1):75–81.

20. Tepper RS, Wise RS, Covar R et al. Asthma outcomes: Pulmonary physiology. *J Allergy Clin Immunol.* 2012;129(Suppl. 3):S65–S87.

21. Kaminsky DA, Wang LL, Bates JH et al. Fluctuation analysis of peak expiratory flow and its association with treatment failure in asthma. *Am J Respir Crit Care Med.* 2017;195(8):993–999.

22. Deesomchok A, Webb KA, Forkert L et al. Lung hyperinflation and its reversibility in patients with airway obstruction of varying severity. *COPD.* 2010;7(6):428–437.

23. Tiddens HA, Bogaard JM, de Jongste JC et al. Physiological and morphological determinants of maximal expiratory flow in chronic obstructive lung disease. *Eur Respir J.* 1996;9(9):1785–1794.

24. Leaver DG, Tatterfield AE, and Pride NB. Contributions of loss of lung recoil and of enhanced airways collapsibility to the airflow obstruction of chronic bronchitis and emphysema. *J Clin Invest.* 1973;52(9):2117–2128.

25. Hogg JC, Chu F, Utokaparch S et al. The nature of small-airway obstruction in chronic obstructive pulmonary disease. *N Engl J Med.* 2004;350(26):2645–2653.

26. Buist AS, Vollmer WM, Johnson LR et al. Does the single-breath N2 test identify the smoker who will develop chronic airflow limitation? *Am Rev Respir Dis.* 1988;137(2):293–301.

27. Cosio M, Ghezzo H, Hogg JC et al. The relations between structural changes in small airways and pulmonary-function tests. *N Engl J Med.* 1978;298(23):1277–1281.

28. Coe CI, Watson A, Joyce H et al. Effects of smoking on changes in respiratory resistance with increasing age. *Clin Sci (Lond).* 1989;76(5):487–494.

29. Kaminsky DA, Irvin CG, Gurka DA et al. Peripheral airways responsiveness to cool, dry air in normal and asthmatic individuals. *Am J Respir Crit Care Med.* 1995;152(6 Pt 1):1784–1790.

30. Yanai M, Sekizawa K, Ohrui T et al. Site of airway obstruction in pulmonary disease: Direct measurement of intrabronchial pressure. *J Appl Physiol (1985)*. 1992;72(3):1016–1023.

31. Woodruff PG, Couper D, and Han MK. Clinical significance of symptoms in smokers with preserved pulmonary function. *N Engl J Med*. 20116;374(19):1811–1821.

32. Pride NB, Ingram RH Jr, and Lim TK. Interaction between parenchyma and airways in chronic obstructive pulmonary disease and in asthma. *Am Rev Respir Dis*. 1991;143(6):1446–1449.

33. Postma DS and Kerstjens HA. Characteristics of airway hyperresponsiveness in asthma and chronic obstructive pulmonary disease. *Am J Respir Crit Care Med*. 1998;158(5 Pt 3):S187–192.

34. Tashkin DP, Altose MD, Connett JE et al. Methacholine reactivity predicts changes in lung function over time in smokers with early chronic obstructive pulmonary disease. The lung health study research group. *Am J Respir Crit Care Med*. 1996;153(6 Pt 1):1802–1811.

35. Rijcken B, Schouten JP, Mensinga TT et al. Factors associated with bronchial responsiveness to histamine in a population sample of adults. *Am Rev Respir Dis*. 1993;147(6 Pt 1):1447–1453.

36. Smith HR, Irvin CG, and Cherniack RM. The utility of spirometry in the diagnosis of reversible airways obstruction. *Chest*. 1992;101(6):1577–1581.

37. Albert P, Agusti A, Edwards L et al. Bronchodilator responsiveness as a phenotypic characteristic of established chronic obstructive pulmonary disease. *Thorax*. 2012;67(8):701–708.

38. Irvin C. Guide to the evaluation of pulmonary function. In Q Hamid, J Shannon, J Martin, eds. *Physiologic Basis of Respiratory Disease*. Hamilton, Ontario: BC Decker.

39. Gibson PG and McDonald VM. Asthma-COPD overlap 2015: Now we are six. *Thorax*. 2015;70(7):683–691.

40. Global Initiative for Asthma (GINA) and Global Initiative for Chronic Obstructive Lung Disease (GOLD). Diagnosis of diseases of chronic airflow limitation: Asthma, COPD and asthma-COPD overlap syndrome (ACO); 2015. Available at http://www.ginasthma.org/Accessed July 1, 2017.

41. Dixon AE and Irvin CG. Early intervention of therapy in asthma. *Curr Opin Pulm Med*. 2005;11(1):51–55.

42. Stem DA, Morgan WJ, Wright AL et al. Poor airway function in early infancy and lung function by age 22 years: A non-selective longitudinal cohort study. *Lancet*. 2007;370(9589):758–764.

43. Fu JJ, McDonald VM, Gibson PG et al. Systemic inflammation in older adults with asthma-COPD overlap syndrome. *Allergy Asthma Immunol Res*. 2014;6(4):316–324.

44. Neveu WA, Allard JL, Raymond DM et al. Elevation of IL-6 in the allergic asthmatic airway is independent of inflammation but associates with loss of central airway function. *Respir Res*. 2010;11:28.

45. Rincon M and Irvin CG. Role of IL-6 in asthma and other inflammatory pulmonary diseases. *Int J Biol Sci*. 2012;8(9):1281–1290.

46. Calverley PM, Burge PS, Spencer S et al. Bronchodilator reversibility testing in chronic obstructive pulmonary disease. *Thorax*. 2003;58(8):659–664.

47. Calzetta L, Rogliani P, Ora J et al. LABA/LAMA combination in COPD: A meta-analysis on the duration of treatment. *Eur Respir Rev*. 2017;26(143):160043.

48. American Thoracic Society. Lung function testing: Selection of reference values and interpretative strategies. *Am Rev Respir Dis*. 1991;144(5):1202–1218.

49. Lee HY, Kang JY, Yoon HK et al. Clinical characteristics of asthma combined with COPD feature. *Yonsei Med J*. 2014;55(4):980–986.

50. de Marco R, Marcon A, Rossi A et al. Asthma, COPD and overlap syndrome: A longitudinal study in young European adults. *Eur Respir J*. 2015;46(3):671–679.

51. Kitaguchi Y, Yasuo M, and Hanaoka M. Comparison of pulmonary function in patients with COPD, asthma-COPD overlap syndrome, and asthma with airflow limitation. *Int J Chron Obstruct Pulmon Dis*. 2016;11:991–997.

52. Cosio BG, Soriano JB, López-Campos JL et al. Defining the Asthma-COPD Overlap Syndrome in a COPD Cohort. *Chest*. 2016;149(1):45–52.

53. Suzuki T, Tada Y, Kawata N et al. Clinical, physiological, and radiological features of asthma-chronic obstructive pulmonary disease overlap syndrome. *Int J Chron Obstruct Pulmon Dis*. 2015;10:947–954.

54. Paredi P, Goldman M, Alamen A et al. Comparison of inspiratory and expiratory resistance and reactance in patients with asthma and chronic obstructive pulmonary disease. *Thorax*. 2010;65(3):263–267.

55. Miravitlles M, Soriano JB, Ancochea J et al. Characterisation of the overlap COPD-asthma phenotype. Focus on physical activity and health status. *Respir Med*. 2013;107(7):1053–1060.

56. Tai A, Tran H, Roberts M et al. The association between childhood asthma and adult chronic obstructive pulmonary disease. *Thorax*. 2014;69(9):805–810.

57. James AL, Palmer LJ, Kicic E et al. Decline in lung function in the Busselton Health Study: The effects of asthma and cigarette smoking. *Am J Respir Crit Care Med*. 2005;171(2):109–114.

58. Janssens JP. Aging of the respiratory system: Impact on pulmonary function tests and adaptation to exertion. *Clin Chest Med*. 2005;26(3):469–484, vi-vii.

59. MacNee W. Is chronic obstructive pulmonary disease an accelerated aging disease? *Ann Am Thorac Soc.* 2016;13(Suppl. 5):S429–S437.

60. de Marco R, Pesce G, Marcon A et al. The coexistence of asthma and chronic obstructive pulmonary disease (COPD): Prevalence and risk factors in young, middle-aged and elderly people from the general population. *PLOS ONE.* 2013;8(5):e62985.

61. Silva GE, Sherrill DL, Guerra S et al. Asthma as a risk factor for COPD in a longitudinal study. *Chest.* 2004;126(1):59–65.

62. Hanania NA, King MJ, Braman SS et al. Asthma in the elderly: Current understanding and future research needs—A report of a National Institute on Aging (NIA) workshop. *J Allergy Clin Immunol.* 2011;128(Suppl. 3):S4–S24.

63. Hardin M, Cho M, McDonald ML et al. The clinical and genetic features of COPD-asthma overlap syndrome. *Eur Respir J.* 2014;44(2):341–350.

64. Han MK, Kim MG, Mardon R et al. Spirometry utilization for COPD: How do we measure up? *Chest.* 2007;132(2):403–409.

65. Arne M, Lisspers K, Ställberg B et al. How often is diagnosis of COPD confirmed with spirometry? *Respir Med.* 2010;104(4):550–556.

Update on the clinical status, genomics, pathophysiology, and treatment of the asthma-COPD overlap

ARTHUR F. GELB AND JAY A. NADEL

6.1 INTRODUCTION TO ACO

CLINICAL VIGNETTE 6.1

A 52-year-old male patient had recurrent hospitalizations for exacerbations of COPD associated with wheezing. Home medications included inhaled short- and long-acting β_2-agonist (LABA) combined with corticosteroid, inhaled short- and long-acting muscarinic receptor antagonist, antibiotics, and tapering oral corticosteroid as needed. Chest X-ray demonstrated hyperinflation, and high resolution, thin-section lung CT was consistent with mild emphysema, predominantly in the upper lung fields. Expiratory spirometry was consistent with moderate to severe obstruction with significant response to inhaled albuterol. Static lung volumes were increased, and diffusing capacity was normal. Blood eosinophils were mildly elevated, and total IgE remained elevated consistent with Th2 eosinophilic asthma. Measurements of exhaled total airway and alveolar nitric oxide were normal. There was a childhood history of allergic asthma that persisted into adulthood and despite treatment, he continued to experience limited exercise ability. Social history was remarkable for smoking, which began at age 18 with a cumulative smoking history of 42 pack years. Serum alpha 1 antitrypsin level and Pi type were normal.

Many patients with a history of chronic cigarette smoking have persistent expiratory airflow obstruction despite partial reversibility with therapeutic intervention. Furthermore, approximately 15%–20% may have phenotypic clinical features of both asthma and chronic obstructive pulmonary disease (COPD).[1,2] Subgroups of smoking-related COPD patients with preexisting and/or current asthma symptoms may have overlapping immune responses including eosinophilia and T helper cell 2 (Th2) type inflammation. This epiphenomenon is called asthma-COPD overlap (ACO). In some cases, a history of asthma diagnosed before the age of 40 has clearly preceded the onset of cigarette smoking–related COPD. There may be variable expiratory airflow limitation and markers of Th2 eosinophilic inflammation noted initially. This includes increased blood and/or sputum eosinophils, increased serum total IgE, and hyperresponsive airways.[1,2] Subsequently, these asthmatics may develop a COPD phenotype, with relatively fixed expiratory airflow limitation, with eosinophilia and/or neutrophilia in their sputum and peripheral blood. Alternatively, in the absence of an initial diagnosis of asthma, cigarette smoking–related COPD may be diagnosed, with concomitant similar Th2 type eosinophilic phenotypic characteristics as usually seen in asthmatics. Recently ACO has been extensively reviewed elsewhere,[1,2] and our present goal is to update the reader with respect to diagnosis, treatment, pathophysiology, genomics, and markers of inflammation in ACO. Other chapters in this book will also address these issues.

6.2 HISTORICAL OVERVIEW OF ASTHMA-COPD OVERLAP (ACO)

Orie and colleagues hypothesized during the First Bronchitis Symposium held in Groningen, Netherlands, in 1961, that the various forms of airway obstruction—such as asthma, chronic bronchitis, and emphysema—should be considered as different clinical and phenotypic expressions of one common disease origin. Orie et al. named this entity chronic nonspecific lung disease (CNSLD).[2,3] They proposed that multiple exogenous and endogenous factors, including atopy and hyperresponsiveness, influenced pathogenesis.[3] Subsequently, at the Third International Bronchitis Symposium in the Netherlands in 1969, Fletcher and Pride suggested the term "Dutch Hypothesis"[4] to further describe the original proposal of Orie and colleagues.[3] Alternatively, in 1991 Vermeire and Pride[5] emphasized that despite common clinical and phenotypic features in COPD and asthma, the origins of these two obstructive lung disorders were distinctly different with respect to pathophysiologic and inflammatory mechanisms, and they coined the term "British Hypothesis," which postulates that recurrent bronchial infections explained why some smokers developed progressive airway obstruction compared to smokers without recurrent infections.[5] In 2006 Kraft[6] and Barnes[7] debated the clinical and pathophysiologic similarities and differences of the Dutch Hypothesis[6] versus the British Hypothesis[7] with respect to asthma and COPD. Now, we also have to integrate and address the controversial issues of the asthma-COPD overlap.

More recently, Postma and colleagues[8] provided an in-depth analysis of the multiple endogenous and exogenous factors that influence the phenotypic homogeneity and heterogeneity in asthma versus COPD and the asthma-COPD overlap (ACO), and others have addressed controversial aspects of ACO in depth.[9–26] We will further explore the genomics, pathophysiology, inflammatory, diagnostic guidelines, and therapeutic dilemma in COPD patients with presumptive ACO and asthmatics with presumptive ACO. Clinicians should exclude any comorbid illnesses that could obfuscate the ongoing saga of diagnosing ACO. ACO includes previously diagnosed and presumably treated asthmatics with significantly reversible expiratory airflow limitation. Subsequently, they may have smoked >10 pack years and developed COPD with only partially reversible expiratory airflow limitation. Alternatively,

smoking-related COPD patients may have concurrent asthma phenotypes including elevated sputum and/or blood eosinophilia, increased blood IgE, and, in some cases, postinhaled albuterol and significantly reversible expiratory airflow limitation.

6.3 EOSINOPHILIC AND TYPE 2 INFLAMMATION IN COPD

As we previously noted[2]: "genome wide association studies"[27,28] suggest, at most, only a weak shared genetic component to the asthma-COPD overlap (ACO). However, there is evidence that increased sputum and/or blood eosinophils and Type 2 inflammation, typically associated with asthma, may identify therapeutic responders when present in COPD. These studies suggest that ACO is not limited to a clinical phenotype, as there potentially may be a COPD subgroup, or endotype, biologically similar to asthma as well. Saha et al.[29] have emphasized that increased levels of sputum eosinophils are found in 20%–40% of COPD patients. Treatment with oral[30] and/or inhaled corticosteroid (ICS)[31] has been noted to increase FEV_1 (L), improve respiratory symptom scores, and reduce exacerbations in COPD.[32] Increased blood eosinophils, as a surrogate of sputum eosinophils, are markers associated with improvements in exacerbation rates following add-on ICS to a LABA in secondary analyses of two large randomized control trials (RCT).[33] A phase 2a RCT of benralizumab, the anti-IL-5 receptor monoclonal antibody that depletes eosinophils, was recently studied in COPD patients with high sputum eosinophil counts. The primary analysis did not show a difference in acute exacerbations.[34]

Type 2-associated proinflammatory pathways have been studied less thoroughly in COPD, because of the difficulty of obtaining direct measurements of the Type 2 cytokines (IL-4, IL-5, and IL-13) in readily available biospecimens.[2,35] However, in a recent study, airway epithelial gene expression alterations were used to overcome this problem to identify Type 2-associated inflammation in two separate COPD cohorts (n = 237, n = 171).[35] The investigators noted that Type 2-associated gene expression alterations were elevated in a COPD subgroup, and also were associated with increased eosinophil levels, greater bronchodilator reversibility, and improvements in measurements of hyperinflation.[35] This suggests Type 2-associated inflammation, in addition to eosinophilic inflammation, may play a clinical role in COPD pathophysiology in a subset of COPD patients. The authors also found a significant overlap of disease-associated airway epithelial gene expression alterations in asthma and a COPD subset.[35] Furthermore, asthma-derived gene expression signatures of Type 2 inflammation were associated with increased disease severity, eosinophil counts, and good ICS response in COPD.[35] These data suggest that there is a clinically relevant COPD subgroup characterized by asthma-like gene expression alterations.[35] Furthermore, Type 2 related gene expression signatures may serve as biomarkers to predict which patients with COPD will benefit from ICS or other Type 2 targeted treatment.[35]

Ghebre et al.[36] used cluster analysis to identify similarities and differences between asthma and COPD. Severe asthma and moderate-to-severe COPD patients were examined using sputum cell counts and cytokine levels as predictor variables. The patients were clustered into three distinct groups:

- Cluster 1: asthma-predominant with high Type 2 sputum cytokines and eosinophilia
- Cluster 2: asthma-COPD overlap with high proinflammatory sputum cytokines IL-1ß, IL-8, IL-10, TNF-alpha, and neutrophilia
- Cluster 3: COPD predominant with near equal sputum eosinophilia and neutrophilia, and increases in IL-6 and CCL2, 13, and 17[36]

They found evidence for ACO on a biological level, with the largest overlap among subjects in whom non-Type 2 or noneosinophilic driven inflammation predominated. These findings may have been skewed by corticosteroid use in both asthma and COPD subjects, particularly the use of systemic corticosteroid in the asthma subject group. Nonetheless, their results suggest that there may be considerable overlap between asthma and COPD patients, and that this overlap may extend beyond eosinophilic and Type 2 inflammation.[36] GOLD[37] has now incorporated ACO clinical guidelines, and Barnes[38] has suggested options for therapeutic intervention in ACO.

6.4 MECHANISM(S) FOR PERSISTENT EXPIRATORY AIRFLOW LIMITATION IN TREATED, NEVER SMOKED, CHRONIC ASTHMATICS

Until recently, structure-function studies have not specifically addressed the unique pathophysiologic mechanism(s) responsible for persistent expiratory airflow limitation in nonsmoking, treated, chronic asthmatics who develop a COPD phenotype.[1,2,39,40] The sentinel study by Gold, Kaufman, and Nadel[41] identified the reversible loss of lung elastic recoil in acute asthma. Subsequently, it was also noted that the persistent loss of lung elastic recoil in stable nonsmoking moderate-to-severe asthmatics with chronic expiratory airflow limitation occurred despite

treatment.[42] Furthermore, with exacerbations of asthma, there was a nearly parallel further shift to the left of the lung pressure-volume curve.[42] The unexpected superimposed loss of lung elastic recoil in nonsmoking asthmatics, contributes additionally to concurrent expiratory airflow limitation due to peripheral airway intrinsic bronchoconstrictive remodeling.[1,2,39,40] It has been noted that treated, nonsmoking asthmatics with persistent expiratory airflow limitation have loss of lung elastic recoil compared to age-matched controls.[1,2] Furthermore, as shown in Figure 6.1, the extent of loss of lung elastic recoil was similar as to the decrease of intrinsic airway conductance in reducing expiratory airflow.[1,2] An insignificant parenchymal attenuation of lung density was noted on high resolution, thin section lung CT using voxel quantification.[39,40] However, unsuspected microscopic lung tissue breakdown of alveolar attachments surrounding the terminal bronchioles was noted predominantly in upper lung fields. Mild centrilobular emphysema was present in formalin-inflated lungs obtained at autopsy in each of four severe asthma cases, despite normal diffusing capacity and near normal lung CT.[39,40] Furthermore, lung tissue breakdown as noted in Figure 6.2 was not consistent with senile emphysema as originally described.[43]

There were also concurrent microscopic findings of typical asthma changes in both large and small airways, including mucosal goblet cell metaplasia, thickening of both the basement membrane (BM) and airway smooth muscle layers.[39,40] These sentinel pathophysiologic findings extend earlier novel pathologic observations by Thais Mauad et al.[44] who described localized periterminal bronchiolar emphysema with breakdown of alveolar attachments in autopsied fatal asthmatics without lung function

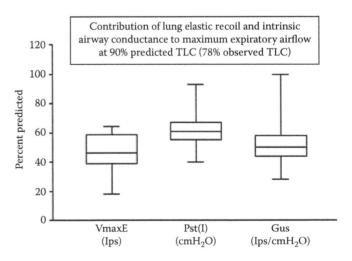

Figure 6.1 This demonstrates that there is a marked reduction in maximal expiratory airflow (VmaxE). Furthermore, the reduction in lung elastic recoil pressure [Pst(l)] is similar as to the reduction in intrinsic airway conductance (Gus). (Permission to reproduce this diagram we previously published will be obtained from Gelb, A., J Allergy Clin Immunol., 133, 263–265, 2014.)

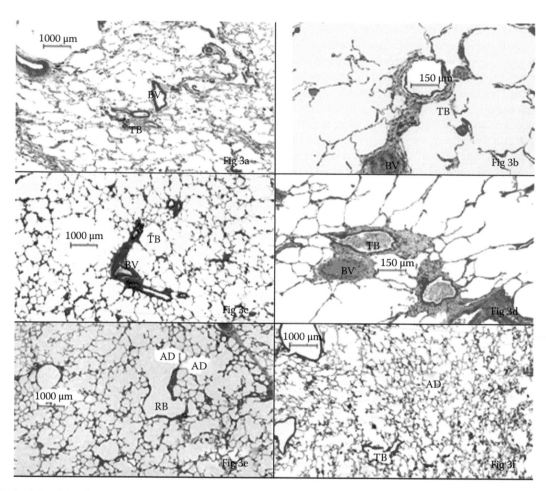

Figure 6.2 Labeled Fig 3 **(a–f)** (H&E stain) reproduced with permission (when obtained) from Chest.[40] Note emphysema observed at autopsy in Fig 3a,b and Fig 3c and d in 2 never smoked asthmatics with moderate to severe asthma with persistent expiratory airflow limitation despite treatment. There was measured loss of lung elastic recoil, normal diffusing capacity, and lung CT showed normal or mild emphysema. There was not only disorganization and unevenly distributed enlarged airspaces, but also disrupted alveolar septa even visible at this magnification as previously reported.[40] In these cases Alcian blue/PAS stain showed mucin in terminal bronchioles (TB) with plugging and the plugs contained 70% recruited neutrophils. Fig 3e is control Case in 82-year-old asthmatic woman with reversible expiratory airflow limitation with treatment. Microscopic morphometry was consistent with "senile lung" with nearly homogenous acinar hyperinflation and alveolar ductal ectasia but without unevenly distributed airspace enlargement, septal disruption, with no free septal fragments detached from the surrounding structures.[40] Fig 3f is a 71-year-old male with normal lung function. TB = terminal bronchiole, BV = blood vessel, RB = respiratory bronchiole, AD = alveolar duct. Scale bar in Fig 3a,c,e,f is 1000 μm and in Fig 3b,d 150 μm.

studies.[44] The inflammatory lung response described in these same subjects included increased eosinophils, mast cells and neutrophils in the peribronchiolar parenchyma.[45,46] The outer wall of small membranous bronchioles was the main site of these inflammatory changes.[46] Recently, Senhorini et al.[47] reported that younger adult fatal asthmatics had thicker BMs, smooth muscle, and outer wall areas, in both small and large airways, compared to both COPD and older asthmatic patients. In older asthmatics, there was an overlap in BM thickness and airway structure in small airways. The inner wall layer in large and small airways and submucosal gland areas were similar among groups. Older fatal asthmatics had overlapping airway structural features with younger adult fatal asthmatics and severe COPD patients.[47]

6.5 MECHANISM(S) RESPONSIBLE FOR THE INFLAMMATORY AND PROTEOLYTIC LUNG TISSUE BREAKDOWN IN CHRONIC NONSMOKING ASTHMATICS

The original description of emphysema by Leopold and Gough suggested that the terminal bronchioles were the nascent sites of lung tissue breakdown that led to centrilobular emphysema.[1,2,39,40,48] Therefore, recurrent asthma attacks may produce bronchiolar inflammation with activation of a predominantly Type 2 associated proinflammatory pathway and subsequent proteolytic cascade leading to lung tissue destruction.[1,2,39,40] This process may be mediated by an autocrine pro-inflammatory, perhaps epidermal growth factor receptor (EGFR)-initiated, signaling cascade stimulated by inhaled invaders in epithelial cells.[1,2,39,40,49] Subsequently, protective mucociliary responses occur in the airway epithelium via interleukin IL-17 and IL-18, which activate IL-8 to induce mucin production and neutrophil recruitment, especially in mild-to-moderate asthma.[1,2,39,40,49] Moreover, proteases, such as neutrophil elastase and cathepsin G, and membrane metalloproteases, activated eosinophils, macrophages, and mast cells, may all induce mucin production via proteolytic activation of the EGFR ligand-initiated signaling cascade.[1,2,39,40,49] In addition, neutrophil elastase and cathepsin G are potent secretagogues for submucosal gland epithelial cells.[1,2,39,40,47] This observation is likely relevant in those mild-to-moderate treated chronic asthmatics who have noneosinophilic and predominantly neutrophilic inflammation,[50] resulting in excessive neutrophil elastase secretion in lung tissue. Together with activated matrix metalloproteinases, this proteolytic cascade has the potential to cleave and disrupt the normal connective tissue integrity of the attachments linking the lung parenchyma to adjacent terminal bronchioles (centrilobular emphysema), resulting in the potential loss of anatomic and physiologic interdependence.[1,2,39,40]

6.6 SEVERITY AND TREATMENT RESPONSE AS A PHENOTYPIC CHARACTERISTIC OF ACO

The identification and treatment of ACO patients has been recently addressed in a joint publication issued by members of the GINA and GOLD guidelines.[37] This document emphasizes that a number of studies have reported ACO is associated with more frequent respiratory exacerbations and hospitalizations compared to COPD patients without ACO.[8-25] Moreover, this in-depth combined GINA/GOLD guideline review,[37] as well as other published guidelines for treatment of ACO,[26,38] recognize the conflicting data on how to diagnose, manage, and treat these varying obstructive lung phenotypes. A significant limitation is that most of the ACO studies to date[8-25] are cross-sectional and lack a randomized controlled therapeutic intervention design. It is reasonable to speculate that ACO patients would most likely benefit from directed therapies, such as combination therapy with ICS, LABA, and a long-acting muscarinic antagonist (LAMA), with or without intermittent short courses of oral corticosteroids as needed. However, it is clear that these patients may not be easily identified by clinical characteristics alone.[37] The complexity of ACO will likely require more specific therapies that may target ACO-relevant inflammatory pathways or a proteolytic cascade with a goal of preventing irreversible structural changes.[8-26,38] Such therapies may be relevant to eosinophilic and Type 2 inflammation, including monoclonal antibodies against interleukin IL-5,

IL-13, IL-33, and TSLP, and the prostaglandin D2 receptor on Th2 cells, CRTH2.[38] In addition, antineutrophil interventions may be more relevant to ACO than asthma given the role of neutrophilic inflammation in COPD including macrolides, CXCR2 antagonists, PDE-4 inhibitors, p38 MAP kinase inhibitors, and antibodies against IL-1 and IL-17.[38] However, these therapies, which have potential mechanistic benefits in ACO, will require further research to confirm their relevance.

The clinical differentiation between ACO, asthma, and COPD phenotypes/endotypes emphasizes the need for a precision medicine strategy specific for chronic obstructive airway diseases.[19] In this setting, phenotypes can be used for hypothesis generation and probabilistic prediction of treatment outcomes, whereas endotypes are the result of hypothesis testing, being more suitable for correctly selecting treatment choices.[19] In the postgenomic era, human diseases will require reclassification beginning with well-defined causal molecular pathways (i.e., endotypes) that correlate with the disease phenotype.[19] The therapy of the ACO patient will thus be based on the presence of clinical characteristics that are not mutually exclusive from other chronic obstructive lung diseases.[19]

6.7 CONCLUSION

A subset of smoking-related COPD patients with hyper-responsive airways with and without a history of asthma has been identified and referred to as ACO. Eosinophilic, Type 2, and neutrophilic immune responses may all potentially play a role in the overlap between asthma and COPD. Therapeutic intervention for ACO should reflect the asthma paradigm. However, how to best characterize this subgroup of obstructive lung disease patients to maximize therapeutic benefit is still unclear. Furthermore, the mechanism(s) responsible for expiratory airflow limitation in nonsmoking, moderate-to-severe asthmatics with persistent expiratory airflow limitation who develop a COPD phenotype is similar to ACO in smokers. Despite normal diffusing capacity and near normal lung CT, microscopic mild emphysema has been noted in lungs obtained at autopsy.[1,2,39,40] Therefore, it is probable that a proinflammatory pathway and proteolytic cascade are key contributors leading to lung tissue breakdown and unsuspected autopsy proven centrilobular emphysema in these patients. Further investigation into the pathophysiologic and inflammatory mechanisms in ACO are required to understand the transition from asthma to COPD in smokers and in nonsmokers.

ACKNOWLEDGMENT

Roxanna Moridzadeh, BS, and Diem Tran, BS, for manuscript preparation.

REFERENCES

1. Gelb A and Nadel J. Understanding the pathophysiology of the asthma–COPD overlap syndrome. *J Allergy Clin Immunol.* 2015;136(3):553–555.

2. Gelb A, Christenson S, and Nadel J. Understanding the pathophysiology of the asthma–COPD overlap syndrome (ACOS). *Curr Opin Pulmon Med.* 2016;22(2):100–105.

3. Orie NGM, Sluiter HJ, De Vries K et al. The host factor in bronchitis. In: Orie NGM, Sluiter HJ, editors, *Bronchitis.* Assen, the Netherlands: Royal Van Gorcum; 1961. pp. 43–59.

4. Fletcher C and Pride N. Definitions of emphysema, chronic bronchitis, asthma, and airflow obstruction: 25 years on from the Ciba symposium. *Thorax.* 1984;39(2):81–85.

5. Vermeire P and Pride N. "Splitting" look at chronic nonspecific lung disease (CNSLD): Common features but diverse pathogenesis. *Eur Respir J.* 1991;4:490–496.

6. Kraft M. Asthma and chronic obstructive pulmonary disease exhibit common origins in any country!. *Am J Respir Crit Care Med.* 2006;174(3):238–240.

7. Barnes P. Against the Dutch hypothesis: Asthma and chronic obstructive pulmonary disease are distinct diseases. *Am J Respir Crit Care Med.* 2006;174(3):240–243.

8. Postma D, Weiss S, van den Berge M et al. Revisiting the Dutch hypothesis. *J Allergy Clin Immunol.* 2015;136(3):521–529.

9. Gibson P and McDonald V. Asthma–COPD overlap 2015: Now we are six. *Thorax.* 2015;70(7):683–691.

10. Cosio B, Soriano J, López-Campos J et al. Defining the asthma–COPD overlap syndrome in a COPD cohort. *Chest.* 2016;149(1):45–52.

11. Postma D and Rabe K. The asthma–COPD overlap syndrome. *N Engl J Med.* 2015;373(13):1241–1249.

12. Barrecheguren M, Esquinas C, and Miravitlles M. The asthma–chronic obstructive pulmonary disease overlap syndrome (ACOS)–opportunities and challenges. *Curr Opin Pulmon Med.* 2015;21(1):74–79.

13. Bujarski S, Parulekar A, Sharafkhaneh A et al. The asthma COPD overlap syndrome (ACOS). *Curr Allergy Asthma Rep.* 2015;15(3):509.

14. Bateman E, Reddel H, van Zyl-Smit R et al. The asthma–COPD overlap syndrome: Towards a revised taxonomy of chronic airways diseases? *Lancet Respir Med.* 2015;3(9):719–728.

15. Yamasaki A, Harada T, Fukushima T et al. Causes of death in patients with asthma and asthma–chronic obstructive pulmonary disease overlap syndrome. *Int J Chron Obstruct Pulmon Dis.* 2015;10:595–602.

16. Fingleton J, Travers J, Williams M et al. Treatment responsiveness of phenotypes of symptomatic airways obstruction in adults. *J Allergy Clin Immunol.* 2015;136(3):601–609.

17. Menezes A, Montes de Oca M, Pérez-Padilla R, et al. Increased risk of exacerbation and hospitalization in subjects with an overlap phenotype COPD–asthma. *Chest.* 2014;145(2):297–304.

18. Barnes P. Asthma–COPD overlap. *Chest.* 2016;149(1):7–8.

19. Agusti A, Bel E, Thomas M et al. Treatable traits: Toward precision medicine of chronic airway diseases. *Eur Respir J.* 2016;47(2):410–419.

20. Sin DD, Miravitlles M, Mannino DM et al. What is asthma-COPD overlap syndrome? Towards a concensus definition from a round table discussion. *Eur Respir J.* 2016;48: 664–673.

21. Lange P, Çolak Y, Ingebrigtsen T et al. Long-term prognosis of asthma, chronic obstructive pulmonary disease, and asthma–chronic obstructive pulmonary disease overlap in the Copenhagen City Heart study: A prospective population-based analysis. *Lancet Respir Med.* 2016;4(6):454–462.

22. Alshabanat A, Zafari Z, Albanyan O et al. Asthma and COPD overlap syndrome (ACOS): A systematic review and meta-analysis. *PLOS ONE.* 2015;10(9):e0136065.

23. FitzGerald JM and Sadatsafavi M. Less chaos in the prognosis of asthma–chronic obstructive lung disease overlap. *Lancet Respir Med.* 2016;4(6):421–422.

24. Aalbers R and van den Berge M. The asthma–COPD overlap syndrome: How is it defined and what are its clinical implications? *J Asthma Allergy.* 2016;9:27–35.

25. Rabe K. Elastic recoil revisited. *Chest.* 2015;148(2): 297–298.

26. Reddel H. Treatment of overlapping asthma–Chronic obstructive pulmonary disease: Can guidelines contribute in an evidence-free zone? *J Allergy Clin Immunol.* 2015;136(3):546–552.

27. Smolonska J, Koppelman G, Wijmenga C et al. Common genes underlying asthma and COPD? Genome-wide analysis on the Dutch hypothesis. *Eur Respir J.* 2014;44(4):860–872.

28. Hardin M, Cho M, McDonald M et al. The clinical and genetic features of COPD–asthma overlap syndrome. *Eur Respir J.* 2014;44(2):341–350.

29. Saha S and Brightling C. Eosinophilic airway inflammation in COPD. *Int J COPD.* 2006;1(1):39–47.

30. Brightling C, Monteiro W, Ward R et al. Sputum eosinophilia and short-term response to prednisolone in chronic obstructive pulmonary disease: A randomised controlled trial. *Lancet.* 2000;356(9240):1480–1485.

31. Brightling C, McKenna S, Hargadon B et al. Sputum eosinophilia and the short term response to inhaled mometasone in chronic obstructive pulmonary disease. *Thorax.* 2005;60(3):193–198.

32. Siva R, Green R, Brightling C et al. Eosinophilic airway inflammation and exacerbations of COPD: A randomised controlled trial. *Eur Respir J.* 2007;29(5):906–913.

33. Pascoe S, Locantore N, Dransfield M et al. Blood eosinophil counts, exacerbations, and response to the addition of inhaled fluticasone furoate to vilanterol in patients with chronic obstructive pulmonary disease: A secondary analysis of data from two parallel randomised controlled trials. *Lancet Respir Med.* 2015;3(6):435–442.

34. Brightling C, Bleecker E, Panettieri R et al. Benralizumab for chronic obstructive pulmonary disease and sputum eosinophilia: A randomised, double-blind, placebo-controlled, phase 2a study. *Lancet Respir Med.* 2014;2(11):891–901.

35. Christenson S, Steiling K, van den Berge M et al. Asthma–COPD overlap. Clinical relevance of genomic signatures of type 2 inflammation in chronic obstructive pulmonary disease. *Am J Respir Crit Care Med.* 2015;191(7):758–766.

36. Ghebre M, Bafadhel M, Desai D et al. Biological clustering supports both "Dutch" and "British" hypotheses of asthma and chronic obstructive pulmonary disease. *J Allergy Clin Immunol.* 2015;135(1):63–72. e10.

37. Global Initiative for Chronic Obstructive Lung Disease - Global Initiative for Chronic Obstructive Lung Disease - GOLD [Internet]. Global Initiative for Chronic Obstructive Lung Disease - GOLD; 2016. Available at http://www.goldcopd.org. Accessed May 28, 2016.

38. Barnes P. Therapeutic approaches to asthma—Chronic obstructive pulmonary disease overlap syndromes. *J Allergy Clin Immunol.* 2015;136(3):531–545.

39. Gelb A, Yamamoto A, Mauad T et al. Unsuspected mild emphysema in nonsmoking patients with chronic asthma with persistent airway obstruction. *J Allergy Clin Immunol.* 2014;133(1):263–265. e3.

40. Gelb A, Yamamoto A, Verbeken E et al. Unraveling the pathophysiology of the asthma–COPD overlap syndrome: Unsuspected mild centrilobular emphysema is responsible for loss of lung elastic recoil in never smokers with asthma with persistent expiratory airflow limitation. *Chest.* 2015;148(2):313–320.

41. Gold W, Kaufman H, and Nadel J. Elastic recoil of the lungs in chronic asthmatic patients before and after therapy. *J Appl Physiol.* 1967;23(4):433–438.

42. Woolcock A and Read J. The static elastic properties of the lungs in asthma. *Am Rev Respir Dis.* 1968;98(5):788–794.

43. Verbeken E, Cauberghs M, Mertens I et al. The senile lung. Comparison with normal and emphysematous lungs. 1. Structural aspects. *Chest.* 1992;101(3):793–799.

44. Mauad T, Silva L, Santos M et al. Abnormal alveolar attachments with decreased elastic fiber content in distal lung in fatal asthma. *Am J Respir Crit Care Med.* 2004;170(8):857–862.

45. Dolhnikoff M, da Silva L, de Araujo B et al. The outer wall of small airways is a major site of remodeling in fatal asthma. *J Allergy Clin Immunol.* 2009;123(5):1090–1097.e1.

46. De Magalhaes Simoes S, dos Santos M, da Silva Oliveira M et al. Inflammatory cell mapping of the respiratory tract in fatal asthma. *Clin Exp Allergy.* 2005;35(5):602–611.

47. Senhorini A, Ferreira D, Shiang C et al. Airway dimensions in fatal asthma and fatal COPD: Overlap in older patients. COPD. *J Chron Obstruct Pulmon Dis.* 2013;10(3):348–356.

48. Leopold J and Gough J. The centrilobular form of hypertrophic emphysema and its relation to chronic bronchitis. *Thorax.* 1957;12(3):219–235.

49. Burgel P and Nadel J. Epidermal growth factor receptor-mediated innate immune responses and their roles in airway diseases. *Eur Respir J.* 2008;32(4):1068–1081.

50. McGrath K, Icitovic N, Boushey H et al. A large subgroup of mild-to-moderate asthma is persistently noneosinophilic. *Am J Respir Crit Care Med.* 2012;185(6):612–619.

Tobacco: Active and passive smoke exposure

NEIL C. THOMSON

CLINICAL VIGNETTE 7.1: POOR RESPIRATORY SYMPTOM CONTROL IN A HEAVY CIGARETTE SMOKER

A 42-year-old male was referred by his primary care physician to a hospital respiratory clinic because of increased symptoms of wheezing and dyspnea. The patient had previously received short courses of broad-spectrum antibiotics and oral corticosteroids, which had only partially resolved his symptoms. His current drug treatment was an inhaled corticosteroid (400 mcg, once daily) in combination with a long-acting β_2-agonist and an inhaled short-acting β_2-agonist (taken as required). The patient had a more than 25-year history of episodic wheezing. His respiratory symptoms were not precipitated by exposure to allergens and there was no seasonal variability in his symptoms. Furthermore, the patient gave a 10-year history of a chronic cough associated with daily expectoration of mucoid sputum. He had been smoking for approximately 20 years, currently around 15 cigarettes per day. His occupation was a shopkeeper. There was no family history of asthma. Both of his parents were lifelong cigarette smokers, and his wife was also a smoker. On examination of the chest, there was mild bilateral wheeze.

Pulmonary function before and after treatment with an inhaled short-acting β_2-agonist.

	Predicted	Measured	Measurements after short-acting β_2-agonist	
–	–	–	Measured	Percent change
Forced expiratory volume in 1 second (FEV₁) (L)	3.8	2.2	2.6	18%
Forced vital capacity (FVC) (L)	4.4	4.2	4.3	–
FEV₁/FVC ratio	86%	52%	60%	–

The patient's chest X-ray appeared normal. Peak expiratory flow (PEF) readings, taken twice daily, were performed over a 2-week period and showed an average variability of 16%.

Questions

- Does the patient have asthma, COPD, or overlap?
- Can exposure to active and passive tobacco smoke cause the development of chronic airway disease?
- What are the prevalence rates for active and passive tobacco smoke exposure in chronic airway disease?
- Are clinical outcomes worse in smokers with asthma?
- Do clinical outcomes differ in current and former smokers with COPD?
- Does exposure to passive smoke worsen clinical outcomes in asthma and COPD?
- Does smoking status or exposure to passive smoke influence clinical outcomes in overlap syndrome?

7.1 INTRODUCTION

Worldwide, more than 1 billion people are estimated to use tobacco products, mainly through smoking cigarettes. In 2014 the prevalence of current cigarette smoking among the general population in the United States and United Kingdom was 16.8% and 19% respectively.[1] Adults living in low-income and middle-income countries have high prevalence rates for cigarette smoking and account for more than three-quarters of all smokers worldwide. In the United States, exposure to passive smoke has reduced by half since 2000.[2] Nevertheless, approximately 25% of nonsmokers are exposed to passive smoke on a regular basis, with higher exposure levels in children, non-Hispanic blacks, and people living in poverty.[2] Homes and workplaces are the main locations for passive-smoke exposure.[3]

Active and passive cigarette smoke exposure cause an enormous burden of disease, including cancer, cardiovascular disorders, and respiratory disease.[3,4] In most developed countries,

around half the adult asthmatic population and most people with COPD are current or former cigarette smokers, and a quarter of children and adults with asthma are exposed to passive smoke. Higher rate of active smoking and exposure to passive smoke are found in developing countries. Exposure to active and passive smoking has a major adverse impact on the health of people with asthma and COPD. In this chapter, the following topics are reviewed: the evidence that active smoking and exposure to passive smoke contribute to the development of asthma, COPD, and overlap; prevalence rates for active and passive tobacco smoke exposure in asthma, COPD, and overlap; and the effects of active and passive tobacco smoke exposure on clinical outcomes and inflammatory variables in people with asthma and COPD.

7.2 ACTIVE SMOKING AND ASTHMA

7.2.1 DEVELOPMENT OF ASTHMA IN ACTIVE SMOKERS

In the 2014 U.S. Surgeon General Report on the Health Consequences of Smoking, the overall evidence is considered suggestive, but not sufficient to infer a causal relationship between active cigarette smoking and the incidence of asthma in adolescents and adults.[4] The U.S. Black Women's Health Study recently reported that a history of current or former smoking increased the risk of asthma by around 40%, and the increased risk was associated with a higher pack-year history.[5]

7.2.2 PREVALENCE OF CIGARETTE SMOKING IN ASTHMA

The World Health Survey of smoking rates among people with asthma in different countries found that more than 23% were current smokers, with smoking rates ranging from 13% to 35%.[6] In many countries, the proportion of cigarette smokers in people with asthma is similar to rates in the general population.[6] In the United States, however, a higher proportion of people with asthma smoke (21%) compared to the general population (16.8%).[1] The U.S. National Survey on Drug Use and Health between 2005 and 2013 found no decline in cigarette smoking among people with asthma.[7] In contrast, the European Community Respiratory Health Survey (ECRHS) II reported that cigarette smoking was less frequent in people with asthma (26%) than in the general population (31%).[8] The prevalence of cigarette smoking differs in certain subgroups of asthma, with increased rates among people visiting emergency rooms with exacerbations of asthma in the United States[9] and with reduced rates in people with severe disease.[10] In Australia, women with asthma during pregnancy are more likely to smoke (34%) than those without asthma (15%).[11] Former smokers account for 25%–43% of the adult asthmatic population.[8–12] In summary, approximately half the population of adults with asthma living in developed countries are either current or former cigarette smokers.

7.2.3 CLINICAL OUTCOMES AND INFLAMMATORY VARIABLES IN CURRENT AND FORMER SMOKERS WITH ASTHMA

Current smoking in asthma is associated with a wide range of adverse health outcomes[13,14] (Table 7.1, Figure 7.1). Differences between people in factors associated with asthma—such as phenotype, severity, and drug treatment—and factors associated with cigarette smoking—such as intensity, duration, and pack-year history—may explain some of the discrepancies in the findings between studies investigating the effects of smoking status on clinical outcomes and inflammatory variables in asthma.

7.2.3.1 Current symptom control and quality of life

Surveys of people with asthma, including those with severe forms of the disease or during pregnancy, demonstrate that current smoking is an important risk factor for poor symptom control.[10,12–15] In some studies, smokers with asthma have worse levels of asthma-specific quality of life,[16] although other surveys report similar levels of health status.[8]

7.2.3.2 Chronic mucus hypersecretion

Chronic mucus hypersecretion occurs more frequently in smokers with asthma than nonsmokers with asthma[8,10–17]), particularly in severe disease, and is associated with worse current symptom control.[18] Computed tomography (CT) large airway luminal area is reduced in smokers with severe asthma who gave a history of chronic mucus hypersecretion,[18] possibly due to mucus accumulation in the large airways and to structural changes to airway luminal size.

7.2.3.3 Exacerbations and health care utilization

The 2014 U.S. Surgeon General's Report considered the evidence sufficient to infer a causal relationship between active cigarette smoking and exacerbations in adults with asthma.[4] Current smoking is a risk factor for severe exacerbations during pregnancy[11] and in severe asthma.[10] In some studies, cigarette smoking is associated with a greater risk of hospitalization for asthma,[16] more visits to the emergency room for asthma,[19] and increased numbers of life-threatening asthma attacks. In contrast to these results, the Copenhagen General Population Study found the risk of exacerbations was similar between never smokers, former smokers, and current smokers with asthma.[12]

Table 7.1 Summary of the reported effects of smoking status on clinical outcomes in asthma*

Clinical outcome	Asthma	
	Current smoker compared with never smoker	Former smoker compared with never smoker
Respiratory symptoms associated with asthma	Increased	Increased or similar
Asthma quality of life	Decreased or similar	Decreased or similar
Chronic mucus hypersecretion	Increased	Similar
Exacerbations	Increased or similar	Similar
Health care utilization	Increased	Increased or similar
Therapeutic response to inhaled corticosteroids		
• Short- to medium-term treatment	Decreased	Decreased or similar
• Long-term treatment	Decreased or similar	Similar
Lung function		
• Proportion with $FEV_1/FVC < 0.7$	Increased	Increased
• Increased decline in FEV_1	Increased or similar	-
• Small airway dysfunction	Increased	-
• Bronchial challenge		-
– AMP	Increased or similar	-
– Methacholine	Similar	
Smoking-related comorbidities	Increased	Similar
All-cause mortality	Increased	Similar

* *Note:* Refer to the main text for information on the published studies used to summarize the effects of smoking status on clinical outcomes in asthma.
Abbreviation and symbol: AMP, adenosine 5′-monophosphate; -, not known

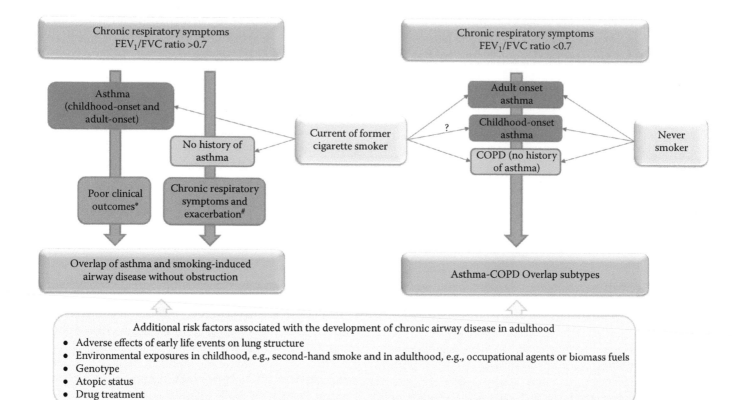

Figure 7.1 Effects of smoking status, history of asthma and age of onset of asthma as well as other risk factors on potential pathways leading to the development in adulthood of chronic respiratory symptoms associated with or without spirometric evidence of chronic airflow obstruction (FEV$_1$/FVC ratio <0.7).

* Compared to never-smokers with asthma

\# Compared to healthy never smokers

? A history of active cigarette smoking in adulthood may not be associated with lower FEV$_1$/FVC ratios in people with childhood-onset persistent asthma. (From Hancox RJ., *Am J Resp Crit Care Med.*, 94, 276–284, 2016.)

7.2.3.4 Corticosteroid insensitivity

Cigarette smokers with mild to moderate asthma are less sensitive to the short- and medium-term beneficial effects of inhaled corticosteroids on symptoms and lung function compared to nonsmokers with asthma.[13,20,21] Smokers with chronic stable asthma are also less sensitive to short-term oral corticosteroid therapy[22] and have an impaired cutaneous vasoconstrictor response to topical corticosteroids. Whether the long-term therapeutic effects of inhaled corticosteroids are impaired in smokers with asthma is less certain.[23] In the Gaining Optimal Asthma Control (GOAL) trial, which compared the efficacy of inhaled fluticasone alone or combined with inhaled salmeterol over 1 year, asthma exacerbation rates were increased in smokers with asthma receiving inhaled fluticasone compared to never-smokers.[24] The effect of inhaled corticosteroids on the rate of decline in lung function is impaired in heavy smokers with asthma,[25] but not in lighter smokers.[25] In an observational study, the decline in lung function in smokers with asthma was lower for those who were receiving inhaled corticosteroids (31 mL/year) compared to for those who were not (58 mL/year).[26] In support of these findings, the

benefits of therapy with inhaled budesonide on preventing lung function decline are similar in light smokers and non-smokers with mild persistent asthma.[27] Taken together, the results of clinical studies in smokers with chronic asthma suggest that most individuals are less sensitive to short and medium treatment with inhaled corticosteroids compared to nonsmokers with asthma, but that a small proportion of smokers may respond adequately to this treatment and that long-term treatment may have beneficial effects. Thus, inhaled corticosteroids should be prescribed to symptomatic smokers with asthma, because of potential short-term and long-term benefits.

7.2.3.5 Lung function

Smoking a cigarette causes acute bronchoconstriction in smokers with asthma, particularly in those with reduced baseline spirometry.[28] Lung function tests, such as FEV$_1$/FVC ratio and FEV$_1$, are often reduced in smokers with asthma compared with never-smokers with asthma.[10,12,29] Several longitudinal population-based studies report accelerated decline in lung function in adult smokers with asthma,[17,30,31] although other studies report a similar decline in FEV_1 in asthma irrespective of smoking status.[8] A greater proportion of smokers with asthma develop persistent airflow obstruction. Tests of small airway function are reduced in asthmatic smokers.[29] Air trapping induced by the indirect bronchial challenge adenosine 5'-monophosphate (AMP) is increased in smokers with asthma, whereas the response to a direct challenge with methacholine is similar to nonsmokers with asthma.[32]

7.2.3.6 Comorbidities

Comorbidities occur frequently in people with asthma who smoke, with higher rates of cardiovascular disease, pneumonia, and lung cancer compared to never-smokers without asthma.[12] Cigarette smoking in the general population is a risk factor for diseases that can impact the health of smokers with asthma, such as anxiety and depression, chronic rhinitis, and osteoporosis. The U.S. National Health and Nutrition Examination Survey Epidemiologic Follow-Up Study (NHEFS) reported an increased risk of respiratory mortality and all-cause mortality in asthma that may be explained by the confounding effect of cigarette smoking.[33]

7.2.3.7 Clinical outcomes in former smokers with asthma

There is limited published information on clinical outcomes in former smokers with asthma compared with never-smokers or current smokers with asthma (Table 7.1). In U.K. general practice, former smokers with mild asthma receiving inhaled corticosteroids have worse symptom control than nonsmokers with asthma and better control than current smokers with asthma.[15] A Canadian general population survey of patients with asthma[34] and data from the British Thoracic Society (BTS) severe asthma registry,[10] both found better symptom control in former smokers compared to current smokers. In contrast, the Copenhagen General Population Study found that among individuals with asthma (2304 never-smokers, 2467 former smokers, and 920 current smokers), the frequency of any respiratory symptom was similar between groups.[12] In some studies, former smokers with asthma have worse asthma-specific quality of life scores than never-smokers with asthma,[16] whereas in the BTS severe asthma registry asthmatics, quality of life was similar in former and never-smokers.[10] The prevalence of chronic mucus hypersecretion is similar in former smokers and never-smokers with asthma (42%) and higher in current smokers with asthma (52%).[8] The frequency of severe exacerbations is similar in former smokers with asthma and current smokers with asthma during pregnancy.[11] In people with asthma recruited to the Copenhagen General Population Study, airflow obstruction (FEV_1/FVC < 70%) was less frequent in never-smokers (23%) than former smokers (38%) or current smokers (47%).[12] In the BTS severe asthma registry population, a range of clinical outcomes in

former smokers with severe asthma were similar to never-smokers with severe asthma, except for anxiety and depression scale scores, which were higher in former smokers.[10] A study in Finland reported an increased risk of emergency room visits for former smokers with asthma,[19] whereas a prospective U.S. study found that the risk of hospitalization for asthma and emergency room visits in former smokers with asthma was similar to never-smokers with asthma.[16] Rates of cardiovascular disease, pneumonia, lung cancer, and all-cause mortality in former smokers with asthma are similar to never-smokers and current smokers with asthma.[12] Although some published information is conflicting, taken together, the findings suggest that clinical outcomes in former smokers with asthma are either similar or worse than never-smokers with asthma and generally better than current smokers with asthma.

7.2.3.8 Phenotypes

Cluster analysis has been used to identify phenotypes of asthma associated with cigarette smoking. A cluster analysis performed in two South Korean cohorts of patients with asthma that included current smokers, identified four asthma subtypes, one of which was termed a "smoking asthma" group. The smoker cluster was the smallest group, subjects were predominately male, one third where atopic, and they had well-preserved FEV_1.[35]

7.2.3.9 Inflammatory variables

Active cigarette smoking in asthma can influence inflammatory variables (Table 7.2). There is limited information on whether smoking-induced airway inflammation persists after smoking cessation.

7.2.3.9.1 TOTAL AND SPECIFIC IgE

In the BTS severe asthma cohort(10) and the Copenhagen General Population Study of asthma,[12] total IgE concentrations are not altered by smoking status, although total IgE concentrations are increased in asthma compared with never-smokers without asthma.[12] Specific IgE sensitization to some common environmental allergens is reduced in current smokers and former smokers with severe asthma compared to never-smokers with severe asthma.[10]

7.2.3.9.2 BLOOD EOSINOPHILS

In the Copenhagen General Population Study, never, former, and current smokers with asthma had similar blood eosinophil count concentrations, although levels were increased in asthma compared with never smokers without asthma.[12] In a U.K. general practice study of people with asthma, the likelihood of a blood eosinophil count greater than 400 cells per microliter was lower in current smokers and former smokers with asthma compared

Table 7.2 Summary of the reported effects of smoking status on inflammatory variables in asthma*

| Inflammatory variable | Asthma | |
	Current smoker compared with never smoker	Former smoker compared with never smoker
Total IgE	Similar	Similar
Specific IgE	Decreased	Decreased
Blood eosinophils	Decreased or similar	Decreased or similar
Exhaled nitric oxide	Decreased or similar	Similar
Airway inflammation and remodeling		
• Sputum eosinophils	Decreased or similar	Decreased or similar
• Sputum neutrophils	Increased or decreased or similar	Increased or similar
Bronchial biopsy changes:		
• Eosinophils	Decreased	Decreased
• Neutrophils	Decreased	Similar
• Mast cells	Increased	Similar
• CD8+ T lymphocytes	Increased	-
• Bronchial epithelial changes: increased goblet cells, proliferation, thickness	Increased	Similar

* *Note:* Refer to the main text for information on the published studies used to summarize the effects of smoking status on clinical outcomes in asthma.
Symbol: -, not known

to nonsmokers with asthma.[36] In the BTS severe asthma cohort, blood eosinophil counts were similar in former and current smokers compared to never-smokers with severe asthma,[10] whereas blood eosinophils were reduced in a study of former and current smokers with mild to moderate asthma.[23]

7.2.3.9.3 EXHALED NITRIC OXIDE

Exhaled nitic oxide concentration is lowered by cigarette smoking.[37] In the BTS severe asthma cohort, exhaled nitic oxide concentration is reduced in current smokers and similar in former and never-smokers.[10]

7.2.3.9.4 SYSTEMIC INFLAMMATORY BIOMARKERS

Among individuals with asthma, former and current smokers have higher levels of inflammatory biomarkers, including C-reactive protein, fibrinogen, whole blood leukocyte count, and whole blood neutrophils compared to never-smokers without asthma.[12] Serum periostin concentrations are reduced in smokers with asthma compared to never-smokers with asthma, are weakly associated sputum eosinophil count in smokers with asthma and are not influenced by disease severity or atopic status.[38]

7.2.3.9.5 AIRWAY INFLAMMATION AND REMODELING

In several studies of smokers with asthma, sputum airway inflammation is often noneosinophilic associated with neutrophilic or paucigranulocytic inflammation.[13,14] In contrast, a recent Belgian study found that proportion

of sputum inflammatory phenotypes was similar between nonsmokers, former smokers, and current smokers with asthma,[39] and that eosinophilic inflammation occurred in approximately one third of the current smoker group. In the BTS severe asthma cohort, sputum eosinophil count was reduced in current smokers and similar in former and never-smokers.[10] Smoking cessation in asthma is associated with a reduction in sputum neutrophils.[40] Bronchial biopsy studies in smokers with asthma compared to never-smokers with asthma have reported reduced eosinophil numbers, increased submucosal mast cell numbers,[41] and increased CD8+ T lymphocytes.[42] In the bronchial epithelium of smokers with asthma, there are increased goblet cell numbers, more proliferation, and greater thickness of the epithelium.[41] Bronchial biopsy airway smooth muscle mass, basement membrane thickness, and submucosal gland area are similar.[41,43] Quantitative computed tomography (CT) measures of segmental airway wall thickness are similar in smokers and never-smokers with asthma in those with mild to severe disease.[29]

7.3 ACTIVE SMOKING AND COPD

7.3.1 DEVELOPMENT OF COPD

Cigarette smoking is the major risk factor for the development of COPD in both men and women in the United States and other developed countries.[4] The prevalence of COPD in women has increased in the last few decades, and although the intensity of cigarette smoking is lower than among men, women are considered more susceptible to the development of smoking-related COPD. Not all cigarette smokers develop COPD, in part due to differences in genetic and gender susceptibility, and to environmental exposures.[44] Exposure to other types of tobacco, such as pipe and cigar smoking are also associated with an increased risk of developing COPD.[44] Greater than 20% of cases of COPD are not attributable to cigarette smoking.[45] COPD in nonsmokers develops due to exposure to environmental factors, such as burning biomass fuels in developing countries, occupational agents, and air pollution, as well as impaired lung growth in childhood, poverty, and asthma.[44,45] In the Copenhagen General Population Study, the majority of symptomatic never-smokers with COPD did not have self-reported asthma, suggesting that airflow limitation was caused by risk factors other than asthma.[46] Cigarette smoking is one of the strongest risk factors for the development of chronic mucus hypersecretion in individuals with and without airflow limitation.[47]

7.3.2 PREVALENCE OF CIGARETTE SMOKING IN COPD

Thirty to fifty percent of people with smoking-related COPD are current smokers and the remainder are former smokers.[48,49] In the U.S. COPDGene study, GOLD D patients (high risk, more symptoms) have a lower proportion of current smokers, approximately 30%, than COPD A patients (low risk, less symptoms), approximately 50%.[49] Prevalence rates for current smoking are higher in COPD than in asthma or in the general population.

7.3.3 CLINICAL OUTCOMES AND INFLAMMATORY VARIABLES

Clinical outcomes in smoking-related COPD are usually described in populations made up of current smokers and former smokers that exclude people with less than 10 pack years and who have a high total exposure to tobacco smoke, usually greater than 40 pack years.[48,49] There is limited information on the similarities and differences in clinical outcomes and inflammatory variables in former smokers with COPD compared with current smokers with COPD.

7.3.3.1 Current smokers and former smokers with COPD

Clinical features experienced by people with smoking-related COPD include progressive dyspnea, chronic mucus hypersecretion, and impaired health status, and these individuals are at increased risk of exacerbations, accelerated decline in lung function, and adverse health effects associated with comorbidities.[44] Female smokers with severe COPD have more hospital admissions, a higher COPD associated mortality, and more small-airway disease and less emphysema than men. In the Evaluation of COPD

Longitudinally to Identify Predictive Surrogate End-points (ECLIPSE) study, continuous smoking was a risk factor for excessive decline in FEV_1 (21 mL/year), as was the presence of CT-defined emphysema.[50] Tobacco smoking is a common risk factor for some comorbidities associated with COPD, such as cardiovascular disease, osteoporosis, and lung cancer.[44-51] Chronic mucus hypersecretion in COPD is associated with continued or resumed cigarette smoking and worse clinical outcomes.[52]

In the Subpopulations and Intermediate Outcome Measures in COPD Study (SPIROMIC) population, current and former smokers without spirometric evidence of COPD, often have chronic respiratory symptoms and exacerbations.[53] Symptomatic current and former smokers, irrespective of a history of asthma, have greater CT airway wall thickening without emphysema compared with asymptomatic individuals.[53] In the COPDGene cohort, smokers without spirometric COPD had more respiratory symptoms, worse overall health status, exercise limitation, and greater CT airway wall thickening or emphysema than never-smokers.[54] These two studies suggest that symptomatic smoking-induced airway disease occurs frequently in people without spirometric evidence of COPD (Figure 7.1). Future research needs to establish the mechanisms of disease in these individuals, what proportion have undiagnosed asthma, and how best to manage these individuals beyond smoking cessation.

A wide range of different inflammatory biomarkers have been measured in smoking-related COPD,[55] and, of these, plasma fibrinogen is identified as a potential marker of all-cause mortality and of increased risk of cardiovascular disease and exacerbations. Blood eosinophil count is a potential marker of corticosteroid responsiveness in preventing and treating exacerbations. Detailed overviews of inflammatory variable in smoking-related COPD have been published.[44,55,56]

7.3.3.2 Former smokers with COPD

Former smokers with COPD compared with current smokers with COPD are less likely to have symptoms of chronic bronchitis (13% versus 32% respectively), and all-cause mortality is lower, whereas the risk of hospital admission due to COPD, pneumonia, and lung cancer, as well as cardiovascular comorbidities, are similar[57] (Table 7.3). The rate of change in FEV_1 varies considerably among people with COPD, with increased rates of decline among current smokers compared to former smokers for all GOLD stages.[50-58] Cumulative exposure to tobacco smoke (pack-year history) does not influence future decline.[50]

Smokers with COPD who stop smoking experience improvements in respiratory symptoms such as dyspnea, wheeze, and chronic mucus hypersecretion, with the greatest decrease occurring in the first year of smoking cessation.[58-60] After smoking cessation, there is a modest initial increase in FEV_1, and persistent smoking abstinence is associated with the

Table 7.3 Summary of the reported effects of smoking status on clinical outcomes and inflammatory variables in COPD*

Clinical outcome	Former smoker with COPD compared with current smoker with COPD
Respiratory symptoms	Decreased
Chronic mucus hypersecretion	Decreased
Hospital admissions due to COPD	Similar
Lung function: decline in FEV_1	Decreased
Smoking-related cardiovascular comorbidities	Similar
All-cause mortality	Decreased
Systemic inflammatory biomarkers	Similar
CT emphysema	Increased
Bronchial biopsy changes	
• Eosinophils	Similar
• Neutrophils	Similar
• Mast cells	Similar
• CD8+ T lymphocytes	Similar
• Bronchial epithelial goblet cells	Decreased

* Note: Refer to the main text for information on the published studies used to summarize the effects of smoking status on clinical outcomes and Inflammatory variables in COPD.

largest benefit in lung function. CT measures of emphysema and air trapping are higher in former smokers than in current smokers with COPD with varying degrees of disease severity.[61]

Inflammatory biomarker levels of C-reactive protein, fibrinogen, and leucocyte count are similar in former smokers and current smokers with COPD.[57] Smoking cessation is the only proven intervention that reduces the pathogenic processes leading to COPD.[4] Based on limited published data, airway inflammation in bronchial biopsies appears to persist in former smokers with COPD, except for a reduction in goblet cell hyperplasia and inflammatory biomarker levels in bronchoalveolar lavage and blood are reduced after smoking cessation.[58–62]

7.4 ACTIVE SMOKING AND THE OVERLAP SYNDROME

7.4.1 DEVELOPMENT OF THE OVERLAP SYNDROME

Active and passive cigarette smoke exposure have an important role in the development of the overlap syndrome (Figure 7.1). Chronic airflow obstruction (FEV_1/FVC ratio <0.7) in adults with asthma can develop through different pathways, such as active cigarette smoking, previous severe childhood-onset asthma, or severe adult-onset asthma in never-smokers. Smoking-related COPD is association in some individuals with "asthma-like" inflammatory features, such as eosinophilic/type-2 inflammation or airway hyper-responsiveness. Other risk factors may contribute to the development of chronic airway disease in adulthood, such as early-life events that affect the structure of the airways, environmental exposures in childhood (such as passive smoke),

or environmental exposures in adulthood (such as occupational agents or biomass materials, as well as other variables, such as genotype, atopic status, and drug treatment).

Age of onset of asthma may be an important factor that influences the effect of active cigarette smoking on the development chronic airflow limitation. In the Dunedin Multidisciplinary Health and Development Study, active smoking history and childhood-onset asthma were both associated with reduced FEV_1/FVC ratios at 38 years of age.[63] Of interest, a history of cigarette smoking was not associated with lower FEV_1/FVC ratios in the group with childhood-onset persistent asthma unlike the subgroup with late-onset asthma (after 13 years of age) in whom cumulative smoking history was associated with lower FEV_1/FVC ratios. Approximately one third of participants with childhood-onset asthma had persistent airflow obstruction irrespective of a history of cigarette smoking. In keeping with the finding that active smoking does not increase the risk of persistent airflow obstruction in young adults whose asthma started in childhood, children with persistent asthma recruited to the Melbourne Asthma Cohort who smoked as adults had a similar decline in lung function at 50 years of age as never-smokers with asthma.[64] The Tucson Epidemiological Study of Airway Obstructive Disease[65] and the European Community Respiratory Health Survey (ECRHS)[30] found that cigarette smokers with late-onset asthma had an increased risk of developing persistent airflow obstruction and had a greater decline in lung function compared to smokers with early-onset asthma. The Tasmanian Longitudinal Health Study, which included participants with both early-onset and late-onset asthma, found a synergistic effect on the development of persistent airflow obstruction of smoking, atopy, and current asthma.[31] In people with the overlap syndrome associated with late-onset asthma (after 40 years of age) recruited to the Copenhagen City Heart Study, the decline FEV_1 is greater than in individuals with the overlap syndrome associated with early-onset asthma (before 40 years of age).[66] Taken together, these findings suggest that active cigarette smoking in people with asthma is an important risk factor for the development of chronic airflow obstruction, particularly in those with late-onset asthma.

7.4.2 PREVALENCE OF CIGARETTE SMOKING IN THE OVERLAP SYNDROME

A systematic review of studies of people with the overlap syndrome or smoking-related COPD found no difference in smoking status between the two groups, although the overlap group had a lower pack-year history.[67] In agreement with these findings, the U.S. Behavioral Risk Factor Surveillance System (BRFSS) survey found that smoking status prevalence rates in individuals with the overlap syndrome or COPD were similar (current smokers, 31% and 34% respectively; former smokers, 43% and 46% respectively; never-smokers, 26% and 20% respectively).[68] Smoking status and smoking exposure in the ECLIPSE and COPDGene studies are in agreement with these findings.[69,70] In a Finnish primary health care population of smokers with asthma, but with no previous diagnosis of COPD, a smoking history of more than 20 pack years and age over 60 years were the best predictors of the overlap syndrome.[71]

7.5 PASSIVE SMOKE EXPOSURE AND ASTHMA

Active smokers inhale mainstream cigarette smoke and when they are not inhaling, the smoldering end of the cigarette produces side-stream smoke. Passive smoke consists mainly of side-stream smoke with the addition of smaller amounts of mainstream exhaled smoke. Exposure to passive smoke can be assessed by a variety of methods. Questionnaires can be influenced by recall bias. More objective means of assessing passive smoke exposure include measurement of cotinine, the primary metabolite of nicotine in urine, serum, and saliva; nicotine in hair; or nicotine badges. Exposure to tobacco smoke has been implicated as a risk factor for the development of asthma as well as a factor adversely affecting clinical outcomes and inflammation variables in asthma.

7.5.1 DEVELOPMENT OF ASTHMA

7.5.1.1 Children and adolescents

The 2006 U.S. Surgeon General Report on the Health Consequences of Involuntary Exposure to Tobacco Smoke concluded that the evidence is sufficient to infer a causal relationship between passive smoke exposure from parental smoking and the onset of wheeze illnesses in early childhood, but the evidence although suggestive is not sufficient to infer a causal relationship between parental smoking and the onset of childhood asthma.[3] Maternal smoking increases the risk of asthma among children[72,73] particularly during pregnancy or following early life exposure to tobacco smoke.[74] Exposure to tobacco smoke during the first trimester is reported to be a risk factor for the development of asthma in some,[73] although not in all studies. The increased risk for asthma associated with maternal smoking during pregnancy persists into adolescence independent of the effects on lower lung function, immune function, or allergic sensitization.[75] Paternal smoking is also a risk factor for asthma, although the strength of the effect is less than for maternal smoking.[76] Maternal passive smoke exposure during pregnancy is associated with an increased risk of childhood asthma even if the mother is a nonsmoker during pregnancy.[77] The Norwegian Mother and Child Cohort Study reported that if a grandmother smoked during the mother's pregnancy, the risk of asthma is increased in the grandchild independent of the smoking status of the mother suggesting that *in utero* exposure to cigarette smoke might have a transgenerational effect on the development of asthma.[78]

Several mechanisms are proposed to explain the increased risk of asthma from *in utero* exposure to tobacco smoke including genetic predisposition, for example, genotypes of glutathione S transferases, impaired lung development, bronchial hyperreactivity, impaired *in utero* immune responses, and augmented allergic inflammation. In particular, the nicotine component of tobacco smoke has been implicated as a potentially important mediator inducing adverse effects on lung function *in utero*.[79]

7.5.1.2 Adults

The 2006 U.S. Surgeon General Report considered that the evidence is suggestive but not sufficient to infer a causal relationship between exposure to passive smoke and the development of asthma in adult life.[3] A systematic review performed by the California Environmental Protection Agency, however, concluded that there is sufficient evidence to support a causal relationship between passive exposure and development of asthma in adolescents and adults.[80] In the U.S. Black Women's Health Study, passive smoke exposure increases the risk of adult-onset asthma by 20% among nonsmokers.[5] There is a dose-dependent synergism between passive smoke exposure and family history of asthma for the risk of adult-onset asthma.[81]

7.5.2 PREVALENCE OF EXPOSURE TO PASSIVE SMOKE

The U.S. National Health and Nutrition Examination Survey (NHANES) reported a decrease in passive exposure among children and adolescents with current asthma in the United States from 1988–1994 to 2005–2010, but that many children and adolescents with asthma are still exposed to passive smoke.[82] Serum and salivary cotinine is commonly found among children admitted for asthma and is associated with readmission.[83]

7.5.3 CLINICAL OUTCOMES AND INFLAMMATORY VARIABLES

Children and adults with asthma exposed to tobacco smoke experience worse clinical outcomes (Table 7.4).

7.5.3.1 Children

Children with asthma exposed to passive smoke have increased asthma symptoms, greater frequency of exacerbations, and greater use of reliever medication, as well as more hospital admissions and a higher number of life-threatening attacks.[84,85] (Table 7.4). In the United States, passive smoke exposure is associated with increased risk of adverse outcomes among children with asthma aged 6–11 years and in non-Hispanic white children aged 6–19 years.[86] Exposure to passive smoke is associated with a reduced therapeutic response to inhaled corticosteroids in children with asthma. Smoke-free legislation is associated with reductions in hospital admissions for asthma in children.[87]

7.5.3.2 Adults

The 2006 U.S. Surgeon General Report considered that the available evidence is suggestive but not sufficient to infer a causal effect between exposure to passive smoke and worsening asthma control in adults.[3] The 2006 California Environmental Protection Agency report, however,

Table 7.4 Potential effects of exposure to passive smoke on clinical outcome in children and adults with asthma*

Children
Increased
Symptoms
Exacerbations
Medication use
School absenteeism
Doctor visits
Hospital admissions
Decreased
Response to corticosteroids
Adults
Increased
Exacerbations
Emergency department visits
Hospital admissions
Decreased
Lung function

* Note: Refer to the main text for information on the studies used to summarize the effects of exposure to passive smoke on clinical outcomes in asthma

concluded that passive smoke exposure is causally associated with exacerbations of asthma.[80] Exposure to passive smoke is associated with worse lung function, greater bronchial hyperreactivity, more exacerbations, and increased health care utilization.[88,89]

7.5.3.3 Inflammatory variables

Exposure to passive smoke has been associated with increased total IgE levels in some but not all studies. Parents smoking during childhood is associated with lower exhaled nitric oxide concentration in adults with asthma. Passive smoking impairs histone deacetylase-2 function through the activation of phosphoinositide-3-kinase signaling, which could contribute to corticosteroid insensitivity in children with severe asthma.[90]

7.6 PASSIVE SMOKE EXPOSURE AND COPD

7.6.1 DEVELOPMENT OF COPD

The 2006 U.S. Surgeon General Report considered that the evidence is suggestive but not sufficient to infer a causal relationship between passive smoke exposure in nonsmokers and risk of COPD.[3] An Official American Thoracic Society Public Policy Statement on novel risk factors and the global burden of COPD concluded that there is strong suggestive evidence of a link between exposure to passive smoke and the development of COPD.[45]

7.6.2 EXPOSURE TO PASSIVE SMOKE

People with COPD, including active smokers, have significant exposure to passive smoke. Of participants with COPD recruited to the SPIROMICS cohort, 27% reported exposure to passive smoke in the past week, and 20% reported living with a smoker.[91]

7.6.3 CLINICAL OUTCOMES AND INFLAMMATORY VARIABLES

In nonsmokers with COPD, exposure to passive smoke is associated with poorer health status and an increased risk of exacerbations resulting in hospital-based care.[92] In participants with COPD recruited to SPIROMICS study, nonsmokers who lived with a smoker had worse symptoms, poorer health status, and increased risk for severe exacerbations.[91] Exposure to passive smoke in the past week is associated with worse symptoms of wheeze, chronic mucus hypersecretion, and with increased airway wall thickness on CT, but not emphysema.[91] Interestingly, active smokers with COPD, have worse clinical outcomes associated with exposure to passive smoke.[91]

7.7 CONCLUSIONS

Exposure to active and passive tobacco smoke has a major adverse impact on the health of people with asthma, COPD, and the overlap. The management of the adverse health effects resulting from active and passive exposure to tobacco smoke in people with asthma, COPD, and the overlap involves interventions ranging from public health measures to control exposure, personal advice on smoking cessation and the use of appropriate targeted therapies.

A summary of the main conclusions of the data reviewed in this chapter is as follows:

1. Does exposure to active and passive tobacco smoke cause the development of chronic airway disease?

Active cigarette smoking is a risk factor for the development of asthma in adolescents and adults and is the major risk factor for the development of COPD in developed countries. Smokers with asthma are at risk of developing the overlap syndrome, particularly in those with late-onset asthma. Exposure to passive smoke from parental smoking and by adolescents and adults increases the risk of developing asthma. There is strong suggestive evidence of a link between exposure to passive smoke and the development of COPD.

2. What are the prevalence rates for active and passive tobacco smoke exposure in chronic airway disease?

In most developed countries, around half the adult asthmatic population and most people with COPD are current or former cigarette smokers, and a quarter of children and adults with asthma are exposed to passive smoke. Cigarette smoking rates are similar in the overlap syndrome and smoking-related COPD, although the overlap group have a lower pack- year history.

3. Are clinical outcomes worse in smokers with asthma?

Adults with asthma who smoke have worse clinical outcomes compared to never-smokers with asthma including worse symptoms, poorer asthma related quality of life, increased exacerbations, worse chronic mucus hypersecretion, increased use of health care resources for asthma, reduced sensitivity to inhaled corticosteroids, greater decline in lung function, increased smoking-related comorbidities, and heightened all-cause mortality.

4. Do clinical outcomes differ in current and former smokers with COPD?

Symptomatic smoking-induced airway disease occurs in people with and without spirometric evidence of COPD. Former smokers with COPD compared with current smokers with COPD have less respiratory symptoms, decreased mucus hypersecretion, reduced decline in lung function, and lower all-cause mortality rates, whereas the risk of hospital admission due to COPD, pneumonia, and lung cancer, as well cardiovascular comorbidities, are similar.

5. Does exposure to passive smoke worsen clinical outcomes in asthma and COPD?

Exposure to passive smoke in children with asthma is associated with increased symptoms and more exacerbations and hospital admissions due to asthma. Exposure to passive smoke in adults with asthma is associated with poor symptom control, worse quality of life, lower lung function and greater health care utilization. In nonsmokers with COPD, exposure to passive smoke is associated with poorer health status and an increased risk of exacerbations resulting in hospital-based care.

6. Does smoking status or exposure to passive smoke influence clinical outcomes in the overlap syndrome?

To date, information is lacking on the effects of smoking status or exposure to passive smoke on clinical outcomes and inflammatory variables in different subtypes of the overlap syndrome.

REFERENCES

1. Percentage of People with Asthma Who Smoke: Centers for Disease Control and Prevention; 2016. Available at http://www.cdc.gov/asthma/asthma_stats/people_who_smoke.htm. Accessed October 10, 2016.
2. Homa D, Neff L, King B et al. Vital signs: Disparities in nonsmokers' exposure to secondhand smoke—United States, 1999–2012. *MMWR Morb Mortal Wkly Rep.* 2015;66(4):103–108.
3. The Health Consequences of Involuntary Exposure to Tobacco Smoke: A Report of the Surgeon General. Atlanta, GA: U.S. Department of Health and Human Services, Centers for Disease Control and Prevention, Coordinating Center for Health Promotion, National Center for Chronic Disease Prevention and Health Promotion, Office on Smoking and Health; 2006.
4. The Health Consequences of Smoking: 50 Years of Progress. A Report of the Surgeon General. Atlanta, GA: U.S. Department of Health and Human Services, Centers for Disease Control and Prevention, Coordinating Center for Health Promotion, National Center for Chronic Disease Prevention and Health Promotion, Office on Smoking and Health; 2014.
5. Coogan PF, Castro-Webb N, Yu J et al. Active and passive smoking and the incidence of asthma in the black women's health study. *Am J Resp Crit Care Med.* November 11, 2015, January 1, 2015;191(2):168–176.
6. To T, Stanojevic S, Moores G et al. Global asthma prevalence in adults: Findings from the cross-sectional world health survey. *BMC Public Health.* 2012;12(1):204. doi:10.1186/1471-2458-12-204.
7. Stanton CA, Keith DR, Gaalema DE et al. Trends in tobacco use among US adults with chronic health conditions: National survey on drug use and health 2005–2013. *Prev Med.* 2016;92:160–168.

8. Cerveri I, Cazzoletti L, Corsico A et al. The impact of cigarette smoking on asthma: A population-based international cohort study. *Int Arch Allergy Immunol.* 2012;158:175–183.

9. Hasegawa K, Sullivan AF, Tsugawa Y et al. Comparison of US emergency department acute asthma care quality: 1997–2001 and 2011–2012. *J Allergy Clin Immunol.* 2015;135(1):73–80. e7.

10. Thomson NC, Chaudhuri R, Heaney LG et al. Clinical outcomes and inflammatory biomarkers in current smokers and exsmokers with severe asthma. *J Allergy Clin Immunol.* April 1, 2013;131(4):1008–16. PubMed PMID: S0091–6749(13)00090–0.

11. Murphy VE, Clifton VL, and Gibson PG. The effect of cigarette smoking on asthma control during exacerbations in pregnant women. *Thorax.* August 1, 2010;65:739–744.

12. Çolak Y, Afzal S, Nordestgaard BG et al. Characteristics and prognosis of never-smokers and smokers with asthma in the copenhagen general population study. A prospective cohort study. *Am J Resp Crit Care Med.* July 15, 2015;192(2):172–181.

13. Thomson NC and Chaudhuri R. Asthma in smokers: Challenges and opportunities. *Curr Opin Pulm Med.* 2009;15(1):39–45.

14. Polosa R and Thomson NC. Smoking and asthma: Dangerous liaisons. *Eur Respir J.* March 1, 2013;41(3):716–726.

15. Clatworthy J, Price D, Ryan D et al. The value of self-report assessment of adherence, rhinitis and smoking in relation to asthma control. *Prim Care Resp J.* 2009;18(4):300–305.

16. Eisner MD and Iribarren C. The influence of cigarette smoking on adult asthma outcomes. *Nicotine Tob Res.* 2007;9(1):53–56.

17. Lange P, Parner J, Vestbo J et al. A 15-year follow-up study of ventilatory function in adults with asthma. *N Engl J Med.* October 22, 1998;339(17):1194–1200.

18. Thomson N, Chaudhuri R, Messow CM et al. Chronic cough and sputum production are associated with worse clinical outcomes in stable asthma. *Respir Med.* 2013;107(10):1501–1508.

19. Kauppi P, Kupiainen H, Lindqvist A et al. Long-term smoking increases the need for acute care among asthma patients: A case control study. *BMC Pulm Med.* 2014;14:119.

20. Chalmers GW, Macleod KJ, Little SA et al. Influence of cigarette smoking on inhaled corticosteroid treatment in mild asthma. *Thorax.* 2002;57(3):226–230.

21. Tomlinson JEM, McMahon AD, Chaudhuri R et al. Efficacy of low and high dose inhaled corticosteroid in smokers versus non-smokers with mild asthma. *Thorax.* 2005;60(4):282–287.

22. Chaudhuri R, Livingston E, McMahon AD et al. Cigarette smoking impairs the therapeutic response to oral corticosteroids in chronic asthma. *Am J Respir Crit Care Med.* 2003;168(11):1308–1311.

23. Telenga E, Kerstjens H, ten Hacken N et al. Inflammation and corticosteroid responsiveness in ex-, current- and never-smoking asthmatics. *BMC Pulm Med.* 2013;13(1):58.

24. Pedersen SE, Bateman ED, Bousquet J et al. Determinants of response to fluticasone propionate and salmeterol/fluticasone propionate combination in the Gaining Optimal Asthma control study. *J Allergy Clin Immunol.* 2007;120(5):1036–1042.

25. Dijkstra A, Vonk JM, Jongepier H et al. Lung function decline in asthma: Association with inhaled corticosteroids, smoking and sex. *Thorax.* 2006;61(2):105–110.

26. Lange P, Scharling H, Ulrik CS et al. Inhaled corticosteroids and decline of lung function in community residents with asthma. *Thorax.* 2006;61(2):100–104.

27. O'Byrne PM, Lamm CJ, Busse WW et al. The effects of inhaled budesonide on lung function in smokers and nonsmokers with mild persistent asthma. *Chest.* December 2009;136(6):1514–1520.

28. Jensen E, Dahl R, and Steffensen F. Bronchial reactivity to cigarette smoke; Relation to lung function, respiratory symptoms, serum-immunoglobulin E and blood eosinophil and leukocyte counts. *Respir Med.* 2000;94:119–127.

29. Thomson NC, Chaudhuri R, Spears M et al. Poor symptom control is associated with reduced CT scan segmental airway lumen area in smokers with asthma. *Chest.* 2015;147(3):735–744.

30. Aanerud M, Carsin A-E, Sunyer J et al. Interaction between asthma and smoking increases the risk of adult airway obstruction. *Eur Respir J.* March 1, 2015;45(3):635–643.

31. Perret JL, Dharmage SC, Matheson MC et al. The interplay between the effects of lifetime asthma, smoking, and atopy on fixed airflow obstruction in middle age. *Am J Respir Crit Care Med.* January 1, 2013;187(1):42–48.

32. Prieto L, Palop J, Llusar R et al. Effects of cigarette smoke on methacholine- and AMP-induced air trapping in asthmatics. *J Asthma.* 2015;52(1):26–33.

33. Savage JH, Matsui EC, McCormack M et al. The association between asthma and allergic disease and mortality: 30-year follow-up study. *J Allergy Clin Immunol.* 2014;133(5):1484–1487.

34. Boulet L, FitzGerald J, McIvor R et al. Influence of current or former smoking on asthma management and control. *Can Respir J.* 2008;15 (5):275–279.

35. Kim TB, Jang AS, Kwon HS et al. Identification of asthma clusters in two independent Korean adult asthma cohorts. *Eur Respir J.* June 1, 2013;41(6):1308–1314.

36. Price DB, Rigazio A, Campbell JD et al. Blood eosinophil count and prospective annual asthma disease burden: A UK cohort study. *Lancet Respir Med.* 2015;3(11):849–858.

37. McSharry C, McKay I, Chaudhuri R et al. Short and long-term effects of cigarette smoking independently

influence exhaled nitric oxide concentration in asthma. *J Allergy Clin Immunol.* 2005;116(1):88–93.

38. Thomson NC, Chaudhuri R, Spears M et al. Serum periostin in smokers and never smokers with asthma. *Respir Med.* 2015;109(6):708–715.

39. Demarche S, Schleich F, Henket M et al. Detailed analysis of sputum and systemic inflammation in asthma phenotypes: Are paucigranulocytic asthmatics really non-inflammatory? *BMC Pulm Med.* 2016;16(1):1–13.

40. Chaudhuri R, Livingston E, McMahon AD et al. Effects of smoking cessation on lung function and airway inflammation in smokers with asthma. *Am J Respir Crit Care Med.* 2006;174(2):127–133.

41. Broekema M, ten Hacken NHT, Volbeda F et al. Airway epithelial changes in smokers but not in ex-smokers with asthma. *Am J Respir Crit Care Med.* December 15, 2009;180(12):1170–1178.

42. Ravensberg AJ, Slats AM, van Wetering S et al. CD8+ T cells characterize early smoking-related airway pathology in patients with asthma. *Respir Med.* July 1, 2013;107(7):959–966.

43. St-Laurent J, Bergeron C, Pagé N et al. Influence of smoking on airway inflammation and remodelling in asthma. *Clin Exp Allergy.* 2008;38(10):1582–1589.

44. Global Strategy For The Diagnosis, Management and Prevention of Chronic Obstructive Pulmonary Disease; 2016. Available at http://www.goldcopd.org. Accessed October 10, 2016.

45. Eisner MD, Anthonisen N, Coultas D et al. An official American thoracic society public policy statement: Novel risk factors and the global burden of chronic obstructive pulmonary disease. *Am J Respir Crit Care Med.* 2010;182(5):693–718.

46. Çolak Y, Afzal S, Nordestgaard BG et al. Majority of never-smokers with airflow limitation do not have asthma: The copenhagen general population study. *Thorax.* 2016;71(7):614–623.

47. Forey BA, Thornton AJ, and Lee PN. Systematic review with meta-analysis of the epidemiological evidence relating smoking to COPD, chronic bronchitis and emphysema. *BMC Pulm Med.* 2011;11:36.

48. Agusti A, Edwards LD, Celli B et al. Characteristics, stability and outcomes of the 2011 GOLD COPD groups in the ECLIPSE cohort. *Eur Respir J.* 2013;42(3):636–646.

49. Han MK, Muellerova H, Curran-Everett D et al. GOLD 2011 disease severity classification in COPDGene: A prospective cohort study. *Lancet Respir Med.* March 1, 2013;1(1):43–50.

50. Vestbo Jr, Edwards LD, Scanlon PD et al. Changes in forced expiratory volume in 1 second over time in copd. *N Engl J Med.* 2011;365(13):1184–1192.

51. Chen W, Thomas J, Sadatsafavi M et al. Risk of cardiovascular comorbidity in patients with chronic obstructive pulmonary disease: A systematic

review and meta-analysis. *Lancet Respir Med.* 2015;3(8):631–639.

52. Kim V, Zhao H, Boriek AM et al. Persistent and newly developed chronic bronchitis are associated with worse outcomes in chronic obstructive pulmonary disease. *Ann Am Thorac Soc.* 2016;13(7):1016–1025.

53. Woodruff PG, Barr RG, Bleecker E et al. Clinical significance of symptoms in smokers with preserved pulmonary function. *New Engl J Med.* 2016;374(19):1811–1821.

54. Regan EA, Lynch DA, Curran-Everett D et al. Clinical and radiologic disease in smokers with normal spirometry. *JAMA Intern Med.* 2015;175(9):1539–1549.

55. Faner R, Tal-Singer R, Riley JH et al. Lessons from ECLIPSE: A review of COPD biomarkers. *Thorax.* 2014;69(7):666–672.

56. Sin DD, Hollander Z, DeMarco ML et al. Biomarker development for chronic obstructive pulmonary disease from discovery to clinical implementation. *Am J Resp Crit Care Med.* 2015;192(10):1162–1170.

57. Thomsen M, Nordestgaard BG, Vestbo J et al. Characteristics and outcomes of chronic obstructive pulmonary disease in never smokers in Denmark: A prospective population study. *Lancet Respir Med.* September 1, 2013;1(7):543–550.

58. Willemse BWM, Postma DS, Timens W et al. The impact of smoking cessation on respiratory symptoms, lung function, airway hyperresponsiveness and inflammation. *Eur Respir J.* 2004;23(3):464–476.

59. Lange P and Vestbo J. Chronic mucus hypersecretion and the natural history of chronic obstructive pulmonary disease. *Am J Respir Crit Care Med.* 2016;193(6):602–603.

60. Allinson JP, Hardy R, Donaldson GC et al. The presence of chronic mucus hypersecretion across adult life in relation to chronic obstructive pulmonary disease development. *Am J Respir Crit Care Med.* 2016;193(6):662–672.

61. Zach JA, Williams A, Jou SS et al. Current smoking status is associated with lower quantitative ct measures of emphysema and gas trapping. *J Thorac Imaging.* 2016;31(1):29–36.

62. Gamble E, Grootendorst DC, Hattotuwa K et al. Airway mucosal inflammation in COPD is similar in smokers and ex-smokers: A pooled analysis. *Eur Respir J.* 2007;30(3):467–471.

63. Hancox RJ, Gray AR, Poulton R et al. The effect of cigarette smoking on lung function in young adults with asthma. *Am J Resp Crit Care Med.* 2016;94(3):276–284.

64. Tai A, Tran H, Roberts M et al. The association between childhood asthma and adult chronic obstructive pulmonary disease. *Thorax.* 2014;69(9):805–810.

65. Guerra S, Sherrill DL, Kurzius-Spencer M et al. The course of persistent airflow limitation in subjects with and without asthma. *Respir Med.* 2008;102(10):1473–1482.

66. Lange P, Çolak Y, Ingebrigtsen TS et al. Long-term prognosis of asthma, chronic obstructive pulmonary disease, and asthma-chronic obstructive pulmonary disease overlap in the Copenhagen City Heart study: A prospective population-based analysis. *Lancet Respir Med.* 2016;4(6):454–462.

67. Alshabanat A, Zafari Z, Albanyan O et al. Asthma and COPD overlap syndrome (ACOS): A systematic review and meta analysis. *PLOS ONE.* 2015;10(9):e0136065.

68. Kumbhare S, Pleasants R, Ohar JA et al. Characteristics and prevalence of asthma/chronic obstructive pulmonary disease overlap in the United States. *Ann Am Thorac Soc.* 2016;13(6):803–810.

69. Hardin M, Silverman E, Barr RG et al. The clinical features of the overlap between COPD and asthma. *Respir Res.* 2011;12(1):127.

70. Wurst KE, Rheault TR, Edwards L et al. A comparison of COPD patients with and without ACOS in the ECLIPSE study. *Eur Respir J.* 2016;47:1559–1562.

71. Kiljander T, Helin T, Venho K et al. Prevalence of asthma–COPD overlap syndrome among primary care asthmatics with a smoking history: A cross-sectional study. *NPJ Prim Care Respir Med.* 2015;16(25):15047.

72. Burke H, Leonardi-Bee J, Hashim A et al. Prenatal and passive smoke exposure and incidence of asthma and wheeze: Systematic review and meta-analysis. *Pediatrics.* 2012;129(4):735–744.

73. Neuman Å, Hohmann C, Orsini N et al. Maternal smoking in pregnancy and asthma in pre-school children. *Am J Resp Crit Care Med.* 2012;186(10):1037–1043.

74. den Dekker HT, Sonnenschein-van der Voort AMM, de Jongste JC et al. Tobacco smoke exposure, airway resistance, and asthma in school-age children: The generation r study. *Chest.* 2015;148(3):607–617.

75. Hollams EM, de Klerk NH, Holt PG et al. Persistent effects of maternal smoking during pregnancy on lung function and asthma in adolescents. *Am J Resp Crit Care Med.* 2014;189(4):401–407.

76. Mitchell EA, Beasley R, Keil U et al. The association between tobacco and the risk of asthma, rhinoconjunctivitis and eczema in children and adolescents: Analyses from Phase Three of the ISAAC programme. *Thorax.* 2012;67(11):941–949.

77. Vardavas CI, Hohmann C, Patelarou E et al. The independent role of prenatal and postnatal exposure to active and passive smoking on the development of early wheeze in children. *Eur Respir J.* 2016;48(7):115–1124.

78. Magnus MC, Håberg SE, Karlstad Ø et al. Grandmother's smoking when pregnant with the mother and asthma in the grandchild: The norwegian mother and child cohort study. *Thorax.* 2015;70(3):237–243.

79. Spindel ER and McEvoy CT. The role of nicotine in the effects of maternal smoking during pregnancy on lung development and childhood respiratory disease. implications for dangers of E-cigarettes. *Am J Resp Crit Care Med.* 2016;193(5):486–494.

80. Proposed Identification of Environmental Tobacco Smoke as Toxic Air Contaminant. Part B: Health Effects; 2006. Available at https://www.arb.ca.gov /regact/ets2006/app3partb.pdf. Accessed October 10, 2016.

81. Lajunen TK, Jaakkola JJK, and Jaakkola MS. The synergistic effect of heredity and exposure to second-hand smoke on adult-onset asthma. *Am J Resp Crit Care Med.* 2013;188(7):776–782.

82. Kit BK, Simon AE, Brody DJ et al. US Prevalence and trends in tobacco smoke exposure among children and adolescents with asthma. *Pediatrics.* 2013;131(3):407–414.

83. Howrylak JA, Spanier AJ, Huang B et al. Cotinine in children admitted for asthma and readmission. *Pediatrics.* 2014;133(2):e355–e362.

84. Cook D and Strachan D. Summary of effects of parental smoking on the respiratory health of children and implications for research. *Thorax.* 1999;54:357–366.

85. Jin Y, Seiber EE, and Ferketich AK. Secondhand smoke and asthma: What are the effects on healthcare utilization among children? *Prev Med.* 2013;57(2):125–128.

86. Akinbami LJ, Kit BK, and Simon AE. Impact of environmental tobacco smoke on children with asthma, united states, 2003–2010. *Acad Pediatr.* 2013;13(6):508–516.

87. Been JV, Nurmatov UB, Cox B et al. Effect of smoke-free legislation on perinatal and child health: A systematic review and meta-analysis. *Lancet.* May 3, 2014;383(9928):1549–1560.

88. Eisner MD, Klein J, Hammond SK et al. Directly measured second hand smoke exposure and asthma health outcomes. *Thorax.* 2005;60(10):814–821.

89. Comhair SAA, Gaston BM, Ricci KS et al. Detrimental effects of environmental tobacco smoke in relation to asthma severity. *PLOS ONE.* 2011;6(5):e18574.

90. Kobayashi Y, Bossley C, Gupta A et al. Passive smoking impairs histone deacetylase-2 in children with severe asthma. *Chest.* 2014;145(2):305–312.

91. Putcha N, Barr RG, Han MK et al. Understanding the impact of second-hand smoke exposure on clinical outcomes in participants with COPD in the SPIROMICS cohort. *Thorax.* 2016;71(5):411–420.

92. Eisner MD, Iribarren C, Yelin EH et al. The impact of SHS exposure on health status and exacerbations among patients with COPD. *Inter J COPD.* 2009;4:169–176.

Indoor and outdoor pollutants and allergens

CHARLES S. BARNES

8.1 INTRODUCTION

Pollution is a normal result of human activity. It is the unwanted introduction of something into the environment that causes harm. In a comparative risk assessment of the global burden of disease, both ambient air pollution and indoor air pollution were among the most significant factors. They ranked alongside factors such as childhood malnutrition, tobacco smoke, and alcohol consumption in global disability adjusted life years reduced.[1] Throughout the history of humans, exposure to pollution has been constant and pervasive. Just to list the names of documented pollution events that have dramatically impacted human health would not be possible in the space allowed. Since the formation of the U.S. Environmental Protection Agency (EPA) in 1970, there have been continuing efforts to monitor and improve air quality throughout the United States. But, there is probably no absolutely safe level of air pollution.[2,3] The interests of health are constantly colliding with the interests of economic development, which further confound issues related to air quality. Regardless of one's perspective, having an essential understanding of the impact of environmental determinants on respiratory conditions such as asthma and COPD is necessary for effective management of these patients.

CLINICAL VIGNETTE 8.1

Because indoor air quality cases are unique and tend to make local news reports, this vignette is necessarily fictitious based on several similar published reports.[4–7]

A 25-year-old female (AB) presents with episodic epistaxis. The occurrence seems to be more frequent on Thursdays and Fridays. She is concerned that there might be some relation to her immunotherapy. AB has been seen by you previously for seasonal allergic rhinitis and has been on allergy shots for ragweed allergy for 16 months. You are aware that AB is a schoolteacher. Upon questioning concerning her environment, you find that she has just moved into a new classroom with carpeted floors and walls to reduce classroom noise. The room has also been decorated for the start of school by the school's Parent Teacher Organization. Upon further questioning, AB relates that some of her students have also had episodes of nosebleeds. You and AB approach her principal concerning the epistaxis episodes, and an air-quality assessment is conducted. The mean indoor formaldehyde level was 0.125 +/− 0.05 ppm, with a minimum of 0.06 ppm and a maximum of 0.25 ppm.

8.2 AIR POLLUTION BACKGROUND

Particulate matter exposure in the form of smoke from fires used for cooking and heating was ubiquitous for ancient man and still a major issue for many underdeveloped regions in the world that use solid fuels for cooking and heating in inadequately ventilated homes.[8–10,11] As cities formed and societies developed the sewage pollution related to crowding, the toxic pollution related to early manufacturing impacted those societies.[12] When the industrial revolution took hold in recent centuries,[13] the air pollution problem expanded to an industrial scale. Overpopulation has restricted the ability to just move away from a polluted area to a cleaner environment. As a result, many regions around the world have been significantly impacted by the long-lasting effects of humanmade pollution. For example, the great forests of the ancient Middle East are essentially gone,[14] and the forests of Britain have been destroyed for shipbuilding and fuel needs.[15] Air pollution is an especially notable human activity because it spreads rapidly and can be difficult to detect and avoid. It is now to the point where humanmade pollution threatens to produce irreversible environmental and climatic changes to our planet.[16,17]

The health effects of the industrial revolution in Europe were most noticeable by physicians in London. In fact, the *Medical Times and Gazette* wrote "The genuine London fog which wrapped the metropolis in *thick darkness* on Saturday may be considered from very different stand-points. Some look upon it as a curiosity,...—but the Medical man knows it to be a terrible scourge, and to many a patient it makes all the difference between life and death. Very many of us could, we doubt not, give instances of phthisis and bronchitis hurried to a fatal close by those hours of fog."[18] One of the earliest studies that evaluated the possible association between air pollution and mortality was related to the Mosa Valley in Belgium. In 1930 the city of Donora along the Meuse River in a heavily industrialized area experienced a toxic killer fog where 60 deaths were documented.[19] One of the best known incidents of a killer fog episode was in London (1952). Over a four-day period, the number of deaths registered in London more than doubled the daily registered deaths for those days in preceding years.[20]

Since those early days of blackened skies and yellow fogs, governmental efforts to reduce and control air pollution have frequently been successful. In one study conducted over a 20-year period in a pollution-prone area of California, it appears that the health related effects of pollution are improving with efforts to improve air quality. In this longitudinal study of 4602 children (age range of 5–18 years) conducted in separate cohorts from 1993 to 2012, investigators estimated the association of changes in pollution levels with bronchitic symptoms. Findings demonstrated that reductions in levels of ambient air pollution over the past 20 years were associated with reductions in symptoms in children with and without asthma, which were proportionally greater in children with asthma.[21] However, it is possible that the more subtle health effects of air pollution are yet to be understood. One of the most prominent efforts to monitor and improve air quality is the ozone monitoring and reporting system for air quality that is active in many U.S. cities. This color-coded system (Figure 8.1) provides daily air quality indices (AQI), and a historical report of these air quality levels provides outdoor pollution trends for most U.S. cities (https://www3.epa.gov/airdata/ad_rep_aqi.html). This information has been vital for implementing air quality interventions, and, as a result, in many U.S. cities this has resulted in vastly improved air quality over the past 50 years.

Individuals susceptible to the respiratory health effects of air pollution need to avoid being outdoors when the AQI is high. Although ozone is essential to protecting life by lining the upper atmosphere, it can have dramatic health impact when increased in the lower atmosphere. Pollutants can come in the form of gasses, toxic liquids, heavy metals, microbial sewage, heat, light, and noise. The big four outdoor airborne pollutants are particulate matter (PM), ozone (O_3), nitrogen dioxide (NO_2), and sulfur dioxide (SO_2). If these outdoor pollutants diffuse into the indoor ambient airspace, they become major indoor air pollutants. The relationship of indoor pollutants to outdoor pollutants is not well studied, likely because there remain significant gaps in our understanding of the health effects of outdoor air pollutants. Progress is being made in our understanding related to the direct health effects of outdoor air pollutants and aeroallergens, as well as the synergistic impact of these environmental determinants in combination. Air pollution has been directly associated with causing increased bronchial hyperresponsiveness, increased airway inflammation, decreased lung function, increased hospitalizations, and emergency room visits. Air pollution has also been demonstrated to enhance airway inflammation induced by allergen exposure and priming the lower airways to elicit allergic responses. High air pollution exposure has also been found to be an independent risk factor for wheezing during infancy and early childhood.[22-24]

8.3 COMMON AIR POLLUTANTS

Our understanding of the complex interactions of the major constituents that make up the air pollution mixture has improved over the past 50 years. The atmospheric concentration of NO_2 gas associated with high-compression automobiles of the 1960s has decreased. However, even low-polluting internal combustion engines produce some nitrogen dioxides, and these combustion processes are also associated with other primary pollutants, including particles and volatile organic compounds (VOCs) that are either not fully consumed in the combustion process, dumped into the atmosphere by evaporation, or just expelled when

Air Quality Index	Who Needs to Be Concerned?	What Should I Do?
Good (0–50)	It is a great day to be active outside.	
Moderate (51–100)	Some people who may be unusually sensitive to ozone.	Unusually sensitive people: *Consider reducing* prolonged or heavy outdoor exertion. Watch for symptoms such as coughing or shortness of breath. These are signs to take it easier. Everyone else: It is a good day to be active outside.
Unhealthy for Sensitive Groups (101–150)	Sensitive groups include people with lung disease such as asthma, older adults, children, and teenagers, and people who are active outdoors.	Sensitive groups: *Reduce* prolonged or heavy outdoor exertion. Take more breaks, do less intense activities. Watch for symptoms such as coughing or shortness of breath. Schedule outdoor activities in the morning when ozone is lower. People with asthma should follow their asthma action plans and keep quick-relief medicine handy. Everyone else: Maintain their normal activities without harm.
Unhealthy (151–200)	Everyone	Sensitive groups: *Avoid* prolonged or heavy outdoor exertion. Schedule outdoor activities in the morning when ozone is lower. Consider moving activities indoors. People with asthma, keep quick-relief medicine handy. Everyone else: *Reduce* prolonged or heavy outdoor exertion. Take more breaks, do fewer intense activities. Schedule outdoor activities in the morning when ozone is lower.
Very Unhealthy (201–300)	Everyone	Sensitive groups: *Avoid all* physical activity outdoors. Move activities indoors or reschedule to a time when air quality is better. People with asthma, keep quick-relief medicine handy. Everyone else: *Avoid* prolonged or heavy outdoor exertion. Schedule outdoor activities in the morning when ozone is lower. Consider moving activities indoors.
Hazardous (301–500)	Everyone	Everyone: *Avoid all* physical activity outdoors.

Figure 8.1 U.S. EPA Air Quality Guide for Ozone

an empty gas tank is filled. After reacting with other airborne gasses under the influence of UV light on sunny days, nitrogen combustion products exist as an array of oxidized compounds generally referred to as NOX. NOX compounds are toxic and typically coexist with ozone and other oxidizing agents. Since NO_2 can be measured relatively easily, its measurement is often used as a surrogate indication of how much of this toxic group of gases is in the air.

NO_2 guidelines recommend that the annual mean levels be kept below 40 $\mu g/m^3$ and that any one-hour mean be maintained below 200 $\mu g/m^3$. Since these levels are set to reduce NOX exposure as well as ozone and particulate matter, values are set lower than they would be to reduce direct toxic effects. Epidemiological studies have indicated that asthmatic symptoms and lung function growth in children is linked to increases in NO_2 concentration.[21,25] Recent indoor studies have reported symptoms in infants associated with NO_2 concentrations below the recommended level of 40 $\mu g/m^3$. This observation must take into consideration the impact of coexposures to PM and other indoor pollutants, such as organic carbon and nitrous acid vapor.

In the presence of sunlight pollutants, NOX, and VOCs, ozone is formed by photochemical reactions. This is an equilibrium process as ozone is also consumed by reactions with NO_2. Ozone is an air toxin that exists in the atmosphere in equilibrium with various other toxic photochemical oxidants arising through several sources. These include substances as peroxyacyl nitrates, nitric acid, and hydrogen peroxide. Whereas ozone is beneficial in the upper atmosphere, in the breathable atmosphere it is harmful.

Measures to control these tropospheric ozone levels focus on controllable pollutant gasses like NOX and transportation-related VOCs. Hemispheric background concentrations of tropospheric ozone vary with uncontrollable factors like temperature and naturally occurring VOCs from plants and sunlight. Ozone concentrations are not considered to be high until they exceed an eight-hour average level of 80 $\mu g/m^3$. Of concern is that many communities in the United States fail to meet mandated ozone levels on a regular basis (Figure 8.1).

Sulfur dioxide guidelines recommend that SO2 be maintained below 20 $\mu g/m^3$ for a 24-hour mean and below 500 $\mu g/m^3$ for any 10-minute mean exposure. Short-term exposures from localized sources can be especially detrimental to breathing. Long-term exposure levels are based on epidemiological studies that rely on multipollutant exposure.[26] Studies from Hong Kong,[27] where they achieved strong SO2 reductions related to rapid reduction in the sulfur content of fuels, demonstrated substantial improvements in childhood respiratory disease and mortality for all age groups. However, elevated SO2 also exists in association with particulate matter and other pollutants. This makes it difficult to ascertain whether the impact on respiratory health is related to SO2, NOX, fine particulates, or the combination of these air pollutants.

Particulate matter is increasingly recognized as the most devastating airborne pollutant. A World Health Organization (WHO) burden of disease assessment attributes more than 4.3 million premature deaths each year to outdoor and indoor particulate pollution (http://www.who.int/mediacentre/factsheets/fs292/en/). In the United States, most routine air quality particulate monitoring measures coarse particles (between 2.5 and 10 μm) and fine particles (less than 2.5 μm). The allowed U.S. daily average for PM10 in a 24-hour period is 150 $\mu g/m^3$, and for PM2.5, it is 35 $\mu g/m^3$ (http://www.baaqmd.gov/research-and-data/air-quality-standards-and-attainment-status). Most particulate monitoring is conducted in metropolitan areas. If airborne PM values exceed allowable limits more than one day a year, then the region does not meet air quality standards and must implement some remediation activities. In the United States, due to geographical, industrial, and population factors, about 100 urban areas mostly on the East and West Coasts fail to maintain the desired air quality every year. Although governments set air quality levels for particulates, there is probably no truly safe level of airborne particulate exposure. In a European epidemiology study of 312,944 people in nine countries, for every increase of 10 $\mu g/m^3$ in PM10, the lung cancer rate rose 22%, and for the smaller PM2.5, cancer rates increased 36% for every 10 $\mu g/m^3$.[28] From a government perspective, setting and enforcing PM levels is mostly a matter of economic considerations, weighing the cost of industrial activity with the health consequences in the general population. This is in contrast for physicians, who are primarily concerned with the health of their patients.

Diesel exhaust particles (DEP) are a major component of airborne particulates, and they are the largest single source of airborne PM. Diesel engines are much dirtier than gasoline engines, emitting up to 100 times more PM. DEP are very complex consisting of a carbon core with a surface coated with chemicals and metals. Much of the health effects associated with DEP are due to chemicals absorbed onto the carbon core surface. Increased DEP levels have been linked to cardiopulmonary mortality.[29] There is an association between DEP levels and cough, bronchitis, asthma, and COPD. Healthy volunteers exposed to 300 $\mu g/m^3$ of DEP for 1 hour were found to have increased immune reactive cells in sputum and increased IL-6, IL-8, and growth-related oncogene levels. Similar studies in patients with mild asthma show increased methacholine-induced airway hyperresponsiveness and airway resistance.[30] Similar to other pollutants, DEP exposure does not occur alone but as part of a complex mixture of airborne pollutants. This makes it very difficult to determine the relative health effect contributions of each pollutant source.

8.4 HEALTH EFFECTS

The primary concern with air pollutants is their resultant health effects. In recent years, there has been increased concern with particulate pollution in urban areas. There is a plethora of studies that have related air pollution to respiratory health. A PubMed search linking the two topics results in more than 12,000 references. In many studies, particulate matter < 2.5 μm in diameter (PM2.5), and associated traffic-related air pollutant concentrations have been linked with cardiovascular risk. Numerous studies document an association between PM 10 levels and ER visits for asthma.[31] In a Seattle study, an increase of 11 $\mu g/m^3$ in fine PM was associated with an 11% increase in asthma ER visits.[32] Ozone and SO2 have been associated with ER visits for asthma in Mexico.[33] One recent study examined the joint associations between particulate air pollution, ambient temperature, and respiratory morbidity. Using data from 50,356 adult Asthma call-back survey respondents and estimates of daily averages of PM2.5 and maximum air temperature, they found that for adults with active asthma, a 14-day average PM2.5 ≥ 7.07 $\mu g.m^3$ was associated with an estimated 4%–5% higher asthma symptom prevalence. The results of this study suggest that each unit increase in PM2.5 may be associated with an increase in the prevalence of asthma symptoms, even at levels normally encountered in many community settings.[34]

Other studies have related air pollution to its impacts on the immune system. Fine particulate matter is emerging as a factor in glucose dysregulation. In a recently reported study of particulate air pollution and fasting blood glucose in nondiabetic individuals,[35] authors investigated whether PM2.5 is associated with increase in fasting blood glucose and explored possible epigenetic roles. Fasting blood glucose levels and DNA methylation of four inflammatory genes (IFN-γ, IL-6, ICAM-1, and TLR-2) was measured sequentially up to four times over 10 years in 551 nondiabetic subjects. PM2.5 levels at each participant's address was evaluated prior to each measurement using a validated hybrid land-use regression/satellite-based model. Of note, increase in PM2.5 was associated with a significant increase in fasting blood glucose. Further analysis indicated that part of this association was mediated by ICAM-1 promoter methylation.

8.5 AEROALLERGENS AS POLLUTANTS

Allergen exposure that occurs indoors and outdoors is an integral component of the overall air pollution problem. Pollen grains released from plants and spores released from fungal colonies both provide a small but noticeable contribution to coarse airborne particulate levels. The most noticeable contribution is in the >30 micron range. On a clear day, typical nonpollen-related particulates in the air measured by light scattering range between 100 and 1000 particles per m^3. During certain seasons the airborne pollen grain levels will increase to 5000 per m^3. Thus during certain times of the year, pollen grains can comprise over half of the total large airborne particulates. However, when total particles smaller than 30 microns are considered, light scattering results of outdoor air rarely yields counts below 1 million and levels of 30 million particles per m^3 are common. On this background of millions of particles, total airborne spore counts of 10,000 cannot be statistically detected. In addition, light-scattering methods cannot distinguish between pollen grains and moisture droplets, which is one reason airborne particulate levels are reported in gravimetric units (milligrams per m^3) and not in particles.

It is now well accepted that under certain conditions pollen grains like grass can rupture and disburse hundreds of small amorphous granules into the air. Each of these granules is coated with grass allergen proteins, which have the ability to reach deep into the airways.[36] The contribution of these micron-sized aeroallergen particles to the overall particulate burden is unknown, but are believed to be substantial.[37] In the indoor environment where total small particles can be more closely controlled, a spore release of 50,000 per m^3 of air can contribute to a significant portion of the overall particulate level.[38] However, except for smoke particulate exposure related to indoor cooking fires, the relationship between indoor airborne particulate levels and respiratory disease has been poorly investigated.

8.6 OUTDOOR POLLEN, SPORES, AND HAY FEVER

Outdoor ambient pollen levels are probably the environmental determinants most frequently associated with respiratory disease. The term "hay fever" was coined initially in relation to the seasonal production of grass pollen.[39]

Numerous studies have linked hospital admissions, emergency room visits, and unscheduled medical appointments with annual pollen peak levels for various pollen types. In the Bronx, New York City, where population density is high and tree pollen exposure comes from local parks and green spaces, tree pollen counts significantly correlated with total asthma related emergency room visits (rho = 0.3639, $p < 0.001$), and pediatric (rho = 0.33, $p < 0.001$) and adult asthma related emergency room visits (rho = 0.28, $p < 0.001$). Asthma-related hospitalizations positively correlated with tree pollen counts (rho = 0.2389, $p < 0.001$).[40] Another group of investigators from New York using the same aerobiological data, collected through the auspices of the New York Department of Health, pharmacy records for allergy medication use as well as ED visits from 58 area hospitals. They found that midspring pollen counts (maple, birch, beech, ash, oak, and sycamore/London planetree) showed the strongest significant associations with medication sales and ER visits. The reported associations were strongest in children ages 5–17. The investigators concluded that tree pollen peaking in midspring, has a substantive impact on allergy and asthma exacerbations, particularly in children.[41]

An often-cited example of increased respiratory disease related to short-term increases in aeroallergens is thunderstorm asthma. Examples have been documented in England in 1994 when a thunderstorm over southern and castern England produced a 10-fold increase in acute asthma attacks documented in emergency departments.[42] Similarly, in Australia where one severe but brief asthma epidemic occurred, the onset coincided with a thunderstorm outflow and a 4–12-fold increase in airborne grass pollen concentration.[43] In a geographically larger study of the relationship of airborne allergens and respiratory disease covering 11 large cities in Canada, the effects of aeroallergens on hospitalization for asthma was examined in relationship to high and low air pollution days. The relative risk of admission for a given increase in tree pollen levels was greater with higher PM2.5 levels. Therefore, the association between aeroallergens and hospitalizations for asthma was enhanced on days with higher air pollution.[44] More recently airborne grass pollen levels have been linked with seasonal increases of other allergic diseases like eosinophilic esophagitis (EoE).[45]

Outdoor fungi are also an important component of airborne PM, especially from their aeroallergen content. In a Japanese study investigating the association between outdoor fungi and pulmonary function in children with and without asthma, morning peak expiratory flow (PEF) rates were measured daily for 339 schoolchildren during the winter of 2015. They reported an increase in the airborne fungal concentration, measured as colony forming units (CFUs), led to decreased spirometry measurements in all children but to a greater degree in children with asthma.[46] Although spores alone are important aeroallergens, they are typically considered in conjunction with airborne pollen as a total natural exposure. In one recent study of outdoor aeroallergens and their link with disease morbidity over several years, researchers examined aeroallergen counts and health insurance data-sets between 2005 and 2011. The relative risk of buying allergy medications increased with increasing aeroallergen levels of grasses and trees.[47] In a large study of air-borne pollen concentrations and emergency room visits for myocardial infarction (MI) in Ontario, Canada, 17,960 cases of MI were studied between the months of April and October 2004–2011. The risk of MI was 5.5% higher (95% confidence interval [CI]: 3.4, 7.6) on days with the highest tertile of total pollen concentrations compared with days with the lowest tertile, and a significant concentration-response trend was observed ($P < 0.001$).[48]

Synergy between air pollution and allergens has been increasingly investigated. It is logical to assume that lungs irritated by traditional air pollution would be more suscep-tible to sensitization by aeroallergens, and vice versa, air-ways sensitized by aeroallergen exposure would be much more likely to become symptomatic when exposed to irri-tating triggers like ozone and nitrogen oxides. Evidence supporting this relationship is that urbanized people in industrialized countries are more affected by allergic respi-ratory diseases than those living in rural areas.[49] For exam-ple, Austrian farm children were reported to have less hay fever and allergic sensitization than urban children.[50] In another example, a study of Amish and Hutterite popula-tions in the United States whose farming practices are dis-tinct shows striking disparities in the prevalence of asthma. Studies in humans and mice indicate the Amish who eschew industrialized farming practices have a degree of environ-mental protection against asthma related to innate immune response.[51] In another crop-related example, analysis of the circumstances related to repeated outbreaks of asthma epi-sodes in Barcelona, Spain, identified soybean dust gener-ated by unloading ships as the etiological agent. Airborne soybean allergen levels depended upon weather conditions, including wind speed and direction, altitude, and vertical turbulence of the air-mixing layer.[52] When pollutant and allergen exposures are combined, there is the possibility for an enhanced IgE-mediated response to aeroallergens, as well as enhanced airway inflammation accounting for more severe allergic rhinitis and asthma. When nanoscale particulates and chemicals adsorbed to their surfaces attach to plant-derived pollen grains, the allergenic potential of the pollen can be enhanced. Through airway inflamma-tion associated with aeroallergen exposure, airway per-meability is increased resulting in enhanced pollutant exposure.[53] Likewise, pollutants can serve to prime the air-ways to respond to aeroallergens as has been demonstrated in animal models sensitized to ragweed pollen.[54] The actual change on allergen protein structure and immunogenicity induced by high concentrations of air pollutants is begin-ning to be investigated. There is evidence that nitrogen oxides can impact the structure and immunogenicity of the major birch pollen,[55] and that high environmental ozone levels can induce enhanced allergenicity of birch pollen.[56]

Genetic variation and epigenetic changes are mechanisms whereby early life air pollution exposures might influence adult phenotypes. As discussed, exposure to ambient air pollutants is known to increase cardiovascular disease risk in adults. More recently it has been demonstrated that pre-natal exposure to NO2 in the third trimester of pregnancy was associated with higher systolic BP in 11-year-old chil-dren, and that prenatal exposure to multiple air pollut-ants in the first trimester was associated with altered DNA methylation in Long Interspersed Nuclear Elements. These epigenetic alterations could have long-term consequences not only in cardiovascular development but also in immune system development.[57] Recent studies related to epigenetic markers have demonstrated a significant interaction effect relating global DNA methylation levels, asthma severity, race/ethnicity, and socioeconomic status.[58]

8.7 CLIMATE CHANGE

It is impossible to separate air pollution from climate change. Indeed as an overwhelming preponderance of scientific evi-dence indicates, humanmade pollution of greenhouse gas-ses and black carbon particulates are the primary factors responsible for observed and expected climate change.[59] One of the best analogies for the inevitability of climate change is comparing the earth's atmosphere to the "village green" scenario. Instead of grass disappearing because of overgrazing of this public resource, the atmosphere is fill-ing up with carbon dioxide because of excessive public use of fossil fuels for energy. Many studies have been published regarding the interrelationship between climate change and pollution[60] and the effect climate change has already had[61] and is expected to have on aeroallergens.[17] However, the impact of increased climate warming and the results of attempts to cope with this warming has the potential to produce serious consequences. As the outdoor environment becomes hotter and more polluted, humans are likely to retreat indoors to artificially cleaned and cooled air. This increased reliance on air-conditioned spaces will produce an increased demand for the energy necessary to produce indoor clean air. Thus, a vicious cycle to produce energy from readily available easy sources such as oil and coal will result in increased outdoor air pollution, further contribut-ing to climate warming.

8.8 INDOOR AIR POLLUTANTS AND ALLERGENS

The EPA and its Science Advisory Board have ranked indoor air pollution among the top five environmental risks to pub-lic health.[62,63] The contribution to pollution-related respira-tory disease made by the protein allergens associated with dust mites, animals, and mold is well appreciated. Airborne particles in the home include biological particles contain-ing bacteria, mold fragments and spores, a small amount of pollen from the outdoors, cat and dog dander, dust mite/cockroach body parts and droppings, and human skin scales. Other particles come from cigarette smoke, burned food, aerosols like hair spray, and deodorizers and particles from hobby or home workshops. The most carefully controlled studies of indoor allergens as air pollutants are in animal facilities. Subjects exposed to laboratory animals are reported to be at a heightened risk of developing asthma and other allergic diseases. Several studies have reported the prevalence of allergic diseases in laboratory animal workers, and that the routine use of preventive measures can mitigate these problems.[64-66]

The typical method for reducing indoor pollution is to dilute it with outdoor fresh air. When increased energy costs during the late 1970s led the American Society of Heating, Refrigeration and Air Conditioning Engineers to reduce the recommended outside air added to air-conditioned and heated spaces, indoor air quality problems became increasingly reported. This standard was reversed by 1983, but the practice of simply diluting indoor pollution with polluted outdoor air has continued.[67] However, this method is becoming increasingly supplemented by active cleaning of indoor air. There is an ever-increasing market for improved indoor air filtration on the heating, ventilation, and air-conditioning (HVAC) system of many homes, and for portable and installed HVAC filtration units. Unfortunately, the field of indoor air quality has developed more rapidly than the development of standards for good indoor air quality practices. Working with well qualified indoor air quality professionals to address complex indoor environmental issues is recommended by environmental guidelines.[38,68]

Indoor allergens from dogs, cats, rodents, dust mites, cockroaches, and fungi are ubiquitous in indoor environments. There is abundant research documenting the relationships between these indoor environmental exposures and human health effects. There are numerous recent practice parameters and review articles focused on these exposures and respiratory health impact. Indoor exposure to these allergen pollutants appear to be associated with an increased risk of developing asthma in young children and asthma morbidity in individuals with asthma.[69-74] For all of these indoor biological exposures, there is ample evidence that specific environmental interventions can reduce exposure and symptoms related to chronic rhinitis and asthma.

8.9 CONCLUSION

There are numerous links between the quality of the air we breathe and the maintenance of good respiratory health. Furthermore, there is emerging evidence that indoor and outdoor air quality issues are related to medical problems beyond respiratory conditions, such as cardiac and gastrointestinal disorders. There is increased recognition for the health impact of household air pollution. Many large

epidemiological studies have confirmed the link between air pollution and a number of public health issues in children including acute lower respiratory infections, low birth weight, stillbirth, preterm birth, stunting, and all-cause mortality.[75] Many studies have investigated the effects of automobile-related pollutants in heavily traveled expressways on asthma symptoms in allergic children. Numerous studies have associated living near highways with high vehicle traffic and either the development of allergic disease or increased asthma symptoms in persons with known allergen sensitization.[76-80] Thus, developing approaches for improving the quality of air we breathe and especially avoiding those factors already recognized to be associated with air pollution will provide immeasurable benefits for improving many areas of human health.

REFERENCES

1. Lim SS, Vos T, Flaxman AD et al. A comparative risk assessment of burden of disease and injury attributable to 67 risk factors and risk factor clusters in 21 regions, 1990-2010: A systematic analysis for the Global Burden of Disease Study 2010. *Lancet.* December 15, 2012;380(9859):2224–2260.

2. Schwartz J, Bind MA, Koutrakis P. Estimating causal effects of local air pollution on daily deaths: Effect of low levels. *Environ Health Perspect.* May 20, 2016;125(1):23–29.

3. Heroux ME, Braubach M, Korol N, Krzyzanowski M, Paunovic E, Zastenskaya I. The main conclusions about the medical aspects of air pollution: The projects REVIHAAP and HRAPIE WHO/EC. *Gig Sani.* November-December 2013;(6):9–14.

4. Yuan WM, Lu YQ, Wei Z et al. An epistaxis emergency associated with multiple pollutants in elementary students. *BES.* December 2016;29(12):893–897.

5. Szyszkowicz M, Shutt R, Kousha T et al. Air pollution and emergency department visits for epistaxis. *Clin Otolaryngol.* December 2014;39(6):345–351.

6. Wantke F, Focke M, Hemmer W et al. Formaldehyde and phenol exposure during an anatomy dissection course: A possible source of IgE-mediated sensitization? *Allergy.* November 1996;51(11):837–841.

7. Wantke F, Demmer CM, Tappler P. Exposure to gaseous formaldehyde induces IgE-mediated sensitization to formaldehyde in school-children. *Clin Exp Allergy.* March 1996;26(3):276–280.

8. Sigsgaard T, Forsberg B, Annesi-Maesano I et al. Health impacts of anthropogenic biomass burning in the developed world. *Eur Respir J.* December 2015;46(6):1577–1588.

9. Tielsch JM, Katz J, Thulasiraj RD et al. Exposure to indoor biomass fuel and tobacco smoke and risk of adverse reproductive outcomes, mortality,

respiratory morbidity and growth among newborn infants in south India. *Int J Epidemiol.* October 2009;38(5):1351–1363.

10. Rehfuess EA, Tzala L, Best N et al. Solid fuel use and cooking practices as a major risk factor for ALRI mortality among African children. *J Epidemiol Community Health.* November 2009;63(11):887–892.

11. Adler J. Why fire makes us human. June 2013. Available at http://www.smithsonian-mag.com/science-nature/why-fire-makes-us-human-72989884/#MZA6iSDWyG1zmcjF.99

12. Gannon M. Workers at Biblical Copper Mines Ate Quite Well. 2014. Available at http://www.livescience.com/48908-metalworkers-diet-biblical-mines.html). Accessed July 7, 2016.

13. Simmons IG. *An Environmental History of Great Britain.* Edinburgh, UK: Edinburgh University Press; 2001.

14. Masri R. The Cedars of Lebanon: Significance, Awareness and Management of the Cedrus libani in Lebanon. 1995. Available at http://almashriq.hiof.no/lebanon/300/360/363/363.7/cedars2.html.

15. van der Zee B. England's forests: A brief history of trees. July 26, 2013. Available at http://www.the-guardian.com/travel/2013/jul/27/history-of-englands-forests. Accessed July 30, 2016.

16. Pachauri R, Meyer L. *IPCC, 2014: Climate Change 2014: Synthesis Report. Contribution of Working Groups I, II and III to the Fifth Assessment Report of the Intergovernmental Panel on Climate Change IPCC, Geneva, Switzerland, 151 pp.* Geneva, Switzerland: IPCC;2014.

17. Barnes C, Alexis NE, Bernstein JA et al. Climate change and our environment: The effect on respiratory and allergic disease. *J Allergy Clin Immunol Pract.* March 2013;1(2):137–141.

18. Churchill J. The Medical Times and Gazette. January 28, 1865. Available at https://babel.hathitrust.org/cgi/pt?q1=fog;id=hvd.32044103089082;view=image;seq=131;start=1;sz=10;page=root;num=93;size=100;orient=0. Accessed July 30, 2016.

19. Nemery B, Hoet PH, and Nemmar A. The Meuse Valley fog of 1930: An air pollution disaster. *Lancet.* March 3, 2001;357(9257):704–708.

20. Logan WP. Mortality in the London fog incident, 1952. *Lancet.* February 14, 1953;1(6755):336–338.

21. Berhane K, Chang CC, McConnell R et al. Association of changes in air quality with bronchitic symptoms in children in California, 1993-2012. *JAMA.* April 12, 2016;315(14):1491–1501.

22. Bernstein DI. Traffic-related pollutants and wheezing in children. *J Asthma.* February 2012;49(1):5–7.

23. Peden DB, Setzer RW, Jr., and Devlin RB. Ozone exposure has both a priming effect on allergen-induced responses and an intrinsic inflammatory action in the nasal airways of perennially allergic asthmatics. *Am J Respir Crit Care Med.* May 1995;151(5):1336–1345.

24. Molfino NA, Wright SC, Katz I et al. Effect of low concentrations of ozone on inhaled allergen responses in asthmatic subjects. *Lancet.* July 27 1991;338(8761):199–203.

25. Schultz ES, Hallberg J, Gustafsson PM et al. Early life exposure to traffic-related air pollution and lung function in adolescence assessed with impulse oscillometry. *J Allergy Clin Immunol.* May 6, 2016;138(3):930–932.

26. World Health Organization. Air quality guidelines for Europe. *WHO Reg Publ Eur Ser.* 2000;(91):V–X, 1–273.

27. Lai HK, Hedley AJ, Thach TQ. A method to derive the relationship between the annual and short-term air quality limits—Analysis using the WHO Air Quality Guidelines for health protection. *Environ Int.* September 2013;59:86–91.

28. Raaschou-Nielsen O, Andersen ZJ, Beelen R et al. Air pollution and lung cancer incidence in 17 European cohorts: Prospective analyses from the European Study of Cohorts for Air Pollution Effects (ESCAPE). *Lancet Oncol.* August 2013;14(9):813–822.

29. Samet JM, Dominici F, Curriero FC. Fine particulate air pollution and mortality in 20 U.S. cities, 1987-1994. *N Engl J Med.* December 14, 2000;343(24):1742–1749.

30. Nordenhall C, Pourazar J, Ledin MC et al. Diesel exhaust enhances airway responsiveness in asthmatic subjects. *Eur Respir J.* May 2001;17(5):909–915.

31. Tramuto F, Cusimano R, Cerame G et al. Urban air pollution and emergency room admissions for respiratory symptoms: A case-crossover study in Palermo, Italy. *Environ Health.* 2011;10:31.

32. Norris G, YoungPong SN, Koenig JQ et al. An association between fine particles and asthma emergency department visits for children in Seattle. *Environ health Perspect.* June 1999;107(6):489–493.

33. Romieu I, Meneses F, Sienra-Monge JJ et al. Effects of urban air pollutants on emergency visits for childhood asthma in Mexico City. *Am J Epidemiol.* March 15, 1995;141(6):546–553.

34. Mirabelli MC, Vaidyanathan A, Flanders WD et al. Outdoor PM2.5, Ambient Air Temperature, and Asthma Symptoms in the Past 14 Days among Adults with Active Asthma. *Environ Health Perspect.* July 6, 2016;124(12):1882–1890.

35. Peng C, Bind MC, Colicino E et al. Particulate air pollution and fasting blood glucose in non-diabetic individuals: Associations and epigenetic mediation in the normative aging study, 2000-2011. *Environ Health Perspect.* May 24, 2016;124(11):1715–1721.

36. Taylor PE, Flagan RC, Valenta R et al. Release of allergens as respirable aerosols: A link between grass pollen and asthma. *J Allergy Clinical Immunol.* January 2002;109(1):51–56.

37. Taylor PE, Jacobson KW, House JM et al. Links between pollen, atopy and the asthma epidemic. *Int Arch Allergy Immunol.* 2007;144(2):162–170.

38. Barnes CS, Horner WE, Kennedy K et al. Home assessment and remediation. *Journal Allergy Clin Immunol Pract.* May-June 2016;4(3):423–431 e415.

39. Scott RW. Case of Bronchorrhoea AEstiva, or Hayfever: With remarks. *Prov Med J Retros Med Sci.* May 21, 1842;4(86):123–124.

40. Jariwala S, Toh J, Shum M et al. The association between asthma-related emergency department visits and pollen and mold spore concentrations in the Bronx, 2001-2008. *J Asthma.* February 2014;51(1):79–83.

41. Ito K, Weinberger KR, Robinson GS et al. The associations between daily spring pollen counts, over-the-counter allergy medication sales, and asthma syndrome emergency department visits in New York City, 2002-2012. *Environ Health.* 2015;14:71.

42. Venables KM, Allitt U, Collier CG et al. Thunderstorm-related asthma—The epidemic of 24/25 June 1994. *Clin Exp Allergy.* July 1997;27(7):725–736.

43. Marks GB, Colquhoun JR, Girgis ST et al. Thunderstorm outflows preceding epidemics of asthma during spring and summer. *Thorax.* June 2001;56(6):468–471.

44. Cakmak S, Dales RE, Coates F. Does air pollution increase the effect of aeroallergens on hospitalization for asthma? *Journal Allergy Clin Immunol.* January 2012;129(1):228–231.

45. Fahey L, Robinson G, Weinberger K et al. Correlation between aeroallergen levels and new diagnosis of eosinophilic esophagitis in NYC. *J Pediatr Gastroenterol Nutr.* April 21, 2016; 64(1):22–25.

46. Watanabe M, Noma H, Kurai J et al. Association between Outdoor Fungal Concentrations during Winter and Pulmonary Function in Children with and without Asthma. *Int J Environ Res Public Health.* 2016;13(5):E452.

47. Guilbert A, Simons K, Hoebeke L et al. Short-term effect of pollen and spore exposure on allergy morbidity in the Brussels-Capital eegion. *EcoHealth.* May 12, 2016;13(2):303–315.

48. Weichenthal S, Lavigne E, Villeneuve PJ, Reeves F. Airborne pollen concentrations and emergency room visits for myocardial infarction: A multicity case-crossover study in Ontario, Canada. *Am J Epidemiol.* April 1, 2016;183(7):613–621.

49. Riedler J, Eder W, Oberfeld G et al. Austrian children living on a farm have less hay fever, asthma and allergic sensitization. *Clin Exp Allergy.* February 2000;30(2):194–200.

50. Braun-Fahrlander C, Gassner M, Grize L et al. Prevalence of hay fever and allergic sensitization in farmer's children and their peers living in the same rural community. SCARPOL team. Swiss Study on Childhood Allergy and Respiratory Symptoms with Respect to Air Pollution. *Clin Exp Allergy.* January 1999;29(1):28–34.

51. Stein MM, Hrusch CL, Gozdz J et al. Innate immunity and asthma risk in amish and hutterite farm children. *N Engl J Med.* August 04, 2016;375(5):411–421.

52. Villalbi JR, Plasencia A, Manzanera R et al. Epidemic soybean asthma and public health: New control systems and initial evaluation in Barcelona, 1996-98. *J Epidemiol Community Health.* Jun 2004;58(6):461–465.

53. D'Amato G, Liccardi G, D'Amato M, Holgate S. Environmental risk factors and allergic bronchial asthma. *Clin Exp Allergy.* September 2005;35(9):1113–1124.

54. Fukuoka A, Matsushita K, Morikawa T et al. Diesel exhaust particles exacerbate allergic rhinitis in mice by disrupting the nasal epithelial barrier. *Clin Exp Allergy.* January 2016;46(1):142–152.

55. Ackaert C, Kofler S, Horejs-Hoeck J et al. The impact of nitration on the structure and immunogenicity of the major birch pollen allergen Bet v 1.0101. *PLOS ONE.* 2014;9(8):e104520.

56. Beck I, Jochner S, Gilles S et al. High environmental ozone levels lead to enhanced allergenicity of birch pollen. *PLOS ONE.* 2013;8(11):e80147.

57. Breton CV, Yao J, Millstein J et al. Prenatal air pollution exposures, DNA methyl transferase genotypes, and associations with newborn LINE1 and alu methylation and childhood blood pressure and carotid intima-media thickness in the children's health study. *Environ Health Perspect.* May 24 2016;124(12):1905–1912.

58. Chan MA, Ciaccio CE, Gigliotti NM et al. DNA methylation levels associate with race and childhood asthma severity. *Journal Asthma.* December 8, 2016;54(8):825–832.

59. Stocker T,. *Climate Change 2013: The Physical Science Basis.* TF. Stocker ed. New York;2013. Available at http://www.climatechange2013.org/.

60. Shea KM, Truckner RT, Weber RW et al. Climate change and allergic disease. *Journal Allergy Clin Immunol.* September 2008;122(3):443–453; quiz 454–445.

61. Ziska L, Knowlton K, Rogers C et al. Recent warming by latitude associated with increased length of ragweed pollen season in central North America. *Proc Natl Acad Sci USA.* March 8, 2011;108(10):4248–4251.

62. US-EPA. *Unfinished Business: A Comparative Assessment of Environmental Problems.* Washington DC: U.S. Environmental Protection Agency; 1990.

63. US-EPA. *Reducing Risk: Setting Priorities and Strategies for Environmental Protection.* Washington DC: U.S. Environmental Protection Agency; 1990.

64. Jones M. Laboratory animal allergy in the modern era. *Curr Allergy Asthma Rep.* December 2015;15(12):73.

65. North ML, Soliman M, Walker T et al. Controlled allergen challenge facilities and their unique contributions to allergic rhinitis research. *Curr Allergy Asthma Rep.* April 2015;15(4):11.

66. Ferraz E, Arruda LK, Bagatin E et al. Laboratory animals and respiratory allergies: The prevalence of allergies among laboratory animal workers and the need for prophylaxis. *Clinics (Sao Paulo).* June 2013;68(6):750–759.

67. Robert C and Brandys GMB. *Worldwide Exposure Standards for Mold and Bacteria with Assessment Guidelines for Air, Water, Dust, Ductwork, Carpet and Insulation.* 8th ed. Hinsdale, IL OEHCS; 1983.

68. Chew GL, Horner WE, Kennedy K et al. Procedures to assist health care providers to determine when home assessments for potential mold exposure are warranted. *J Allergy Clin Immunol Pract.* May-June 2016;4(3):417–422 e412.

69. Baxi SN, Portnoy JM, Larenas-Linnemann D et al. Exposure and health effects of fungi on humans. *Journal Allergy Clin Immunol Pract.* May-June 2016;4(3):396–404.

70. Portnoy J, Miller JD, Williams PB et al. Environmental assessment and exposure control of dust mites: A practice parameter. *Ann Allergy Asthma Immunol.* December 2013;111(6):465–507.

71. Portnoy J, Chew GL, Phipatanakul W et al. Environmental assessment and exposure reduction of cockroaches: A practice parameter. *J Allergy Clin Immunol.* October 2013;132(4):802–808 e801–825.

72. Phipatanakul W, Matsui E, Portnoy J et al. Environmental assessment and exposure reduction of rodents: A practice parameter. *Ann Allergy Asthma Immunol.* December 2012;109(6):375–387.

73. Portnoy J, Kennedy K, Sublett J et al. Environmental assessment and exposure control: A practice parameter—Furry animals. *Ann Allergy Asthma Immunol.* April 2012;108(4):223 e221–215.

74. Moller HU. Granular corneal dystrophy Groenouw type I (GrI) and Reis-Bucklers' corneal dystrophy (R-B). One entity? *Acta Ophthalmologica.* December 1989;67(6):678–684.

75. Bruce NG, Dherani MK, Das JK et al. Control of household air pollution for child survival: Estimates for intervention impacts. *BMC Public Health.* 2013;13(Suppl. 3):S8.

76. Brunekreef B, Beelen R, Hoek G et al. Effects of long-term exposure to traffic-related air pollution on respiratory and cardiovascular mortality in the Netherlands: The NLCS-AIR study. *Res Rep Health Eff Inst.* March 2009(139):5–71; discussion 73–89.

77. Janssen NA, Brunekreef B, van Vliet P et al. The relationship between air pollution from heavy traffic and allergic sensitization, bronchial hyper-responsiveness, and respiratory symptoms in Dutch schoolchildren. *Environ Health Perspect.* September 2003;111(12):1512–1518.

78. Nicolai T, Carr D, Weiland SK et al. Urban traffic and pollutant exposure related to respiratory outcomes and atopy in a large sample of children. *Eur Respir J.* June 2003;21(6):956–963.

79. Venn AJ, Lewis SA, Cooper M, Hubbard R, Britton J. Living near a main road and the risk of wheezing illness in children. *Am J Respir Crit Care Med.* December 15 2001;164(12):2177–2180.

80. Wyler C, Braun-Fahrlander C, Kunzli N et al. Exposure to motor vehicle traffic and allergic sensitization. The Swiss Study on Air Pollution and Lung Diseases in Adults (SAPALDIA) Team. *Epidemiology.* July 2000;11(4):450–456.

The microbiome in asthma, COPD, and asthma-COPD overlap

STEPHANIE CHRISTENSON

9.1 INTRODUCTION

The "microbiome" has been defined as "a community of microorganisms (such as bacteria, fungi, and viruses) that inhabit a particular environment, and especially the collection of microorganisms living in or on the human body."[1] We are just beginning to understand how the microbiome interacts with the human host, and how this interaction contributes to health and disease. The microbiome has traditionally been investigated using culture-based methods.

However, the advent of culture-free techniques to probe microbial sequences in recent years has vastly improved our ability to evaluate the microbiome. Much of the effort in humans has concentrated on the bacterial microbiome, the focus of this chapter. Yet, related to the advances in high-throughput technologies, viral and fungal communities are beginning to be analyzed as well. There is ever-increasing evidence that the microbial environment on human mucosal surfaces, specifically the airways and gastrointestinal tract, shape the development, maintenance, and heterogeneity of acute and chronic responses in airway disease.

CLINICAL VIGNETTE 9.1

Ms. A is a 64-year-old female with a history of COPD, previous smoking (20 pack years, quit 10 years ago), childhood asthma, and seasonal allergies, who presents to pulmonary clinic in follow-up after hospitalization for a COPD exacerbation 1 week ago. She notes that she had developed an upper respiratory infection approximately 1 week prior to admission and had become increasingly dyspneic with worsening wheezing over the course of the week. She was hospitalized for 1 week during which time she received a seven-day course of prednisone and levofloxacin. Her chest radiograph did not show an opacity to suggest pneumonia but her sputum culture grew *Haemophilus influenzae*. She feels her symptoms of dyspnea, wheezing, and cough have improved since discharge but are not quite back to baseline. At baseline, she notes dyspnea after walking one block, and wheezing intermittently throughout the day for which she takes albuterol at least a few times per week. She takes Budesonide 160 μg/Formoterol 4.5 μg combo inhaler 2 puffs BID and umeclidinium 62.5 mcg inhaled daily. She has now had two exacerbations of her symptoms requiring oral corticosteroids this year, but this is the first time she has required hospitalization. Her FEV_1 is 60% predicted, and she is bronchodilator responsive. Given her history of exacerbations and symptoms despite triple inhaler therapy, adjunctive therapy with daily azithromycin is considered. She has no ECG abnormalities and denies hearing deficits.

This case highlights important questions when considering the role of microorganisms and antibiotic therapy in obstructive airway disease:

1. How do microorganisms contribute to the pathogenesis of asthma, COPD, and asthma-COPD overlap?
2. How is the contribution of microorganisms to obstructive airway disease pathogenesis modified by acute exacerbations of the disease?
3. Does this patient have asthma, COPD, or asthma-COPD overlap, and how important is it to make this distinction when considering chronic macrolide therapy?
4. Which patient populations benefit from antibiotic therapy during stable disease and acute exacerbations?
5. How does chronic macrolide therapy mitigate exacerbation risk?

9.2 CONTEMPORARY MICROBIOME ANALYTICAL METHODS

Culture-based techniques are highly inadequate for studying the microbiome given their high degree of insensitivity.[2] This has necessitated the development of culture-free techniques. Methods based on polymerase chain reaction (PCR) amplification of the 16S ribosomal RNA (rRNA) gene have led the way for contemporary microbiome analysis.[3] The 16S rRNA gene is exclusive to and universal among bacteria. It is composed of regions highly conserved across all bacteria that flank hypervariable regions. Investigators have exploited the conserved regions of the 16S gene to generate universal primers that then allow for the amplification of this gene in the majority of known bacteria.[4] The hypervariable regions, which display significant diversity across bacteria, are amplified as well. The taxon-specificity of these hypervariable regions can then be leveraged to classify bacteria into taxonomic units so that microbial community composition can be investigated.

Next-generation microarray and sequencing technologies have led to advancements in the microbiome field by offering exponentially increasing throughput. 16S rRNA gene analysis is now most often carried out via sequencing. As the sequencing technology improves, read depths increase and costs decrease. With these developments, shotgun sequencing is now starting to be used for microbiome analysis as well. In shotgun sequencing, all sequences in a given sample are sequenced. When evaluating samples from a host organism (e.g., humans), shotgun sequencing will often require tremendous sequencing depth for microbiome analysis.[4] This is a technical limitation due to a large proportion of the sequencing reads being dedicated to host sequences. This large sequencing depth is thus required to adequately sequence the small proportion of reads that cover the microbiome. Nevertheless, this type of analysis, "metagenomics," provides some benefits over 16S rRNA gene sequencing. These benefits include the ability to evaluate genes beyond the 16S rRNA gene, some of which may be functionally relevant. Shotgun sequencing also allows for the study of other organisms in a sample, including fungi and viruses. Techniques for microbiome analysis using RNA, proteins, and metabolites (metatranscriptomics, metaproteomics, and meta-metabolomics, respectively) are being developed as well. These techniques may be used in tandem with DNA-based methods to investigate transcriptional, translational, and metabolic correlates of the microbes identified in a sample. See Table 9.1 for microbiome analysis definitions.

9.3 THE GUT MICROBIOME AND THE DEVELOPMENT OF AIRWAY DISEASE

The highest bacterial burden in the human body resides in the lower gastrointestinal tract.[5] Immediately after birth, an infant's mucosal surfaces are colonized by the first bacterial species he/she is exposed to.[6,7] As such, early environmental exposures and diet greatly affect the infant's microbial composition. In healthy individuals, gut microbial composition is highly variable in early life,[8] but progressively stabilizes with an adult-like community developing by 3 years of age.[9]

The study of germ-free mice has been leveraged to understand how the microbiome contributes to the development of the immune system. Comparisons between germ-free mice and those colonized with microbiota show that the microbiome is crucial to the structural and functional development of the immune system, including the development of lymphoid tissues.[10,11] Allergic airway inflammation is exaggerated in germ-free mice, when compared to specific pathogen-free mice (i.e., mice free from a pre-specified list of pathogens that may affect research outcomes or are known to not cause disease in mice). This inflammation is reversed when the gut microbiota from specific pathogen-free mice are transferred to the germ-free mice in early life.[12] Consequently, it appears that the gut microbiota in particular may be important for the development of allergic disease, even at other mucosal surfaces.

Further studies in murine models have supported this "gut-lung inflammatory axis" hypothesis, with the early life gut microbiome playing an important role in asthma development.

Table 9.1 Glossary of microbiome analysis terms

Microbiome	A community of microorganisms (such as bacteria, fungi, and viruses) that inhabit a particular environment, and especially the collection of microorganisms living in or on the human body.
Metagenome	All the genetic material present in an environmental sample, consisting of the genomes of multiple individual organisms. Derivations of this term are used in regards to RNA ("metatranscriptome") and protein ("metaproteome").
16S rRNA gene	Component of the 30S subunit of prokaryotic ribosomes used for phylogenetic studies as it is highly conserved between different species of bacteria and archaea. The bacterial 16S gene contains nine hyper-variable regions (V1–V9) that flank the highly conserved regions. Conservation of hyper-variable regions vary across taxonomies and are used for classification.
Dysbiosis	A microbial imbalance inside the body categorized into one of three types: 1. Loss of beneficial organisms, 2. Expansion of potentially harmful organisms, 3. Loss of microbial diversity.
Taxonomy	Rank-based classification of organisms: domain -> phylum -> class -> order -> family -> genus -> species.
Shotgun sequencing	A method for sequencing long DNA strands. The long strands are fragmented ("shotgunned") into shorter transcripts and sequenced. These sequence fragments are then reassembled into a complete sequence using their overlap. When a sample containing host and microbial cells (e.g., a human sputum sample) is sequenced, all sequences will be fragmented (human and microbial) and reassembly will require assigning fragments to both host and microbial genomes.
DNA microarray	A 2D grid of oligonucleotide probes against known DNA sequences used to detect thousands of genes at the same time. For microbiome classification, the 16S rRNA is targeted.

Mice fed *Helicobacter pylori* had an increase in systemic T regulatory cells (Tregs) as well as a decrease in airway hyperresponsiveness, airway tissue inflammation, and goblet cell metaplasia.[13] Similar findings have been demonstrated after feeding mice a mix of *Clostridium* (which promoted Treg accumulation and reduced systemic IgE) and *Lactobacillus reuteri* (which promoted Treg accumulation and decreased the allergic response to OVA challenge).[14,15] Altering diet appears to have an effect on the gut microbiome and systemic inflammation as well. Feeding mice a diet high in fermentable fiber increased the relative abundance of *Bacteroidetes* in comparison to *Firmicutes*, increased circulating short-chain fatty acid levels, and suppressed allergic lung disease in the setting of decreased Th2 cell effector function.[16]

The importance of the microbiome in the early development of the immune system and atopy has given rise to the "hygiene hypothesis." The hygiene hypothesis suggests that a reduction in early life microbial exposures leads to impaired immune system maturation and an increased susceptibility to the development of allergic diseases. A major notion of this hypothesis is that a relative lack of exposure to microbes has led to the increased prevalence of asthma and atopy in Westernized nations.[17] This theory was first tested in epidemiologic studies in humans by showing that asthma susceptibility in childhood is decreased when, in the first year of life, the child is exposed to environments high in bacterial burden and diversity. These environments include growing up with dogs in the home, multiple older siblings, or on farms with high exposure to livestock.[17–22] Work in murine models also supports the hygiene hypothesis. One study showed that chronic low-dose exposure to bacterial endotoxin or farm dust leads to suppression of Type 2 immunity and protection from house dust mite–induced asthma.[23]

Epidemiologic studies further go on to suggest that early life gastrointestinal tract microbial exposures specifically are important to the development of allergic disease. Childhood asthma prevalence is higher in bottle-fed vs. breast-fed infants and vs. those fed pasteurized milk.[24] Multiple studies have shown that microbial dysbiosis in the stool of infants is associated with greater asthma or allergy risk in childhood. These studies generally showed that lower abundance of *Bifidobacteria*, *Lactobacilli*, and *Bacteriodetesi*, and higher abundance of *Enterococci* and *Clostridia*, are associated with increased allergic risk.[25–28]

While the role of the gut microbiome in childhood asthma development has been well-studied, its role in the development of COPD, adult-onset asthma, and asthma-COPD overlap (ACO) is poorly understood. Studying the microbiome in cohort studies that follow at-risk adults to the development of airway disease is a much more daunting task than following infants to the development of childhood asthma. Longer follow-up times and large sample sizes will likely be required. Nonetheless, an association between aberrant alterations in microbial composition, dysbiosis, in the gut and cigarette smoking, the main risk factor for COPD development, has been found.[29] Ten participants undergoing smoking cessation had increases in bacterial diversity and a shift toward the *Firmicutes* and *Actinobacteria* phyla following smoking cessation. While this was a very limited study with potential confounders, it does suggest a role for smoking in gut microbial dysbiosis that could potentially contribute to systemic inflammation. In COPD, many patients have evidence of systemic inflammation with increased circulating cytokine and chemokine levels.[30] Whether gastrointestinal microbial dysbiosis in response to cigarette smoking may lead to or potentiate systemic inflammation and the development of airway disease is still unknown.

9.4 THE HEALTHY LUNG MICROBIOME

Investigation of the human airway microbiome has lagged substantially behind investigation of the gut microbiome. This is partially due to the considerably lower bacterial burden in the airways compared to the gastrointestinal tract. Only within the past several years has culture-free technology to study this lower bacterial burden advanced enough to allow for this line of inquiry. Indeed, as culture-based techniques were previously unable to sample this lower bacterial load, it was commonly thought that the healthy airways were sterile until as recently as this last decade.[31]

The lung microbiome is significantly more dynamic than the gut microbiome. Gut microbes migrating from the mouth through the digestive tract must endure the chemical barrier of differing pHs along their passage.[32] Microbial immigration into the distal airways does not confront these same physical barriers. Furthermore, contrary to the unidirectional movement along the gastrointestinal tract, the movement of microbes in the airways is bidirectional. Even during healthy states microbes immigrate into the airways through inhalation, subclinical microaspiration of upper respiratory or gastrointestinal contents, and direct movement along the airways. The human airways, however, have many defenses against this continuous introduction of microbes. Microbes are eliminated through mucociliary clearance, cough, and host mucosal immune defense.

In health, the airway microbiome most closely resembles that of the oral cavity albeit with a 2–4 log lower bacterial burden.[33] The *Bacteroidetes* phylum (particularly *Prevotella*) and *Firmicutes* phylum (particularly *Streptococci*) are most prevalent. In contrast, the nasal mucosa is generally populated by microbial communities more closely resembling skin flora. As microbiota in the lower airways are sampled via bronchoscopy, there has been a concern that the flora detected in the lower airways are due to contamination tracked down from the oral cavity with introduction of the bronchoscope. However, the finding that the healthy lower airway microbiome most closely resembles the oral microbiome remains even when brushes protected against oral contamination are used for sampling or when the bronchoscope is introduced through the nose.[33] It is hypothesized, although not proven, that the similarity between oral and lower airway microbiomes may be a consequence of chronic microaspiration.[32] Saliva accounts for a much greater volume of the host secretions than is normally produced by the nasal mucosa. In disease (e.g., respiratory infection or allergic rhinitis), the contribution of other airway mucosal surfaces to production of secretions, including the nasal mucosa, increases and, in turn, may alter the airway microbiome.

Although the lower airway microbiome most closely resembles the oral microbiome, regional differences do exist. Composition varies by region of the lung studied, likely due to a combination of factors. The compartment studied (e.g., epithelium, bronchoalveolar lavage, sputum, or parenchyma) appears to be associated with differences in composition.[34,35] Additionally, the lung is comprised of microenvironments. Growth conditions, such as temperature, pH, and oxygen concentration, vary throughout the lung and likely influence survival and growth of specific microbes.[36] For example, members of the *Bacteroidetes* phylum are anaerobic and thus are at a disadvantage in oxygen-rich environments. In addition, inflammation at the mucosal surface may lead to changes in microenvironment conditions.[37] Thus, type of sample and regional variation must be taken into account when studying the lung microbiome.

9.5 THE LUNG MICROBIOME IN CHRONIC AIRWAY DISEASE

It has been shown across many studies that the microbial composition of the airways changes during both acute and chronic airway disease. In health immigration of microbiota into the lower respiratory tract and subsequent elimination are the primary factors that determine the microbiome of the lower airways (Figure 9.1). Reproduction of resident bacteria contributes little in the healthy state. However, during acute and chronic airway disease the host conditions change such that reproduction of resident bacteria contributes more to the microbiome.[38] For example, chronic airway diseases are often associated with decreases in mucociliary clearance and increases in mucin production. These alterations, in turn, can lead to alterations in the environmental conditions of the lower respiratory tract. This new environment can then provide a better opportunity for bacterial growth.

9.5.1 ASTHMA

The link between asthma and chronic colonization of the airways with pathogenic bacteria or outright infection has long been suggested. This hypothesis formed well before the widespread use of the more modern high-throughput methods. Both serologic testing and PCR-based methods have shown that *Chlamydophila pneumoniae* and *Mycoplasma pneumoniae* are found more frequently in the airways of asthma patients than healthy controls.[39–42] *M. pneumoniae* and *C. pneumoniae* may even be involved in the onset of adult asthma in a subset of patients, although a causal link has not been established.[41,42] Culture-based methods also showed that identification of *Streptococcus pneumoniae*, *Haemophilus influenzae*, or *Moraxella catarrhalis* in the oropharynx of one-month-old infants is associated with greater risk of childhood asthma.[43] These findings are only associations. Consequently, it is still unclear if the microbes themselves are increasing asthma risk or are just an indicator of an altered immune system.

Contemporary high-throughput methods have commonly shown that the relative abundance of the *Proteobacteria* phylum is increased in at least a subset of asthmatics across a range of severity.[31,44–46] This phenomenon has even

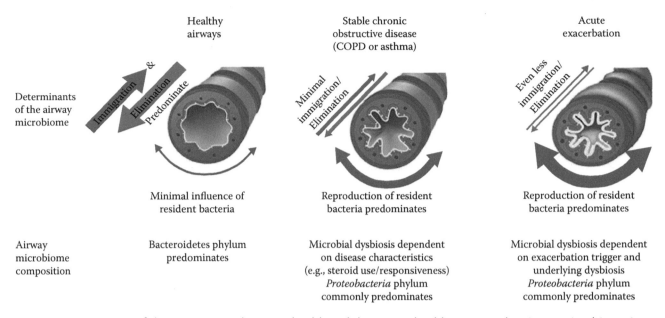

Figure 9.1 Determinants of the airway microbiome in health and disease. In healthy airways the airway microbiome is primarily determined by immigration into and elimination out of the distal airways with little contribution from the resident population. In disease, conditions within the airways have changed such that reproduction of resident bacteria is favored, and thus this contributes more to the microbial population in the airways.

been shown in corticosteroid naive participants, suggesting it is not just a medication effect.[45] Studies have further found that asthma is usually characterized by a greater bacterial burden and diversity.[44]

Both the clinical characteristics and immunologic responses in asthma are heterogeneous. Thus, most studies of the microbiome in stable asthma have gone beyond evaluating the association between disease state and microbial composition to look at specific phenotypic characteristics. In a study of 65 suboptimally controlled asthmatics and 10 healthy controls, bronchial epithelial brushings were collected. Bronchial hyperresponsiveness was found to be associated with increased bacterial diversity and an increase in multiple families within the *Proteobacteria* phylum. This increase in bacterial diversity was particularly high among participants who demonstrated a significant reduction in bronchial reactivity in response to macrolide antibiotic treatment.[44] A subset of corticosteroid-resistant asthmatics has been shown to have an increased proportion of *Proteobacteria* and *Actinobacteria* in bronchoalveolar lavage samples.[47] Lung-function decrements and increased neutrophils have been shown to be associated with *M. Catarrhalis*, *Haemophilus*, and *Streptococcus*. Increased sputum leukocyte counts and worse asthma control measured on the Asthma Control Questionnaire have been related to increases in *Proteobacteria*.[46] That same study showed that steroid responsiveness, as measured by FK506 gene expression, and increased asthma severity are associated with increased *Actinobacteria*. Thus exists substantial evidence that microbial dysbiosis is associated with phenotypic variation in asthma. Most of these studies are, however, correlative. Further investigation into the causative relationships between microbial and clinical variability is still needed.

9.5.2 COPD

Several small studies have been done to examine the airway microbiome in COPD with mixed results. The first study compared eight healthy controls, 11 participants with asthma, and five with COPD using samples obtained from airway brushings.[31] Similar to asthma, they identified a shift in microbial composition toward the pathogenic *Proteobacteria* phylum and away from the *Bacteroidetes* phylum that dominates the healthy airways. This has not, however, been consistently replicated across studies. While one other study showed similar results,[34] others have instead shown a shift toward the *Firmicute* phylum.[35,48,49] Furthermore, one study showed a decrease in microbial diversity with increasing airway obstruction,[34] while others have shown no change or increased diversity in COPD compared to health or with increasing disease severity.[35,48,49]

Unfortunately, the studies of the airway microbiome in COPD were done using different sample types (e.g., bronchoalveolar lavage, airway brushings, and parenchymal samples) with small sample sizes. Thus, some of the inconsistencies may be due to a difference in the compartment sampled. Another plausible explanation is that, similar to COPD itself, the microbial communities that dominate the COPD airways are heterogeneous. One study found that additional host factors, including age and medication use (inhaled steroids or bronchodilators), significantly influenced the composition of the microbiome in COPD.[48] Larger studies that can more appropriately examine the contribution of host response to microbial composition, and whether the heterogeneity that exists across studies also exists within a study, must be done. Based on these preliminary studies it is, however, clear that stable COPD is associated with an alteration in microbial composition when compared to the healthy airway.

9.6 THE LUNG MICROBIOME DURING ACUTE EXACERBATIONS

As is the case with obstructive diseases overall, acute exacerbations of obstructive lung diseases are heterogeneous. Viruses are considered the predominant trigger for asthma exacerbations,[50] and are an important trigger for COPD exacerbations as well.[51,52] However, alterations in the bacterial communities in the airways and environmental exposures (e.g., allergens) also trigger a significant number of exacerbations in obstructive lung disease.

As in stable obstructive disease, culture-based techniques have proven inadequate in investigating the contribution of dysbiosis during exacerbations. Culture is often negative at the time of exacerbation. In one study, 51% of cases of COPD exacerbation were culture negative.[53] Furthermore, the same pathogens cultured during exacerbation can be cultured during periods of stability, raising concern that the long-held belief that pathogenic bacteria are causing the exacerbation may be untrue or oversimplified.

Importantly, studies of the microbiome to date have found that episodes of acute exacerbations of lung disease are different from acute lung infections in several key ways.[38] First, exacerbations only occur in patients with underlying lung disease. Bacterial diversity is also not necessarily decreased in acute exacerbations as it is during acute infection, where it indicates that one type of bacteria predominates. Furthermore, as explained below, antibiotics are not indicated for all obstructive lung disease exacerbations as they are for acute infections. It is hypothesized instead that an acute trigger (e.g., viral infection) initiates an alteration in host inflammation that leads to a shift in regional microbial growth conditions in abnormal airways. This leads to further microbial dysbiosis with a positive feedback loop leading to further host inflammation and acute symptoms (Figure 9.1). Thus, as opposed to an acute infection where one pathogen is often the culprit, in exacerbations it is the interaction between a dysregulated microbiome and altered host response in chronically abnormal airways that likely leads to symptoms.

9.6.1 ASTHMA EXACERBATIONS

While viral infections appear to be the predominant trigger for asthma exacerbations in children, the same microbes that are associated with increased risk of developing asthma are associated with an increased exacerbation risk as well. Identifying *M. catarrhalis*, *H. influenzae*, or *S. pneumoniae* in the airways, either by culture or PCR, is associated with wheezing episodes and asthma exacerbations.[43,54,55] These

associations were found both in the presence and absence of concomitant respiratory virus infection. However, a theory exists that the microbial composition of the airway may affect the response of the airways to a viral infection. While *Haemophilus*, *Moraxella*, and *Streptococcus* are associated with exacerbations on their own, rhinovirus infection is associated with an increased abundance of these pathogenic bacteria. Furthermore, in the presence of these pathogenic bacteria, rhinovirus is more likely to lead to exacerbations.[55]

9.6.2 COPD EXACERBATIONS

The microbiome of COPD exacerbations has been studied more thoroughly than that of stable COPD or asthma exacerbations. A study using bronchoscopic sampling and culture methods found that 54% of COPD exacerbations were associated with abnormal culture results.[56] Culture techniques have also found that acquisition of new strains of *H. influenzae*, *Moraxella catarrhalis*, *Streptococcus pneumoniae*, or *Pseudomonas aeruginosa* are all associated with increased exacerbation occurrence.[57] However, the majority of participants in that study did not have a new strain isolated during exacerbation, suggesting that a newly acquired pathogen is not the sole reason for exacerbations.

With the advent of 16s techniques, more comprehensive analyses of the COPD exacerbation microbiome have been completed. The first study was a longitudinal analysis of 12 participants in which sputum samples were collected before, during, and after exacerbation.[49] The investigators found that the microbial composition shifted toward an increase in *Proteobacteria* during the exacerbation, with a decrease in *Actinobacteria*, *Clostridia*, and *Bacteroidetes*. They further identified a "like will to like" phenomenon in which they found that both *H. influenzae* and phylogenetically related bacteria increased in abundance in tandem. Less related bacteria decreased in abundance. Another small study (16 participants) also showed increases in abundance of specific phyla during exacerbation compared to stable disease, although these phyla varied.[58] These small studies thus suggest that COPD exacerbations are associated with microbial dysbiosis, and that similarity of bacteria introduced into the airway ecosystem may influence their intrusion success.

As noted previously, COPD exacerbations are thought to occur in the setting of various triggers. A larger study evaluated the association between suspected COPD exacerbation phenotype and alterations in microbial composition. Sputum samples were collected from 87 participants at baseline, during exacerbation, 2 weeks after therapy, and at 6 weeks recovery.[59] Investigators found that there was an overall reduction in diversity with a slight, although insignificant, relative increase in *Proteobacteria* abundance. They then went on to phenotype participants by type of exacerbation based on prespecified criteria. They found that participants in the group classified as "bacterial" exacerbation had a significant increase in *Proteobacteria*, particularly *Haemophilus*, and a decrease in *Firmicutes*, particularly *Streptococcus*, compared to a group classified as "eosinophilic" exacerbation. This study suggests that microbe-specific alterations are heterogeneous across COPD exacerbations and are likely related to the exacerbation trigger.

Another study went even further, evaluating the microbiome alterations associated specifically with virus-induced exacerbation. The investigators used an experimental human model in which COPD participants and healthy controls were inoculated with human rhinovirus.[60] In the COPD participants, viral infection was associated with an increase in the relative abundance of *Proteobacteria*. There was not a similar change in healthy controls. Thus, virus-induced exacerbation specifically can contribute to bacterial microbiome dysbiosis in the airways.

These longitudinal studies also demonstrate that treatment at the time of exacerbation influences the postexacerbation microbial composition.[49,59] Antibiotic treatment resulted in diminished bacterial burden, particularly of *Proteobacteria*, while steroid treatment resulted in the reverse results. Hence, the effects of the exacerbation and associated treatment type on the airway microbiome may last far beyond the exacerbation. The importance of these alterations on the severity of symptoms in chronic disease and future exacerbation risk are important areas for future study.

9.7 THE AIRWAY MICROBIOME AND ASTHMA-COPD OVERLAP

To date, minimal work has been done relating the microbiome to ACO. One study clustered 75 participants with moderate-to-severe COPD and 86 participants with severe asthma based on sputum cytokine levels.[61] They then evaluated the clinical and biological characteristics associated with these clusters. They identified three clusters: (1) asthma-predominant; (2) COPD-predominant; and (3) overlap of participants with asthma or COPD. They noted that this asthma-COPD overlap group had more neutrophilia; had increased sputum IL-1β, IL-8, IL-10, and TNF-α levels; and was more likely to have sputum bacterial colonization (based on culture). Upon stratification by disease state though, most of the bacterial colonization in this group was seen in the COPD participants. What this work does suggest is that there are similarities in host response between asthma and COPD, and that there is some evidence that this may be related to bacterial colonization. Further work will be necessary in larger studies, with more advanced technologies, to study these relationships in more depth.

Any further understanding of the microbiome in ACO must be extrapolated from our understanding of the microbiome in asthma and COPD. It does appear that chronic airway disease and acute exacerbations of that disease are associated with significant microbial dysbiosis in the airways. This appears true of both asthma and COPD, and, thus, is likely

true of ACO. As asthma, COPD, and ACO involve heterogeneous patient populations, further understanding of how this heterogeneity interacts with the microbiome is needed.

9.8 THE LUNG MICROBIOME AS A THERAPEUTIC TARGET IN CHRONIC AIRWAY DISEASE

Despite the lack of an established causative relationship between airway dysbiosis and worse outcomes in obstructive lung diseases, the effect of chronic antibiotic therapy, particularly macrolide therapy, on outcomes in both asthma and COPD, has been studied repeatedly. Macrolides have been shown to exert not only antimicrobial effects, but also immunomodulatory and potentially antiviral effects. While it does appear that there is a role for macrolide therapy in the treatment of exacerbation-prone asthma and COPD, it is unclear whether the derived benefit is due to an alteration in the microbiome, the host immune response, or both (Figure 9.2).

In COPD, several RCTs have examined the effect of macrolide therapy on exacerbations and/or symptom control. The largest of these studies, the multicenter MACRO study evaluated the effect of azithromycin 250 mg daily versus placebo over 12 months in 1142 participants with moderate to severe COPD at risk for COPD exacerbations (hospitalization or oral steroids received for COPD exacerbation in the past year, or use of continuous oxygen supplementation).[62] This study showed a modest 17% reduction in exacerbation rates as well as a significant increase in time to first exacerbation and reduction in symptom scores. A Cochrane review of macrolide RCTs, including the MACRO study, determined that chronic macrolide therapy was associated with a significant decrease in patients experiencing exacerbations (number needed to treat to prevent one exacerbation = 8, high-quality evidence).[63] They also found a significant decrease in exacerbation rates and improvement in quality of life. There was no effect on hospital admissions, serious adverse events, or all-cause mortality. Importantly, they noted that the data only applies to frequent exacerbators.

In asthma, the effectiveness of macrolides is not as well-established, although the studies have historically been limited by low sample sizes. Meta-analyses have suggested that macrolides improve symptoms and quality of life, but their effect on exacerbations has been inconclusive.[64] However, the recently published Australian multicenter AMAZES trial addresses the sample-size limitations of the previous studies, and indicates the potential benefit of macrolides in asthma exacerbation prevention.[65] AMAZES randomized 421 participants to Azithromycin 500 mg or placebo for 48 weeks. They limited their study population to those with uncontrolled symptoms despite maintenance therapy with medium- to high-dose inhaled corticosteroids and a long-acting bronchodilator. They found that azithromycin

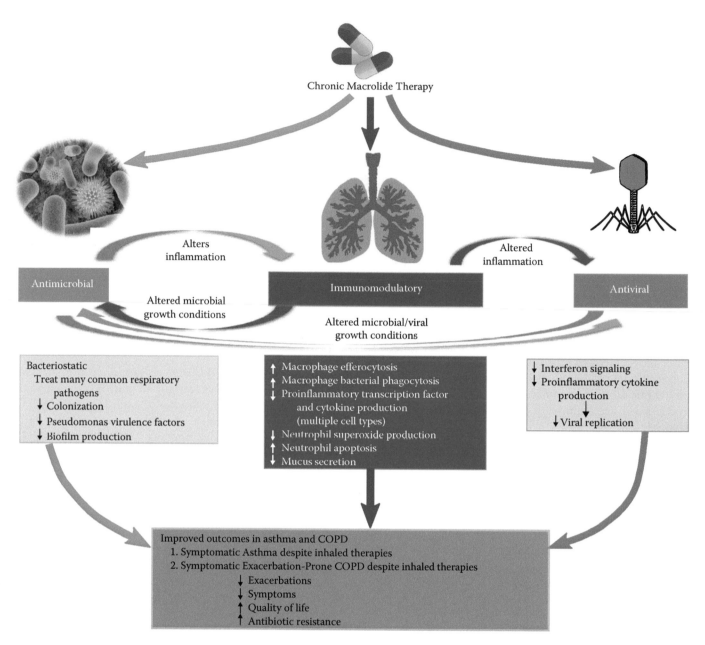

Figure 9.2 The effect of chronic macrolide therapy ion airway biology and asthma and COPD outcomes. Chronic macrolide therapy has been shown to have antimicrobial, immunomodulatory, and antiviral effects. Alterations in the microbial communities, host response, and response to virus can then interact with each other to amplify the direct effects of the macrolide. Although still unclear how these effects interact to improve clinical outcomes, chronic macrolide therapy has been shown to decrease exacerbation rates and symptoms in obstructive lung diseases.

reduced the rate of total exacerbations and severe exacerbations, number of antibiotic courses used, and participants reporting respiratory infections. Azithromycin also improved quality of life and symptom scores. While a previous smaller study showed an effect of azithromycin on exacerbations only on those participants without eosinophilia,[66] AMAZES showed an effect in both eosinophilic and noneosinophilic disease. AMAZES generally included older adults (median age 60) and included former smokers (38% overall) in addition to never-smokers. Caution should be applied when generalizing these findings outside of this older uncontrolled asthma population.

The use of chronic macrolide therapy should be approached with hesitancy given concerns for adverse effects, in particular antibiotic resistance. There is evidence of higher rates of macrolide resistance in those treated with chronic macrolides.[62] As concerns regarding antibiotic resistance as a public health crisis grow, special attention should be paid to ensure that only those patients who may derive most benefit from macrolide therapy are prescribed these medications. Further, chronic azithromycin use is associated with a significant increase in hearing loss,[62] of particular concern in the older COPD and ACO populations. Macrolides are also known to prolong the QTc, thus prolonged QTc at baseline was an exclusion criteria for both MACRO and AMAZES.[62,65] This should be considered when selecting patients for macrolide therapy as well.

Macrolide therapy has not yet been included as a treatment option in asthma guidelines given the previous inconclusive evidence. With the publication of AMAZES, macrolides may be added for inhaled therapy-resistant asthma in older patient populations. For COPD, the 2017 GOLD guidelines cautiously recommend that azithromycin or erythromycin be considered as adjunctive therapy in those patients who remain symptomatic and exacerbation prone (history of 2 or more exacerbations in the past year or one requiring hospitalization) despite treatment with inhaled corticosteroids, long-acting beta agonists, and long acting antimuscarinics. They limit their recommendation to former smokers only.

Consideration of chronic macrolide therapy in ACO would need to be extrapolated from the COPD and asthma studies. History of asthma was an exclusion criteria for MACRO.[62] Low-diffusing capacity, as a marker of possible emphysema, was an exclusion criteria for AMAZES.[65] Thus, not all ACO patients were described by either study. However, both RCTs studied older adults and included former smokers. Both found utility in macrolides in patients who remained symptomatic (and in COPD were prone to exacerbations) despite maintenance inhaled therapies. Thus, for ACO, it may be extrapolated, as with other therapies that macrolides may be useful in a symptomatic and inhaled therapy–resistant subgroup. Again, potential adverse reactions, in particular antibiotic resistance, should be strongly considered when contemplating macrolides as a treatment option.

There are multiple potential mechanisms of action for macrolide therapy, although it is still unclear which of these lead to the beneficial effects in chronic obstructive disease (Figure 9.2).[50,67,68] Potential immunomodulatory mechanisms of macrolides include the improved ability of macrophages to phagocytose pathogenic bacteria and apoptotic cells ("efferocytosis"), and the inhibition of proinflammatory cytokine production in several cell types.[50] Macrolides are also clinically effective against three of the four most common bacteria implicated in COPD and neutrophilic asthma exacerbations: nontypeable *Haemophilus influenzae, Moraxella catarrhalis, and Streptococcus pneumoniae.*[67] Long-term treatment with macrolides may provide prophylaxis against these pathogens or may diminish their colonization. Colonization with pathogenic bacteria has been shown to increase chronic inflammation. By diminishing the colonization, macrolides may dampen this chronic inflammation, creating a less hospitable environment for the emergence of new pathogenic bacteria or viruses.[68] Macrolides are not clinically effective against one of the major COPD exacerbation pathogens, Pseudomonas, although they may decrease its virulence.[67] This issue, as well as the fact that two studies found improvement despite macrolide dosing below that which is clinically effective, suggest that more than the antimicrobial effects are leading to improvements. Beyond or related to their immunomodulatory effects, macrolides may also possess antiviral effects, although this has been less well-studied.[50] There is some evidence that they stimulate an interferon response and consequently decrease viral replication. This would be of particular importance in asthma in which exacerbations are predominantly attributed to viral infection.

Altering the microbial communities along the mucosal surfaces in ways that do not require antibiotics is being examined more and more for the treatment of inflammatory disorders. The administration of probiotics or prebiotics as well as fecal microbiota transplant have been shown to alter the gut microbiome and have immunomodulatory effects.[69] As evidence is mounting on the importance of the gut microbiome in asthma development and outcomes, identifying the utility of these therapies in asthma prevention and treatment is essential. Currently, however, there is not enough data to support the use of these therapies in obstructive lung disease.

9.9 ANTIBIOTIC THERAPY IN ACUTE EXACERBATIONS

Antibiotic therapy at the time of an acute asthma exacerbation is not recommended, as a viral trigger is more common. In COPD, however, antibiotic therapy is recommended for acute exacerbations when sputum purulence, and an increase in dyspnea or sputum production are present. These recommendations are based on the evidence that this symptom constellation is associated with a higher bacterial burden in the airways.[70] A Cochrane review of antibiotic therapy for COPD exacerbations found that empiric antibiotics reduced treatment failure in hospitalized patients but not those treated as outpatients.[71] Only one study was done in patients mechanically ventilated in the ICU.[72] This was also the only included study in the review that found a mortality benefit for antibiotics. What these studies suggest is that acute treatment with antibiotics should be used with caution.

9.10 CONCLUSIONS

We are just beginning to understand how the microbiome is contributing to the development and manifestations of chronic airway disease. While improving high-throughput technologies have vastly improved our understanding of the contribution of the bacterial microbiome to airway disease, there are many unanswered questions. Little attention has been paid to the fungal and viral microbiomes to date, and it is quite likely that these play a role in airway disease. Furthermore, most of the research, particularly in humans, has been associative. Thus, much work must be done to understand the causal pathways. Are the alterations in microbial communities leading to alterations in the host immune response, or is the causal pathway in the reverse direction? It is likely that there is a complex interaction between the responses of the viral, bacterial, and fungal microbiomes and the host.

It will also be important to understand how variations in microbial composition contribute to the various heterogeneous host responses in chronic airway diseases, including ACO. In the future, recognizing these variable alterations in the microbiome may inform therapeutic choices in airway disease. Appreciating which patients may benefit from antibiotics, corticosteroids, or other therapies, and how the microbiome informs these decisions, is crucial.

REFERENCES

1. Abraham C and Cho JH. Inflammatory bowel disease. *N Engl J Med.* 2009;361(21):2066–2078.
2. Rappe MS and Giovannoni SJ. The uncultured microbial majority. *Annu Rev Microbiol.* 2003;57:369–394.
3. Woese CR and Fox GE. Phylogenetic structure of the prokaryotic domain: The primary kingdoms. *Proc Natl Acad Sci U S A.* 1977;74(11):5088–5090.
4. Fujimura KE and Lynch SV. Microbiota in allergy and asthma and the emerging relationship with the gut microbiome. *Cell Host Microbe.* 2015;17(5):592–602.
5. Sender R, Fuchs S, and Milo R. Are we really vastly outnumbered? revisiting the ratio of bacterial to host cells in humans. *Cell.* 2016;164(3):337–340.
6. Dominguez-Bello MG, Blaser MJ, Ley RE et al. Development of the human gastrointestinal microbiota and insights from high-throughput sequencing. *Gastroenterology.* 2011;140(6):1713–1719.
7. Dominguez-Bello MG, Costello EK, Contreras M et al. Delivery mode shapes the acquisition and structure of the initial microbiota across multiple body habitats in newborns. *Proc Natl Acad Sci U S A.* 2010;107(26):11971–11975.
8. Palmer C, Bik EM, DiGiulio DB et al. Development of the human infant intestinal microbiota. *PLOS Biol.* 2007;5(7):e177.
9. Yatsunenko T, Rey FE, Manary MJ et al. Human gut microbiome viewed across age and geography. *Nature.* 2012;486(7402):222–227.
10. Sommer F and Backhed F. The gut microbiota–masters of host development and physiology. *Nat Rev Microbiol.* 2013;11(4):227–238.
11. Bauer H, Horowitz RE, Levenson SM et al. The response of the lymphatic tissue to the microbial flora. Studies on germfree mice. *Am J Pathol.* 1963;42:471–483.
12. Herbst T, Sichelstiel A, Schar C et al. Dysregulation of allergic airway inflammation in the absence of microbial colonization. *Am J Respir Crit Care Med.* 2011;184(2):198–205.
13. Arnold IC, Dehzad N, Reuter S et al. Helicobacter pylori infection prevents allergic asthma in mouse models through the induction of regulatory T cells. *J Clin Invest.* 2011;121(8):3088–3093.
14. Atarashi K, Tanoue T, Shima T et al. Induction of colonic regulatory T cells by indigenous clostridium species. *Science.* 2011;331(6015):337–341.
15. Karimi K, Inman MD, Bienenstock J et al. Lactobacillus reuteri-induced regulatory T cells protect against an allergic airway response in mice. *Am J Respir Crit Care Med.* 2009;179(3):186–193.
16. Trompette A, Gollwitzer ES, Yadava K et al. Gut microbiota metabolism of dietary fiber influences allergic airway disease and hematopoiesis. *Nat Med.* 2014;20(2):159–166.
17. Strachan DP. Hay fever, hygiene, and household size. *BMJ.* 1989;299(6710):1259–1260.
18. Ownby DR, Johnson CC, and Peterson EL. Exposure to dogs and cats in the first year of life and risk of allergic sensitization at 6 to 7 years of age. *JAMA.* 2002;288(8):963–972.
19. Fujimura KE, Johnson CC, Ownby DR et al. Man's best friend? the effect of pet ownership on house dust microbial communities. *J Allergy Clin Immunol.* 2010;126(2):410–2, 412. e1–e3.
20. Ege MJ, Mayer M, Normand AC et al. Exposure to environmental microorganisms and childhood asthma. *N Engl J Med.* 2011;364(8):701–709.
21. Heederik D and von Mutius E. Does diversity of environmental microbial exposure matter for the occurrence of allergy and asthma? *J Allergy Clin Immunol.* 2012;130(1):44–50.
22. Riedler J, Braun-Fahrlander C, Eder W et al. Exposure to farming in early life and development of asthma and allergy: A cross-sectional survey. *Lancet.* 2001;358(9288):1129–1133.
23. Schuijs MJ, Willart MA, Vergote K et al. Farm dust and endotoxin protect against allergy through A20 induction in lung epithelial cells. *Science.* 2015;349(6252):1106–1110.
24. Waser M, Michels KB, Bieli C et al. Inverse association of farm milk consumption with asthma and allergy in rural and suburban populations across Europe. *Clin Exp Allergy.* 2007;37(5):661–670.
25. Bjorksten B, Sepp E, Julge K et al. Allergy development and the intestinal microflora during the first year of life. *J Allergy Clin Immunol.* 2001;108(4):516–520.
26. Kalliomaki M, Kirjavainen P, Eerola E et al. Distinct patterns of neonatal gut microflora in infants in whom atopy was and was not developing. *J Allergy Clin Immunol.* 2001;107(1):129–134.
27. Penders J, Thijs C, van den Brandt PA et al. Gut microbiota composition and development of atopic manifestations in infancy: The KOALA birth cohort study. *Gut.* 2007;56(5):661–667.
28. van Nimwegen FA, Penders J, Stobberingh EE et al. Mode and place of delivery, gastrointestinal microbiota, and their influence on asthma and atopy. *J Allergy Clin Immunol.* 2011;128(5):948–55. e1–e3.
29. Biedermann L, Zeitz J, Mwinyi J et al. Smoking cessation induces profound changes in the composition of the intestinal microbiota in humans. *PLOS ONE.* 2013;8(3):e59260.

30. Barnes PJ. Inflammatory mechanisms in patients with chronic obstructive pulmonary disease. *J Allergy Clin Immunol.* 2016;138(1):16–27.

31. Hilty M, Burke C, Pedro H et al. Disordered microbial communities in asthmatic airways. *PLOS ONE.* 2010;5(1):e8578.

32. Dickson RP and Huffnagle GB. The lung microbiome: New principles for respiratory bacteriology in health and disease. *PLOS Pathog.* 2015;11(7):e1004923.

33. Charlson ES, Bittinger K, Haas AR et al. Topographical continuity of bacterial populations in the healthy human respiratory tract. *Am J Respir Crit Care Med.* 2011;184(8):957–963.

34. Erb-Downward JR, Thompson DL, Han MK et al. Analysis of the lung microbiome in the "healthy" smoker and in COPD. *PLOS ONE.* 2011;6(2):e16384.

35. Sze MA, Dimitriu PA, Hayashi S et al. The lung tissue microbiome in chronic obstructive pulmonary disease. *Am J Respir Crit Care Med.* 2012;185(10):1073–1080.

36. West JB. Regional differences in the lung. *Chest.* 1978;74(4):426–437.

37. Duncan SH, Louis P, Thomson JM et al. The role of pH in determining the species composition of the human colonic microbiota. *Environ Microbiol.* 2009;11(8):2112–2122.

38. Dickson RP, Martinez FJ, and Huffnagle GB. The role of the microbiome in exacerbations of chronic lung diseases. *Lancet.* 2014;384(9944):691–702.

39. Martin RJ, Kraft M, Chu HW et al. A link between chronic asthma and chronic infection. *J Allergy Clin Immunol.* 2001;107(4):595–601.

40. Specjalski K and Jassem E. Chlamydophila pneumoniae, mycoplasma pneumoniae infections, and asthma control. *Allergy Asthma Proc.* 2011;32(2):9–17.

41. Hahn DL, Dodge RW, and Golubjatnikov R. Association of chlamydia pneumoniae (strain TWAR) infection with wheezing, asthmatic bronchitis, and adult-onset asthma. *JAMA.* 1991;266(2):225–230.

42. ten Brinke A, van Dissel JT, Sterk PJ et al. Persistent airflow limitation in adult-onset nonatopic asthma is associated with serologic evidence of chlamydia pneumoniae infection. *J Allergy Clin Immunol.* 2001;107(3):449–454.

43. Bisgaard H, Hermansen MN, Buchvald F et al. Childhood asthma after bacterial colonization of the airway in neonates. *N Engl J Med.* 2007;357(15):1487–1495.

44. Huang YJ, Nelson CE, Brodie EL et al. Airway microbiota and bronchial hyperresponsiveness in patients with suboptimally controlled asthma. *J Allergy Clin Immunol.* 2011;127(2):372–381.e1–e3.

45. Marri PR, Stern DA, Wright AL et al. Asthma-associated differences in microbial composition of induced sputum. *J Allergy Clin Immunol.* 2013;131(2):346–52.e1–e3.

46. Huang YJ, Nariya S, Harris JM et al. The airway microbiome in patients with severe asthma: Associations with disease features and severity. *J Allergy Clin Immunol.* 2015;136(4):874–884.

47. Goleva E, Jackson LP, Harris JK et al. The effects of airway microbiome on corticosteroid responsiveness in asthma. *Am J Respir Crit Care Med.* 2013;188(10):1193–1201.

48. Pragman AA, Kim HB, Reilly CS et al. The lung microbiome in moderate and severe chronic obstructive pulmonary disease. *PLOS ONE.* 2012;7(10):e47305.

49. Huang YJ, Kim E, Cox MJ et al. A persistent and diverse airway microbiota present during chronic obstructive pulmonary disease exacerbations. *OMICS.* 2010;14(1):9–59.

50. Wong EH, Porter JD, Edwards MR et al. The role of macrolides in asthma: Current evidence and future directions. *Lancet Respir Med.* 2014;2(8):657–670.

51. Seemungal T, Harper-Owen R, Bhowmik A et al. Respiratory viruses, symptoms, and inflammatory markers in acute exacerbations and stable chronic obstructive pulmonary disease. *Am J Respir Crit Care Med.* 2001;164(9):1618–1623.

52. Papi A, Bellettato CM, Braccioni F et al. Infections and airway inflammation in chronic obstructive pulmonary disease severe exacerbations. *Am J Respir Crit Care Med.* 2006;173(10):1114–1121.

53. Monso E, Ruiz J, Rosell A et al. Bacterial infection in chronic obstructive pulmonary disease. A study of stable and exacerbated outpatients using the protected specimen brush. *Am J Respir Crit Care Med.* 1995;152(4 pt 1):1316–1320.

54. Bisgaard H, Hermansen MN, and Bonnelykke K. Association of bacteria and viruses with wheezy episodes in young children: Prospective birth cohort study. *BMJ.* 2010;341:c4978.

55. Kloepfer KM, Lee WM, Pappas TE et al. Detection of pathogenic bacteria during rhinovirus infection is associated with increased respiratory symptoms and asthma exacerbations. *J Allergy Clin Immunol.* 2014;133(5):1301–1307, 1307. e1–e3.

56. Rosell A, Monso E, Soler N et al. Microbiologic determinants of exacerbation in chronic obstructive pulmonary disease. *Arch Intern Med.* 2005;165(8):891–897.

57. Sethi S, Evans N, Grant BJ et al. New strains of bacteria and exacerbations of chronic obstructive pulmonary disease. *N Engl J Med.* 2002;347(7):465–471.

58. Millares L, Ferrari R, Gallego M et al. Bronchial microbiome of severe COPD patients colonised by pseudomonas aeruginosa. *Eur J Clin Microbiol Infect Dis.* 2014;33(7):1101–1111.

59. Wang Z, Bafadhel M, Haldar K et al. Lung microbiome dynamics in COPD exacerbations. *Eur Respir J.* 2016;47(4):1082–1092.

60. Molyneaux PL, Mallia P, Cox MJ et al. Outgrowth of the bacterial airway microbiome after rhinovirus exacerbation of chronic obstructive pulmonary disease. *Am J Respir Crit Care Med.* 2013;188(10):1224–1231.

61. Ghebre MA, Bafadhel M, Desai D et al. Biological clustering supports both "dutch" and "british" hypotheses of asthma and chronic obstructive pulmonary disease. *J Allergy Clin Immunol.* 2015;135(1):63–72.

62. Albert RK, Connett J, Bailey WC et al. Azithromycin for prevention of exacerbations of COPD. *N Engl J Med.* 2011;365(8):689–698.

63. Herath SC and Poole P. Prophylactic antibiotic therapy in chronic obstructive pulmonary disease. *JAMA.* 2014;311(21):2225–2226.

64. Kew KM, Undela K, Kotortsi I et al. Macrolides for chronic asthma. *Cochrane Database Syst Rev.* 2015;15(9):CD002997.

65. Gibson PG, Yang IA, Upham JW et al. Effect of azithromycin on asthma exacerbations and quality of life in adults with persistent uncontrolled asthma (AMAZES): A randomised, double-blind, placebo-controlled trial. *Lancet.* 2017;390(10095):659–668.

66. Brusselle GG, Vanderstichele C, Jordens P et al. Azithromycin for prevention of exacerbations in severe asthma (AZISAST): A multicentre randomised double-blind placebo-controlled trial. *Thorax.* 2013;68(4):322–329.

67. Parameswaran GI and Sethi S. Long-term macrolide therapy in chronic obstructive pulmonary disease. *CMAJ.* 2014;186(15):1148–1152.

68. Dickson RP and Morris A. Macrolides, inflammation and the lung microbiome: Untangling the web of causality. *Thorax.* 2017;72(1):10–12.

69. West CE, Renz H, Jenmalm MC et al. The gut microbiota and inflammatory noncommunicable diseases: Associations and potentials for gut microbiota therapies. *J Allergy Clin Immunol.* 2015;135(1):3–13; quiz 14.

70. Anthonisen NR, Manfreda J, Warren CP et al. Antibiotic therapy in exacerbations of chronic obstructive pulmonary disease. *Ann Intern Med.* 1987;106(2):196–204.

71. Vollenweider DJ, Jarrett H, Steurer-Stey CA et al. Antibiotics for exacerbations of chronic obstructive pulmonary disease. *Cochrane Database Syst Rev.* 2012;12:CD010257.

72. Nouira S, Marghli S, Belghith M et al. Once daily oral ofloxacin in chronic obstructive pulmonary disease exacerbation requiring mechanical ventilation: A randomised placebo-controlled trial. *Lancet.* 2001;358(9298):2020–2025.

Exercise in asthma, COPD, and asthma-COPD overlap

LOUIS-PHILIPPE BOULET AND FRANÇOIS MALTAIS

CLINICAL VIGNETTE 10.1: ASTHMA

An 18-year-old man with allergic rhinitis complains of exercise-induced breathlessness and cough, one half hour following exercise. He denies respiratory symptoms at night or on other occasions, except when he is exposed to a cat. His forced expiratory volume in one second (FEV_1) was 88% of the predicted value and chest radiograph was normal. He was prescribed a short-acting β_2-agonist (SABA) to be used 15 minutes before exercise, and this reduced his exercise-induced respiratory symptoms, but he continued to require this treatment before each exercise session. Allergy skin-prick tests revealed sensitization to animal dander and tree pollen. He had no pets at home. His physician recommended he use a low dose of inhaled corticosteroid (ICS) daily. After 1 month, his FEV_1 improved to 96%, and he rarely required his SABA before exercise, unless he trained intensely in cold weather. His symptoms of exercise-induced rhinitis were also controlled with a nasal corticosteroid.

Comment: This case illustrates a typical example of exercise-induced asthma in an atopic mild asthma patient. He required use of an inhaled β_2-agonist before exercise, but when asthma was better controlled with an ICS, symptoms in response to exercise decreased, as did the need for a preventive SABA.

CLINICAL VIGNETTE 10.2: COPD

A 62-year-old woman with established chronic obstructive pulmonary disease (COPD) (FEV_1 = 1.4 L, 60% predicted value) was seen in a COPD clinic. Despite having quit smoking five years earlier and being on optimal bronchodilation therapy, she continued to complain of fatigue, exercise intolerance, and poor quality of life. Her physical exam was unremarkable except for a low body mass index of 19 kg/m². An incremental cycle exercise showed a peak oxygen consumption (VO_2) of 12 mL/kg/min and a peak work capacity of 60 watts. Peak ventilation was 41 L/min, representing 84% of the estimated maximum voluntary ventilation (MVV). A constant-work-rate cycling exercise was performed at a work rate of 80% of her peak capacity (Figure 10.1). Dyspnea and leg fatigue Borg score rose rapidly during the test, leading to early exercise termination at the sixth minute of exercise. This was accompanied by an exhaustion of her ventilatory reserve, while her heart rate only reached 130 beats/min, well below the predicted maximum heart rate (160 beats/min) for a woman of her age. Results from the exercise evaluation were deemed consistent with a diagnosis of COPD. She was subsequently referred to a pulmonary rehabilitation program for a 12-week aerobic and muscle-strengthening exercise program.

This patient felt remarkably improved after 12 weeks of pulmonary rehabilitation despite the fact that her lung function was not modified by the intervention. She reported less fatigue and better exercise tolerance after the program. She completed 30 sessions of exercise training during this program. A typical session for her consisted of 30–40 minutes of aerobic exercises (cycling and walking) and four muscle-strengthening exercises involving the upper and lower extremities. To document the magnitude and mechanisms of improvement, a constant-work-rate cycling exercise test at the same workload that was used during the pre-rehabilitation testing was used. While exercise duration on the bicycle was limited to six minutes before the program, she had to stop at 20 minutes after the program (the maximum duration of the test in the laboratory). At any given exercise time, she reported much less dyspnea and leg fatigue after the training program (Figure 10.1). Consistent with a physiological adaptation to training, ventilatory requirements were reduced during exercise.

Comment: This case illustrates the multifactorial nature of exercise limitation in COPD, including mechanisms such as early dyspnea and ventilatory limitation that are typical in this disease. Also, in a significant proportion of patients such as in this example, limb-muscle fatigue contributes to exercise limitation. Pulmonary rehabilitation that includes exercise training improves exercise tolerance in COPD by addressing several mechanisms of exercise limitation. In the illustrated case, reduced ventilatory requirement at a given exercise level contributed to less dyspnea perception. Also, this patient perceived less leg fatigue during exercise after the training program, a likely result of limb-muscle adaptation to training.

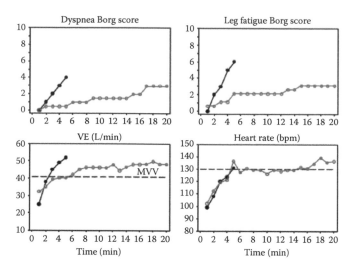

Figure 10.1 Symptomatic (dyspnea and leg fatigue), ventilatory (VE), and heart-rate response in a woman with COPD before (black lines) and after (blue lines) 12 weeks of exercise training. While exercise duration on the bicycle was limited to six minutes before the program, she had to stop at 20 minutes after the program (the maximum duration of the test in the laboratory). The same exercise workload was used on both testing days. At any given exercise time, the patient reported much less dyspnea and leg fatigue after the training program. Her ventilatory requirements were reduced during exercise consistent with a physiological adaptation to exercise training.

CLINICAL VIGNETTE 10.3: ASTHMA-COPD OVERLAP

A 50-year-old woman with a BMI of 32 kg/m², who was diagnosed with allergic asthma since childhood and had smoked approximately 40 pack years, consulted for increasing shortness of breath following exercise. In the past, she only required an occasional bronchodilator when exposed to animals. She was prescribed an ICS but had not been adherent to this treatment. She tried to begin a physical-conditioning program, but in addition to having persistently limited effort tolerance, she often experienced increased dyspnea, chest tightness, and wheezing one half hour following exercise. An inhaled SABA prior to exercise partly relieved her exercise-induced respiratory symptoms. Her FEV_1 was initially 64% predicted (FEV_1/forced vital capacity [FVC]: 54%) with a postbronchodilator FEV_1 improvement of 15% from the prebronchodilator value. Lung volumes showed mild air trapping and carbon monoxide (CO) diffusion capacity was 70% of predicted value. She was prescribed a combination therapy with a moderate dose of ICS and a long-acting β_2-agonist (LABA), which she took regularly for 3 months, and she was referred to an exercise program. On reassessment, her FEV_1 was 72% predicted (FEV_1/FVC: 68%) and she had a significant improvement in exercise tolerance.

Comment: This case illustrates a woman with allergic asthma who developed features of smoking-induced COPD and evidence of significant exercise intolerance that was probably due to her respiratory condition in addition to obesity and deconditioning. Pharmacotherapy in conjunction with an exercise rehabilitation program appeared to be effective at improving her exercise performance.

10.1 INTRODUCTION

Exercise is an essential component of a healthy lifestyle for all, including those with chronic diseases such as respiratory ailments. In asthma, chronic obstructive pulmonary disease (COPD), and asthma-COPD overlap, limitation to perform exercise is a key manifestation of the disease. However, proper management can allow patients afflicted with these conditions to more easily perform regular exercise, resulting in improvement in exercise tolerance and in their general condition. This chapter discusses the prevalence, mechanisms, evaluation, and treatment of exercise intolerance for asthma, COPD, and the overlap.

10.2 ASTHMA

10.2.1 INTRODUCTION

In asthmatic patients, regular exercise improves disease control.[1] However, exercise can also trigger bronchoconstriction. The term "exercise-induced bronchoconstriction" (EIB) is commonly used to describe the narrowing of the airways induced by exercise, associated with or without respiratory symptoms. In contrast, "exercise-induced asthma" (EIA) is used to describe the occurrence of a transient narrowing of the airways after exercise that is reversible following the inhalation of a bronchodilator in an individual with a previous diagnosis of asthma and who is associated with respiratory symptoms.[2] The magnitude of this response will vary according to the individual's condition and type or duration of exercise. EIB could be considered mild if the maximal fall in forced expiratory volume in one second (FEV_1) after exercise is $\geq 10\%$ but $< 25\%$, moderate if $\geq 25\%$ but $< 50\%$, and severe if $\geq 50\%$ for corticosteroid-naive patients or $\geq 30\%$ for corticosteroid-treated patients.[3] According to guidelines, asthma will be considered controlled if patients can perform exercise without limitations or significant symptoms.[4]

10.2.2 PREVALENCE AND DIFFERENTIAL DIAGNOSIS

The majority of subjects with asthma can experience EIA/EIB, depending on their degree of airway responsiveness and the intensity of exercise.[5] The prevalence of EIA, but not necessarily its magnitude, correlates with the severity of asthma, particularly in children.[6] Subjects can present with EIB, which can manifest without a diagnosis of asthma, but EIB can also manifest in unrecognized, undiagnosed cases of asthma, especially in young athletes.[7,8] EIB and EIA should be differentiated from dysfunctional breathing such as exercise-induced laryngeal obstruction (EILO) and its vocal cord dysfunction (VCD) variant, hyperventilation syndrome, other heart and lung diseases, deconditioning in a sedentary person, nasal dyspnea, and a variety of less common conditions (Table 10.1).

10.2.3 MECHANISMS OF AIRWAY RESPONSES IN ASTHMA

When asthma is controlled with normal baseline expiratory flows and airway resistance, the cardiorespiratory demand generated by exercise is similar to that of nonasthmatic

Table 10.1 Conditions associated with exercise-induced symptoms

Condition	Characteristics	Diagnosis	Treatment	Other features
ASTHMA	Dyspnea, cough, wheeze, chest tightness, usually lasting after exercise	Demonstration of variable airway obstruction/ hyperresponsiveness	Bronchodilators and bronchial anti-inflammatory agents	Can be minimized with preventative measures
Vocal cord dysfunction*	Dyspnea, inspiratory stridor Develops during exercise—quickly disappears after exercise	Clinical features: Laryngoscopy (at rest or during exercise/EVH)	Respiratory maneuvers, referral to speech therapist, medications	May be transient. Often associated with psychogenic causes or GERD**
Deconditioning	Dyspnea with low-intensity exercise	Exercise test	Training	Often associated with obesity
Hyperventilation syndrome	High ventilatory rates during exercise or at rest	Clinical features: Often associated with dizziness and paresthesia	Psychological intervention	Low CO_2 during episodes Stress/anxiety contributory

Note: * Also called exercise-induced laryngeal obstruction. ** Gastroesophageal reflux disease.

individuals. However, some asthma patients who are not exercising regularly, sometimes because they are afraid of inducing respiratory symptoms, have a limited exercise capacity amplified by a deconditioning process. When asthma is uncontrolled, expiratory flow obstruction increases the work of breathing. Furthermore, exercise can trigger bronchoconstriction. The main underlying mechanism responsible for this transient airway obstruction induced by exercise is considered to be dehydration of the airways. This is due to water loss from evaporation from the airway surface, following increased ventilation required to meet the metabolic demand imposed by exertion, while large volumes of air are warmed and humidified.[9] The postexercise increase in airway-lining-fluid osmolarity from dehydration may otherwise cause transfer of water out of epithelial cells through aquaporins (water channels), resulting in shrinkage of these cells and increased intracellular ion content. This may then trigger bronchoconstriction through the release of inflammatory mediators, such as histamine and cysteinyl leukotrienes, and possibly neurogenic stimulation of cholinergic pathways. Airway cooling during exercise and postexercise rewarming of the airways following increased blood flow in the airway vasculature, may also contribute to the fall in expiratory flows, but this process does not seem mandatory for inducing EIB. Patients with COPD do not typically experience EIB, probably because they are unable to ventilate large volumes of air and as such, are prevented from dehydrating the airways. In addition, most COPD patients do not characteristically exhibit airway hyperresponsiveness (AHR).

EIA/EIB usually does not begin during exercise. In fact, at the early phase of exercise, there is a reduction in airway resistance, possibly from airway smooth-muscle stretching, reducing airway smooth-muscle tone and/or adrenergic-induced bronchodilatation. The magnitude of fall in expiratory flow is usually a maximum of 10–15 minutes following exercise, and there is a progressive recovery in the next 30–60 minutes or within 5–10 minutes if a rapid-acting SABA or LABA is used. The airway response will be more marked after 6–8 minutes of intense exercise, compared to a more prolonged, less strenuous effort. During exercise, the arterial partial pressure of carbon dioxide (PaO_2) increases, and it decreases during bronchoconstriction while $PaCO_2$ usually remains within normal limits. If exercise is accompanied by exaggerated hyperventilation, $PaCO_2$ may be low however.

Factors that may increase the severity of EIB, other than increased AHR, include poor pulmonary function, dryness of inspired air, short/intense exercise, and the presence of eosinophilic airway inflammation. Previously, a correlation between eosinophilic inflammation and magnitude of EIB has been described.[10]

10.2.4 EVALUATION OF EIA/EIB

An investigation algorithm for EIA/EIB is proposed in Figure 10.2. In the presence of increased variations in expiratory flows or AHR confirmed by bronchoprovocation tests (both indicating the presence of variable airway

Evaluation of exercise-induced asthma

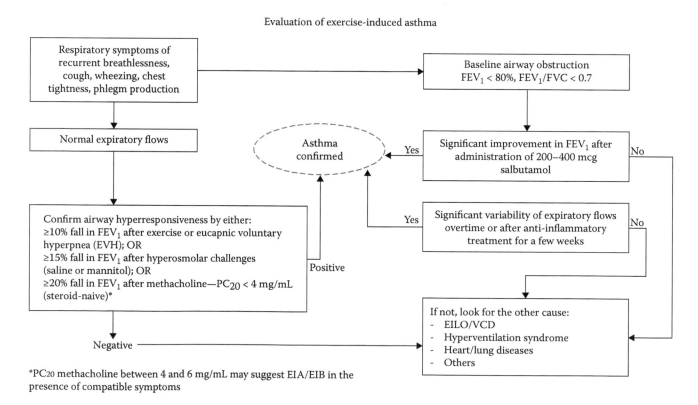

*PC20 methacholine between 4 and 6 mg/mL may suggest EIA/EIB in the presence of compatible symptoms

Figure 10.2 Algorithmic approach for confirming a diagnosis of exercise-induced asthma.

obstruction), exercise-induced symptoms can be generally attributed to asthma. A direct test, acting on airway smooth muscle, such as methacholine challenge, is often used to identify AHR in subjects with normal expiratory flows, but indirect bronchoprovocation tests, acting through the release of inflammatory mediators, such as laboratory or field exercise tests, eucapnic voluntary hyperpnea (EVH) test, or mannitol/hyperosmolar challenge, can also be used.[11] These last two tests mimic the exercise-induced increase in airway-fluid osmolarity. Although less sensitive than methacholine, exercise testing is also used for this purpose, although EVH is increasingly available, in addition to mannitol, in some countries.[12]

If a laboratory exercise test is conducted on either a treadmill or an ergocycle, temperature and humidity conditions should be controlled.[13] A target workload of at least 60%, ideally achieving an increase in heart rate close to 95% of predicted maximum, should be sustained for at least 6–8 minutes.[14] When EVH is used (particularly in young athletes), the subject inhales dry air containing 5% CO_2 for 6 minutes at a ventilation usually at least $21xFEV_1$ if untrained, or higher if in better physical condition. The test is positive when a 10% reduction in FEV_1 or more is observed at least twice after EVH.[15] Finally, a field test reproducing the type of exercise responsible for inducing symptoms can be useful if other tests are negative and suspicion of EIB/EIA is high.[16]

10.2.5 PREVENTION AND TREATMENT

As for the general population, asthmatic subjects should exercise regularly to improve general health and asthma control, but they ideally need to take some preventative measures. It is better to avoid exercising during periods of asthma exacerbations (e.g., following a viral respiratory infection) or during conditions of poor outdoor air quality (e.g., during episodes of high pollutant concentrations, close to traffic-related diesel emission, etc.), in very cold air, or in presence of high levels of airborne allergens to which the subject is sensitized. Indoor pollutants such as NO_2 or ultrafine particles produced by gas-propelled resurfacers in arenas or smoky environments can also affect asthmatic airways. Adequate chlorine levels in pools should be ensured, and swimmers hygiene should be optimized to reduce formation of chloramines.[17] Measures to prevent EIA/EIB should be applied (Table 10.2). A low-intensity, short-duration exercise warmup is suggested; this can help induce a two-hour refractory period to EIB that allows the subject to complete the exercise session.

In addition, various medications can prevent or inhibit exercise-induced symptoms related to EIB/EIA.[18] Inhaled β_2-agonists are highly efficient.[13] The duration of prevention of a SABA against EIB is about 4–6 hours. However, tolerance to the bronchoprotective effects of β_2-agonists develop with regular use, probably in part from downregulation of β_2 receptors on the mast cell, thereby not preventing mediator release as effectively.[19] Thus, SABAs should ideally not be used on a daily basis but intermittently, as a short-term prophylaxis to prevent

Table 10.2 Measures to prevent EIA/EIB

1) Ensure good control of asthma
2) Avoid exercising in the presence of high airborne allergen levels to which the subject is sensitized or if there is a high level of outdoor air pollution
3) Perform warm-up exercises to attenuate responses to exercising outdoors to attenuate responses to environmental determinants
4) Use a SABA one half hour before exercise
5) Use a face mask to prevent cold air–induced asthma if tolerated
6) Consider chronic inhaled corticosteroid use for long-term prevention of exercise-induced symptoms

EIB/EIA. Other drugs such as sodium cromoglycate, leukotriene receptor antagonists (LTRAs), and anticholinergics can reduce the effects of exercise on the airways but β_2-agonists are more potent. Furthermore, sodium cromoglycate in a hydrofluoroalkane metered-dose inhaler, although available in some countries, is not available in the United States. Long-acting β_2-agonists should not be used as monotherapy for prevention of EIB/EIA as there is a risk of deterioration of underlying asthma when not used in conjunction with an ICS.

When improving asthma control with an ICS, airway responses to various stimuli, including exercise, can decrease, and reduce or eliminate the need for preventative short-acting β_2-agonists when the asthmatic person exercises regularly.[20] Antihistamines may help associated rhinitis but are not effective in the prevention of EIB/EIA.

Other measures that have been studied to help reduce EIB include dietary changes and supplements, such as low-salt diet, fish oil, ascorbic acid, and omega 3. Although some reports have shown beneficial effects, more evidence is needed before recommending their use.

10.2.6 ASTHMA IN THE HIGH-LEVEL ATHLETE: A SPECIFIC PHENOTYPE

High-level athletes, especially those participating in endurance sports, despite their equal or superior performances to nonasthmatic subjects when competing, show an increased prevalence of asthma, EIB/EIA, allergic or nonallergic rhinitis, chronic cough, dysfunctional breathing, vocal cord dysfunction, and recurrent respiratory infections.[2] The prevalence of AHR is particularly high in chlorinated-pool swimmers and winter sports athletes, but this does not always translate into physician-diagnosed asthma.

Although the prevalence of atopy is high in athletes, it does not explain entirely the increased prevalence of airway diseases, suggesting that other factors, such as indoor/outdoor pollutants and cold air exposure, play a role. These latter factors may contribute to increased airway mechanical stress and marked dehydration of airway epithelial cells, which may cause airway damage by inducing inflammatory and remodeling processes, as has been observed in athletes without AHR or asthma.[2,21] Although athletes have an increased parasympathetic activity, hypercholinergic responsiveness seems only to modulate AHR.

Specific issues should be considered in the athlete with respect to airway responses induced by exercise (Table 10.3), and these have recently been reviewed extensively elsewhere.[21] Objective measurements, such as those obtained from broncho-provocation tests, are usually required to confirm the diagnosis, and should ideally be conducted during a period of training, as airway responsiveness can normalize out of training season.[22] In athletes, atypical symptoms or poor treatment response should prompt the clinician to revisit the diagnosis of asthma and consider other possible diagnoses including EILO or VCD, which are associated with asthma in up to 50% of individuals. Treatment should be offered according to general asthma guidelines, however World Anti-Doping Agency (WADA) regulations should be adhered to by athletes.[23] Most drugs used to treat asthma except terbutaline and vilanterol are authorized by anti-doping agencies (https://www.wada-ama.org).

10.2.7 CONCLUSION

In asthmatic patients, EIA/EIB may reflect an insufficient control of asthma. These patients should ideally perform regular exercise to improve their general health and asthma control, but preventative measures should be observed. Optimal asthma control will reduce the effects of exercise on the airways. In high-level athletes, EIA/EIB may be considered by many as an occupational disease, and appropriate recommendations and management in this context should be offered. The effects of exercise on asthma are summarized in Table 10.4. For comparative purposes, the effects of exercise on COPD and ACO are also provided.

Table 10.3 Management of asthma in athletes: Special consideration

Difficulties in making the diagnosis Baseline expiratory flows often normal	Usually requires a bronchoprovocation test (sometimes more than one type)—ideally during competition season (may normalize out of training).
Confounding or comorbid conditions	Vocal cord dysfunction, rhinitis-associated symptoms, GERD, or hyperventilation syndrome should be recognized.
Adjustment of asthma therapy	Undertreatment and overtreatment seem common in the athlete—objective tests are required.
Tolerance to β_2-agonists may develop	Use of rescue β_2-agonists should be minimized in ensuring good asthma control (usually with ICS).
Environmental control may be difficult	Whenever possible, should avoid exercising in periods of poor air quality, in very cold air, or if there is a risk of intense exposure to airborne allergens.
Requirements by sports authorities	These should be checked (WADA website).

Table 10.4 Comparative effects of exercise on asthma, COPD, and ACO

Feature	ASTHMA	COPD	ACO
Effect			
- short-term	Possible bronchoconstriction	Variable dyspnea	Variable dyspnea
- long-term (regular exercise)	Improved control and exercise tolerance	Improved exercise tolerance	Improved exercise tolerance
Main mechanism	Dehydration of airways	Reduced lung function/gas exchange abnormalities	Undetermined—probably a mixture of both
Preventative measures	Ensure good asthma control (regular ICS*) Warmup before exercise Short-acting β_2-agonist before exercise Avoid exercising during pollutants/relevant allergen exposure	Regular bronchodilator use	Regular bronchodilator/controller medication
Treatment of acute episodes	Short-acting β_2-agonist	Short-acting β_2-agonist	Short-acting β_2-agonist
Contraindications	Preferably to avoid during acute exacerbations/intense pollutant or allergen exposures	Avoid during acute exacerbations	Avoid during acute exacerbations

* May reduce airways response to exercise over time

10.3 COPD

10.3.1 INTRODUCTION

Exercise intolerance is almost universal in chronic obstructive pulmonary disease (COPD), and it has been reported even in mild disease.[24] Exercise intolerance results from a complex and variable interaction between symptoms, ventilatory and respiratory mechanics impairment, gas-exchange limitations, and peripheral muscle fatigue.[25-27] In this section, we will use a clinical vignette to discuss the mechanisms of exercise intolerance and show how to approach this consequence of COPD from a therapeutic standpoint.

10.3.2 SYMPTOM PERCEPTION DURING EXERCISE

From the patient's perspective, poor functional status can be explained by the discomfort experienced while performing various activities of daily living. The two symptoms most commonly cited by COPD patients as the main reason for exercise termination are dyspnea and leg fatigue.[28,29] However, the intensity of symptom perception for a given exercise level is higher in COPD compared to controls.[30] Limiting symptoms are thus reached at a lower intensity in COPD patients[28,30] and are described differently than in healthy individuals.[31,32] Phrases denoting an "increased work/effort of breathing" and "heaviness of breathing" are commonly used by both healthy and diseased individuals to describe exertional dyspnea, but descriptors of "increased inspiratory difficulty," "unsatisfied inspiratory effort," and "shallow breathing" appear to be specific to patients with COPD.[31,32] This qualitatively distinct sensation of exertional dyspnea is believed to be linked to the presence of hyperinflation in these patients.[32] Indeed, the intensity of exertional dyspnea correlates with the degree of dynamic hyperinflation experienced by COPD patients. In general, the perception of dyspnea is more intense than that of leg fatigue in patients with moderate to severe COPD, while the reverse is often seen in milder disease.[28,33]

10.3.3 VENTILATORY LIMITATION

Expiratory flow limitation in COPD is the hallmark feature of COPD and is related to reduced airway caliber and loss of lung elastic recoil. Ventilatory capacity, which is largely determined by expiratory flow rates,[34] is therefore reduced in patients with COPD. In contrast to healthy individuals, ventilation ($\dot{V}_E$) frequently reaches maximum voluntary ventilation as estimated from resting FEV_1 in this population.[34,35] In addition to reduced ventilatory capacity, ventilatory requirements are often increased at submaximal exercise in patients with COPD, due to higher dead space ventilation and inefficient gas exchange. The unfortunate combination of reduced ventilatory capacity and increased ventilatory requirement correlate with premature

exhaustion of the ventilatory reserve, an important factor in early exercise termination in COPD.

10.3.4 PHYSIOLOGICAL DETERMINANTS OF DYSPNEA

The intensity of dyspnea is intimately linked to the pressure generated by respiratory muscles during tidal breathing as a function of the maximum pressure available.[36] In COPD, this ratio could be increased by greater airway resistances or alternatively, by intrinsically or functionally weakened respiratory muscles, which would work at a higher proportion of their capacity even if normal efforts are made during tidal breathing. Dynamic hyperinflation and its related consequences on respiratory muscles are involved in the pathogenesis of dyspnea and exercise intolerance in COPD, which will be discussed further in Section 10.3.5.

10.3.5 DYNAMIC HYPERINFLATION

At rest and during exercise, healthy individuals breathe within the maximal envelope of the flow-volume relationship such that inspiratory and expiratory flows can be easily increased to accommodate the ventilatory requirements of exercise. In these individuals, end-expiratory volume remains stable or decreases during exercise,[37,38] as reflected by an increased inspiratory capacity with exercise. The physiological benefits of this reduction in end-expiratory lung volume could be to place the diaphragm in a more advantageous position in terms of its length-tension relationship and to store elastic energy in the chest wall during expiration, which when released during inspiration could assist the respiratory muscles.[39] In patients with COPD, the ability to increase inspiratory and expiratory flows is compromised because patients are often already breathing on some parts of the maximum flow-volume loop envelope at rest, in mild to moderate to advanced diseases.[40-42] This problem can be overcome, at least temporarily, by breathing at higher lung volumes, thereby permitting greater expiratory flows to be generated.[40-42] In fact, an increase in end-expiratory lung volume is seen in the majority of patients with COPD, translating into a progressive reduction in inspiratory capacity as exercise proceeds.[38] This one positive consequence of dynamic hyperinflation (i.e., to allow patients to increase ventilation) is not without important disadvantages.

Dynamic hyperinflation limits the expansion in tidal volume once end-inspiratory lung volume reaches a critical zone in the vicinity of 500 mL of total lung capacity.[43,44] At such high end-inspiratory volume, dyspnea rises exponentially leading to rapid exercise termination.[43,44] Breathing at high lung volumes also implies that a portion of tidal breathing will occur on the flat portion of the lung volume-pressure relationship thereby increasing work of breathing. An important concept is that dynamic hyperinflation uncouples the relationship between respiratory effort and the resulting tidal volume.[43] In other words, respiratory efforts will not be rewarded appropriately in terms of the tidal volume generated during the breath, as indicated by a marked increase in esophageal pressure excursion to tidal volume ratio in patients with COPD compared to healthy controls.[43] This phenomenon, referred to as neuromechanical uncoupling, is a strong determinant of dyspnea.[43] Dynamic hyperinflation also places the diaphragm in an unfavorable portion of its length-tension relationship, further compromising its role as the main pressure generator during inspiration. As a result of both the increased work of breathing and the weakened respiratory muscles, a higher fraction of the respiratory muscle strength will be used to generate tidal breathing, another contributor to dyspnea.[43]

These physiological concepts have been tested in clinical trials evaluating the impact of long acting bronchodilation on exercise tolerance.[45,46] In these studies, the impact of bronchodilation on operating lung volumes and dyspnea during exercise, as well as on the endurance to constant-work-rate cycling exercise was assessed. Bronchodilation markedly reduced end-expiratory lung volume at rest allowing patients to tolerate the exercise stimulus for a longer period of time. In these trials, the reduction in operational lung volumes, the decrease in dyspnea, and the improvement in exercise tolerance were all tightly interrelated, providing a strong clinical validation of physiological concepts supporting the role of dynamic hyperinflation on functional status in COPD.

10.3.6 LIMB MUSCLE FATIGUE

Despite the presence of ventilatory limitation and dynamic hyperinflation, up to a third of patients with COPD are limited by leg fatigue and not by dyspnea during exercise.[28,29] The COPD case study described in this chapter exemplifies this situation where leg fatigue Borg score was superior to the dyspnea score. This information is relevant because the response to bronchodilation may be suboptimal in patients complaining of leg fatigue as their main exercise limiting symptom.[47,48] In these patients, treatment of the peripheral muscles in combination with pharmacological interventions should be incorporated into the management plan. Muscle fatigue in COPD has been linked to certain peripheral muscle alterations, such as poor oxidative capacity, muscle atrophy, and muscle weakness, which are commonly observed in this disease and which increase susceptibility to contractile fatigue.[49]

10.3.7 INTERACTIONS BETWEEN LIMB MUSCLES AND THE RESPIRATORY SYSTEM

An appealing concept is that the peripheral and central components of exercise limitation may interact with each other to further reduce exercise tolerance. As of now, only indirect evidence exists to support this notion in patients with COPD, and research is this field is needed. One obvious possible mechanism for this interaction between the peripheral muscles and the respiratory system is that metabolic changes occurring in the fatiguing muscles lead to early acidosis[50,51] and likely contribute to the increase ventilatory requirement during exercise.[52] This imposes an additional burden on the respiratory muscles already facing increased impedance to breathing.

Moreover, there could be a steal phenomenon of blood from the peripheral muscles toward the respiratory muscles that would leave both muscle groups with insufficient perfusion and oxygenation during exercise. This competition for blood flow between the respiratory and contracting peripheral muscles has been described elegantly in athletes in whom unloading the respiratory muscles using noninvasive ventilatory support improved blood flow and oxygen transport to the contracting locomotor muscles[53,54] while reducing quadriceps fatigability.[55] Only indirect proofs of this phenomenon are currently available in patients with COPD. Consistent with these notions, Amann and colleagues reported that unloading the respiratory muscles during constant-work-rate cycling exercise was associated with reduced quadriceps fatigue in patients with COPD.[56] Although limb-muscle blood flow was not measured in this study, this report is consistent with a redirection of blood flow from the respiratory muscles with unloading toward the contacting limb muscles, thereby reducing the degree of muscle fatigue.

During fatiguing exercise, feedback from the lower limb muscle mechano- and metabo-sensitive receptors modulates central motor output via the activation of group III and IV muscle afferents.[57,58] One important role of this neural pathway that detects the changes in muscle metabolism and the accumulation of several chemical products in the extracellular environment during exercise is to modulate the level of muscle fatigue.[57,58] This pathway is also implicated in the regulation of the ventilatory and cardiovascular responses to exercise.[57,58] In patients with COPD, spinal anesthesia, presumably blocking group III/IV sensory afferents from the lower limb muscles, was associated with improved exercise tolerance during constant-work-rate cycling exercise by reducing the perception of leg fatigue and attenuating the ventilatory response during exercise.[59] Thus, there are several interrelated mechanisms by which muscle fatigue can contribute to exercise limitation in COPD patients. Some act directly on the muscle contraction process and others through their effects on both the cardiorespiratory and nervous systems. This discussion highlights the importance of considering exercise intolerance in COPD from an integrative perspective, considering the interplay between the ventilatory and cardiovascular systems, the limb muscles, and the central nervous system.

10.3.8 RELATIVE CONTRIBUTION OF EXERCISE-LIMITING FACTORS

The relative contribution of ventilatory mechanics and peripheral muscle fatigue as limiting factors to exercise tolerance varies according to individual factors. As described earlier, the locus of symptom limitation is not uniform among patients with COPD. Likewise, the physiological response to exercise is not homogeneous in this disease. For example, although dynamic hyperinflation may occur in as many as 80% of patients with moderate-to-severe airflow obstruction[38] the increase in end-expiratory lung volumes during exercise varies in magnitude from patient to patient.[60] Contractile leg fatigue occurs in approximately 60% of COPD patients after cycling exercise.[29,61] Apart from the individual factors, the relative contribution of peripheral and central factors of exercise limitation is also influenced by the exercise modality used for testing.[29,62] Leg fatigue, alone or in combination with dyspnea, is predominant during both incremental and constant-load cycling exercise,[29] while dyspnea outweighs leg fatigue as a limiting symptom during walking protocols.[29]

10.3.9 EVALUATION OF EXERCISE INTOLERANCE

Considering the key role of exercise intolerance in the pathophysiology and course of COPD, the evaluation of exercise tolerance should now be included in the assessment of this disease.[63] Exercise testing can be used to document the functional impact of the disease and to better understand the physiopathological mechanisms involved in exercise intolerance. This functional characterization is crucial; the relationship between resting indices of respiratory function and exercise tolerance is, at best, modest. Exercise testing can also be used to quantify the impact of pharmacological and nonpharmacological interventions to improve exercise tolerance[64–66] or dyspnea,[67,68] and in the preoperative assessment of patients.[69]

Several exercise protocols are available for the evaluation of patients with COPD, and they have been reviewed extensively elsewhere.[63,66,70,71] Incremental exercise-testing protocols involving cycling or walking exercise methodologies (also called cardiopulmonary exercise testing when coupled with physiological measurements) are currently considered as the "gold standard" method for the evaluation of the degree of exercise limitation and to investigate the mechanisms of exercise limitation. One limitation of the incremental exercise protocols is that they are not the ideal methodology as evaluative tools due to their limited responsiveness to intervention.[70]

Cycling or walking constant-work-rate exercise protocols are gaining popularity in clinical and research settings because of their established responsiveness to interventions.[45,65,70] Constant-work-rate endurance protocols are based on externally imposed and constant cycling or walking cadence that the patient has to maintain until exhaustion. The primary endpoint of these protocols is thus the endurance time (or the distance which is a product of the speed and time). These tests are usually performed at a high fraction of peak exercise capacity, typically 75%–85% of peak capacity.[66]

Due to the constraints relative to incremental exercise testing protocols and their being more representative of the daily activities performed by patients with COPD, field tests have been developed as more simple tools for the evaluation of exercise capacity. The self-paced walking test, particularly the six-minute walking test (6MWT), is the most popular field test when it comes to the evaluation of patients with COPD. The 6MWT is not the most responsive tool to evaluate the effects of interventions (pulmonary rehabilitation and bronchodilation) on exercise tolerance in patients with COPD.[70] However, it has good discriminative properties, particularly to quantify the functional consequences of COPD, a good predictive value in estimating vital prognosis.[71]

10.3.10 PREVENTION AND TREATMENTS

10.3.10.1 Pharmacotherapy

Optimal bronchodilation is the foundation of COPD pharmacological therapy. LABA and long-acting muscarinic antagonists are effective in improving cycling exercise tolerance in COPD.[45,46,72–74] In well-designed clinical trials, bronchodilators have been convincingly shown to reduce operating lung volume at rest and during exercise and to improve the endurance time to submaximal cycling exercise in COPD.[45,46,72–74] Breathing at lower operative lung volumes will allow larger expansion in tidal volume (VT), a major determinant of exercise tolerance in COPD.[75] This ability to expand VT reflects a lesser mechanical ventilatory constraint in relation to the increased resting and exercising inspiratory capacity and inspiratory reserve volume.[43] From the patient perspective, breathing at lower operative volumes, farther from total lung capacity, has a tremendous impact in reducing the perception of dyspnea.[45,46,72–74]

10.3.10.2 Exercise training and pulmonary rehabilitation

Despite optimal bronchodilation, exercise intolerance persists in most patients with COPD and there is a need to further improve this component of the disease. Exercise training, delivered in the context of pulmonary rehabilitation is the most effective therapy to improve exercise tolerance in COPD.[76] It typically involves a combination of aerobic exercises, such as walking or cycling, in addition to muscle-strengthening exercises.[77] Program duration ranges from 8 to 12 weeks, at a rate of 2–3 weekly sessions. Exercise training enhances exercise tolerance through different mechanisms other than bronchodilation. Exercise training does not modify lung function, as least in the short term. The improvement in exercise tolerance seen after exercise training in patients with COPD is related to a multitude of factors, including desensitization to dyspnea, improved limb-muscle function and oxidative capacity, and reduced fatigue susceptibility.[78–80] In addition to treating peripheral muscles, exercise training may also alleviate the central component of exercise intolerance in COPD. In fact, a reduced ventilatory requirement at a given exercise level is one of the first-reported evidence of physiological adaptation following exercise training in COPD.[52] As a result, exercise-induced dynamic hyperinflation is diminished,[81,82] an important consideration given its negative impact on exercise tolerance in COPD. The synergistic interactions between pharmacotherapy and rehabilitation are interesting to consider, and it is only through combination therapy that optimization of the functional status will occur.[83] On one hand, optimal bronchodilation facilitates the tolerance to higher training intensities during the rehabilitation program while patients may be enabled to take full advantage of bronchodilation with exercise training, which addresses the peripheral component of exercise intolerance. Despite the indisputable efficacy of exercise training and pulmonary rehabilitation, there are still too few patients who are enrolled in these programs.[84] Additionally, translating the gains in exercise capacity seen during the program into more participation in daily life remains an important challenge for the future.

10.3.11 CONCLUSION

Exercise intolerance is a ubiquitous clinical manifestation of COPD, and it negatively impacts quality of life and survival in this disease. The causes and mechanisms of exercise intolerance in patients with COPD are complex and involve symptoms, ventilatory and respiratory mechanics impairment, gas-exchange limitations, and limb-muscle impairment. The mechanisms of exercise limitation are heterogeneous within the COPD population, highlighting the importance of comprehensive exercise testing (assessing cardiopulmonary and muscular contributions to exercise limitation) in this patient population. Consistent with its multifactorial origins, it is only through combination therapy that includes bronchodilation and exercise training that optimization of the functional status can be obtained in COPD.

10.4 ASTHMA-COPD OVERLAP

10.4.1 INTRODUCTION

The term "asthma-COPD overlap (ACO)" is often used when features of asthma and COPD are present in the same patient.[85] There has recently been a marked interest in this condition as it became evident that we needed data on the population that is usually excluded from clinical trials and that is associated with frequent health care utilization, as well as marked morbidity and mortality. However, there are limited data on optimal management of ACO. Currently, management of this overlapping condition depends on the

predominant features in a given individual, although with respect to pharmacotherapy, the combined used of an ICS and a long-acting bronchodilator is probably the best initial treatment for most patients. An exhaustive review of possible pharmacotherapy of these patients has been reviewed in Chapter 17 of this book.[86] Prevalence, magnitude, and mechanisms of exercise tolerance in well-phenotyped patients with asthma-COPD overlap remain to be studied.

Data on exercise capacity in patients with ACO is conflicting, with some reports suggesting reduced performance compared to patients with asthma or COPD, whereas others show no significant differences in six-minute walking test (6MWT) nor in the level of physical activity.[87–89] In this last study, the decline over 4 years in exercise capacity, assessed by the 6MWT, was less pronounced in the ACO group compared to the COPD group.[87,89] In a cross-sectional study based on the "COPD Gene Study," Hardin et al. looked at a subgroup of 450 patients classified as ACO.[88] The BODE index (Body Mass Index, Obstruction, Dyspnea, Exercise Capacity) was slightly higher (indicating worse health status) in the ACO group compared to COPD, but this did not approach the clinically minimal important difference (MID) for this variable. This could possibly reflect differences in the MIDs for some subphenotypes of ACO, but this remains to be determined.

10.4.2 MECHANISMS

In ACOS, exertional dyspnea is usually persistent but can show some variability similar to asthma. Exercise intolerance in these patients is probably due to mechanisms that are relevant for asthma and COPD, but this needs to be studied.

10.4.3 MANAGEMENT

The main objective for managing exercise-induced symptoms in ACO is to help improve exercise tolerance in addition to antagonize acute exercise-induced symptoms, similar to asthma and COPD. Although the optimal management of ACO remains to be determined, current pharmacological guidelines suggest a regular dose of ICS/LABA and/or a long-duration anticholinergic can help reduce respiratory symptoms. Furthermore, nonpharmacological measures such as smoking cessation, treatment of comorbidities, environmental measures, regular exercise, and weight loss when overweight or obese, should be recommended. Although further studies on the effects of rehabilitation programs in the ACO population are needed, initial reports suggest a benefit of these programs.[90]

10.4.4 CONCLUSION

ACO shares many features of both diseases, but more research is required to elucidate exercise-induced airway responses in this population.

10.5 GENERAL CONCLUSION

Regular exercise can improve disease control in chronic airway obstructive diseases, but often these patients show exercise intolerance due to various mechanisms elaborated on in this chapter. It is mandatory for the clinician to assess their patients' responses to exercise and then to propose interventions that will improve exercise performance and reduce the effect of exercise on airway function. Although much is known about exercise intolerance in asthma and COPD, more information is required on this topic in patients with ACO.

REFERENCES

1. Eichenberger PA, Diener SN, Kofmehl R et al. Effects of exercise training on airway hyperreactivity in asthma: A systematic review and meta-analysis. *Sports Med.* 2013;43:1157–1170.
2. Fitch KD, Sue-Chu M, Anderson SD et al. Asthma and the elite athlete: Summary of the International Olympic Committee's consensus conference, Lausanne, Switzerland, January 22–24, 2008. *J Allergy ClinImmunol.* 2008;122:254–260.
3. Anderson SD and Kippelen P. Assessment of EIB: What You Need to Know to Optimize Test Results. *Immunol Allergy Clin North Am.* 2013;33:363–380.
4. Global Initiative for Asthma. Global Strategy for Asthma Management and Prevention, 2016. Available from: www.ginasthma.org.
5. Del Giacco SR, Firinu D, Bjermer L et al. Exercise and asthma: An overview. *Eur Clin Respir J.* 2015;2:27984.
6. Cabral AL, Conceicao GM, Fonseca-Guedes CH et al. Exercise-induced bronchospasm in children: Effects of asthma severity. *Am J Respir Crit Care Med.* 1999;159:1819–1823.
7. Ulrik CS, and Backer V. Increased bronchial responsiveness to exercise as a risk factor for symptomatic asthma: Findings from a longitudinal population study of children and adolescents. Eur Respir J: *Official J Eur Society Clin Respir Physiol.* 1996;9:1696–1700.
8. Kukafka DS, Lang DM, Porter S et al. Exercise-induced bronchospasm in high school athletes via a free running test: Incidence and epidemiology. *Chest.* 1998;114:1613–1622.
9. Anderson SD, and Kippelen P. Exercise-induced bronchoconstriction: Pathogenesis. *Curr Allergy Asthma Rep.* 2005;5:116–122.
10. Duong M, Subbarao P, Adelroth E et al. Sputum eosinophils and the response of exercise-induced bronchoconstriction to corticosteroid in asthma. *Chest.* 2008;133:404–411.
11. Anderson SD, Charlton B, Weiler JM et al. Comparison of mannitol and methacholine to predict exercise-induced bronchoconstriction and a clinical diagnosis of asthma. *Respir Res.* 2009;10:4.
12. Pasnick SD, Carlos WG 3rd, Arunachalam A et al. Exercise-induced bronchoconstriction. *Ann Am Thorac Soc.* 2014;11:1651–1652.
13. Parsons JP, Hallstrand TS, Mastronarde JG et al. An official American Thoracic Society clinical practice guideline: Exercise-induced bronchoconstriction. *Am J Respir Crit Care Med.* 2013;187:1016–1027.
14. Weiler JM, Anderson SD, Randolph C et al. Pathogenesis, prevalence, diagnosis, and management of exercise-induced bronchoconstriction: A practice parameter. *Ann Allergy Asthma Immunol.* 2010;105:S1–47.
15. Bougault V, Turmel J, and Boulet LP. Bronchial challenges and respiratory symptoms in elite swimmers and winter sport athletes: Airway hyperresponsiveness in asthma: Its measurement and clinical significance. *Chest.* 2010;138:31S–37S.
16. Rundell KW, Wilber RL, Szmedra L et al. Exercise-induced asthma screening of elite athletes: Field versus laboratory exercise challenge. *Med Sci Sports Exerc.* 2000;32:309–316.
17. Bougault V, Boulet LP. Airways disorders and the swimming pool. *Immunol Allergy Clin North Am.* August 2013;33(3):395–408.
18. Carlsen KH, Anderson SD, Bjermer L et al. Treatment of exercise-induced asthma, respiratory and allergic disorders in sports and the relationship to doping: Part II of the report from the Joint Task Force of European Respiratory Society (ERS) and European Academy of Allergy and Clinical Immunology (EAACI) in cooperation with GA(2)LEN. *Allergy.* 2008;63:492–505.
19. Hancox RJ, Subbarao P, Kamada D et al. Beta2-agonist tolerance and exercise-induced bronchospasm. *Am J Respir Crit Care Med.* 2002;165:1068–1070.
20. Koh MS, Tee A, Lasserson TJ et al. Inhaled corticosteroids compared to placebo for prevention of exercise induced bronchoconstriction. *Cochrane Database Syst Rev.* 2007;3:CD002739.
21. Boulet LP and O'Byrne PM. Asthma and exercise-induced bronchoconstriction in athletes. *N Eng J Med.* 2015;372:641–648.
22. Bougault V, Turmel J, and Boulet LP. Airway hyperresponsiveness in elite swimmers: Is it a transient phenomenon? *J Allergy ClinImmunol.* 2011;127:892–898.
23. World Anti-Doping Agency. World Anti-doping program. Available at https://www.wada-ama.org.
24. Gagnon P, Casaburi R, Saey D et al. Cluster analysis in patients with GOLD 1 chronic obstructive pulmonary disease. *PLOS ONE.* 2015;10:e0123626.
25. O'Donnell DE and Webb KA. The major limitation to exercise performance in COPD is dynamic hyperinflation. *J Appl Physiol (1985).* 2008;105:753–755; discussion 55–57.
26. Aliverti A and Macklem PT. The major limitation to exercise performance in COPD is inadequate energy supply to the respiratory and locomotor muscles. *J Appl Physiol (1985).* 2008;105:749–751; discussion 55–57.

27. Debigare R and Maltais F. The major limitation to exercise performance in COPD is lower limb muscle dysfunction. *J Appl Physiol (1985)*. 2008;105:751–753; discussion 55–57.

28. Killian KJ, Leblanc P, Martin DH et al. Exercise capacity and ventilatory, circulatory, and symptom limitation in patients with chronic airflow limitation. *Am Rev Respir Dis*. 1992;146:935–940.

29. Pepin V, Saey D, Whittom F et al. Walking versus cycling: Sensitivity to bronchodilation in chronic obstructive pulmonary disease. *Am J Respir Crit Care Med*. 2005;172:1517–1522.

30. Hamilton AL, Killian KJ, Summers E et al. Muscle strength, symptom intensity, and exercise capacity in patients with cardiorespiratory disorders. *Am J Respir Crit Care Med*. 1995;152:2021–2031.

31. Mahler DA, Harver A, Lentine T et al. Descriptors of breathlessness in cardiorespiratory diseases. American journal of respiratory and critical care medicine. 1996;154:1357–1363.

32. O'Donnell DE, Bertley JC, Chau LK et al. Qualitative aspects of exertional breathlessness in chronic airflow limitation: Pathophysiologic mechanisms. *Am J RespiCrit Care Med*. 1997;155:109–115.

33. O'Donnell DE, Laveneziana P, Ora J et al. Evaluation of acute bronchodilator reversibility in patients with symptoms of GOLD stage I COPD. *Thorax*. 2009;64:216–223.

34. Hyatt RE, Schilder DP, and Fry DL. Relationship between maximum expiratory flow and degree of lung inflation. *J Applied Physiol*. 1958;13:331–336.

35. Potter WA, Olafsson S, and Hyatt RE. Ventilatory mechanics and expiratory flow limitation during exercise in patients with obstructive lung disease. *J Clin Invest*. 1971;50:910–919.

36. Leblanc P, Bowie DM, Summers E et al. Breathlessness and exercise in patients with cardiorespiratory disease. *Am Rev Respir Dis*. 1986;133:21–25.

37. Babb TG and Rodarte JR. Exercise capacity and breathing mechanics in patients with airflow limitation. *Med Sci Sports Exerc*. 1992;24:967–974.

38. O'Donnell DE, Revill SM, and Webb KA. Dynamic hyperinflation and exercise intolerance in chronic obstructive pulmonary disease. *Am J Respir Crit Care Med*. 2001;164:770–777.

39. Dodd DS, Brancatisano T, and Engel LA. Chest wall mechanics during exercise in patients with severe chronic air-flow obstruction. *Am Rev Respir Dis*. 1984;129:33–38.

40. Grimby G and Stiksa J. Flow-volume curves and breathing patterns during exercise in patients with obstructive lung disease. *Scand J Clinic Lab Invest*. 1970;25:303–313.

41. Stubbing DG, Pengelly LD, Morse JL et al. Pulmonary mechanics during exercise in subjects with chronic airflow obstruction. *J Appl Physiol Respir Environ Exerc Physiol*. 1980;49:511–515.

42. Babb TG, Viggiano R, Hurley B et al. Effect of mild-to-moderate airflow limitation on exercise capacity. *J Appl Physiol (1985)*. 1991;70:223–230.

43. O'Donnell DE, Hamilton AL, and Webb KA. Sensory-mechanical relationships during high-intensity, constant-work-rate exercise in COPD. *J Appl Physiol (1985)*. 2006;101:1025–1035.

44. Casaburi R and Rennard SI. Exercise limitation in chronic obstructive pulmonary disease. The O'Donnell threshold. *Am J Respir Crit Care Med*. 2015;191:873–875.

45. O'Donnell DE, Fluge T, Gerken F et al. Effects of tiotropium on lung hyperinflation, dyspnoea and exercise tolerance in COPD. Eur Respir J. 2004;23:832–840.

46. Maltais F, Hamilton A, Marciniuk D et al. Improvements in symptom-limited exercise performance over 8 h with once-daily tiotropium in patients with COPD. *Chest*. 2005;128:1168–1178.

47. Saey D, Debigaré R, LeBlanc P et al. Contractile leg fatigue after cycle exercise: A factor limiting exercise in patients with chronic obstructive pulmonary disease. *Am J Respir Crit Care Med*. 2003;168:425–430.

48. Deschenes D, Pepin V, Saey D et al. Locus of symptom limitation and exercise response to bronchodilation in chronic obstructive pulmonary disease. *J Cardiopul Rehabil Prev*. 2008;28:208–214.

49. Maltais F, Decramer M, Casaburi R et al. An official American thoracic society/European respiratory society statement: Update on limb muscle dysfunction in chronic obstructive pulmonary disease. *Am J Respir Crit Care Med*. 2014;189:e15–62.

50. Maltais F, Jobin J, Sullivan MJ et al. Metabolic and hemodynamic responses of lower limb during exercise in patients with COPD. *J Appl Physiol (1985)*. 1998;84:1573–1580.

51. Sala E, Roca J, Marrades RM et al. Effects of endurance training on skeletal muscle bioenergetics in chronic obstructive pulmonary disease. *Am J Respir Crit Care Med*. 1999;159:1726–1734.

52. Casaburi R, Patessio A, Ioli F et al. Reductions in exercise lactic acidosis and ventilation as a result of exercise training in patients with obstructive lung disease. *Am Rev Respir Dis*. 1991;143:9–18.

53. Harms CA, Wetter TJ, McClaran SR et al. Effects of respiratory muscle work on cardiac output and its distribution during maximal exercise. *J Appl Physiol (1985)*. 1998;85:609–618.

54. Harms CA, Babcock MA, McClaran SR et al. Respiratory muscle work compromises leg blood flow during maximal exercise. *J Appl Physiol (1985)*. 1997;82:1573–1583.

55. Romer LM, Lovering AT, Haverkamp HC et al. Effect of inspiratory muscle work on peripheral fatigue of locomotor muscles in healthy humans. *J Physiol*. 2006;571:425–439.

56. Amann M, Regan MS, Kobitary M et al. Impact of pulmonary system limitations on locomotor muscle fatigue in patients with COPD. *Am J Physiol RegulIntegr Comp Physiol.* 2010;299:R314–324.

57. Amann M, Proctor LT, Sebranek JJ et al. Opioid-mediated muscle afferents inhibit central motor drive and limit peripheral muscle fatigue development in humans. *J Physiol.* 2009;587:271–283.

58. Rotto DM and Kaufman MP. Effect of metabolic products of muscular contraction on discharge of group III and IV afferents. *J Appl Physiol (1985).* 1988;64:2306–2313.

59. Gagnon P, Bussieres JS, Ribeiro F et al. Influences of spinal anesthesia on exercise tolerance in patients with chronic obstructive pulmonary disease. *Am J Respir Crit Care Med.* 2012;186:606–615.

60. O'Donnell DE, Travers J, Webb KA et al. Reliability of ventilatory parameters during cycle ergometry in multicentre trials in COPD. *Eur Respir J.* 2009;34:866–874.

61. Saey D, Michaud A, Couillard A et al. Contractile fatigue, muscle morphometry, and blood lactate in chronic obstructive pulmonary disease. *Am J Respir Crit Care Med.* 2005;171:1109–1115.

62. Man WD, Soliman MG, Gearing J et al. Symptoms and quadriceps fatigability after walking and cycling in chronic obstructive pulmonary disease. *Am J Respir Crit Care Med.* 2003;168:562–567.

63. American Thoracic S, American College of Chest P. ATS/ACCP Statement on cardiopulmonary exercise testing. *Am J Respir Crit Care Med.* 2003;167:211–277.

64. Aguilaniu B. Impact of bronchodilator therapy on exercise tolerance in COPD. *Int J Chron Obstruct Pulm Dis.* 2010;5:57–71.

65. Laviolette L, Bourbeau J, Bernard S et al. Assessing the impact of pulmonary rehabilitation on functional status in COPD. *Thorax.* 2008;63:115–121.

66. Puente-Maestu L, Palange P, Casaburi R et al. Use of exercise testing in the evaluation of interventional efficacy: An official ERS statement. *Eur Respir J.* 2016;47:429–460.

67. Dyspnea. Mechanisms, assessment, and management: A consensus statement. American Thoracic Society. *Am J Respir Crit Care Med.* 1999;159:321–340.

68. Perrault H, Baril J, Henophy S et al. Paced-walk and step tests to assess exertional dyspnea in COPD. *COPD.* 2009;6:330–339.

69. Brunelli A, Charloux A, Bolliger CT et al. ERS/ESTS clinical guidelines on fitness for radical therapy in lung cancer patients (surgery and chemo-radiotherapy). *Eur Res J.* 2009;34:17–41.

70. Borel B, Provencher S, Saey D et al. Responsiveness of various exercise-testing protocols to therapeutic interventions in COPD. *Pulm Med.* 2013;2013:410748.

71. Singh SJ, Puhan MA, Andrianopoulos V et al. An official systematic review of the European Respiratory Society/American thoracic society: Measurement properties of field walking tests in chronic respiratory disease. *Eur Respir J.* 2014;44:1447–1478.

72. O'Donnell DE, Voduc N, Fitzpatrick M et al. Effect of salmeterol on the ventilatory response to exercise in chronic obstructive pulmonary disease. *Eur Respir J.* 2004;24:86–94.

73. Maltais F, Celli B, Casaburi R et al. Aclidinium bromide improves exercise endurance and lung hyperinflation in patients with moderate to severe COPD. *Respir Med.* 2011;105:580–587.

74. Beeh KM, Korn S, Beier J et al. Effect of QVA149 on lung volumes and exercise tolerance in COPD patients: The BRIGHT study. *Respir Med.* 2014;108:584–592.

75. O'Donnell DE, Lam M, and Webb KA. Spirometric correlates of improvement in exercise performance after anticholinergic therapy in chronic obstructive pulmonary disease. *Am J Respir Crit Care Med.* 1999;160:542–549.

76. McCarthy B, Casey D, Devane D et al. Pulmonary rehabilitation for chronic obstructive pulmonary disease. *Cochrane Database Syst Rev* 2015;2:CD003793.

77. Spruit MA, Singh SJ, Garvey C et al. An official American Thoracic Society/European Respiratory Society statement: Key concepts and advances in pulmonary rehabilitation. *Am J Respir Crit Care Med.* 2013;188:e13–64.

78. Maltais F, LeBlanc P, Simard C et al. Skeletal muscle adaptation to endurance training in patients with chronic obstructive pulmonary disease. *Am J Respir Crit Care Med.* 1996;154:442–447.

79. Bernard S, Whittom F, Leblanc P et al. Aerobic and strength training in patients with chronic obstructive pulmonary disease. *Am J Respir Crit Care Med.* 1999;159:896–901.

80. Casaburi R and ZuWallack R. Pulmonary rehabilitation for management of chronic obstructive pulmonary disease. *N Engl J Med.* 2009;360:1329–1335.

81. Gigliotti F, Coli C, Bianchi R et al. Exercise training improves exertional dyspnea in patients with COPD: Evidence of the role of mechanical factors. *Chest.* 2003;123:1794–802.

82. Porszasz J, Emtner M, Goto S et al. Exercise training decreases ventilatory requirements and exercise-induced hyperinflation at submaximal intensities in patients with COPD. *Chest.* 2005;128:2025–2034.

83. Casaburi R, Kukafka D, Cooper CB et al. Improvement in exercise tolerance with the combination of tiotropium and pulmonary rehabilitation in patients with COPD. *Chest.* 2005;127:809–817.

84. Rochester CL, Vogiatzis I, Holland AE et al. An official American thoracic Society/European respiratory society policy statement: Enhancing implementation, use, and delivery of pulmonary rehabilitation. *Am J Respir Crit Care Med.* 2015;192:1373–1386.

85. Postma DS and van den Berge M. The different faces of the asthma-COPD overlap syndrome. *Eur Respir J.* 2015;46:587–590.

86. Barnes PJ. Therapeutic approaches to asthma-|chronic obstructive pulmonary disease overlap syndromes. *J Allergy Clin Immunol.* 2015;136:531–545.

87. Kumbhare S, Pleasants R, Ohar JA et al. Characteristics and prevalence of Asthma/Chronic obstructive pulmonary disease overlap in the United States. *Ann Am Thorac Soc* 2016.

88. Miravitlles M, Soriano JB, Ancochea J et al. Characterisation of the overlap COPD-asthma phenotype. Focus on physical activity and health status. *Respir Med.* 2013;107:1053–1060.

89. Fu JJ, Gibson PG, Simpson JL et al. Longitudinal changes in clinical outcomes in older patients with asthma, COPD and asthma-COPD overlap syndrome. *Respir.* 2014;87:63–74.

90. Nici L and ZuWallack R. Pulmonary rehabilitation for patients with chronic airways obstruction. *J Allergy Clin Immunol Pract.* 2015;3:512–518.

Occupational-related asthma, COPD, and asthma-COPD overlap

KARIN A. PACHECO AND LISA A. MAIER

11.1 INTRODUCTION

Asthma, chronic obstructive pulmonary disease (COPD), and asthma-COPD overlap syndrome or ACO are not well differentiated in the occupational literature. However, many occupational obstructive lung disease syndromes have a number of features that are suggestive of and meet the current clinical criteria for ACO. The workplace exposures causing occupational asthma and occupational COPD have been intensively investigated and reported, and it is likely that some of these exposures are also responsible for the development of ACO in a subset of susceptible workers. Further, exposures to combinations of particulates, gases, vapors, dusts, irritants, and allergens are known to cause ACO, and many such "mixed" exposures are found in the workplace. In addition, epidemiological studies implicate occupational exposures as risk factors for ACO. Indeed, the many phenotypes of ACO likely reflect the effects of differing exposures modulated by host characteristics. It is important to identify occupations and workplace exposures that are risk factors for ACO, as this not only establishes the etiologies of the disease, but may impact prognosis, recommendations for removal from exposure, and workers' benefits. As an example, workers with ACO have been documented to experience the highest frequency of pulmonary symptoms, use

more respiratory medications, develop more frequent respiratory exacerbations, are more likely to require hospitalization, and report worse quality of life[1] than those with either asthma or COPD alone. Similar to published work on other occupational lung diseases, removal from exposure may be necessary to prevent progression of disease. This makes identification of the source of exposure critical, and most importantly, provides the potential to reduce exposure for other workers, thereby preventing occurrences of future disease. In this chapter, the definition of ACO used is an obstructive airways disease with evidence of partial reversibility via inhaled bronchodilator, along with persistent airflow obstruction. Given the lack of studies that have examined occupational exposure risks specifically for ACO, studies that describe exposures associated with airflow obstruction and/or COPD will be included in this review, as it is likely that some such exposures may also cause ACO that was not considered as a specific outcome at the time. This chapter will review some of the epidemiological studies that identify specific occupations and exposures as risk factors for ACO, as well as general exposures quantified as vapors, dusts, gases, and fumes. We will then proceed to discuss specific workplace exposures with the best documentation for causing potential ACO. Finally, specific jobs and exposures with limited documentation, but nonetheless suggestive of causing ACO, will be examined.

11.2 EPIDEMIOLOGY

The ability of occupational exposures to ozone, grain, cotton, and other vegetable-fiber dust to cause airways obstruction in workers was recognized in a May 1981 review.[2] Another review published in May 1990[3] expanded the array of occupations and exposures capable of causing nonspecific airways obstruction and indicated that many of these exposures were also associated with increases in airways responsiveness, consistent with what we now call ACO. The expanded list of occupations included those working with organic dusts, such as farmers; swine producers; grain workers; and cotton, hemp, flax, and jute workers. Other workers exposed to nonorganic dusts causing obstructive lung disease separate from pneumoconiosis included coal miners and other coal workers, gold miners, and workers exposed to cement dust. Respiratory irritants such as ammonia, nitrogen dioxide, phosgene, chlorine gas, sulfur dioxide, and ozone, were also listed as causative of obstructive lung disease. Other irritant gases associated with the development of airways obstruction include hydrogen chloride, hydrogen bromide and bromine, fluorine, hydrogen fluoride, and fluoride.[4] As a result, it is prudent to identify such exposures to determine whether they cause ACO, initiate direct health surveillance programs, and support efforts to reduce or eliminate these and other harmful exposures, such as cigarette smoking.

More recently, several large cohort studies have further assessed risk factors for obstructive lung disease and ACO. The European Community Respiratory Health Survey characterized a random subsample of young adults with current asthma that included 218 with ACO, 166 with COPD, and 5,659 without a respiratory diagnosis. Occupational exposure to vapors, dust, gas, or fumes was reported by 42% of the healthy group, 46% of the asthma-only group, 44% of the ACO group, and 57% of the COPD-only group ($p < 0.001$ across groups).[5]

The Swiss Cohort Study on Air Pollution and Lung and Heart Disease in Adults (SAPALDIA) evaluated 4,267 non-asthmatic subjects for COPD and noted that the incidence of mild COPD was significantly higher in nonsmokers exposed to mineral dusts compared to nonsmoking, unexposed subjects, while exposure to biological dusts was associated with more severe COPD (forced expiratory volume in one second [FEV_1] < 80% predicted) in ever-smokers.[6] As response to bronchodilator was not measured, it is not possible to determine who among these individuals might have developed ACO, although it is reasonable to assume that some did. A more specific assessment of occupations associated with COPD risk was analyzed in the UK Biobank cohort study of 228,614 participants. Again, because bronchodilator response was not measured, it is not possible to determine which portion of the COPD group had ACO; however, the highest prevalence ratios (PR > 1.5) of COPD were found in seafarers, coal mine operatives, industrial cleaners, roofers, packers and bottlers, and workers in the horticultural trades (Table 11.1).[7] These studies suggest occupations where the presence of ACO should be further investigated. Furthermore, a general review of risk factors for the development of ACO reports exposure to noxious particles and gases, mainly tobacco smoke and biomass fuels.[8] The 2017 monograph jointly published by GINA and GOLD[9] recommends that part of the standard clinical evaluation of patients with ACO should include reviewing exposures to environmental hazards, both occupational and domestic exposures to airborne pollutants.

11.3 BIOLOGICAL DUSTS

Biological dusts and aerosols often contain both allergens and adjuvants that, along with irritants, may trigger a syndrome of increased respiratory inflammation and lead to both fixed and reversible airflow obstruction in susceptible workers. Interestingly, an earlier study of asthmatic patients with a component of irreversible airflow limitation (i.e., patients who would meet the definition of ACO), found that occupational sensitization and continued exposure to the causative agent was associated with more rapid decline in lung function and poorer outcomes.[10,11] A cross-sectional study of 1,232 subjects in Australia found a similar effect of biological dusts on prevalence of respiratory symptoms and obstructive airways disease. The effects of exposure to different categories of dusts, including biological, mineral, gaseous, vapor, and fume, were compared. Biological dusts were found to be significantly associated with morning cough, dyspnea, chronic obstructive bronchitis, and COPD.[12] The associations were similar in ever-smokers and in never-smokers for all conditions and exposures, suggesting that cigarette smoking had at best a minor effect on the observed relationships. The job categories with biological dust exposure included nurses and other health workers, food and textile workers, artists, and cleaners.

11.3.1 COTTON AND OTHER TEXTILE WORKERS

Byssinosis, also known as Monday fever, brown lung disease, mill fever, or cotton workers' lung, is an occupational lung disease that primarily affects workers in cotton processing, as well as hemp and flax industries. Cotton dust–related obstructive lung disease has been shown to demonstrate characteristics of both asthma and COPD consistent with ACO.[13] Specifically, disease that develops early in exposure demonstrates airway hyperresponsiveness and reversible airflow obstruction. Although both atopic and nonatopic workers are affected, atopic workers demonstrate a greater effect. Follow-up over time with continued exposure demonstrates chronic and progressive dyspnea, cough, and sputum production characteristic of COPD and chronic bronchitis. Longitudinal decline in FEV_1 is accelerated compared to unexposed controls, even in nonsmokers and after retirement. Exposures to cotton dust are not trivial, ranging from 0.2 to 1.6 mg/m^3 in Chinese cotton mills, although this

Table 11.1 Overview of individual agents causing occupational asthma and/or COPD

Single Agents		
Agent	**Types**	**Example sources**
Acids	Acetic, hydrochloric, hydrofluoric, nitric, perchloric acids	Mineral analysis lab, chemical spill, lead acid batteries, bleach and ammonia
Acrylates	Alkyl cyanoacrylates, cyanoacrylate glue, methacrylate, methyl 2-cyanoacrylate, methyl methacrylate	Industrial use of adhesives
Aluminum salts	Aluminum fluoride, aluminum sulfate	Soldering aluminum cables
2-Ethanolamine (Amino-ethyl-ethanolamine)	Triethanolamine Monoethanolamine	Metal working fluid, cleaners
3-amino-5-mercapto-1,2,4-triazole	Pharmaceutical and pesticide intermediate	Factory workers
Ammonia	Ammonium chloride, ammonium thioglycolate	Soldering flux, rubber, lacquer, shellac, beauty industries
Anhydrides	Phthalic anhydride, tetrachlorophthalic anhydride, trimellitic anhydride, maleic anhydride	Production of epoxy resins, flame retardant
Polyfunctional aziridine	Water-based crosslinker in two-component paints, paint primers, lacquers, topcoats, and other protective coatings	Painters
Azobisformamide (azodicarbonamide)	Expanding and blowing agent for resins and rubbers	Plastics processing, pigment grinder
Benzalkonium chloride	Fumes	Cleaning solutions
Cadmium	Fumes	Battery workers, pigment manufacture
Chloramine T	Cleaning product/disinfectant	Food industry
Chlorine		Paper and pulp mills, bleaching
Chromate	Also in cement	Stone cutting, electroplating
Cobalt	Multiple	Production workers, hard metal workers, diamond polishers
Ethylenediamine		Color photo development
Formaldehyde	Gas, dust	Production of urea formaldehyde resin, embalming, anatomic dissection labs
Glutaraldehyde	Glutaral	Endoscopy, radiography
Isocyanates, isocyanurate	Diphenylmethane diisocyanate (MDI); Hexamethylene diisocyanate (HDI); Toluene diisocyanate (TDI), isophorone diisocyanate (IPDI), isodurane diisocyanate; methyl isocyanate, prepolymers, polymethyl-methacrylate(Plexiglas powder)	Foundry workers, wood products, polyurethane foam production, spray painters, car repair
Nickel sulfate	Anhydrous hexahydrate	Electroplating
Nitrogen chloride	Nitrogen trichloride, trichloramine	Pool workers
Paraquat	Herbicide	Farm workers
Persulfate	Ammonium, potassium and ammonium peroxydisulfate, diammonium peroxodisulfate	Hairdressers, Persulfate production
Platinum salts		Catalyst production, refineries, pharmaceuticals

(Continued)

Table 11.1 (*Continued*) Overview of individual agents causing OA and/or COPD

Single Agents		
Agent	**Types**	**Example sources**
Polyethylene; Polypropylene		Shrink wrapping, electrical cable repair
Polyvinyl chloride	Fumes	Plastic building and flooring materials
Rosin core solder (colophony)	Thermal decomposition products	Soldering fumes
Sodium iso-nonanoyl oxybenzene sulphonate	Detergents	
Sodium metabisulfite		Fish and prawn processing industry
Styrene monomer		Fiberglass molding
Sulfur dioxide		Sulfite mills, paper and pulp production, antioxidants in food production
Terpene	(3-carene)	Pine resin, sawmills, woodshops
Tetramethrin	(1-(5-tretrazoly)-4-guanly-tetrazene hydrate)	Exterminators, related to Pyrethrin
Uranium hexafluoride	Used in uranium enrichment process	
Vanadium	Divanadium pentoxide	Vanadium pentoxide production, boilers of oil-fired power plants
Zinc	Fumes	Soldering on galvanized metal
Mixed Agents		
Cement		
Chlorofluorocarbons	Degradation products	
Cleaning agents	Detergents not otherwise specified	
Coffee, green		
Cotton, dust, raw		
Cutting oil, lubricants	Not otherwise specified	
Diesel exhaust		
Endotoxin		
Environmental tobacco smoke		
Grain		
Paint	Fumes	
Pesticides	Not otherwise specified	
Potroom aluminum smelting		
Reactive dyes		
Refractory ceramic fibers		
Smoke, fires, pyrolysis products	Oil fire and dust storm, indoor biomass	
Soldering flux fumes	Potassium ammonium tetrafluoride flux	Soldering aluminum cables
Solvents	Not otherwise specified	
Tear gas		
Welding fumes		
Worksite or Profession		
Construction work dust		
Farming	Various crops, livestock, poultry confinement, swine confinement	
Foundry workers		
Health care workers		
World Trade Center disaster 2001		

Source: Modified from Baur X. et al., *J Occup Med Toxicol.*, 7, 19, 2012.

is decreasing over time. Endotoxin exposures, in contrast, have increased over time, with a peak level of 12,038 EU/m^3 in 1992, compared to 2,580 EU/m^3 in 1981.[14]

11.3.2 COTTON TEXTILE WORKER WITH ACO

CLINICAL VIGNETTE 11.1

A 41-year-old woman has worked at a cotton textile company in Huzhou, China, for the past 20 years. Before beginning work, she had no history of asthma, allergies, or cigarette use. She first worked in the carding room, where the carding machines were open to the air, and the room was very dusty. Here, cotton fibers were separated to form a thick, continuous, untwisted strand called sliver, while discarding impurities. After a few months, she noticed occasional episodes of fever and muscle aches at the end of the workday. About 10 years after beginning work, she developed chest tightness and shortness of breath on the first day back to work after 2 days off. Initially, symptoms were intermittent, but then occurred consistently on return to work. About a year later, she developed a chronic cough with occasional sputum production. A methacholine challenge performed at the end of a work shift was positive with a provocative concentration of methacholine causing a 20% fall in the FEV$_1$ (PC20 FEV$_1$) of 1.1 mg/mL. She was treated with an inhaled bronchodilator and continued working in the carding room for a total of 11 years, when she was then able to change jobs to work in the drawing and roving rooms. Here, the cotton sliver was fed through a draw frame machine, which pulled it between rollers to thin the thread, and then twisted and loaded these onto bobbins. These machines had no dedicated ventilation, and the air was filled with cotton dust. Her symptoms worsened, and the chest tightness and shortness of breath began to persist over the six-day work period, although they remitted somewhat during the 2 days off. After 7 years, she was promoted to work in the weaving room, where she continues to work presently. Although the weaving process is mechanized, workers maintain the machines and keep looms supplied with cotton yarn. Although her respiratory symptoms are less severe in this environment, they are constant, and no longer improve away from work on weekends. Current symptoms include cough, wheezing, chest tightness, and mild sputum production. Compared to her baseline spirometry obtained 20 years ago when she began work, her current FEV$_1$ has fallen by 55 mL/year, compared to 25 mL/year expected. She has no plans to change employment.

This case exemplifies the long-term impact of employment in cotton manufacturing, with increased risk for onset of respiratory symptoms, decreases in spirometry, and increases in bronchial hyperreactivity. A study of 85 symptomatic workers from six Lancashire County, England, cotton-spinning mills compared their symptom history and lung function to 84 asymptomatic controls. Workers with byssinosis ($n = 23$) showed the greatest losses of FEV$_1$ and forced vital capacity (FVC) compared to predicted, and were most likely to have bronchial hyperresponsiveness (BHR): 78% compared to 38% of 56 symptomatic workers without byssinosis, and 17% of 84 asymptomatic controls.[15] Other potential factors affecting lung function, including atopy and smoking, were similarly distributed between the groups. Overall, workers with bronchial hyperreactivity were significantly older, had spent a longer time working in the cotton industry, and had higher mean cumulative dust exposure, suggesting a causative relationship. Cotton workers also have accelerated loss of lung function, measured in one longitudinal study at 42 mL/year in FEV$_1$ compared to 25 mL/year in unexposed controls, $p < 0.001$, with smokers demonstrating the highest rates of symptoms and lung-function loss.[16]

Manufacturing hemp and jute rope similarly exposes workers to plant dust mixed with endotoxin, with similar risk for chronic respiratory symptoms and lung-function decline. Airborne dust and endotoxins measured in two jute rope factories between April 1997 and August 1998 found area dust concentrations from 0.06 mg/m^3 to 2.69 mg/m^3 (vs. an Occupational Safety and Health Administration [OSHA] permissible exposure limit [PEL] of 0.2 mg/m^3), and peak endotoxin concentrations estimated at 1,600 EU/m^3. Employees with symptoms consistent with byssinosis and with persistent symptoms after retirement were more likely to have worked in areas of high dust and have lower airflow. In current workers, the highest odds ratios (ORs) for chronic bronchitis (6.1), byssinosis (8.9), and emphysema (12.0) were seen in current smokers who worked in high dust areas, and the effect was multiplicative compared to either risk factor alone.

Retirement, or moving out of cotton dust exposure, does not immediately halt the excess respiratory symptoms and decline in lung function for these workers. A prospective study of 383 cotton textile workers with at least 3 years of exposure at entry found a persistently accelerated decline in FEV$_1$ and FVC, and a significantly higher frequency of respiratory symptoms after retirement ($n = 180$) compared to those remaining in the mills ($n = 101$). Of 71 male cotton workers retired for the 6 years of the study, 53% reported chronic bronchitis, 55% had significant dyspnea, and 59% had partial or total impairment compared to 23%, 18%, and 31% of 51 current male workers ($0.001 \leq p \geq 0.01$).[16] However, the higher rates of lung-function decline in retired cotton workers appear to slow after about 8 years. A 15-year follow-up of 447 Chinese cotton textile workers found that retired cotton workers initially had greater decreases in FEV$_1$ and FVC at initial follow-up compared to active workers, but a smaller decline at the third follow-up visit. After 8 years of retirement, the annual FEV$_1$ decline in cotton workers had slowed to match that of unexposed silk workers. In addition, airflow obstruction resolved in 14% of retired cotton workers compared to 9% of active workers,[17] while risk for respiratory symptoms (chest tightness, chronic bronchitis, chronic cough, and dyspnea) also declined with increasing years away from exposure.[18]

11.3.2.1 Is it cotton dust or endotoxin?

Cotton textile workers are exposed to high levels of cotton dust, bacteria, fungi, and endotoxin contaminating the unprocessed cotton bolls, all of which may affect respiratory symptoms and lung function, begging the question as to which agent(s) are likely causing ACO. In an experimental challenge study, selected cotton workers were exposed to different kinds of cotton while airborne concentrations of viable fungi, total bacteria, gram-negative bacteria, elutriated dust, and endotoxin were measured, and correlated with pre- and postexposure spirometry. Although all exposures, except for fungi, correlated with decreases in FEV_1, endotoxin was the most highly correlated ($r = -0.94$, $p < 0.00001$).[19] Higher past cumulative exposures to endotoxin were associated with reduced levels of FEV_1 in retired cotton workers, although higher recent (within 5 years) endotoxin exposure was most commonly associated with chronic cough, chronic bronchitis, and byssinosis.[20] In contrast, the longitudinal study of Chinese cotton workers described above[18] found that cumulative dust, but not endotoxin, was associated with an 11-year loss in FEV_1.[14] Since cotton dust and endotoxin tend to be correlated, it may be difficult to distinguish their effects.[21]

The mechanisms underlying the endotoxin effects were elucidated in a murine model of persistent airflow obstruction resulting from chronic endotoxin exposure. Similar to workers, all endotoxin-exposed mice developed increased airway hyperresponsiveness compared to control mice. After 8 weeks, the exposed mice also showed increased markers of lung inflammation, including more neutrophils, CD4 + and CD8 + T cells, CD19 + B cells, inflammatory myeloid CD11b + lung dendritic cells, and IL-6.[22] Such animal models may also help us tease apart the complex mechanisms and specific exposures important in the pathogenesis of ACO.

11.4 SWINE CONFINEMENT AND DAIRY WORKERS

Animal confinement workers and dairy farmers are exposed to complex bioaerosols that include animal allergens, grain and other plant feed components, endotoxin and animal waste products, bacteria, and fungi, analogous to textile workers. They similarly demonstrate a high prevalence of respiratory symptoms, airflow limitation, and BHR consistent with ACO.

11.4.1 ACO IN A CATTLE FEEDLOT WORKER

CLINICAL VIGNETTE 11.2

A 44-year-old man presented with worsening severe dyspnea over the past 3–4 years. He had a history of childhood asthma (age 5–8 years) that resolved during his teens and 20s, not requiring medication. In his 30s, he began working on farms; over the past 4 years, he worked exclusively on a large feedlot with roughly 100,000 head of cattle. He noted recurrence of asthma-like symptoms of shortness of breath, cough, wheeze, and dyspnea, and was started on an inhaled corticosteroid (ICS) inhaler and a rescue short-acting bronchodilator (SABA). Despite treatment, he started having "asthma attacks" while working at the feedlot, one requiring air flight evacuation and intubation 1 years prior. In the past year, he had been seen in the emergency room six times for asthma, and for the past 2 years had been treated with a daily prednisone dose of approximately 20 mg, along with high-dose ICS/long-acting bronchodilator (LABA), and an inhaled SABA as needed. He admitted that his breathing was greatly worsened at work. His medical history was also significant for gastroesophageal reflux disease (GERD), joint pain, and obesity. He was a never-smoker, married with three children, and had an outdoor dog and five outdoor cats. His exam only revealed normal to diminished breath sounds without wheezes or crackles. Laboratory evaluation showed an elevated immunoglobulin E (IgE) of 301 kU/L (normal 0–100), positive skin-prick tests to cat and environmental molds, but not to trees, grasses, weeds, cattle, pigs, or horses. The absolute eosinophil count was 800 (> 500 abnormal). Lung function showed airflow obstruction: FEV_1/FVC ratio 60%; FEV_1 2.48 L (60% predicted); FVC 4.12 (71%), with a partial (19%) improvement of the FEV_1 after a SABA. A chest computed tomography (CT) showed air trapping.

He was started on omalizumab, a monoclonal IgG anti-IgE therapy, montelukast, nonsedating long-acting antihistamines, and a nasal corticosteroid. After 3 months, he left livestock work to pursue a higher education degree. One month after quitting the feedlot, he was completely weaned off prednisone. During his last follow-up, the FEV_1 and FVC improved to 2.95 (70%) and 4.92 (85%), respectively but the FEV_1/FVC remained obstructed at 60%.

Farmers directly exposed to animals, for example in swine-confinement facilities and in dairies as exemplified by our case, have a high frequency of respiratory symptoms and BHR, as well as an accelerated decline in FEV_1 and the FEV_1/FVC ratio. Review of the existing research, which has investigated changes in lung function in response to animal organic dust exposure, suggests that overlapping features of COPD and asthma exist in affected workers, and they may represent ACO. Several studies have demonstrated airflow obstruction and increased bronchial hyperreactivity in swine farmers and swine-confinement workers compared to unexposed controls. For example, a comparison of 47 Danish swine farmers reporting asthma (group I) to 63 farmers reporting wheezing, shortness of breath, or dry cough (group II) and 34 farmers without respiratory symptoms (group III) found a higher prevalence of $FEV_1 < 95\%$ predicted in groups I (43%) and II (23%), compared to 0% in group III, although bronchial hyperreactivity was found in all three groups. Pig farmers with symptoms in group II also manifested an accelerated loss of FEV_1 that was predicted by the logPC20 and number of years in pig farming.[23] Influenza-like symptoms, cough, and throat irritation are common in swine and dairy farmers, while chest tightness and eye irritation are mainly reported by swine farmers, as compared to greenhouse workers. In these swine and dairy farmers, the methacholine PC20 FEV_1 was significantly lower and associated with the number of years worked in the trade ($p < 0.05$),[24] although cross-shift changes in FEV_1 were small. Similarly, a comparison of 20 Hutterite swine farmers matched to 20 controls found a higher prevalence of respiratory symptoms, significantly lower FEV_1 (97% vs. 103%, $p < 0.03$), and significantly lower PC20 in the swine farmers.[25]

Signs of COPD and chronic bronchitis are also more frequent in swine-confinement workers and dairy farmers than in comparison populations.[26] A study of 60 swine-confinement workers from Quebec, Canada, found that those with chronic bronchitis symptoms *and* airflow limitation had a significantly lower FEV_1 (89%), lower FEV_1/FVC ratio (82%), signs of hyperinflation (total lung capacity [TLC] 111%) and air trapping (residual volume [RV] 148%), as well as the lowest methacholine PC20 FEV_1 compared to farmers with symptoms only, airflow obstruction only, or neither.[27] Work in swine-confinement buildings also has been shown to cause an accelerated decline in FEV_1 compared to dairy barns, as evidenced by a seven-year longitudinal Danish study demonstrating an annual decline of 54 mL in FEV_1 in swine farmers compared to 42 mL in dairy farmers ($p = 0.045$); this response was more pronounced in the nonsmoking farmers (53 mL vs. 36 mL; $p = -0.018$).[28] Similarly, in a study of 194 French dairy farmers, 13% reported chronic bronchitis, 10% reported acute bronchitis, and 37% reported dyspnea, compared to 7%, 4%, and 14% of 155 controls respectively. A subgroup of 45-year-old male farmers also demonstrated a greater annual decline in mean vital capacity (VC) (−73 mL vs. 53 mL, $p < 0.05$) and FEV_1 (−59 mL vs. −34 mL, $p < 0.01$) compared to unexposed controls,[29] with little evidence of reversibility. Concurrently, the same group reported statistically significant increases in ever-wheezing (OR 2.7; $p < 0.05$), wheezing within the last year (OR 5.2; $p < 0.025$), usual morning cough (OR 5.0; $p < 0.001$), usual morning phlegm (OR 11.3; $p < 0.0001$), and chronic bronchitis (OR 11.8; $p < 0.01$). Cigarette smoking and dairy farm exposure had an additive effect on symptoms.[30] A longitudinal analysis also demonstrated an accelerated decline in FEV_1/VC ($p < 0.025$) in dairy farmers after adjustment for age, smoking, sex, height, log IgE, altitude, and initial respiratory function values.[31] Declines in FEV_1 ($p < 0.05$) and the spO2 ($p < 0.025$) were significantly associated with the mean duration of dairy farming, and especially work on traditional farms that did not dry the hay or heat the barn,[32]

suggesting a potential causative exposure for the observed difference. Taken together, these findings demonstrate a high prevalence of respiratory symptoms, airflow limitation, BHR, and accelerated decline in FEV_1 consistent with ACO in these animal-exposed workers.

11.5 GRAIN WORKERS

Workers in grain processing and the animal feed industry are similarly exposed to a potent mixture of organic dusts that include grain antigens, storage mites and other insect parts, bacteria, fungi, and endotoxins. Not surprisingly, exposed workers have also been shown to have both accelerated declines in FEV_1 consistent with COPD and an increased prevalence of nonspecific BHR consistent with asthma, thus suggesting ACO. One longitudinal analysis of Canadian grain handlers identified specific risk factors for the increased decline in $FEV_1 > 100$ mL/year as being BHR and a fall in the FEV_1 over the course of the work week, which together imply the presence of ACO. Grain workers exposed to the highest dust concentrations, cleaners, and sweepers were most likely to demonstrate these findings.[33] A cross-sectional study of 315 Dutch animal feed workers that found that FEV_1 and FVC were significantly lower (by 70 mL and 64 mL respectively) in those exposed to the highest dust concentrations (> 9 mg/mL), implies a similar effect of exposure on lung function deterioration.[34] Most notably, both respiratory symptoms and airflow were more related to present and historic endotoxin exposure than to the respirable dust fraction.[33] Workers with an overall mean endotoxin level of ≥ 25 ng/m^3 demonstrated an FEV_1 decreased by 122 mL, an FVC lower by 112 mL, and a peak expiratory flow (PEF) lower by 910 mL/s compared to workers in lower endotoxin-exposure categories. A five-year follow-up study of the original participants corroborated the initial findings, noting that the presence of respiratory symptoms in the first survey strongly predicted subsequent loss to follow-up, suggesting that the respiratory effects of grain dust exposure was underrepresented in a longitudinal cohort.[34]

Increased nonspecific bronchial hyperreactivity is also more common in grain handlers compared to unexposed controls. A study of 29 nonsmoking grain handlers with an average of 14 exposure years found that 45% of workers reported cough, sputum, dyspnea, and wheeze compared to 17% of the nonsmoking control subjects, and symptoms were associated with a significantly lower mean histamine PC35 in the exposed group ($p < 0.05$ for both comparisons).[35] Specific inhalational challenge to nebulized corn dust extract reproduced the symptoms and cross-shift decreases in lung function found in grain workers in the workplace. Even nonatopic, nonasthmatic, and nonsmoking grain handlers demonstrated a 15%–20% fall in FEV_1 and FVC, and FEV_1/FVC obstruction to 71% for 5 hours after grain dust challenge, associated with significantly increased neutrophils in blood and bronchoalveolar lavage (BAL), along with increased BAL IL1β, IL-1 RA, IL-6, IL-8, and TNF-α.[36] Taken together, the acute, cross-shift worsening of airflow, accompanied by a decline in baseline airflow over time and increased prevalence of BHR, are characteristic of ACO in long-term exposed grain workers.

11.5.1 OTHER ORGANIC DUST EXPOSURES

Exposure to other organic aerosols in an occupational setting may also be associated with the development of chronic airflow obstruction and BHR characteristic of ACO. A study of Croatian workers exposed to a range of organic dusts such as coffee, tea, spices, soy, fur, or animal food, found that chronic respiratory symptoms, including cough, phlegm, bronchitis, dyspnea, nasal drainage, and sinusitis, were significantly more common compared to unexposed controls ($p < 0.01$), and were aggravated by cigarette smoking. Workers demonstrated both acute and chronic airflow obstruction, and in some, work-related symptoms were more intense at the beginning of the work week or after a long absence from work, suggestive of a Monday-morning effect.[37]

11.6 BIOMASS

The chronic inhalation of biomass fuel is associated with respiratory issues worldwide, with estimates of almost 3 billion exposed people. Biomass fuel refers to plant- and animal-based material that has been recently derived, such as wood, grass, charcoal, crop residues, and dried animal dung, which is burned for energy. Chronic biomass exposures are associated with a number of airways diseases, including chronic bronchitis, COPD, asthma, and ACO. Insofar as biomass fuel exposure may be occupational, the related development of ACO is included in this section.

11.6.1 ACO IN A BIOMASS SMOKE–EXPOSED WORKER

CLINICAL VIGNETTE 11.3

A 75-year-old woman presented with a two-year-history of progressive breathlessness. She recalls wheezing, cough, and episodes of "bronchitis" since her 20s, but the symptoms have become more noticeable over the past 15 years since she moved to Albuquerque, New Mexico, from Mexico. She never smoked cigarettes and had no secondhand tobacco exposure. However, she was exposed to wood smoke for 40 years in Mexico, where she was a housewife with 16 children of her own, for whom she cooked using an open fire woodstove. On average, she spent 4 hours daily in the kitchen since her teenage years, and she describes the kitchen as poorly ventilated, especially in the wintertime. As a young adult, she recalls occasional cough and wheeze especially while cooking. Her symptoms have been worsening in New Mexico, despite no exposure to wood smoke for 15 years. Current medications included an ICS/LABA combination, and she required 20 mg daily of prednisone. A physical exam showed diminished breath sounds without wheeze or crackles.

Spirometry demonstrated profound airflow obstruction: FEV_1 of 0.8L (46% predicted) with partial (32%) improvement after a SABA to 1.1L (60% predicted), an FVC of 1.6L (69% predicted) that improved to 1.9L (81% predicted) after a SABA, and a post-SABA FEV_1/FVC of 57%. Lung volumes demonstrated air trapping, with an residual volume of 2.9 L, 138% predicted. The diffusing capacity of the lungs for carbon monoxide (DLCO) was normal. A chest radiograph revealed hyperinflation and bronchial wall thickening, with subsegmental atelectasis in the right middle lobe (RML). Bronchoscopy was performed, and biopsies showed diffuse anthracofibrosis, which was more severe in the RML. Cultures were negative for an infectious workup including tuberculosis. Laboratory studies including a complete blood count (CBC), metabolic panel, IgE, and antineutrophil cytoplasmic antibodies (ANCA) were normal.

Based on her symptoms and objective testing, the patient was diagnosed with ACO. The bronchial anthracofibrosis was considered a manifestation of past biomass exposure. Her ICS/LABA dose was increased, and she was started on a long-acting muscarinic antagonist (LAMA). She was gradually tapered off her daily prednisone dose. However, she continues to have frequent ACO exacerbations requiring ER visits and treatment with high-dose prednisone. She was also started on supplemental oxygen for exertional hypoxemia. More recently, she reported worsening dyspnea and lower-extremity edema, and she was found to have right-sided heart failure on echocardiogram.

Patients with ACO from biomass exposure have both bronchial hyperreactivity and incomplete reversibility of airflow obstruction as noted in the case above. Such subjects demonstrate a strong Th2-type inflammatory response in the airways.[38] A Spanish study compared the clinical characteristics of patients with obstructive airways disease from biomass fuel to those with COPD from tobacco smoke, and found that subjects with biomass-related COPD were more likely to be women, have a significantly higher BMI and a relatively higher FEV_1 percentage predicted.[39] Biomass-exposed subjects were more likely to demonstrate ACO than the tobacco smoke–exposed subjects (21.3% vs. 5%; $p < 0.0001$), although, when corrected for gender, the difference was no longer significant. Interestingly, although the emphysema phenotype was more frequent in 46% of the tobacco smoke–exposed group, it was still observed in 32% of the ACO group. High-resolution CT (HRCT) chest imaging studies of subjects with biomass fuel–induced ACO show a greater prevalence of airway changes, including ground glass opacities, mosaic air trapping, and peribronchial vascular thickening compared to unexposed subjects.[38] Because exposure to biomass smoke typically begins in early childhood, it likely has an effect on the developing airways, and thus contributes to early onset of disease.[40] Higher hour-years of biomass smoke exposure are associated with a high odds ratio for developing chronic bronchitis. Conversely, similar to the improvement in lung function with the cessation of cigarette smoking, individuals in households that switched to biogas or added kitchen ventilation to biomass stoves demonstrated a slowed and reduced decline in the FEV_1, although not a return to normal.

11.7 DIESEL EXHAUST

Diesel exhaust is a complex mixture of gases, metal oxides, polycyclic hydrocarbons, and fine and ultrafine particulates which are the byproducts of diesel fuel combustion. Approximately 80% of the particulate mass consists of organic and elemental carbon, and 20% is sulfuric acid. Multiple organic compounds are adsorbed to the particulate mass, such as alkanes and alkenes, aldehydes, polycyclic aromatic hydrocarbons (PAHs) and derivative, and heterocyclic compounds. The large surface area of diesel exhaust particulates can adsorb large amounts of organic materials, including mutagens and carcinogens.[41]

Occupations with significant exposures to diesel exhaust are associated with increased risk for both COPD and asthma manifesting as an accelerated decline in lung function, suggestive of ACO.[42] The OR for the development of COPD ranges from 1.2 to 2.0 in more heavily exposed occupations, such as vehicle mechanics, transportation workers, construction workers, and motor vehicle operators. In never-smoker workers in these occupations, the OR ranges from 2.1 to 3.4 for the development of COPD. A population-based study from Kaiser Permanente evaluated the association between diesel exposure and development of COPD in individuals reporting routine weekly exposure to diesel exhaust. Compared to unexposed workers, individuals reporting any diesel exhaust exposure had an OR of 1.9 (1.3, 3.0) for COPD, whereas never-smokers with moderate exposure had an OR of 6.4 (1.3, 31.6).[43]

Railroad workers are a subset of workers with a well-defined increase in COPD mortality risk as one measure of their risk for lung disease. A 2.5% increase in COPD mortality is estimated for each additional year of work, which is only minimally attenuated after adjustment for smoking.[44] New-onset asthma in railroad workers from both acute and chronic diesel exposures has also been reported.[45]

11.7.1 ACO IN A RAIL WORKER EXPOSED TO DIESEL EXHAUST AND IRRITANTS

CLINICAL VIGNETTE 11.4

A 61-year-old man from Cheyenne, Wyoming, started working in the mechanical department of the railroad a year after graduating high school. In 1980 he began working in the engine service, first as a fireman riding with the engineer and then as the engineer. His typical runs were manifest trains, carrying coal, soda ash, grain, and other dusty loads. Because of the hazardous nature of their loads, the train typically moved at only 10 to 15 miles an hour through tunnels, which resulted in significant exposure to diesel exhaust. Working in the yard, he was also exposed to air pollution from an adjacent fertilizer plant. As an engineer, he was required to put out electrical fires on the engine, and he estimates putting out five or six fires resulting in exposure to fire smoke and the fire extinguisher chemicals. During several layoffs, he returned to work in the frog shop, which was a very dusty and smoky job that involved grinding and welding steel switch points. He had a childhood history of asthma and cigarette smoking of 15 pack years. He retired in 2014, in part due to extreme dyspnea and a requirement for supplemental oxygen.

Pulmonary-function tests with lung volumes showed hyperinflation (TLC 9.92 L, 137% predicted), and airflow limitation, with FEV_1 at 1.93 L (50% predicted), which increased partially by 22% to 2.35 (61% predicted) after a SABA. The diffusion capacity was reduced to 24.03 (65% predicted), with over a 2 L volume difference between the TLC and the alveolar volume measured at 7.53 L (102%), consistent with markedly poor gas distribution. A HRCT scan of the chest showed moderate emphysema, mild diffuse airway wall thickening, and diffuse air trapping on expiratory images. The patient was diagnosed with ACO, and treated with a high-dose ICS/LABA, albuterol, and supplemental oxygen at 2 lpm at night. However, his lung function continued to gradually decline.

Extrapolating from other population-based studies, it is possible that exposure to particulates and PAH fractions are the most relevant for the development of ACO in diesel exhaust–exposed workers. A recent study of particulate air pollution found an adjusted hazard ratio (HR) of 2.78 (CI: 1.62–4.78) per 10 $\mu g/m^3$ increase in cumulative exposure to $PM_{2.5}$ for the specific development of ACO.[46] Ultrafine particles <100 nm aerodynamic diameter have been demonstrated to promote allergic sensitization and exacerbate asthma, which could explain their propensity to cause ACO; occupational examples of ultrafine particles include diesel exhaust particles, products of biofuels, and nanotechnology.[47] A potential mechanism may be through the decreased expression of tolerance by means of epigenetic changes. A study of 256 children ages 10–21 years found that a higher average PAH exposure was significantly associated with increased methylation of the forkhead box protein 3 (FOXP3) locus ($p < 0.05$), in a dose-dependent fashion, although this finding was conditional on atopic status. Downstream effects included decreased protein expression of FOXP3 ($p < 0.001$) and IL-10, along with increased total plasma IgE and IFN-gamma.[48] Although such effects have not, as yet, been specifically studied in adults, immune modulation from diesel PAH exposures may similarly contribute to the development of occupational ACO.

11.8 FIREFIGHTERS

Fire smoke also is a complex particulate aerosol of fine and ultrafine particles, vapors, and toxic gases that include carbon monoxide (CO), hydrogen cyanide, formaldehyde, sulfur and nitrogen oxides, and phosgene, along with chemical carcinogens such as PAHs and dioxin. Given the similarity of fire smoke components to other complex aerosols discussed in this chapter, it is reasonable to assume that firefighters are at a similar risk for the development of ACO. Firefighters have been reported to develop increases in BHR and respiratory symptoms, along with cross-shift and cross-season decreases in lung function. A cross-sectional study of metropolitan firefighters in Sao Paulo, Brazil, found a significant increase in asthma symptoms (wheezing, breathlessness, morning chest tightness, and rhinitis) compared to municipal police officers. Risk factors for asthma symptoms included years employed, work as a firefighter, smoking, and rhinitis, but not age or gender.[49] Another survey of 575 metropolitan firefighters identified 10% with chronic respiratory conditions, including 24 (4%) with a physician's diagnosis of asthma or using asthma medications, and 39 (7%) with a physician's diagnosis of COPD, emphysema, or chronic bronchitis. There was an interaction between a chronic respiratory diagnosis and inconsistent use of respiratory protection during fire knockdown ($p < 0.001$).[50]

A study of 63 wildland firefighters from Northern California and Montana[51] showed statistically significant declines of 0.09 L in FVC (0.05, 0.13), 0.15 L in FEV_1 (0.13, 0.17), and 0.44 L in FEF 25–75 (0.26, 0.62) between pre- and postseason spirometry. Methacholine reactivity also increased significantly postseason, $p = 0.02$. Results were not affected by smoking status, history of allergies or asthma, full-time or seasonal employment, or a history of respiratory symptoms. Another study found a significant cross-shift decline of 0.25 L (0.02, 0.48) in FEV_1 of firefighters exposed to high levels of levoglucosan measured by personal-filter cassettes as a marker for fire smoke exposure.[52] Taken together, these epidemiologic and exposure data suggest a high risk of developing ACO.

11.9 WELDING FUMES

Electric arc welding is a process to join different metals and alloys using the heat produced by passing electricity from one conductor or wire rod to another. All of the components, including the base metal, electrode or wire rod, electrode coatings, fluxes, shielding gases, and point or surface coatings may be volatilized during the process and contribute to the welding aerosol. Welding fumes are composed of fine-particulate metal oxides, which form from the reactions of vaporized metal with oxygen. Higher concentrations are created with higher currents and the use of flux. A cross-sectional study of 137 current, former, and nonwelder subjects in New Zealand found that work-related respiratory symptoms were more prevalent in welders (30.7%) compared to nonwelders (15.0%), and these symptomatic workers had significantly lower FEV_1, $p < 0.004$, and FVC, $p = 0.04$.[53] More than 10 years of total welding exposure, as well as a high proportion of time spent welding in confined spaces, was the strongest predictor of chronic bronchitis. A study of South Korean welders with moderate to high cumulative welding exposures found higher rates of COPD with an OR of 3.9 (1.4, 13.3) and 3.8 (1.03, 16.2) respectively, compared to those with low exposures.[54] Welding has also been associated with the development of asthma. A prospective study of 194 apprentice welders demonstrated that their FEV_1 percentage predicted dropped significantly by 8.4% by the end of the study, and 23 (12%) of apprentices had a significant decrease ≥ 3.2 in their PC20. The incidence of occupational asthma was nearly 3% when defined as the new onset of cough, wheeze, or chest tightness.[55] Occupational asthma due to stainless steel–welding fumes by specific challenge has also been demonstrated in 34 Finnish welders, with an immediate reaction in 26%, a delayed reaction in 47%, and a dual reaction in 26%.[56] Based on this literature documenting the development of both COPD and asthma in welders, ACO is a likely outcome of welding-fume exposures.

11.9.1 MINERAL DUSTS

Exposures to mineral dusts, best exemplified by silica and coal dust, are known to contribute to the development of COPD and chronic airways obstruction. For example, a meta-analysis of six studies of workers occupationally exposed to respirable quartz dust (in a granite quarry, potato sorters exposed to diatomaceous earth, cement factory workers, tunnel workers, and foundry workers), found a statistically significant decrease in FEV_1 and FEV_1/FVC consistent with airways obstruction and COPD.[57] Mineral dusts primarily affect the walls of the smaller bronchioles and alveolar ducts, causing chronic inflammation and remodeling of the small airways (bronchitis) and destruction of the alveoli clustered at the end of the airways (emphysema) through the generation of reactive oxygen species and cytotoxicity. Irritation and abrasion of the airway epithelial walls can also facilitate passage of the small particles into the lung parenchyma, and initiate a concurrent process of fibrosis and the development of nodules. The two processes may occur simultaneously or separately, and hence airflow obstruction in miners has been reported in both the presence and absence of radiological silicosis.[58] There is an exposure-response relation between loss of FEV_1 and FEV_1/FVC and cumulative silica dust exposure, although smoking appears to potentiate the effect of silica dust on the airways. Whereas in nonsmokers, silica dust tends to lead to restrictive physiology, smoking and silica exposure are associated with a pattern of airflow obstruction and emphysema. Even in simple radiographic silicosis, it is emphysema, rather than the silicotic nodule, that is associated with an obstructed FEV_1/FVC ratio and reductions in maximum mid-expiratory flow (MMEF) and DLCO.

In contrast to the strong evidence that silica dust causes COPD in a dose-dependent fashion, it is not clear whether it can cause or worsen asthma. Several cross-sectional studies suggest that asthma, atopy, and BHR do not worsen the effect of silica dust on lung-function decline and the development of COPD.[59,60] However, silica dust has known immunogenic effects, such as in the causation of scleroderma and rheumatoid lung, and may similarly affect the development of reactive airways disease.

There is excellent evidence supporting the association of coal mining and COPD. Decline in FEV_1 over time has been related to cumulative exposure to respirable coal mine dust, regardless of smoking status. A large, longitudinal survey of 3,380 British coal miners found that cumulative exposure to respirable coal mine dust was related to risk of three important end points of COPD: $FEV_1 < 80\%$ predicted, symptoms of chronic bronchitis, and $FEV_1 < 65\%$ predicted.[61] Emphysema, too, has been associated with lifetime coal mine dust exposure. Inhalation of coal dust is associated with the accumulation and activation of neutrophils and alveolar macrophages, with increased neutrophil elastase activity, and spontaneous release of superoxide anion and H_2O_2 as potential mechanisms of airways damage.[62] Coal mines also have multiple exposures that may cause or exacerbate asthma,[63] including isocyanates, diesel particulates, and a complex bioaerosol of bacteria and fungi,[64] although it is not clear if coal mine dust in itself can cause asthma. It is plausible to hypothesize that these combined coal mine exposures could also contribute to the development of ACO.

Exposures to other, poorly soluble low-toxicity particles referred to as biopersistent granular dust, such as Portland cement, carbon black, soot, rubber, talcum, and other metal-processing and mining exposures also play a role in the development of occupational COPD. The decline of FEV_1 in these workers is also related to cumulative occupational dust concentrations. In a meta-analysis of 27 studies, there was a very consistent decrease of 1.6 mL (1.24, 1.93) per 1 mg/m³ years of exposure, and the mean FEV_1 of exposed workers was 160 mL lower or 5.7% less than predicted compared to unexposed workers. The risk of COPD, defined as an $FEV_1/FVC < 70\%$, increased by 7% with each increase of 1 mg/m³ respirable biogranular dust.[65] However, there are no studies to date that have looked for the presence of asthma or BHR in these workers, and the possibility of ACO remains unexplored in this population as well.

11.10 SUMMARY AND CONCLUSIONS

Both epidemiological studies and investigations of specific workplaces and professions make it likely that ACO develops in certain occupational exposures. Studies have described ACO in cotton textile workers and in biomass-exposed workers. While asthma and COPD have been individually demonstrated in the exposed workforce, suggesting that the overlap syndrome ACO is also a product of the work exposures, it has not yet been definitively assessed. For example, in welders, firefighters, and farmers, asthma and COPD have been documented separately, but the demonstration of the overlap ACO is still lacking, but likely to be found if sought.

A common characteristic of the occupational exposures that have been demonstrated to cause both asthma and COPD appears to be the combination of an immunologically active component presented together with an irritant particulate(s). In many cases, the exposures are mixed and complex. Well-documented examples include cotton, hemp, and jute exposures that involve plant allergens, animal parts, bacteria, and endotoxin, as well as a particulate dust fraction. Exposures in grain and animal feed workers similarly include plant, mite, and animal allergens; bacteria and endotoxins; fungal antigens; and volatile organic compounds (VOCs), together with an irritant particulate. Biomass smoke contains comparable combinations of organic materials and irritant particles, and might behave in the same way as tobacco smoke. Silica particulates have been demonstrated to have combined irritant and immunological properties, and plausibly may act similarly to other biologically active organic dusts. The exhaust particulates from diesel combustion, which is itself ultimately plant based, are 80% organic and elemental carbon, and 20% are composed mainly of sulfuric acids. Polyaromatic hydrocarbons from diesel exhaust have been shown to enhance the allergic response.[66–71] Lastly, a number of other occupational chemicals with both irritant and immunological properties are known to cause a blend of occupational asthma, COPD, and/or ACO; examples include welding fumes, isocyanates, phthalic anhydrides, glutaraldehyde, and cleaning agents.[4] With this information in mind, it is plausible and likely that other occupational exposures are capable of causing ACO, but are as yet unidentified. Those who develop ACO generally do worse over time, with more frequent and severe exacerbations, need for medication and emergency care, and poorer outcomes. Hence, such workers who develop ACO may need to be restricted or removed from exposure at an earlier stage of disease. However, we need more information to define the exposures, jobs, and host factors that result in ACO, and longitudinal studies to understand the natural history of workplace-related ACO. Only then will we be able to implement the right measures in the workplace to prevent future disease.

ACKNOWLEDGMENTS

We wish to thank Dr. David Christiani (textile worker), Dr. Jill Poole (cattle feedlot worker), and Dr. Nour Ass'ad and Dr. Akshay Sood (biomass exposure) for the contribution of their cases and their helpful discussions regarding these disease processes. We also wish to acknowledge Stephanie Clancy and Megan Marchant for their help in formatting this chapter. Lastly, we would like to thank the patients whose stories are presented here. It is through them that we have gained a better understanding of occupational ACO.

REFERENCES

1. Bujarski S, Parulekar AD, Sharafkhaneh A et al. The asthma COPD overlap syndrome (ACOS). *Curr Allergy Asthma Rep.* 2015;15:509.
2. Dosman JA, Cockcroft DW, and Hoeppner VH. Airways obstruction in occupational pulmonary disease. *Med Clin North Am.* 1981;65:691–706.
3. Dosman JA, Kania J, and Cockcroft DW. Occupational obstructive disorders: Nonspecific airways obstruction and occupational asthma. *Med Clin North Am.* 1990;74:823–835.
4. Baur X, Bakehe P, and Vellguth H. Bronchial asthma and COPD due to irritants in the workplace-an evidence-based approach. *J Occup Med Toxicol.* 2012;7:19.
5. Postma DS and van den Berge M. The different faces of the asthma-COPD overlap syndrome. *Eur Respir J.* 2015;46:587–590.
6. Mehta AJ, Miedinger D, Keidel D et al. Occupational exposure to dusts, gases, and fumes and incidence of chronic obstructive pulmonary disease in the Swiss Cohort Study on Air Pollution and Lung and Heart Diseases in Adults. *Am J Respir Crit Care Med.* 2012;185:1292–1300.
7. De Matteis S, Jarvis D, Hutchings S et al. Occupations associated with COPD risk in the large population-based UK Biobank cohort study. *Occup Environ Med.* 2016;73:378–384.
8. van den Berge M and Aalbers R. The asthma-COPD overlap syndrome: How is it defined and what are its clinical implications? *J Asthma Allergy.* 2016;9:27–35.
9. Asthma, COPD, and asthma-COPD overlap. 2016. Available at http://ginasthma.org/asthma-copd-and-asthma-copd-overlap-syndrome-acos/. Accessed September 20, 2016.
10. Anees W, Moore VC, and Burge PS. FEV$_1$ decline in occupational asthma. *Thorax.* 2006;61:751–755.
11. ten Brinke A. Risk factors associated with irreversible airflow limitation in asthma. *Curr Opin Allergy Clin Immunol.* 2008;8:63–69.
12. Matheson MC, Benke G, Raven J et al. Biological dust exposure in the workplace is a risk factor for chronic obstructive pulmonary disease. *Thorax.* 2005;60:645–651.
13. Lai PS and Christiani DC. Long-term respiratory health effects in textile workers. *Curr Opin Pulm Med.* 2013;19:152–157.
14. Christiani DC, Ye TT, Zhang S et al. Cotton dust and endotoxin exposure and long-term decline in lung function: Results of a longitudinal study. *Am J Ind Med.* 1999;35:321–331.
15. Fishwick D, Fletcher AM, Pickering CA et al. Lung function, bronchial reactivity, atopic status, and dust exposure in Lancashire cotton mill operatives. *Am Rev Respir Dis.* 1992;145:1103–1108.
16. Beck GJ, Schachter EN, Maunder LR et al. A prospective study of chronic lung disease in cotton textile workers. *Ann Intern Med.* 1982;97:645–651.
17. Wang XR, Zhang HX, Sun BX et al. Is chronic airway obstruction from cotton dust exposure reversible? *Epidemiology.* 2004;15:695–701.
18. Wang XR, Eisen EA, Zhang HX et al. Respiratory symptoms and cotton dust exposure; Results of a 15 year follow up observation. *Occup Environ Med.* 2003;60:935–941.
19. Castellan RM, Olenchock SA, Hankinson JL et al. Acute bronchoconstriction induced by cotton dust: Dose-related responses to endotoxin and other dust factors. *Ann Intern Med.* 1984;101:157–163.
20. Shi J, Mehta AJ, Hang JQ et al. Chronic lung function decline in cotton textile workers: Roles of historical and recent exposures to endotoxin. *Environ Health Perspect.* 2010;118:1620–1624.
21. Christiani DC, Wegman DH, Eisen EA et al. Cotton dust and gram-negative bacterial endotoxin correlations in two cotton textile mills. *Am J Ind Med.* 1993;23:333–342.
22. Lai PS, Fresco JM, Pinilla MA et al. Chronic endotoxin exposure produces airflow obstruction and lung dendritic cell expansion. *Am J Respir Cell Mol Biol.* 2012;47:209–217.
23. Iversen M, Dahl R, Jensen EJ et al. Lung function and bronchial reactivity in farmers. *Thorax.* 1989;44:645–649.
24. Rylander R, Essle N, and Donham KJ. Bronchial hyperreactivity among pig and dairy farmers. *Am J Ind Med.* 1990;17:66–69.

25. Zhou C, Hurst TS, Cockcroft DW et al. Increased airways responsiveness in swine farmers. *Chest.* 1991;99:941–944.

26. Choudat D, Goehen M, Korobaeff M et al. Respiratory symptoms and bronchial reactivity among pig and dairy farmers. *Scand J Work Environ Health.* 1994;20:48–54.

27. Bessette L, Boulet LP, Tremblay G et al. Bronchial responsiveness to methacholine in swine confinement building workers. *Arch Environ Health.* 1993;48:73–77.

28. Iversen M and Dahl R. Working in swine-confinement buildings causes an accelerated decline in FEV$_1$: A 7–yr follow-up of Danish farmers. *Eur Respir J.* 2000;16:404–408.

29. Dalphin JC, Maheu MF, Dussaucy A et al. Six year longitudinal study of respiratory function in dairy farmers in the Doubs province. *Eur Respir J.* 1998;11:1287–1293.

30. Dalphin JC, Dubiez A, Monnet E et al. Prevalence of asthma and respiratory symptoms in dairy farmers in the French province of the Doubs. *Am J Respir Crit Care Med.* 1998;158:1493–1498.

31. Chaudemanche H, Monnet E, Westeel V et al. Respiratory status in dairy farmers in France; Cross sectional and longitudinal analyses. *Occup Environ Med.* 2003;60:858–863.

32. Gainet M, Thaon I, Westeel V et al. Twelve-year longitudinal study of respiratory status in dairy farmers. *Eur Respir J.* 2007;30:97–103.

33. Smid T, Heederik D, Houba R et al. Dust- and endotoxin-related respiratory effects in the animal feed industry. *Am Rev Respir Dis.* 1992;146:1474–1479.

34. Post W, Heederik D, and Houba R. Decline in lung function related to exposure and selection processes among workers in the grain processing and animal feed industry. *Occup Environ Med.* 1998;55:349–355.

35. Mink JT, Gerrard JW, Cockcroft DW et al. Increased bronchial reactivity to inhaled histamine in nonsmoking grain workers with normal lung function. *Chest.* 1980;77:28–31.

36. Clapp WD, Becker S, Quay J et al. Grain dust-induced airflow obstruction and inflammation of the lower respiratory tract. *Am J Respir Crit Care Med.* 1994;150:611–617.

37. Zuskin E, Schachter EN, Kanceljak B et al. Organic dust disease of airways. *Int Arch Occup Environ Health.* 1993;65:135–140.

38. Assad NA, Balmes J, Mehta S et al. Chronic obstructive pulmonary disease secondary to household air pollution. *Semin Respir Crit Care Med.* 2015;36:408–421.

39. Golpe R, Sanjuan Lopez P, Cano Jimenez E et al. Distribution of clinical phenotypes in patients with chronic obstructive pulmonary disease caused by biomass and tobacco smoke. *Arch Bronconeumol.* 2014;50:318–324.

40. Golpe R and Perez de Llano L. Are the diagnostic criteria for asthma-COPD overlap syndrome appropriate in biomass smoke-induced chronic obstructive pulmonary disease? *Arch Bronconeumol.* 2016;52:110.

41. National Toxicology Program. 2016. Report on carcinogens, 14th edition: Diesel exhaust particulates. Available at https://ntp.niehs.nih.gov/ntp/roc/content/profiles/dieselexhaustparticulates.pdf. Accessed September 20, 2016.

42. Hart JE, Eisen EA, and Laden F. Occupational diesel exhaust exposure as a risk factor for chronic obstructive pulmonary disease. *Curr Opin Pulm Med.* 2012;18:151–154.

43. Weinmann S, Vollmer WM, Breen V et al. COPD and occupational exposures: A case-control study. *J Occup Environ Med.* 2008;50:561–569.

44. Hart JE, Laden F, Eisen EA et al. Chronic obstructive pulmonary disease mortality in railroad workers. *Occup Environ Med.* 2009;66:221–226.

45. Wade JF, 3rd, and Newman LS. Diesel asthma. Reactive airways disease following overexposure to locomotive exhaust. *J Occup Med.* 1993;35:149–154.

46. To T, Zhu J, Larsen K et al. Progression from asthma to chronic obstructive pulmonary disease. Is air pollution a risk factor? *Am J Respir Crit Care Med.* 2016;194:429–438.

47. Li N, Georas S, Alexis N et al. A work group report on ultrafine particles (American Academy of Allergy, Asthma & Immunology): Why ambient ultrafine and engineered nanoparticles should receive special attention for possible adverse health outcomes in human subjects. *J Allergy Clin Immunol.* 2016;138:386–396.

48. Hew KM, Walker AI, Kohli A et al. Childhood exposure to ambient polycyclic aromatic hydrocarbons is linked to epigenetic modifications and impaired systemic immunity in T cells. *Clin Exp Allergy.* 2015;45:238–248.

49. Ribeiro M, de Paula Santos U, Bussacos MA et al. Prevalence and risk of asthma symptoms among firefighters in Sao Paulo, Brazil: A population-based study. *Am J Ind Med.* 2009;52:261–269.

50. Schermer TR, Malbon W, Morgan M et al. Chronic respiratory conditions in a cohort of metropolitan fire-fighters: Associations with occupational exposure and quality of life. *Int Arch Occup Environ Health.* 2014;87:919–928.

51. Liu D, Tager IB, Balmes JR et al. The effect of smoke inhalation on lung function and airway responsiveness in wildland fire fighters. *Am Rev Respir Dis.* 1992;146:1469–1473.

52. Gaughan DM, Piacitelli CA, Chen BT et al. Exposures and cross-shift lung function declines in wildland firefighters. *J Occup Environ Hyg.* 2014;11:591–603.

53. Bradshaw LM, Fishwick D, Slater T et al. Chronic bronchitis, work related respiratory symptoms, and pulmonary function in welders in New Zealand. *Occup Environ Med.* 1998;55:150–154.

54. Koh DH, Kim JI, Kim KH et al. Welding fume exposure and chronic obstructive pulmonary disease in welders. *Occup Med (Lond).* 2015;65:72–77.

55. El-Zein M, Malo JL, Infante-Rivard C et al. Incidence of probable occupational asthma and changes in airway calibre and responsiveness in apprentice welders. *Eur Respir J.* 2003;22:513–518.

56. Hannu T, Piipari R, Tuppurainen M et al. Occupational asthma caused by stainless steel welding fumes: A clinical study. *Eur Respir J.* 2007;29:85–90.

57. Bruske I, Thiering E, Heinrich J et al. Respirable quartz dust exposure and airway obstruction: A systematic review and meta-analysis. *Occup Environ Med.* 2014;71:583–589.

58. Hnizdo E and Vallyathan V. Chronic obstructive pulmonary disease due to occupational exposure to silica dust: A review of epidemiological and pathological evidence. *Occup Environ Med.* 2003;60:237–243.

59. Humerfelt S, Eide GE, and Gulsvik A. Association of years of occupational quartz exposure with spirometric airflow limitation in Norwegian men aged 30–46 years. *Thorax.* 1998;53:649–655.

60. Jorna TH, Borm PJ, Koiter KD et al. Respiratory effects and serum type III procollagen in potato sorters exposed to diatomaceous earth. *Int Arch Occup Environ Health.* 1994;66:217–222.

61. Marine WM, Gurr D, and Jacobsen M. Clinically important respiratory effects of dust exposure and smoking in British coal miners. *Am Rev Respir Dis.* 1988;137:106–112.

62. Coggon D and Newman Taylor A. Coal mining and chronic obstructive pulmonary disease: A review of the evidence. *Thorax.* 1998;53:398–407.

63. Go LH, Krefft SD, Cohen RA et al. Lung disease and coal mining: What pulmonologists need to know. *Curr Opin Pulm Med.* 2016;22:170–178.

64. Wei M, Yu Z, and Zhang H. Molecular characterization of microbial communities in bioaerosols of a coal mine by 454 pyrosequencing and real-time PCR. *J Environ Sci (China).* 2015;30:241–251.

65. Bruske I, Thiering E, Heinrich J et al. Biopersistent granular dust and chronic obstructive pulmonary disease: A systematic review and meta-analysis. *PLOS ONE.* 2013;8:e80977.

66. Takenaka H, Zhang K, Diaz-Sanchez D et al. Enhanced human IgE production results from exposure to the aromatic hydrocarbons from diesel exhaust: Direct effects on B-cell IgE production. *J Allergy Clin Immunol.* 1995;95:103–115.

67. Diaz-Sanchez D. The role of diesel exhaust particles and their associated polyaromatic hydrocarbons in the induction of allergic airway disease. *Allergy.* 1997;52:52–56; discussion 57–58.

68. Fujieda S, Diaz-Sanchez D, and Saxon A. Combined nasal challenge with diesel exhaust particles and allergen induces In vivo IgE isotype switching. *Am J Respir Cell Mol Biol.* 1998;19:507–512.

69. Diaz-Sanchez D, Garcia MP, Wang M et al. Nasal challenge with diesel exhaust particles can induce sensitization to a neoallergen in the human mucosa. *J Allergy Clin Immunol.* 1999;104:1183–1188.

70. Devouassoux G, Saxon A, Metcalfe DD et al. Chemical constituents of diesel exhaust particles induce IL-4 production and histamine release by human basophils. *J Allergy Clin Immunol.* 2002;109:847–853.

71. Riedl MA, Diaz-Sanchez D, Linn WS et al. Allergic inflammation in the human lower respiratory tract affected by exposure to diesel exhaust. *Res Rep Health Eff Inst.* 2012;165:5–43; discussion 45–64.

Asthma, COPD, and asthma-COPD overlap in special populations

STEPHEN BUJARSKI, AMIT PARULEKAR, AND NICOLA A. HANANIA

12.1 INTRODUCTION

Asthma and chronic obstructive pulmonary disease (COPD) are common diseases that affect a substantial proportion of individuals worldwide. The structured and formalized definitions and diagnostic criteria for both asthma and COPD have allowed focused analysis and characterization of subgroups or special populations with some standardization and reproducibility.[1,2] However, without a clearly accepted consensus definition and known heterogeneous criteria for defining patients with asthma-COPD overlap (ACO), it is not completely certain how ACO relates to specific patient populations.[3] Available data suggest that ACO reflects a mixture of features, characteristics, and subsequent special-population effects of those seen in individuals with both asthma and COPD. In this chapter, we will explore current knowledge on special populations with asthma, COPD, and ACO.

12.2 ILLUSTRATIVE CLINICAL VIGNETTES

CLINICAL VIGNETTE 12.1

A 76-year-old male presents to a clinic complaining of difficulty breathing for several years. He was diagnosed with heart failure a few years ago after a heart attack and has been seeing his primary care doctor and cardiologist for this. Initially, his breathing improved with an increase in his furosemide dose, but he continued to have limitations due to shortness of breath. More recently, he has also been complaining of an intermittent cough that is worse in the morning, as well as nasal congestion and itchy eyes. He smoked about a half a pack of cigarettes per day from his teens until a few years ago. He never reported any other lung issues. He underwent spirometry with a FEV_1/FVC ratio of 66% and near normalization of the obstruction after administration of albuterol on postbronchodilator study. He was thus started on an inhaled corticosteroid (ICS) and long-acting β_2-agonist (LABA) with improvement in his dyspnea and cough.

Take-home messages:

- Late-onset asthma (LOA) is a well-known entity that is often underdiagnosed and undertreated.
- Other comorbidities may complicate the course and lead to its underdiagnosis.

CLINICAL VIGNETTE 12.2

A 54-year-old male presents with complaints of daily cough and shortness of breath. He reports having a harder time completing his daily activities at work, which include manual labor lifting and carrying heavy objects due to his dyspnea. He denies allergies. He is a current smoker of one pack a day and has done so for the past 20 years. Five years ago, he was diagnosed with asthma and was prescribed a scheduled daily ICS, as well as a rescue albuterol inhaler as needed. He noted some improvement in his symptoms, mostly his cough, but was still not able to tolerate sustained activity at work before needing to rest and was using his rescue albuterol inhaler multiple times throughout the day. Spirometry demonstrated a postbronchodilator FEV_1 65% of predicted, FEV_1/FVC ratio of 62% and 14% (250 mL) improvement in FEV_1 after bronchodilator treatment. He was prescribed a LABA to be used with his ICS, which resulted in significant improvement in his activity tolerance. He was subsequently able to go back to work without limitations with only minimal utilization of his rescue inhaler.

Take-home messages:

- COPD should be suspected in any patient who is 40 years of age or older with respiratory symptoms and a history of exposure to smoke.
- The diagnosis of COPD is confirmed with the presence of postbronchodilator FEV_1/FVC < 0.7.
- Significant acute bronchodilator response (>12% and 200 mL change in FEV_1 or FVC) does not differentiate asthma from COPD.
- Symptoms of asthma and COPD may overlap. The mainstay of treatment of COPD is long-acting bronchodilator administration and when appropriate and ICS.

CLINICAL VIGNETTE 12.3

A 26-year-old female with difficult-to-control childhood asthma presents to the emergency room complaining of wheezing, chest tightness, and difficulty breathing. She is 26 weeks pregnant and stopped her daily asthma maintenance medications, which included an ICS, LABA, and a leukotriene receptor antagonist, after finding out she was pregnant because she was fearful they may harm her baby. Recently, she has been requiring her albuterol inhaler more frequently due to daily wheezing, and the morning of her office visit woke up with the inability to breathe well. Her pregnancy has been otherwise uncomplicated except for worsening heart burn. She was treated appropriately for her asthma exacerbation, and she was sent home to restart her asthma-controller medications including the ICS and LABA. She was also advised to take antacids and to sleep on a slight incline to reduce her GERD symptoms. On reevaluation in a clinic a few weeks later, her asthma was controlled.

Take-home messages:

- Asthma during pregnancy should be managed the same as in nonpregnant women.
- Pregnancy can complicate the course of asthma, and poorly controlled asthma is associated with poor maternal and fetal outcomes.

12.3 EFFECT OF AGE ON ASTHMA, COPD, AND ACO

The population of older people is growing by 2% per year, a rate which is faster than the growth of the total world population.[4] By 2030, it is estimated that 20% of the population of the United States will be over the age of 65.[5] Although morbidity and mortality from many diseases have either declined or been stable over time, morbidity and mortality from lung diseases have increased with the increasing average age of the population.[6] Aging leads to a decline of the structure and function of organs, including the airways and lungs. One mechanism by which this may occur is through loss of adaptive immunity and increase in nonspecific tissue inflammation.[7] Traditionally, asthma has been thought of as a disease of young individuals and COPD a disease of old individuals. Although this may be generally true, age-related differences should be recognized within each of these two disease states. ACO appears to affect individuals in between the usual age ranges of those with asthma and COPD alone. Its impact on younger and older individuals is not clearly understood and has not been examined.

12.3.1 AGE AND ASTHMA

Unlike COPD or ACO, asthma is usually thought of as a disease of the young. In fact, it often starts in childhood or at least has its first clinical signs and symptoms prior to age 40. It is estimated that 8%–10% of school-aged children have asthma, and it is considered the leading chronic disease in children as well as the top reason for missed school days.[8] Furthermore, children are more likely to need acute care due to asthma than adults. In addition, some children with asthma have reduced lung growth resulting in lower levels of maximal lung function, as well as early lung function decline as adults. Subsequently, individuals with a history of childhood asthma are indeed at greater risk to develop COPD and commonly do so at an earlier age.[9]

Although not traditionally considered as often, asthma has a significant impact in the older population as well. With the aging population, asthma in older adults is a rapidly growing public health problem.[10–12] In the United States, 10.4% (8.0% of men, 12.2% of women) of adults 65 and older reported lifetime asthma, and 7.6% (5.7% of men, 9.1% of women) reported current asthma in 2011.[13] However, this may be an underestimate as the diagnosis of asthma in this population is often overlooked because of comorbidities, underreporting of symptoms, insufficient use of lung-function testing, and overlap with other diseases such as COPD.[14–18]

Asthma in the older population is associated with high disease burden and leads to a major impairment in quality of life, poor general health, symptoms of depression, and significant limitation of daily activity. Of note, the highest death rate in adults with asthma is reported for those age 65 and older (0.58 per 1000 persons).[19] This accounts for more than 50% of the total annual deaths from this disease, and it increases with age. Despite its high public health impact, asthma in older adults has not been systematically studied, as patients are often excluded from participating in clinical trials because of age restriction. Furthermore, asthma guidelines are generally based on evidence collected from studies in younger populations and do not take into consideration the elderly, who often suffer from multiple comorbidities. Two distinct presentations for asthma in older adults based on the onset and duration of the disease have been described. Patients with LOA start having asthma symptoms for the first time when they are 40 years of age or older. It has been suggested that patients belonging to this group tend to have fewer atopic manifestations, higher baseline FEV_1, and a more-pronounced bronchodilator response than those with long-standing asthma (LSA), who start having asthma symptoms early in life. Those with LSA usually have their initial symptoms prior to age 40, have more atopic manifestations, and have a greater degree of obstruction.[20,21] (Table 12.1).

Aging is associated with changes in organs, tissues, and cells that diminish functional reserve and confer vulnerability to stressors and/or disease. Both aging and asthma may affect patients' well-being, including symptoms, functionality, and health status. The interactions between aging-related effects and asthma on functionality and health status, lung function, and airway and systemic inflammation have not been examined. Furthermore, there is no current uniform consensus on the definition of the clinical and physiologic characteristics or phenotypes of asthma in the older population. An exploratory workshop of experts of asthma in older adults sponsored by the National Institute on Aging was organized by the applicants and highlighted the need for studies to better understand the pathophysiologic mechanisms of asthma in this population.[22] More recently, an American Thoracic Society workshop also highlighted unmet research needs in this population.[23]

Symptoms of asthma in older adults may mislead clinicians to consider causes other than asthma, such as old age, COPD, and heart failure. Furthermore, atopic diseases are often not considered in older patients with asthma because of the myth that these diseases only exist in the younger population. At the same time, older people with asthma tend to attribute breathlessness to their aging process as opposed to their disease.[1] Alterations in the perception of airway obstruction due to aging often lead to underestimation of the disease severity and thus the delay in seeking advice.[24] Although this delayed diagnosis may also be aggravated by the susceptibility of this population to deterioration of cognitive and physical functions and memory loss, these effects have not been fully evaluated in this population of patients with asthma.

Therapeutic and management concerns also exist for older individuals with asthma. Data on efficacy of asthma medications are limited, as many of the trials excluded elderly individuals. However, the risk of treatment failure increases with increasing age, especially in regards to response to ICS.[25] Furthermore, limited inspiratory flows and comorbid diseases, such as arthritis, general weakness, and impaired vision or cognition, may negatively impact the proper utilization of inhaler medications. Side effects, such as bruising, osteoporosis, cataracts, cardiotoxicity,

Table 12.1 Potential mechanisms for the asthma phenotypes in the elderly

	Age of onset	Genetic role	Infection	Atopy	Inflammation	Environment
Long-standing asthma	*Child or young adult (≤45)*	*Likely gene by environment*	*Viral: rhinovirus and RSV*	*Likely*	*T_2 High, eosinophilic*	*Allergens, day care and school, workplace*
Late-onset asthma	*Adult (>45)*	*Likely epigenetic including oxidative stress, shortened telomeres*	*Viral: RSV, influenza, and bacterial (e.g., Chlamydia pneumoniae, microbial superantigens)*	*Unlikely*	*T_2 High or Low, neutrophilic and/or eosinophilic, innate immunity, TH-17*	*Workplace, dwelling type (house, apartment, institutional)*

and drug-interaction profiles of the common asthma medications, are also of concern and must be considered when prescribing these medications to older individuals.[26] In addition, cost is often an obstacle in this population, who are often on a fixed income and cannot afford their medication, which frequently results in either not taking their prescribed dosage or decreasing the frequency and dose in order to make it last longer.

12.3.2 AGE AND COPD

Even though COPD has usually been considered a disease of the older population, any individual at risk above age 40 can be affected, especially if exposed to noxious stimuli such as tobacco smoke. Indeed, there is a tremendous growing interest in COPD in the younger population as these patients may have worse quality of life (QOL) and more progressive course of disease.[27]

COPD may accelerate the aging process and the prevalence of COPD exponentially increases with age. While the estimated cumulative prevalence of COPD is 3.1% in people less than 40 years of age and 8.2% in people ages 40–64, it is 14.2% in people over the age of 65.[28] In 2010 the Global Burden of Disease Study estimated that 23.1% of total disease burden was attributable to disorders in people age 60 years and older, and COPD accounted for 43.3 million disability adjusted life years (DALYs) in older people.[29] Comorbidities, which are part of the definition of the disease, are a significant contributor to the burden of disease, particularly in older people, since multimorbidity also increases with age. Analysis of Medicare data from 2008 found that 67% of people age 65 and older had multiple chronic conditions, and the prevalence of multiple comorbid conditions increased with age.[30] Multimorbidity in the elderly leads to increased functional impairment, poor QOL, inpatient hospitalizations, and high health care utilization and costs.[31,32] Despite the strong associations between COPD, comorbidities, and aging, little is understood about the impact of age in the COPD population. Many studies have investigated physiologic parameters, functional capacity, and QOL in middle-aged COPD patients[33–37]; however, limited data exist detailing COPD patients over the age of 65.[38–41]

12.3.3 AGE AND ASTHMA-COPD OVERLAP

Classically, COPD causes an accelerated rate of decline in FEV_1 due to continuous and progressive toxic effects of cigarette or other irritants. However, emerging data suggests that reduced lung development resulting in lower-than-expected maximal FEV_1 early in life may be a strong and very important factor in individuals who develop fixed airway obstruction later in life. In addition, these individuals develop a fixed airway obstruction earlier than those with the more classically defined COPD. This is especially true for individuals who were born prematurely, are

malnourished, who experienced early respiratory illnesses, who were exposed to airborne contaminants, and those with childhood asthma.[9,42] Existing evidence suggests that ACO is usually encountered in individuals slightly younger than those with COPD alone but older than those with asthma alone.[43,44] Most data report individuals with ACO are between 60–68 years of age, but some information suggests that the incidence of ACO increases as age continues to advance.[45–47] Whether this is due to normal physiologic changes related to aging or represents a separate pathophysiologic process such as reduced lung growth is uncertain.

Interestingly, the prevalence of asthma decreases with increasing age while COPD prevalence increases with increasing age. Traditionally, individuals were labeled as COPD once spirometry demonstrated a fixed airway obstruction. It is very possible that as individuals age, changes in lung function make it more likely that individuals with asthma develop fixed airway obstruction and are later diagnosed as COPD.[48] This may account for some of the increase in COPD prevalence with subsequent reduction in asthma prevalence, especially in the elderly population. One can speculate that many of these individuals, many of whom will be older, have findings consistent with ACO and should be diagnosed as such.[46]

12.4 EFFECT OF GENDER ON ASTHMA, COPD, AND ACO

12.4.1 GENDER AND ASTHMA

Gender disparities exist in asthma, but they also change with age (Figure 12.1).[49] This variation is believed to reflect the changes in sex hormones, as well as the variable effects of these hormones on airway inflammation and physiology women experience as they age.[50,51] As children, more boys than girls have asthma and are also more likely to be hospitalized due to asthma. During adolescence, the prevalence drops in males and increases in females, so that by the time of adulthood, more women are affected by asthma than men. A subset of women has variations in symptom control, lung function, and subsequent severity of asthma based on the menstrual cycle stage. In addition, more adult women have severe asthma and are more likely to be hospitalized for asthma-related events than adult men.[52] Eventually, the prevalence and severity of asthma begins to decrease in women as they reach postmenopausal age.

12.4.2 GENDER AND COPD

Traditionally, COPD was considered a disease of older male smokers. However, this perception is outdated. Although men still likely account for a larger proportion of those with COPD, the prevalence of COPD is increasing more rapidly in women. In addition, COPD-related deaths are higher in women compared to men in several countries.[53,54] These

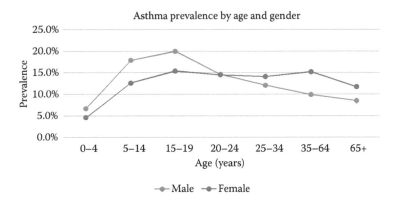

Figure 12.1 Lifetime asthma prevalence (percent) stratified by age and gender, United States. (Adapted from CDC. National Health Interview Survey (NHIS) Data; 2015. Available at http://www.cdc.gov/asthma/nhis/2015/table2-1.htm.)

facts account for the urgent need for providers to recognize the burden COPD has in women. Recognizing some of the differences in how and why COPD presents in women can heighten provider awareness to better recognize this disease in women (Table 12.2).

Although personal susceptibility and exposure-related factors determine an individual's risk for developing COPD, some evidence suggests that women may be more susceptible to developing COPD and have more rapid progression of disease compared with men. Women appear to have worse lung function for comparative tobacco-related exposure.[54] Also, women with COPD are generally younger, smoke less in general, have a lower BMI, and come from lower socioeconomic status than men. Physiologically, women have more small-airway disease (bronchiolitis), greater airway hyperresponsiveness, and less of an emphysematous phenotype compared with men.[55] In addition, women more commonly have COPD not related to just smoking, but due to other exposures, such as biomass and occupational exposures, especially when looked at globally. Therefore, an evaluation of potential exposures beyond just smoking should be actively pursued in women with COPD. These findings highlight why women represent the majority of individuals

Table 12.2 Gender differences in COPD (women in comparison to men)

- Disease more often misdiagnosed
- More susceptible to COPD with same amount of smoke exposure
- Higher prevalence of nonsmoking-related COPD
- Younger
- Lower smoke exposure
- Lower BMI
- Lower socioeconomic class
- Higher prevalence of small airways disease
- Higher prevalence of severe exacerbations
- Report worse dyspnea and quality of life
- Higher airway hyperresponsiveness
- Greater physiologic impact with smoking cessation but less likely to achieve cessation

with COPD who have never smoked. Even symptom presentation may be slightly different in women when compared to men. Women have been reported to have higher rates of exacerbations and more severe exacerbations, both of which likely account for the increased death rate seen in some countries. Women also seem to have greater dyspnea compared to men for similar level of lung function.

Currently, gender-specific treatment and management guidelines do not exist. Although asthma and COPD treatment recommendations should not differ based on gender, response to certain targeted strategies may be different.[53] Some evidence suggests smoking cessation has more of an impact on lung function in women compared with men. However, it appears women are overall less successful in achieving cessation. Differences in response to pharmacological therapies, pulmonary rehabilitation, and long-term oxygen supplementation may be different but remain unknown.

12.4.3 GENDER AND ACO

Conflicting data currently exist in regards to gender specifics in ACO; some reports suggest a higher prevalence of ACO in females, while others suggest that males are more affected.[48,56-60] The heterogeneous definitions and diagnostic criteria utilized in much of the current ACO data largely accounts for this variability.[3] The reported gender differences in ACO populations likely depend on how the ACO cohorts were gathered and analyzed, as well as the ACO diagnostic criterion utilized. Cohorts generated from clinics or pools with more asthma patients will likely identify more women, while cohorts generated from individuals with more COPD will likely identify more male patients with ACO.[46] Since women seem to have greater airway hyperresponsiveness than men,[53] it could be inferred that more women would fit within the bronchodilator criteria for ACO, but this is not clear from existing data. Until further information emerges, it is unknown how gender affects rates of ACO in addition to how it may affect therapeutic or management strategies.

12.5 EFFECTS OF PREGNANCY

Asthma is one of the most common potentially serious conditions that affect pregnancy. It is estimated that approximately 4%–8% of childbearing women have asthma.[61,62] Women who have asthma and become pregnant typically follow a "one-third rule": one-third experience an improvement in their symptom control, one-third will remain unchanged, and one-third will have worsening control of asthma symptoms.[63] Although it is not completely predictable, those women with more severe and poorly controlled asthma prior to pregnancy tend to experience worsening control during pregnancy, and those with milder and/or stable disease remain stable or improve. Whatever change is experienced, the same response is often encountered in subsequent pregnancies. About 20% of pregnant women with asthma will experience exacerbations that need medical intervention, and about 6% of these will require hospitalization. The exacerbations tend to occur during the late second or early third trimester, but improvement in the last month of pregnancy is often noted. Although uncommon, some women do experience exacerbations during the labor and delivery process. Prepregnancy level of control often returns several months after delivery.[63]

The variability and changes seen in asthma control during pregnancy is speculated to be secondary to fluctuations and changes in hormones that occur during pregnancy.[64] It has also been speculated that despite guideline recommendations to continue asthma medications during pregnancy, worsening control is often due to poor adherence or stoppage of asthma-control medications due to concerns about whether the medication is safe for the fetus.[1,65–67] Though not well studied, available information suggests that most medications commonly used for asthma treatment, both in acute and maintenance settings, are safe to use during pregnancy. More importantly, the advantages of actively treating asthma markedly outweigh any potential risks.[1,68] Use of ICS, β_2-agonists, montelukast, or theophylline is not associated with an increased incidence of fetal abnormalities. Stopping maintenance drugs that have helped achieve adequate control is likely more dangerous, as this can precipitate acute exacerbations resulting in hypoxia, leading to a substantial risk to both mother and fetus. In fact, cessation of ICS during pregnancy is a significant risk factor for exacerbations.[69] However, since not all side effects or complications with asthma medications are completely known in regards to maternal-fetal safety, it is prudent to have an informed discussion with expecting mothers on risks and benefits of asthma medications before any changes are made, as well as close clinical monitoring, especially during the final trimester and delivery phases. In addition, other factors such as maternal smoking, and worsening or uncontrolled comorbid conditions (such as perinatal GERD and rhinitis, as well as increased acute respiratory infections, especially viral) likely account for some proportion of worsening asthma control and exacerbations during pregnancy, and should be managed accordingly.[64,69–71]

Maternal and fetal outcomes in women with asthma are conflicted. Some studies report pregnant women with asthma have increased risk for pregnancy-induced hypertension, preeclampsia, gestational diabetes, and delivery by caesarean section, whereas other have found no such associations. Some studies, but not all, report asthma is associated with worse neonatal outcomes, including low birth weight, preterm labor or delivery, congenital malformations, and neonatal sepsis.[70]

Since COPD and ACO typically do not occur until at least 40 years of age, there is very little knowledge on these issues as the usual child-bearing age has often been passed prior to them becoming clinically significant.

12.6 EFFECTS OF RACE AND ETHNICITY

12.6.1 RACE, ETHNICITY, AND ASTHMA

Minorities, including African Americans and Hispanics, especially Puerto Ricans, have a higher prevalence of asthma when compared to Caucasian populations in the United States.[72,73] Whether this disparity is secondary to an inherent predisposition; differences in physiology, behaviors, or environmental exposures; variations in socioeconomic class and health care disparities; or a combination of several variables is uncertain.[74] However, it also seems evident that minorities with asthma have worse control of their symptoms, greater acute health-care utilization, and worse morbidity and mortality compared to Caucasians. Both African Americans and Puerto Rican Hispanics have an estimated 3 to 1 mortality ratio due to asthma when compared to Caucasians in the United States. In addition, the impact of racial and ethnic disparities is even more evident in minority children with asthma.[72,73,75,76]

There are several proposed factors to consider that may account for the disparities among different races and ethnicities. There are likely some genetic variations that account for susceptibility to the disease and that influence response to asthma medications. Currently, however, data suggests that LABA add-on to ICS is just as efficacious and safe as a long-acting anticholinergic add-on to ICS for black adults with asthma.[77] Environmental factors may also play a role. Asthma risk in minorities is often attributable to allergen and irritant exposures, which are typically more prevalent due to poorer living conditions. Poor health-care access and underutilization of asthma medications, most notably controller medications, are evident, which are the result of poor access to providers, underprescribing by health-care providers, nonadherence with visits and treatment recommendations, and poor inhaler technique. Mental health factors, such as depression, anxiety, and bipolar disorder, play an important role with adherence of treatment plans as well. Minorities have a greater dependence or reliance on acute and emergency care systems, which impacts overall asthma care. Lower education and poor understanding of asthma likely further impacts these behavioral issues. Asthma education is often lacking for minorities and those with lower levels of education. Targeted programs for asthma education have demonstrated improvement in minorities dealing with asthma and certainly provides direction for caretakers and policymakers to implement changes that can improve asthma outcomes and reduce associated costs across socioeconomic strata.[74]

12.6.2 RACE AND ETHNICITY AND COPD

Data demonstrate an increasing prevalence of COPD, as well as an increase in death rates due to COPD, among African Americans. Some information suggests racial and ethnic differences in tobacco susceptibility as African Americans and Hispanics often demonstrate similar lung function despite lower levels of smoke exposure.[78,79] This is believed to be in part the result of differences in the rates of nicotine metabolism. Response to inhaled medications seem to be different for African Americans as well. This may account for differences in symptom control and rates of exacerbations. Overall, African Americans exhibit asthma symptoms at a younger age and have fewer smoking pack years than Caucasians; but African Americans generally have worse symptoms, more dyspnea, decreased activity tolerance (measured as distance during a six-minute walking test), and an increased rate of exacerbations that require hospitalization.[78,80] These differences are clearly multifactorial again, including socioeconomic status and behavioral factors, but are also in part due to an increased rate of confounding comorbidities in African Americans with COPD.[81]

12.6.3 RACE, ETHNICITY, AND ASTHMA-COPD OVERLAP

Although limited, available data from the United States suggest that African Americans make up a higher percentage of individuals with ACO than they do for COPD alone.[82] While there is not enough evidence to definitively comment on this disparity, it is reasonable to assume that some of the higher prevalence of asthma in this subpopulation accounts for some of the increased prevalence of ACO, based on how studies have defined ACO as individuals with a history of reported asthma or an asthma diagnosis based on ICD-9 coding. In addition, a subanalysis of the COPDGene study demonstrated that African Americans have less emphysema but similar amounts of air trapping and airway-wall thickness compared to Caucasians. This analysis also demonstrated that despite having less smoking exposure and higher FEV_1 values, African Americans had more reported pulmonary symptoms and less distance endurance during a six-minute

walking test. These differences may be in part explained by the fact that African Americans in this analysis had a much higher reported history of asthma.[83] Given the fact that bronchial-wall thickness has been associated with more frequent COPD exacerbations and chronic bronchitis, one may infer that African Americans may be more likely to present with phenotypic characteristics consistent with ACO. Ultimately, more research is needed to fully understand and determine whether race and ethnicity impact ACO.

12.7 SUMMARY

Asthma, COPD, and ACO are common disorders. The impact, clinical course, and outcomes of these disorders may be different in special populations based on age, gender, race, and ethnicity. However, our knowledge is limited to a few published studies. Future research is needed to evaluate mechanisms, as well as clinical and therapeutic implications of these disorders, in these special populations.

REFERENCES

1. Global Initiative for Asthma. Global Strategy for Asthma Management and Prevention; 2015. Available at www.ginasthma.org.
2. Global Initiative for Chronic Obstructive Lung Disease. Global Strategy for the Diagnosis, Management, and Prevention of Chronic Obstructive Pulmonary Disease; 2017. Available at www.gold-copd.org.
3. Bujarski S, Parulekar AD, Sharafkhaneh A et al. The asthma COPD overlap syndrome (ACOS). *Curr Allergy Asthma Rep.* 2015;15(3):509.
4. Divo MJ, Martinez CH, and Mannino DM. Ageing and the epidemiology of multimorbidity. *Eur Respir J.* 2014;44(4):1055–1068.
5. Vincent GK, Velkoff VA, and U.S. Census Bureau. *The Next Four Decades: The Older Population in the United States: 2010–2050.* Washington, DC: U.S. Department of Commerce, Economics and Statistics Administration, U.S. Census Bureau; 2010. 14 p.
6. Thannickal VJ, Murthy M, Balch WE et al. Blue journal conference. Aging and susceptibility to lung disease. *Am J Respir Crit Care Med.* 2015;191(3):261–269.
7. Weyand CM and Goronzy JJ. Aging of the immune system. Mechanisms and therapeutic targets. *Ann Am Thorac Soc.* 2016;13(Suppl. 5):S422–S428.
8. Centers for Disease Control and Prevention. Asthma's impact on the nation factsheet; 2014. Available at www.cdc.gov/asthma/impacts_nation/asthmafactsheet.pdf.
9. McGeachie MJ, Yates KP, Zhou X et al. Patterns of growth and decline in lung function in persistent childhood asthma. *N Engl J Med.* 2016;374(19):1842–1852.

10. King MJ and Hanania NA. Asthma in the elderly: Current knowledge and future directions. *Curr Opin Pulm Med*. 2010;16(1):55–59.

11. Tsai CL, Lee WY, Hanania NA et al. Age-related differences in clinical outcomes for acute asthma in the United States, 2006–2008. *J Allergy Clin Immunol*. 2012;129(5):1252–1258. e1.

12. Tsai CL, Delclos GL, Huang JS et al. Age-related differences in asthma outcomes in the United States, 1988–2006. *Ann Allergy Asthma Immunol*. 2013;110(4):240–246, 6. e1.

13. Centers for Disease Control and Prevention. Asthma: National Health Interview Survey (NHIS) Data; 2011, Tables 2-1 & 4-1. Available at https://www.cdc.gov /asthma/nhis/default.htm.

14. Parameswaran K, Hildreth AJ, Chadha D et al. Asthma in the elderly: Underperceived, underdiagnosed and undertreated; A community survey. *Respir Med*. 1998;92(3):573–577.

15. Enright PL. The diagnosis and management of asthma is much tougher in older patients. *Curr Opin Allergy Clin Immunol*. 2002;2(3):175–181.

16. Enright PL, McClelland RL, Newman AB et al. Underdiagnosis and undertreatment of asthma in the elderly. Cardiovascular health study research group. *Chest*. 1999;116(3):603–613.

17. Bellia V, Battaglia S, Catalano F et al. Aging and disability affect misdiagnosis of COPD in elderly asthmatics: The SARA study. *Chest*. 2003;123(4):1066–1072.

18. Oraka E, Kim HJ, King ME et al. Asthma prevalence among US elderly by age groups: Age still matters. *J Asthma*. 2012;49(6):593–599.

19. Akinbami LJ, Moorman JE, Bailey C et al. Trends in asthma prevalence, health care use, and mortality in the United States, 2001–2010. *NCHS Data Brief*. 2012(94):1–8.

20. Braman SS, Kaemmerlen JT, and Davis SM. Asthma in the elderly. A comparison between patients with recently acquired and long-standing disease. *Am Rev Respir Dis*. 1991;143(2):336–340.

21. Braman SS, Corrao WM, and Kaemmerlen JT. The clinical outcome of asthma in the elderly: A 7-year follow-up study. *Ann N Y Acad Sci*. 1991;629:449–450.

22. Hanania NA, King MJ, Braman SS et al. Asthma in the elderly: Current understanding and future research needs—A report of a national Institute on Aging (NIA) workshop. *J Allergy Clin Immunol*. 2011;128 (Suppl. 3):S4–S24.

23. Skloot GS, Busse PJ, Braman SS et al. An official American thoracic society workshop report: Evaluation and management of asthma in the elderly. *Ann Am Thorac Soc*. 2016;13(11):2064–2077.

24. Ekici M, Apan A, Ekici A et al. Perception of bronchoconstriction in elderly asthmatics. *J Asthma*. 2001;38(8):691–696.

25. Dunn RM, Lehman E, Chinchilli VM et al. Impact of age and sex on response to asthma therapy. *Am J Respir Crit Care Med*. 2015;192(5):551–558.

26. Song WJ, and Cho SH. Challenges in the management of asthma in the elderly. *Allergy Asthma Immunol Res*. 2015;7(5):431–439.

27. Martinez CH, Diaz AA, Parulekar AD et al. Age-related differences in health-related quality of life in COPD: An Analysis of the COPDGene and SPIROMICS cohorts. *Chest*. 2016;149(4):927–935.

28. Raherison C, and Girodet PO. Epidemiology of COPD. *Eur Respir Rev*. 2009;18(114):213–221.

29. Prince MJ, Wu F, Guo Y et al. The burden of disease in older people and implications for health policy and practice. *Lancet*. 2015;385(9967):549–562.

30. Salive ME. Multimorbidity in older adults. *Epidemiol Rev*. 2013;35:75–83.

31. Marengoni A, Angleman S, Melis R et al. Aging with multimorbidity: A systematic review of the literature. *Ageing Res Rev*. 2011;10(4):430–439.

32. Wolff JL, Starfield B, and Anderson G. Prevalence, expenditures, and complications of multiple chronic conditions in the elderly. *Arch Intern Med*. 2002;162(20):2269–2276.

33. Killian KJ, Leblanc P, Martin DH et al. Exercise capacity and ventilatory, circulatory, and symptom limitation in patients with chronic airflow limitation. *Am Rev Respir Dis*. 1992;146(4):935–940.

34. Mahler DA, Tomlinson D, Olmstead EM et al. Changes in dyspnea, health status, and lung function in chronic airway disease. *Am J Respir Crit Care Med*. 1995;151(1):61–65.

35. McGavin CR, Artvinli M, Naoe H et al. Dyspnoea, disability, and distance walked: Comparison of estimates of exercise performance in respiratory disease. *Br Med J*. 1978;2(6132):241–243.

36. McSweeny AJ, Grant I, Heaton RK et al. Life quality of patients with chronic obstructive pulmonary disease. *Arch Intern Med*. 1982;142(3):473–478.

37. Prigatano GP, Wright EC, and Levin D. Quality of life and its predictors in patients with mild hypoxemia and chronic obstructive pulmonary disease. *Arch Intern Med*. 1984;144(8):1613–1619.

38. Peruzza S, Sergi G, Vianello A et al. Chronic obstructive pulmonary disease (COPD) in elderly subjects: Impact on functional status and quality of life. *Respir Med*. 2003;97(6):612–617.

39. van Durme Y, Verhamme KMC, Stijnen T et al. Prevalence, incidence, and lifetime risk for the development of COPD in the elderly: The rotterdam study. *Chest*. 2009;135(2):368–377.

40. Vaz Fragoso CA, Concato J, McAvay G et al. Chronic obstructive pulmonary disease in older persons: A comparison of two spirometric definitions. *Respir Med.* 2010;104(8):1189–1196.

41. Yohannes AM, Roomi J, Waters K et al. Quality of life in elderly patients with COPD: Measurement and predictive factors. *Respir Med.* 1998;92(10):1231–1236.

42. Martinez FD. Early-life origins of chronic obstructive pulmonary disease. *N Engl J Med.* 2016;375(9):871–878.

43. de Marco R, Pesce G, Marcon A et al. The coexistence of asthma and chronic obstructive pulmonary disease (COPD): Prevalence and risk factors in young, middle-aged and elderly people from the general population. *PLOS ONE.* 2013;8(5):e62985.

44. Global Initiative for Asthma. Diagnosis of diseases of chronic airflow limitation: Asthma, COPD, and asthma-COPD overlap syndrome (ACOS); 2014. Available at www.ginasthma.org.

45. Gibson PG and Simpson JL. The overlap syndrome of asthma and COPD: What are its features and how important is it? *Thorax.* 2009;64(8):728–735.

46. Zeki AA, Schivo M, Chan A et al. The asthma-COPD overlap syndrome: A common clinical problem in the elderly. *J Allergy (Cairo).* 2011;2011:861926.

47. van Boven JF, Roman Rodriguez M, Palmer JF et al. Comorbidome, pattern, and impact of asthma-COPD overlap syndrome in real life. *Chest.* 2016;149(4):1011–1020.

48. Postma DS and Rabe KF. The asthma-COPD overlap syndrome. *N Engl J Med.* 2015;373(13):1241–1249.

49. CDC. National Health Interview Survey (NHIS) data. Available at http://www.cdc.gov/asthma/nhis/2015/table2-1.htm.

50. Fuseini H and Newcomb DC. Mechanisms driving gender differences in asthma. *Curr Allergy Asthma Rep.* 2017;17(3):19.

51. Zein JG and Erzurum SC. Asthma is different in women. *Curr Allergy Asthma Rep.* 2015;15(6):28.

52. Kynyk JA, Mastronarde JG, and McCallister JW. Asthma, the sex difference. *Curr Opin Pulm Med.* 2011;17(1):6–11.

53. Jenkins CR, Chapman KR, Donohue JF et al. Improving the management of COPD in women. *Chest.* 2017;151(3):686–696.

54. Rycroft CE, Heyes A, Lanza L et al. Epidemiology of chronic obstructive pulmonary disease: A literature review. *Int J Chron Obstruct Pulmon Dis.* 2012;7:457–494.

55. Han MK, Postma D, Mannino DM et al. Gender and chronic obstructive pulmonary disease: Why it matters. *Am J Respir Crit Care Med.* 2007;176(12):1179–1184.

56. Cosio BG, Soriano JB, Lopez-Campos JL et al. Defining the asthma-COPD overlap syndrome in a COPD cohort. *Chest.* 2016;149(1):45–52.

57. Cosentino J, Zhao H, Hardin M et al. Analysis of asthma-chronic obstructive pulmonary disease overlap syndrome defined on the basis of bronchodilator response and degree of emphysema. *Ann Am Thorac Soc.* 2016;13(9):1483–1489.

58. Barrecheguren M, Roman-Rodriguez M, and Miravitlles M. Is a previous diagnosis of asthma a reliable criterion for asthma-COPD overlap syndrome in a patient with COPD? *Int J Chron Obstruct Pulmon Dis.* 2015;10:1745–1752.

59. Kumbhare S, Pleasants R, Ohar JA et al. Characteristics and prevalence of asthma/chronic obstructive pulmonary disease overlap in the United States. *Ann Am Thorac Soc.* 2016;13(6):803–810.

60. Wurst KE, Rheault TR, Edwards L et al. A comparison of COPD patients with and without ACOS in the ECLIPSE study. *Eur Respir J.* 2016;47(5):1559–1562.

61. Kwon HL, Belanger K, and Bracken MB. Asthma prevalence among pregnant and childbearing-aged women in the United States: Estimates from national health surveys. *Ann Epidemiol.* 2003;13(5):317–324.

62. Kwon HL, Triche EW, Belanger K et al. The epidemiology of asthma during pregnancy: Prevalence, diagnosis, and symptoms. *Immunol Allergy Clin North Am.* 2006;26(1):29–62.

63. Schatz M, Harden K, Forsythe A et al. The course of asthma during pregnancy, post partum, and with successive pregnancies: A prospective analysis. *J Allergy Clin Immunol.* 1988;81(3):509–517.

64. Gluck JC and Gluck PA. The effect of pregnancy on the course of asthma. *Immunol Allergy Clin North Am.* 2006;26(1):63–80.

65. Lim AS, Stewart K, Abramson MJ et al. Asthma during pregnancy: The experiences, concerns and views of pregnant women with asthma. *J Asthma.* 2012;49(5):474–479.

66. Enriquez R, Wu P, Griffin MR et al. Cessation of asthma medication in early pregnancy. *Am J Obstet Gynecol.* 2006;195(1):149–153.

67. Lim AS, Stewart K, Abramson MJ et al. Management of asthma in pregnant women by general practitioners: A cross sectional survey. *BMC Fam Pract.* 2011;12:121.

68. Lim A, Stewart K, Konig K et al. Systematic review of the safety of regular preventive asthma medications during pregnancy. *Ann Pharmacother.* 2011;45(7–8):931–945.

69. Murphy VE, Clifton VL, and Gibson PG. Asthma exacerbations during pregnancy: Incidence and association with adverse pregnancy outcomes. *Thorax.* 2006;61(2):169–176.

70. Murphy VE and Gibson PG. Asthma in pregnancy. *Clin Chest Med.* 2011;32(1):93–110, ix.

71. Murphy VE, Clifton VL, and Gibson PG. The effect of cigarette smoking on asthma control during exacerbations in pregnant women. *Thorax.* 2010;65(8):739–744.

72. Centers for Disease Control and Prevention. Most recent asthma data. 2015. Available at www.cdc.gov.

73. United States Environmental Protection Agency (EPA). Asthma facts. 2016. Available at https://www.epa.gov/sites/production/files/2016-05/documents/asthma_fact_sheet_english_05_2016.pdf.

74. Asthma and Allergy Foundation of America. Ethnic disparities in the burden and treatment of asthma; 2005. Available at http://www.aafa.org/media/Ethnic-Disparities-Burden-Treatment-Asthma-Report.pdf.

75. Centers for Disease Control and Prevention. QuickStats: Asthma death rates, by race and age group – United States, 2007–2009. Morbidity and Mortality Weekly Report (MMWR). 2012;61(17):315.

76. American Lung Association. Trends in asthma morbidity and mortality. 2012. Available at http://www.lung.org/assets/documents/research/asthma-trend-report.pdf.

77. Wechsler ME, Yawn BP, Fuhlbrigge AL et al. Anticholinergic vs long-acting beta-agonist in combination with inhaled corticosteroids in black adults with asthma: The BELT randomized clinical trial. *JAMA.* 2015;314(16):1720–1730.

78. Han MK, Curran-Everett D, Dransfield MT et al. Racial differences in quality of life in patients with COPD. *Chest.* 2011;140(5):1169–1176.

79. Adams SG, Anzueto A, Pugh JA et al. Mexican American elders have similar severities of COPD despite less tobacco exposure than European American elders. *Respir Med.* 2006;100(11):1966–1972.

80. Foreman MG, Zhang L, Murphy J et al. Early-onset chronic obstructive pulmonary disease is associated with female sex, maternal factors, and African American race in the COPDGene study. *Am J Respir Crit Care Med.* 2011;184(4):414–420.

81. Putcha N, Han MK, Martinez CH et al. Comorbidities of COPD have a major impact on clinical outcomes, particularly in African Americans. *Chronic Obstr Pulm Dis.* 2014;1(1):105–114.

82. Hardin M, Silverman EK, Barr RG et al. The clinical features of the overlap between COPD and asthma. *Respir Res.* 2011;12:127.

83. Hansel NN, Washko GR, Foreman MG et al. Racial differences in CT phenotypes in COPD. *COPD.* 2013;10(1):20–27.

History and physical examination of asthma, COPD, and asthma-COPD overlap

MARK H. ALMOND AND KIAN FAN CHUNG

CLINICAL VIGNETTE 13.1: LATE-ONSET, CORTICOSTEROID-DEPENDENT EOSINOPHILIC ASTHMA

A 43-year-old Caucasian female with a confirmed diagnosis of late-onset, corticosteroid-dependent eosinophilic asthma presented to a respiratory outpatient clinic with a five-day history of increasing chest tightness, nocturnal awakening, and exertional dyspnea. Her asthma control questionnaire (ACQ) in the clinic was > 4 and comorbidities included allergic rhinitis, confirmed previously by allergy skin testing that correlated with her exposure history, morbid obesity (BMI 42.2 kg/m^2), anxiety disorder, vertebral osteopenia, and vitamin D deficiency. Her treatment regimen included maximal inhaled corticosteroid, a combination of long-acting β-agonist (LABA) and long-acting muscarinic antagonist (LAMA) therapy, modified release aminophylline, and prednisolone 40 mg (increased from a baseline dose of 10 mg, daily). She had been hospitalized once since her previous outpatient consultation for an asthma exacerbation, which required intravenous hydrocortisone, magnesium, and short-acting β-agonist (SABA) nebulizer therapy. Examination revealed widespread, expiratory multiple monophonic wheeze but was otherwise unremarkable. Her peak expiratory flow rate (PEFR) and forced expiratory volume in 1 second (FEV$_1$) were both decreased by 20%. Further enquiry revealed that she had been under considerable stress due to the threat of being fired from her job following repeated absences from work. Notably, her eosinophil count was elevated at 1.3 on the day of her consultation.

Learning point: Adherence to therapy should be evaluated at every consultation; in this instance, the elevated eosinophil count, despite 40 mg of corticosteroid therapy, should alert the physician to a potential issue with adherence to treatment; this was confirmed by the absence of expected serum prednisolone levels and suppressed levels of serum cortisol. On further questioning, the patient acknowledged her poor adherence and explained it was secondary to the anxiety surrounding her employment status and concerns about further weight gain and worsening osteopenia. Clinical improvement was promptly observed with reinitiation of corticosteroid therapy and discussion regarding other potential treatment approaches to improve asthma control and reduce or discontinue oral corticosteroids was initiated. The recent availability of anti-IL5 antibody treatment should be considered in this patient with severe eosinophilic asthma if she continues to need maintenance oral corticosteroid therapy.[1]

CLINICAL VIGNETTE 13.2: SUSPECTED COPD

A 41-year-old Caucasian male office worker with a 10 pack-year smoking history presented to the outpatient clinic with a three-month history of exertional dyspnea while playing with his seven-year-old son. Further questioning revealed a nonproductive cough present for 2 months, but no other significant respiratory symptoms. His past medical history revealed three lower respiratory-tract infections requiring antibiotics over the previous 10 years. His father, also a smoker, had died at age 55 from "bronchitis." He had no significant occupational exposures. Physical examination was unremarkable, and no stigmata of pulmonary hypertension were evident.

Subsequent pulmonary function testing at presentation revealed airflow obstruction with insignificant bronchodilator reversibility. High-resolution computed tomography (HRCT) of the chest revealed bilateral lower-lobe predominant emphysema and a serum alpha-1 anti-trypsin assay indicated a PiZZ phenotype, consistent with a diagnosis of alpha-1 anti-trypsin deficiency. The importance of smoking cessation was emphasized, and inhaled bronchodilator therapy administered.

Learning point: Alpha-1 antitrypsin deficiency should be considered in all younger individuals presenting with dyspnea and a smoking history or appropriate occupational history.

CLINICAL VIGNETTE 13.3: ASTHMA-COPD OVERLAP

A 62-year-old Caucasian, male, ex-metalworker presented to a respiratory outpatient clinic with a six-month history of exertional dyspnea and productive cough. On a good day, his exercise tolerance was unlimited and he was asymptomatic. However, on a bad day, he experienced wheezing, chest tightness, and exercise intolerance after a few meters. He was an exsmoker (25 pack-year history) and had been labeled with asthma by his general practitioner 12 years previously. He had required three courses of antibiotics and prednisolone for exacerbations of his asthma over the previous 12 months. He recalls frequent chest infections as a child, and his family history revealed that his mother had asthma. Examination revealed evidence of hyperinflation and bilateral, diffuse, expiratory wheeze. Spirometry revealed airflow obstruction (post-bronchodilator forced expiratory volume in 1 second [BD FEV_1] 62% predicted, post-BD FEV_1/FVC ratio 0.5), bronchodilator reversibility, gas trapping, and hyperinflation. A high-resolution CT scan of the thorax revealed widespread emphysema. His peripheral eosinophil count was elevated at 2.4, and serum-specific IgE to aeroallergens were positive for grass pollen and house dust mites. His total IgE was only slightly elevated at 160 kU/L, and specific IgE and precipitating IgG antibodies to Aspergillus fumigatus were both negative. He was commenced on prednisolone and combination ICS/LABA therapy, which resulted in significant symptomatic benefit.

Learning point: When syndromic assessment favors a diagnosis of asthma-COPD overlap (ACO), the recommended default position is to start treatment for asthma until further investigations have been performed, thus recognizing the pivotal role of ICS in preventing morbidity and mortality in patients with uncontrolled asthma symptoms.[2] The diagnosis of ACO in this patient was based upon his obstructive spirometry and features consistent with both asthma (symptomatic variability, previous physician diagnosis, positive family history, atopy, eosinophilia, bronchodilator reversibility) and chronic obstructive pulmonary disease (COPD) (gradual onset exertional dyspnea, hyperinflation on examination, significant smoking history, emphysema on HRCT thorax).

Such patients are likely to need follow-up in specialist respiratory clinics, since they experience an increased number of comorbidities and are at increased risk for hospitalization or emergency room visits more so than COPD-only patients.[3]

13.1 INTRODUCTION

Despite improvements in our understanding of the pathophysiology of asthma and COPD, and technological advances in diagnostic techniques such as high-resolution thoracic CT imaging and fractional exhaled nitric oxide (FeNO), a thorough medical history and physical examination remain of paramount importance in the diagnosis of both conditions, especially when diagnostic uncertainty exists.

When contemplating a diagnosis of asthma or COPD, as applies for all clinical presentations, the presenting symptoms should be fastidiously characterized and evaluated in the context of the predisposing risk factors for each condition. Once the differential diagnosis has been considered (Table 13.1),[4,5] and a working diagnosis of asthma or COPD established, the severity of the condition should be determined, and the impact on the patient's quality of life and their capacity to perform their daily activities evaluated. Furthermore, symptoms and signs of potential secondary complications, such as malignancy or pulmonary hypertension in the case of COPD, should be actively sought at each consultation.

The aim of this chapter is to provide a practical, guideline-based framework for performing thorough-yet-focused clinical assessments of adults with asthma, COPD, and ACO. The chapter has three sections, each

Table 13.1 Differential diagnostic possibilities for asthma and COPD in adults

Asthma	COPD
– COPD	– Asthma
– Congestive heart failure	– Congestive heart failure
– Pulmonary embolism	– Bronchiectasis
– Mechanical obstruction of the airways (benign and malignant tumors)	– Tuberculosis
– Pulmonary infiltration with eosinophilia	– Obliterative bronchiolitis
– Cough secondary to drugs (e.g., angiotensin-converting enzyme [ACE] inhibitors)	– Diffuse panbronchiolitis
– Vocal cord dysfunction	

Source: Derived from GINA. Global strategy for asthma management and prevention; 2015. Available at www.ginasthma.org; GOLD. Global strategy for the diagnosis, management, and prevention of chronic obstructive pulmonary disease; 2016. Available at www.goldcopd.org.

corresponding to a common scenario in which individuals with these conditions are likely to be encountered: the initial outpatient consultation in which a diagnosis of asthma, COPD, or ACO is suspected; the routine outpatient follow-up consultation; and the acute presentation of the exacerbating patient in the emergency room.

Initial consultation – suspected asthma

13.1.1 MEDICAL HISTORY

The classical presenting symptoms of asthma are episodic wheeze, dyspnea, chest tightness, and cough that occur following exposure to characteristic triggers and are relieved by bronchodilator medications.[4] However, these symptoms are nonspecific, and the definitive diagnosis of asthma requires the presence of both typical respiratory symptoms and signs *and* the clinical demonstration of variable expiratory airflow obstruction[4] (Table 13.2).[6] Asthma may develop, or reemerge, at any age, although new-onset asthma is less frequent in older adults.

When assessing an individual with suspected asthma one should weigh the clinical features that heighten or reduce the probability of asthma.[4] The classical symptoms listed above are characteristically variable in both intensity and time course, and are often worse at night or in the early morning. The probability of asthma is increased, especially in adults, if more than one of these symptoms is present. Conversely, features that reduce the probability that the symptoms are due to asthma include the presence of an isolated cough in the absence of other respiratory symptoms, a lack of improvement in symptoms following the administration of antiasthma medications, such as inhaled bronchodilators or oral glucocorticoids, age of onset over the age of 50, a significant smoking history (>20 pack years), chronic sputum production, dyspnea associated with dizziness, light-headedness and peripheral tingling, chest pain, syncope, and exercise-induced dyspnea with noisy inspiration.[4]

The history should include questions that allow characterization of exacerbating factors; typical triggers include viral infections, exercise, changes in weather, emotions (e.g., laughter), and exposure to cold air, irritants, or aeroallergens. Respiratory viral infections (e.g., rhinovirus) are common triggers, but not specific for asthma as they may also

Table 13.2 Key indicators for considering a diagnosis of asthma

Consider a diagnosis of asthma and perform spirometry if any of these indicators is present.[a] These indicators are not diagnostic by themselves, but the presence of multiple key indicators increases the probability of a diagnosis of asthma. Spirometry is needed to establish a diagnosis of asthma.

Wheezing

– high-pitched whistling sounds when breathing out—especially in children. (Lack of wheezing and a normal chest examination do not exclude asthma.)

History of any of the following:

– Cough, worse at night
– Recurrent wheeze
– Recurrent difficulty breathing
– Recurrent chest tightness

Symptoms occur or worsen in the presence of

– Exercise
– Viral infection
– Animals with fur or hair
– House-dust mites (in mattresses, pillows, upholstered furniture, carpets)
– Mold
– Smoke (tobacco, wood)
– Pollen
– Changes in weather
– Strong emotional expression (laughing or crying hard)
– Airborne chemicals or dust
– Menstrual cycles

Symptoms occur or worsen at night, awakening the patient.

Source: Adapted from the NHLBI. Expert Panel Report 3 (EPR-3): Guidelines for the Diagnosis and Managment of Asthma - Summary Report; 2007. Available at http://www.nhlbi .nih.gov/health-pro/guidelines/current/asthma -guidelines/summary-report-2007.
[a] Eczema, hay fever, or a family history of asthma or atopic diseases are often associated with asthma, but they are not key indicators.

result in exacerbations of other respiratory diseases such as COPD or bronchiectasis. Classical aeroallergens that may trigger asthma include house dust mites, molds, cats, dogs, cockroaches, and pollens, and atopy can be confirmed by either skin-prick testing or serum-specific IgE immunoassays (e.g., ImmunoCAP). Notably, symptoms brought on by irritant-type exposures (e.g., cigarette smoke, strong fumes, and changes in weather and airborne chemicals/dusts are not specific to asthma). Nonsteroidal anti-inflammatory drug (NSAID) sensitivity is unique to asthma, with the onset of classic symptoms 30 to 120 minutes following aspirin or COX-1 inhibitor exposure. Although specific, aspirin-exacerbated respiratory disease (AERD), also known as aspirin triad (classically described as chronic rhinosinusitis and nasal polyposis, followed by the onset of asthma, and finally by aspirin or NSAID intolerance, manifesting as a severe asthma exacerbation) is seen only in a minority (7%) of asthmatic individuals.[7] Other potential, less-common triggers that may be reported include ingestion of sulphites (used in the production of most wines) and certain food dyes. Exercise-induced symptoms in asthma usually occur 5–15 minutes after a short period of exertion or 15 minutes into exercise, and typically resolve with rest within an hour.

To help confirm the diagnosis of asthma, it is important to determine an individual's predisposing risk factors. The medical history should therefore include questions to determine whether the patient has a personal or family history of atopic diseases, such as atopic dermatitis, seasonal allergic rhinitis, or conjunctivitis. Furthermore, enquiry into childhood asthmatic symptoms should be made (e.g., chronic cough or recurrent bronchitis). Using the Asthma Predictive Index, a combination of three or more episodes of recurrent wheeze before the age of three, either physician-diagnosed eczema or a family history of parental asthma, two of either physician-diagnosed allergic rhinitis or wheezing without colds, or peripheral eosinophilia > 4%, was associated with a very high chance of developing active asthma between the ages of 6 and 13.[8] Other risk factors that increase the probability of developing asthma should therefore be documented, include prematurity, early menarche, smoke exposure, and obesity. It is important to document a thorough occupational history at the initial consultation, as approximately 10% of adult-onset new cases are employment related; in occupational asthma, the characteristic symptoms in most cases are temporally associated with variable airflow obstruction after a work shift, sometimes hours later reflecting a late-phase reaction.

A detailed past medical history is important, as comorbidities associated with asthma may contribute to symptom burden, poor asthma control, impaired quality of life, and polypharmacy, which can lead to medication interactions. Obesity, gastroesophageal reflux disease (GERD), rhinitis, and rhinosinusitis are commonly seen in individuals with asthma, and these comorbidities should be actively assessed and managed from the outset. Furthermore, a detailed medication and allergy history should be obtained, as asthma may be exacerbated by certain medications. Deaths continue to be reported following inappropriate beta blocker or NSAID prescriptions, and, therefore, all asthma patients should be asked about past reactions to these agents.[9,10]

Once a likely diagnosis of asthma based on presenting symptoms, triggers, and risk factors has been established, it is important to evaluate the current level of asthma control and the impact on quality of life. It is important to emphasize that determination of asthma control requires careful assessment of both current symptoms and the future risk of adverse outcomes.[4]

13.1.2 PHYSICAL EXAMINATION

When assessing an individual with suspected asthma it should be emphasized that the physical examination may be entirely normal in between exacerbations. Examination should focus on the chest; however, evidence of chronic rhinitis (pale or erythematous, swollen nasal membranes with cobblestoning suggestive of postnasal drainage) or nasal polyposis may be evident upon inspection of the upper respiratory tract. In atopic patients with asthma, eczema suggestive of atopic dermatitis is more commonly identified and may be evident, especially in the flexure areas of the skin.

Inspection, palpation, and percussion of the chest is usually normal in an individual with stable asthma. However, in individuals with long-standing, severe asthma, signs of hyperinflation (e.g., increased anterior-posterior [AP] thoracic diameter and reduced sternocricoid distance) may be evident and the expiratory phase of the respiratory cycle may be prolonged. The most frequent positive finding on auscultation of the chest is wheeze, an adventitious, continuous musical sound thought to be produced by oscillation of opposing walls of an airway that is narrowed almost to the point of closure.[11]

The differential diagnosis of wheeze is extensive, and it should be noted that wheeze is not specific to asthma and that not all asthma results in wheeze (Table 13.3).[12] It is useful to determine the phase of the respiratory cycle in which the wheeze occurs (expiratory/inspiratory or both), the distribution (localized or widespread), the location (extrathoracic or intrathoracic), and the timbre (polyphonic or monophonic), as these features may help narrow the differential. However, the sensitivity and specificity of physical examination in determining the location and severity of airflow obstruction is limited.

As the airways are inflamed and narrowed in asthma, wheeze is more commonly heard during expiration, as the airways normally narrow during this phase of the respiratory cycle. However, wheeze may be heard during both the inspiratory and expiratory phases, and this may suggest more severe airway obstruction. Nevertheless, the presence or absence of wheezing is a poor predictor of the severity of airflow obstruction, as it may alert one to the presence of airway narrowing, but it does not indicate its severity. Indeed, the absence of wheezing in an asthma patient may indicate either improvement of the bronchoconstriction or severe, widespread airflow obstruction.

Table 13.3 Differential diagnosis of wheeze according to anatomic site of obstruction

Extrathoracic upper-airway obstruction		Intrathoracic upper-airway obstruction	Lower-airway obstruction
Postnasal drip syndrome	Obesity	Tracheal stenosis	Asthma
Paroxysmal vocal cord motion	Klebsiella rhinoscleroma	Foreign body aspiration	COPD
Hypertrophied tonsils	Mobile supraglottic soft tissue	Benign airway tumors	Pulmonary edema
Supraglottitis	Relapsing polychondritis	Malignancies	Aspiration
Laryngeal edema	Laryngocele	Intrathoracic goiter	Pulmonary embolism
Laryngostenosis	Abnormal arytenoid movement	Tracheobronchomegaly	Bronchiolitis
Postextubation granuloma		Acquired tracheomalacia	Cystic fibrosis
Retropharyngeal abscess	Vocal cord hematoma	Herpetic tracheobronchitis	Carcinoid syndrome
Benign airway tumors	Bilateral vocal cord paralysis	Right-sided aortic arch	Bronchiectasis
Anaphylaxis	Cricoarytenoid arthritis		Lymphangitic carcinomatosis
Malignancy	Granulomatosis with polyangiitis (Wegener's)		Parasitic infections

Source: Adapted from Irwin RS. Evaluation of wheezing illnesses other than asthma in adults. *UpToDate*. Available at www.uptodate.com: UptoDate, Waltham, MA; 2016.

The timbre or resonance of audible wheeze may be monophonic (single or multiple) or polyphonic. Polyphonic wheezing is confined to the expiratory phase and comprises multiple musical notes/pitches that start and end at the same time (like a musical chord); it is typically produced by dynamic compression of the large centralized airways, and the pitch of the polyphonic wheeze increases at the end of expiration as the equal pressure point moves toward the periphery.[13] Monophonic wheezing comprises single musical notes/pitches that start and end at different times. If the obstruction is rigid, then wheeze may be heard throughout the respiratory cycle, whereas if it is flexible, it may vary throughout the respiratory cycle. Widespread, expiratory, multiple, monophonic wheezes are typical of asthma,[13] whereas a persistent focal wheeze may indicate the presence of a foreign body, an obstructing tumor, or a congenital abnormality.[12,14]

13.1.2.1 Clinical assessment of individuals with confirmed asthma in the outpatient setting

The history and examination performed during routine outpatient follow-up consultations of individuals with confirmed diagnoses of asthma should focus on determining the level of asthma control, identifying any issues with the current therapeutic regimen, and evaluating any changes in associated comorbidities.[4] At each consultation the question of whether treatment can be de-escalated should always be considered.

The level of asthma control is defined as the extent to which manifestations of asthma are evident in the patient, or have been reduced or removed by treatment. As mentioned earlier, determination of asthma control requires careful evaluation of both current symptoms and the future risk of adverse outcomes. Direct questioning about asthma symptoms for 1 to 4 weeks prior to the

appointment should be asked to assess symptom control. Specific enquiry into the frequency of asthma symptoms (days per week), night waking, exercise limitation, and frequency of reliever use (excluding prior to exercise) should be determined. The patient should also be asked about the nature and frequency of any exacerbations, unanticipated medical office visits, courses of antibiotics or corticosteroids, and emergency room visits with or without hospitalizations. In U.K. primary care, simple tools such as the Royal College of Physicians three questions (RCP3Q)[15] can be used to identify individuals who require more detailed assessment (Table 13.4). Numerical or categorical questionnaires, such as the ACQ[16] or asthma control test (ACT)[17] may also be used to determine asthma control, and can be completed by patients while waiting in the office for their appointments.

The second domain of the assessment of asthma control is to identify whether the patient is at increased risk of

Table 13.4 The Royal College of Physicians three questions (RCP3Q)

In the last month	
1 Have you had difficulty sleeping because of asthma symptoms (including cough)?	Yes/No
2 Have you had your usual asthma symptoms during the day (cough, wheeze, chest tightness, or breathlessness)?	Yes/No
3 Has your asthma interfered with your usual activities (e.g., housework, work, school, etc.)?	Yes/No

Source: Adapted from Pearson MG and Bucknell CE., *Measuring Clinical Outcomes in Asthma: A Patient Focused Approach*, London, Royal College of Physicians, Clinical Effectiveness and Evaluation Unit, 1999.

Note: The "yes/no" responses are scored with 1 for each positive answer giving a total score between 0 and 3.

adverse asthma outcomes, including exacerbations, fixed airflow limitation, and medication side effects as mentioned in GINA[4] (Table 13.5). In the National Heart, Lung, and Blood Institute (NHLBI) guidelines in the United States, these are framed as both impairment and risk.[6]

The control-based asthma management cycle recommended by GINA (Figure 13.1) advocates adjustment of pharmacological and nonpharmacological treatments in a continuous fashion that involves assessment, treatment, and review. Therefore, following evaluation of asthma control, the current therapeutic regimen, and the patient's comprehension of it should be reviewed, including adherence, dosages, side effects, inhaler technique, and effectiveness of any changes in the regimen at controlling symptoms. It should be noted that poor inhaler technique leads to poor asthma control, increased risk of exacerbations, and increased adverse effects, and that the majority of patients (up to 70%–80%) are unable to use their inhaler correctly; furthermore, most people with incorrect technique are unaware that they have a problem.[18] Poor adherence is defined as the failure of treatment to be taken correctly as agreed upon by the patient and the health-care provider, and it is a common reason for poor asthma control. Approximately, 50% of individuals on long-term therapy for asthma fail to take medications as directed at least part of the time. In clinical practice, poor adherence may be identified by an empathetic question that acknowledges the likelihood of incomplete adherence and encourages an open discussion to address social, mental, cultural, and economic barriers that may contribute to poor compliance. Checking the date of the last prescription or the date on the inhaler may also assist in identifying poor adherence.[19]

Comorbidities associated with asthma may contribute to symptom burden, poor asthma control, and impaired quality of life, and may lead to polypharmacy resulting in medication interactions. It is therefore important that comorbidities, including obesity, diabetes, rhinitis/rhinosinusitis, GERD, VCD, and heart issues (e.g., CHF), are actively assessed and managed at each outpatient appointment. Obesity confers a significant negative impact upon the health status of individuals with asthma and has been reported to be associated with poorer asthma control, impaired response to inhaled corticosteroid therapy, increased exacerbation frequency, increased healthcare utilization, and diminished asthma-specific quality of life relative to normal-weight asthmatics.[20] Therefore, BMI should be recorded at each outpatient visit. In addition, patients with a confirmed diagnosis of asthma, GERD should be considered as a possible cause of dry cough. Since, psychiatric disorders, particularly depression and anxiety disorders, are more prevalent among individuals with asthma, it is important to be alert to these conditions, especially where there has been a previous history. Rhinitis and rhinosinusitis frequently coexist with asthma and may contribute to poor asthma control. Therefore, these conditions should be assessed at each outpatient consultation with specific questions that address nasal blockage, obstruction, anterior and posterior discharge, facial pain/pressure, and/or a reduction or loss of smell.[21]

Table 13.5 Risk factors for poor asthma outcomes

Risk factors for exacerbations	Risk factors for developing fixed airflow limitation	Risk factors for medication side effects
Ever intubated or in intensive care for asthma	Lack of ICS treatment	*Systemic:* Frequent OCS; long-term, high-dose, and/or potent ICS; taking P450 inhibitors
≥1 severe exacerbation in the last month	*Exposures:* Tobacco smoke, noxious chemicals, occupational exposures	*Local:* High-dose or potent ICS, poor inhaler technique
Uncontrolled asthma symptoms	Low initial FEV$_1$	–
High SABA use	Chronic mucus hypersecretion	–
Inadequate ICS: Not prescribed, poor adherence, incorrect inhaler technique	Sputum or blood eosinophilia	–
Low FEV$_1$, especially if <60% is predicted	–	–
Major psychological or socioeconomic problems	–	–
Exposures: Smoking, allergen exposure if sensitized	–	–
Comorbidities: Obesity, rhinosinusitis, confirmed food allergy	–	–
Sputum or blood eosinophilia	–	–
Pregnancy	–	–

Source: Adapted from GINA. Global Strategy for Asthma Management and Prevention; 2015. Available at www.ginasthma.org.

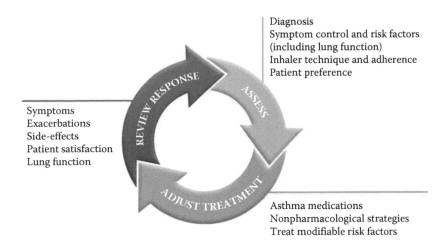

Figure 13.1 The control-based asthma management cycle.

13.1.2.2 Asthma in the emergency room: Clinical assessment of an asthma exacerbation

An asthma exacerbation is a deterioration in symptoms and lung function relative to the patient's usual baseline status. Respiratory viruses cause approximately 90% of asthma exacerbations, with rhinovirus being the most common culprit. Exacerbations are an important cause of asthma mortality, and they result in frequent hospitalizations and considerable socioeconomic cost.[4] It is especially important to recognize signs of worsening asthma and to initiate appropriate treatment as early as possible.

Severe exacerbations of asthma are life-threatening medical emergencies. Therefore, in the context of an individual with asthma presenting to the emergency room, a brief focused history and relevant physical examination should be conducted concurrently with the prompt initiation of therapy. It is important to note that in a minority of patients (predominantly male or patients with a history of near-fatal asthma) symptoms may be perceived poorly, and a significant decrease in lung function may occur without a perceptible change in symptoms.

On arrival of a known asthma patient to the emergency room, the initial assessment should evaluate the individual's airway, breathing, and circulation (ABC) and determine whether any features of life-threatening asthma (drowsiness, confusion, or silent chest) are present. If any of these latter signs are evident, the intensive care unit should be consulted, SABA and oxygen therapy initiated, and the patient prepared for intubation. If these signs of a life-threatening exacerbation are not present, then the patient may be triaged by clinical status. An asthma patient who is experiencing a mild/moderate exacerbation is able to talk in sentences, prefers sitting to lying, and is not agitated. Examination may reveal tachypnea or tachycardia (100–120 bpm), and simple bedside observations may reveal oxygen saturations 90%–95% on air and PEF > 50% predicted or best. Conversely, individuals experiencing

severe exacerbations are often only able to talk in words and are agitated. These patients often sit hunched forward, are tachypneic (RR > 30), tachycardic (>120 bpm), and use accessory muscles of respiration. Oxygen saturations may be < 90% on air and the PEF < 50% predicted of historical best effort.

Following the initial assessment and determination of asthma severity, the focused history performed in conjunction with initiation of appropriate therapy should prioritize the timing of onset and precipitating cause of the present exacerbation, the severity of asthma symptoms (including any limiting exercise or disturbance in sleep), any risk factors for asthma-related death, and all current reliever and preventer medications (including doses and devices prescribed, adherence pattern, any recent dose changes, and response to current therapy). It should be noted that an asthma exacerbation thought to be occurring as part of an anaphylaxis event requires prompt administration of intramuscular epinephrine in conjunction with other therapies being used to manage the asthma exacerbation.

Health-care professionals should be aware that patients with severe asthma and one or more adverse psychosocial factors are at risk of death. The risk factors for near-fatal asthma are the same as for asthma-related death and are outlined in Table 13.6. Notably, asthma patients who die are significantly more likely to have learning difficulties, a history of psychosis requiring antipsychotic medications, financial and/or employment problems, repeated missed medical appointments, self-discharges from the emergency room or hospital against medical advice, drug/alcohol abuse, obesity, and previous near fatal asthma.

The focused physical examination during an asthma exacerbation should include assessment of vital signs (level of consciousness, temperature, pulse, heart rate, respiratory rate, blood pressure), signs of exacerbation severity (including ability to complete sentences, use of accessory muscles), complicating factors (anaphylaxis, pneumonia, pneumothorax), and signs of alternative conditions that could explain acute breathlessness (e.g., cardiac failure,

Table 13.6 Factors that increase the risk of asthma-related death

- A history of near-fatal asthma requiring intubation and mechanical ventilation
- Hospitalization or emergency care visit for asthma in the past year
- Currently using or having recently stopped using oral corticosteroids (a marker of event severity)
- Not currently using inhaled corticosteroids
- Overuse of SABAs, especially use of more than one canister of SABA (or equivalent) monthly
- A history of psychiatric disease or psychosocial problems
- Poor adherence with asthma medications and/or poor adherence with (or lack of) a written asthma action plan
- Food allergy in a patient with asthma

Source: Adapted from GINA. Global Strategy for Asthma Management and Prevention; 2015. Available at www .ginasthma.org.

upper airway dysfunction, inhaled foreign body, or pulmonary embolism). Systolic paradox (pulsus paradoxus) is an inadequate indicator of asthma severity and should not be assessed.[22]

13.1.2.3 Initial consultation: Suspected COPD

COPD is a common, preventable, and treatable disease characterized by persistent airflow limitation that is usually progressive and associated with an enhanced chronic inflammatory response in the airways and the lung to noxious particles and gases.[5] COPD is an umbrella term that encompasses both chronic bronchitis and emphysema. Chronic bronchitis is defined clinically as a chronic productive cough for 3 months in each of two successive years in a patient in whom other causes of chronic cough have been excluded, whereas emphysema, a pathological term, describes the abnormal and permanent enlargement of the airspaces distal to the terminal bronchioles that is accompanied by destruction of the airspace walls, without obvious fibrosis.[5] A diagnosis of COPD should be considered and spirometry performed in individuals over the age of 40 years (35 years in some guidelines[23]), if one or more symptoms of dyspnea, chronic cough, or chronic sputum production exists; if there is a history of exposure to risk factors for COPD; or if there is a family history of COPD.

Dyspnea is the major cause of disability and anxiety in COPD; it is often progressive, presenting on exertion initially, but subsequently occurring at rest in end-stage disease. The severity of dyspnea should be formally graded using a tool such as the Medical Research Council (MRC) dyspnea scale[24] (see Table 13.7) and reevaluated at each consultation, along with exercise tolerance and the impact of dyspnea on the individual's quality of life and ability to perform their activities of daily living (ADLs).

Chronic cough is often the first symptom to develop in COPD, although it is frequently discounted by the patient as an expected consequence of smoking or environmental exposures. The cough, which may be unproductive, is frequently worse in the morning and may initially be intermittent, but later becomes present on a daily basis and often persists throughout the day. Cough syncope may be reported and is a consequence of rapid increases in intrathoracic pressure during prolonged coughing attacks; furthermore, vigorous coughing may also result in rib fractures and severe, and localized chest pain. The differential diagnosis of chronic cough is shown in Table 13.8.

Any pattern of chronic sputum production may indicate COPD. It is common for individuals with COPD to expectorate small quantities of tenacious, thick sputum following coughing bouts. However, this is often difficult to evaluate as patients frequently swallow sputum rather than expectorate it. The sputum is often mucoid but the quality may change with exacerbations. Wheezing and chest tightness are nonspecific symptoms that may vary across the course

Table 13.7 The Medical Research Council (MRC) dyspnea scale

Grade	Degree of breathlessness related to activity
1	Not troubled by breathlessness except on strenuous exercise
2	Short of breath when hurrying on a level or when walking up a slight hill
3	Walks slower than most people on the level, stops after a mile or so, or stops after 15 minutes walking at own pace
4	Stops for breath after walking 100 yards, or after a few minutes on level ground
5	Too breathless to leave the house, or breathless when dressing/undressing

Source: Fletcher CM., Br Med J., 2, 1665, 1960.

Table 13.8 Differential diagnosis of chronic cough

Intrathoracic	Extrathoracic
COPD	Chronic rhinitis with postnasal drainage
Asthma	Upper airway cough syndrome (UACS)
Lung cancer	Gastroesophageal reflux
Tuberculosis	Medication (e.g., ACE inhibitors)
Bronchiectasis	–
Left heart failure	–
Interstitial lung disease	–
Cystic Fibrosis	–
Idiopathic cough	–

Source: Adapted from GOLD. Global Stategy for the Diagnosis, Management, and Prevention of Chronic Obstructive Pulmonary Disease; 2016. Available at www.goldcopd.org.

of several days or over a single day. It is important to note, as with asthma, their absence does not exclude a diagnosis of COPD. Chest pain and hemoptysis are uncommon in COPD and should alert the health care provider as to the possibility of alternative diagnoses, such as ischemic heart disease, pulmonary embolism, or bronchogenic carcinomas.

Similar to asthma, in addition to determining the presenting symptoms and the pattern of their development, predisposing risk factors for developing COPD should be formally evaluated. Cigarette smoking is the major risk factor for the development of COPD, and, consequently, current smoking status and the number of pack years smoked (number of pack years = [packs smoked per day] × [years as a smoker] should be established). In the absence of genetic, environmental, or occupational factors, a pack-year history of < 15 years is unlikely to result in COPD, whereas the single best variable for predicting which adults will have airflow obstruction on spirometry is a pack-year history > 40. However, it should be emphasized that up to 20% of patients with COPD have never smoked. Current and previous occupations and environmental history should be determined to establish any potential occupational or environmental exposures to fumes and organic/inorganic dusts. A family history of COPD should be obtained, as it is a strong risk factor for developing subsequent COPD, independent of family history of smoking, personal lifetime smoking, or childhood environmental tobacco smoke exposure.[25] Furthermore, any factor that affects lung growth during gestation and childhood has the potential for increasing the risk of COPD. Therefore, it is useful to enquire about prematurity, and childhood or adolescent exposures.

Following clinical assessment of the presenting complaints, risk factors, and comorbidities, symptoms suggestive of secondary complications of COPD should actively be pursued. Fatigue, anorexia, and weight loss may occur in severe disease, but may also herald the development of pulmonary malignancy. Symptoms suggestive of the development of secondary pulmonary hypertension, such as ankle swelling, fatigue, dizziness, syncope, chest pain, and palpitations should also be sought. The impact of COPD on mental health is often underestimated and symptoms of both depression and anxiety should be evaluated, as both are common in severe COPD and are associated with increased risk of exacerbations and poorer overall health status. Finally, it is important for future planning that the social and family support networks available to the patient are determined.

Since clinical signs are not usually elicited in COPD until significant impairment of lung function has occurred, it is not surprising that, in early stage disease, physical examination may be entirely normal.[5] Numerous signs may be observed in individuals with more advanced disease simply by inspection at the bedside. Individuals with severe COPD may breathe through pursed lips (in an attempt to generate autoPEEP), exhibit tachypnea at rest, and adopt a "tripod" position to relieve dyspnea, leaning forward with arms outstretched and weight supported on palms or elbows (calluses or swollen bursas on the extensor surfaces of the forearms may even be seen). The expiratory phase of the respiratory cycle may be prolonged, and audible wheeze on forced expiration may be evident. Use of the accessory muscles of respiration, especially the sternocleidomastoids, may be present (due to increased work of breathing), and the anterior-posterior thoracic diameter may be increased due to hyperinflation, giving the impression of a barrel-shaped chest. Indeed, paradoxical retraction of the lower interspaces during inspiration (Hoover's sign) may be present. Body mass index may be increased due to decreased activity levels or decreased due to increased work of breathing. The patient may be cyanotic, a feature diminished by anemia but accentuated by polycythemia, and exhibit peripheral edema as a consequence of secondary pulmonary hypertension (cor pulmonale).[26]

Examination of the peripheral extremities and digits may reveal tar staining of the fingers and stigmata of hypercapnia, such as asterixis, warm hands and feet, and bounding pulses. It should be noted that digital clubbing is not a feature of COPD, and its presence, in the clinical context of COPD, should raise suspicion of pulmonary malignancy or other chronic pulmonary and nonpulmonary conditions.[27] Closer examination of the neck may reveal a reduced sternocricoid distance and an elevated jugular venous pressure (JVP); neck veins may be distended due to increased intrathoracic pressures or the JVP may be elevated if pulmonary hypertension is present. The presence of cervical lymphadenopathy should again alert one to the possibility of malignancy.

As discussed, inspection of the chest may reveal an increased antero-posterior diameter and Hoover's sign. Palpation may reveal diminished thoracic expansion and possibly a right ventricular heave if pulmonary hypertension is present. Hyperresonance may be observed upon percussion. Auscultation may elicit diminished breath sounds and diffuse, multiple monophonic wheezes due to small airways obstruction. Crackles or rales suggest concurrent infection. Cardiac auscultation may reveal further signs of pulmonary hypertension, such as a systolic murmur of tricuspid regurgitation and a loud pulmonary component to the second heart sound. Tender, pulsatile hepatomegaly and peripheral edema secondary to right heart failure may also be present.

13.1.2.4 Clinical assessment of individuals with COPD in the outpatient clinic

Routine follow-up is essential in COPD as lung function worsens with time, even with the best of care. The average rate of FEV_1 decline in nonsmoking, healthy adults is 15–20 mL/year, so the progression to clinically overt COPD can be insidious and progressive similar to the natural course of asthma.[28] Follow-up visits should reevaluate symptoms, particularly any new or worsening symptoms, and include a physical examination. Questionnaires such as the COPD Assessment Test (CAT)[29] (Figure 13.2) or the St. George's

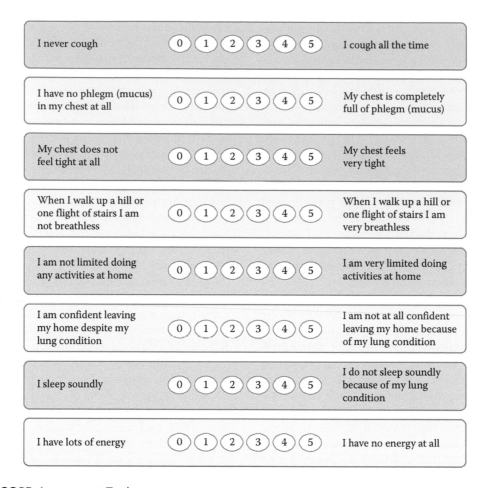

Figure 13.2 The COPD Assessment Tool.

Respiratory Questionnaire (SGRQ)[30] are particularly useful for assessing trends in symptom changes.

Cough, sputum quality and production, dyspnea, fatigue, activity limitation, and sleep disturbance should be assessed, quantified (where possible), and recorded at each consultation. Smoking status and smoke exposure should also be revisited at each appointment, and participation in programs to reduce and eliminate exposure to COPD risk factors promoted at every opportunity. The current therapeutic regimen and the patient's comprehension of it should be reviewed, including adherence, dosages, side effects, inhaler technique, and effectiveness of the current regimen at controlling symptoms (Table 13.9).

It is important to note the frequency, severity, and likely causes of any exacerbations that may have occurred between consultations. Specific inquiry into unscheduled visits to providers, telephone calls for assistance, and use of urgent or emergency care facilities is important. In addition, any hospitalizations should be documented, including the facility, duration of stay, and any use of critical care or mechanical ventilatory support. The dose and duration of any corticosteroid or antibiotic therapy should also be recorded, in addition to any available microbiology culture results. Naturally, increased sputum volume, worsening

Table 13.9 Questions to determine symptomatic response to clinical treatment

- Have you noticed a difference since starting this treatment?
- If you are better:
  - Are you less breathless?
  - Can you do more?
  - Can you sleep better?
- Describe what difference it has made to you.
- Is that change worthwhile to you?

Source: Adapted from GOLD. Global strategy for the diagnosis, management, and prevention of chronic obstructive pulmonary disease; 2016. Available at www.goldcopd.org.

dyspnea, and the presence of purulent sputum revealed during the course of an outpatient consultation should alert one to the presence of a current exacerbation.

Status of comorbidities (e.g., ischemic heart disease, diabetes mellitus) should also be reviewed, as they may amplify the disability of COPD patients and can potentially complicate their management. The psychological morbidity associated with COPD should not be underestimated, and, therefore, changes in social isolation and social support networks should also be addressed. Furthermore, each individual's ability to cope in their usual environment and their capacity to carry out physical activity and their ADLs should be reviewed. Finally, one should constantly be alert for symptoms and signs suggestive of the development of new malignancy or pulmonary hypertension when reviewing COPD patients in outpatient clinics.

13.1.2.5 Clinical assessment of COPD in the emergency room

Acute exacerbations are a common occurrence for many COPD patients, and the diagnosis relies on an acute change of symptoms (baseline dyspnea, cough, and/or sputum production) that is beyond normal day-to-day variation.[5] Several etiological factors have been associated with COPD exacerbations, including changes in air temperature and pollutant levels. However, the majority of COPD exacerbations are thought to be triggered by respiratory infection (both viral and bacterial).[5] In addition to negatively impacting individual patients' quality of life and lung function, COPD exacerbations are a common cause of hospitalization and death, and thus confer considerable socioeconomic costs to the patient and society.[5] Similar to asthma exacerbations, a focused clinical history and examination should be performed with concurrent initiation of appropriate treatment if a COPD exacerbation is suspected (Table 13.10).

The medical history should focus on careful characterization of the presenting complaints (typically increasing dyspnea, cough, sputum production), establishment of baseline status, COPD severity, determination of the treatment regimen, and comorbidities. When assessing baseline status, it is useful to determine typical daily symptoms when healthy, smoking status, degree of airflow limitation, exacerbation frequency (including hospitalizations and use of invasive/noninvasive ventilation [NIV]), use of long-term oxygen therapy or domiciliary NIV, previous or current malignancy, and whether a diagnosis of pulmonary hypertension has been made. Enquiry into the potential trigger for the exacerbation (e.g., coryzal symptoms, exposures to air pollutants) should be made and the current, and previous, treatment regimen documented, including change in metered-dose inhaler or nebulizer usage, recent courses of antibiotics and corticosteroids, change in oxygen requirements, and previous pulmonary rehabilitation. It is important to determine performance status, ability to cope at home and whether the patient has made any prior wishes regarding invasive and NIV. Naturally, it is essential that conditions that may mimic and/or aggravate exacerbations, including pneumonia, pulmonary embolism, congestive heart failure, cardiac arrhythmia, pneumothorax, and pleural effusion should be considered and excluded.

When performing a physical examination of an individual with a suspected COPD exacerbation, both the work of breathing and the general physical condition of the individual should be determined. Signs indicative of increased work of breathing may be readily evident, including tachypnea, use of accessory muscles, inability to complete sentences, pursed lip breathing with a prolonged expiratory phase, paradoxical retraction of the lower interspaces during inspiration (Hoover's sign), and adoption of postures to relieve dyspnea (such as the tripod position). Furthermore, the patient may display evidence of peripheral and central cyanosis and signs of hypercapnia manifested as decreased conscious level, asterixis (neither sensitive nor specific), warm peripheral extremities with bounding, high-volume pulses, and, rarely, papilledema. In addition to respiratory acidosis, severe dyspnea with clinical signs suggestive of respiratory muscle fatigue, increased work of breathing, or both, such as use of respiratory accessory muscles, paradoxical motion of the abdomen, or retraction of the intercostal spaces, are indications for commencing NIV.[31]

Regarding the general physical condition of the patient, it is important to determine whether the patient is displaying signs of fatigue, sepsis, hemodynamic instability, cardiac failure, or general cachexia suggestive of either advanced disease or potential concurrent malignancy. If the patient has a productive cough, sputum purulence should be established, bearing in mind that its presence during an exacerbation can be sufficient indication for starting empirical antibiotic treatment. Examination of the chest typically reveals signs of hyperinflation, with increased AP diameter, hyperresonance to percussion, and diminished breath sounds; however, auscultation of the chest may reveal crepitations or bronchial breathing suggestive of concurrent pneumonia. Expiratory wheeze may be evident; however, this is neither sensitive nor specific for a COPD exacerbation. The JVP may be difficult to assess in COPD exacerbations due to a combination of prominent respiratory muscle activity and wide swings during respiration. However, other signs of pulmonary hypertension including a loud P2, peripheral edema, pulsatile liver, right ventricular heave and pansystolic murmur may still be evident and should be sought.

Table 13.10 Assessment of COPD exacerbations

Medical history	Signs of severity
Severity of COPD based on degree of airflow limitation	Use of accessory respiratory muscles
Duration of worsening or new symptoms	Paradoxical chest wall movements
Number of previous episodes (total/hospitalizations)	Worsening or new onset central cyanosis
Comorbidities	Development of peripheral edema
Present treatment regimen	Hemodynamic instability
Previous use of mechanical ventilation	Deteriorated mental status

Source: Adapted from GOLD. Global stategy for the diagnosis, management, and prevention of chronic obstructive pulmonary disease; 2016. Available at www.goldcopd.org.

13.1.2.6 Clinical assessment of an individual with suspected ACO

Asthma and COPD are the most common diagnoses in the patient with breathlessness and airway obstruction presenting to the physician, but some of these patients may share characteristics of each condition. This has been defined as ACO characterized by the presence of persistent airflow limitation and clinical features of *both* asthma and COPD.[2] The ACO is a common condition, with an estimated prevalence ranging between 1.8% and 4.5% individuals, based on receiving a diagnosis of COPD and asthma by their healthcare professional.[3,32,33]

An algorithmic approach to the diagnosis of this condition is recommended[2] (Table 13.11). The initial step comprises clinical history, physical examination, and imaging with the aim of identifying patients who have a disease of chronic airflow limitation. Step two involves consolidation and comparison of the clinical features of each airways disease potentially present (asthma, COPD, or ACO), so that a provisional diagnosis may be reached.

As discussed in the sections above for asthma and COPD, the features that should prompt consideration of chronic airways disease include a history of chronic or recurrent cough, sputum production, dyspnea, wheezing, repeated lower respiratory tract infections, report of a previous doctor diagnosis of asthma or COPD, history of prior treatment with inhaled medications, history of smoking tobacco, and/or other substances, and exposure to airborne pollutants and/or allergens in the home and workplace environments.

Physical examination may be normal in between exacerbations and signs of hyperinflation and other features of chronic lung disease, or respiratory insufficiency may not be evident. The key features of the clinical history that may help distinguish between asthma, COPD, and ACO are outlined in Table 13.12.[2]

Table 13.11 Stepwise approach to the diagnosis of patients with respiratory symptoms

Step 1	Does the patient have chronic airways disease?
Step 2	The syndromic diagnosis of asthma, COPD, and ACO in the adult patient
Step 3	Spirometry
Step 4	Commence initial therapy
Step 5	Referral for specialized investigations (if necessary)

Source: Adapted from GINA, GOLD. Diagnosis of diseases of chronic airflow limitation: Asthma, COPD and asthma-COPD overlap (ACO); 2015. Available at www.ginasthma.org.)

Table 13.12 Usual features of asthma, COPD, and ACO

Feature	Asthma	COPD	ACO
Age of onset	Usually childhood onset but can commence at any age.	Usually > 40 years of age.	Usually age > 40 years, but may have had symptoms in childhood or early adulthood.
Pattern of respiratory symptoms	Symptoms may vary over time (day to day, or over longer periods), often limiting activity. Often triggered by exercise, emotions (including laughter), dust, or exposure to allergens.	Chronic usually continuous symptoms, particularly during exercise, with "better" and "worse" days.	Respiratory symptoms including exertional dyspnea are persistent but variability may be prominent.
History or family history	Many patients have allergies and a personal history of asthma in childhood, and/or family history of asthma.	History of exposure to noxious particles and gases (mainly tobacco smoking and biomass fuels).	Frequently a history of doctor-diagnosed asthma (current or previous), allergies, and a family history of asthma, and/or a history of noxious exposures.
Time course	Often improves spontaneously or with treatment, but may result in fixed-airflow limitation.	Generally, slowly progressive over years, despite treatment.	Symptoms are partly but significantly reduced by treatment. Progression is usual and treatment needs are high.
Exacerbations	Exacerbations occur, but the risk of exacerbations can be considerably reduced by treatment.	Exacerbations can be reduced by treatment. If present, comorbidities contribute to impairment.	Exacerbations may be more common than in COPD but are reduced by treatment. Comorbidities can contribute to impairment.

Source: Adapted from GINA, GOLD. Diagnosis of diseases of chronic airflow limitation: Asthma, COPD and asthma-COPD overlap syndrome (ACOS); 2015. Available at www.ginasthma.org.

Clinical features that are particularly favorable toward the diagnosis of asthma include age of onset before age 20, symptom variability over minutes, hours, or days; symptom deterioration during the night; or early morning and characteristic triggers, such as exercise, emotions, dust, or allergen and irritant exposures. Conversely, features that particularly suggest a diagnosis of COPD include onset over the age of 40, persistence of symptoms despite treatment, daily symptoms, exertional dyspnea, chronic cough and sputum-preceded dyspnea, heavy smoking history or biomass fuel exposure, progressive deterioration, limited relief from fast-acting bronchodilators, and severe hyperinflation on imaging.[2]

13.2 SUMMARY

A thorough clinical history and physical examination are essential for establishing an accurate diagnosis of asthma, COPD, or ACO, especially when diagnostic uncertainty exists. Following fastidious characterization of the presenting respiratory symptoms and the predisposing risk factors for each condition should be evaluated. Once the differential diagnosis has been considered, and a working diagnosis of asthma, COPD, or ACO has been established, the severity of the condition should be determined and the impact on the patient's quality of life and on their capacity to perform their daily activities evaluated. Furthermore, symptoms and signs of potential secondary complications for each airways disease and their treatments should be actively sought at each consultation.

REFERENCES

1. Chung KF. Targeting the interleukin pathway in the treatment of asthma. *Lancet.* 2015;386(9998):1086–1096.
2. GINA, GOLD. Diagnosis of Diseases of Chronic Airflow Limitation: Asthma, COPD and Asthma-COPD Overlap Syndrome (ACOS); 2015. Available at www.ginasthma.org.
3. Kumbhare S, Pleasants R, Ohar JA et al. Characteristics and prevalence of asthma/chronic obstructive pulmonary disease overlap in the United States. *Ann Am Thorac Soc.* 2016;13(6):803–810.
4. GINA. Global Strategy for Asthma Management and Prevention; 2015. Available at www.ginasthma.org.
5. GOLD. Global Stategy for the Diagnosis, Management, and Prevention of Chronic Obstructive Pulmonary Disease; 2016. Available at www.goldcopd.org.
6. NHLBI. Expert panel report 3 (EPR-3): Guidelines for the Diagnosis and Managment of Asthma—Summary Report; 2007. Available at http://www.nhlbi.nih.gov/health-pro/guidelines/current/asthma-guidelines/summary-report-2007.
7. Rajan JP, Wineinger NE, Stevenson DD et al. Prevalence of aspirin-exacerbated respiratory disease among asthmatic patients: A meta-analysis of the literature. *J Allergy Clin Immunol.* 2015;135(3):676–681. e1.
8. Castro-Rodriguez JA, Holberg CJ, Wright AL et al. A clinical index to define risk of asthma in young children with recurrent wheezing. *Am J Respir Crit Care Med.* 2000;162(4 Pt 1):1403–1406.
9. Ledford DK, Wenzel SE, and Lockey RF. Aspirin or other nonsteroidal inflammatory agent exacerbated asthma. *J Allergy Clin Immunol Pract.* 2014;2(6):653–657.
10. Raine JM, Palazzo MG, Kerr JH et al. Near-fatal bronchospasm after oral nadolol in a young asthmatic and response to ventilation with halothane. *Br Med J (Clinical research ed).* 1981;282(6263):548–549.
11. Gong H. Wheezing and asthma. In HK Walker, WD Hall, JW Hurst, eds. *Clinical Methods: The History, Physical, and Laboratory Examinations.* Boston, MA: Butterworths; 1990.
12. Irwin RS. Evaluation of wheezing illnesses other than asthma in adults. *UpToDate.* Available at www.uptodate.com: UptoDate, Waltham, MA; 2016.
13. Forgacs P. The functional basis of pulmonary sounds. *Chest.* 1978;73(3):399–405.
14. Daniel SJ. The upper airway: Congenital malformations. *Paediatr Respir Rev.* 2006;7(Suppl. 1):S260–S263.
15. Pearson MG and Bucknell CE. *Measuring Clinical Outcomes in Asthma: A Patient Focused Approach.* London: Royal College of Physicians, Clinical Effectiveness and Evaluation Unit; 1999.
16. Juniper EF, O'Byrne PM, Guyatt GH et al. Development and validation of a questionnaire to measure asthma control. *Eur Respir J.* 1999;14(4):902–907.
17. Nathan RA, Sorkness CA, Kosinski M et al. Development of the asthma control test: A survey for assessing asthma control. *J Allergy Clin Immunol.* 2004;113(1):59–65.
18. Price D, Bosnic-Anticevich S, Briggs A et al. Inhaler competence in asthma: Common errors, barriers to use and recommended solutions. *Respir Med.* 2013;107(1):37–46.
19. Lindsay JT and Heaney LG. Non-adherence in difficult asthma and advances in detection. *Expert Rev Respir Med.* 2013;7(6):607–614.
20. Pradeepan S, Garrison G, and Dixon AE. Obesity in asthma: Approaches to treatment. *Curr Allergy Asthma Rep.* 2013;13(5):434–442.
21. Giavina-Bianchi P, Aun MV, Takejima P et al. United airway disease: Current perspectives. *J Asthma Allergy.* 2016;9:93–100.
22. BTS, SIGN. British Guideline on the Management of Asthma; 2014. Available at www.brit-thoracic.org.uk.

23. NICE, BTS. Chronic Obstructive Pulmonary Disease in Over 16s: Diagnosis and Management; 2010. Available at www.nice.org.uk/guidance/cg101.

24. Fletcher CM. Standardised questionnaire on respiratory symptoms: A statement prepared and approved by the MRC committee on the aetiology of chronic bronchitis (MRC breathlessness score). *Br Med J.* 1960;2:1665.

25. Hersh CP, Hokanson JE, Lynch DA et al. Family history is a risk factor for COPD. *Chest.* 2011;140(2):343–350.

26. MacNee W. Pathophysiology of cor pulmonale in chronic obstructive pulmonary disease. Part One. *Am J Respir Crit Care Med.* 1994;150(3):833–852.

27. Dubrey S, Pal S, Singh S et al. Digital clubbing: Forms, associations and pathophysiology. *Br J Hosp Med (Lond).* 2016;77(7):403–408.

28. Kohansal R, Martinez-Camblor P, Agusti A et al. The natural history of chronic airflow obstruction revisited: An analysis of the Framingham offspring cohort. *Am J Respir Crit Care Med.* 2009;180(1):3–10.

29. Jones PW, Harding G, Berry P et al. Development and first validation of the COPD Assessment Test. *Eur Respir J.* 2009;34(3):648–654.

30. Jones PW, Quirk FH, and Baveystock CM. The st george's respiratory questionnaire. *Respir Med.* 1991;85(Suppl. B):25–31; discussion 3–7.

31. Ramsay M and Hart N. Current opinions on non-invasive ventilation as a treatment for chronic obstructive pulmonary disease. *Curr Opin Pulm Med.* 2013;19(6):626–630.

32. Menezes AM, Montes de Oca M, Perez-Padilla R et al. Increased risk of exacerbation and hospitalization in subjects with an overlap phenotype: COPD-asthma. *Chest.* 2014;145(2):297–304.

33. de Marco R, Pesce G, Marcon A et al. The coexistence of asthma and chronic obstructive pulmonary disease (COPD): Prevalence and risk factors in young, middle-aged and elderly people from the general population. *PLOS ONE.* 2013;8(5):e62985.

Diagnostic testing for asthma, COPD, and asthma-COPD overlap

SVIEN A. SENNE AND KRISTINA L. BAILEY

CLINICAL VIGNETTE 14.1

Mr. W. is a 44-year-old male who presents to your office complaining of increasing shortness of breath and wheezing. He reports feeling wheezy during the day, and has several nocturnal awakenings per week due to wheezing. Upon further questioning, he denies changes in sputum production, fevers, or chills. He has past medical history of obesity, type II diabetes mellitus, tobacco use (quit 12 years ago, 30 pack years), and allergic rhinitis and asthma diagnosed as an adolescent. He takes both long- and short-acting insulin, an angiotensin-converting-enzyme inhibitor (ACEi), an albuterol metered-dose inhaler (MDI) daily. He reports significant relief with his albuterol inhaler.

On physical exam, his temperature is 98.2°F, HR 94, RR 20, height 1.75 m tall, 110 kg, Sa 02 93% on room air. Lungs had scattered expiratory wheezing and prolonged expiratory phase, skin was without rashes, and extremities were without clubbing. A chest radiograph showed moderate hyperinflation. A pulmonary function test (PFT) shows a forced expiratory volume in one second/forced vital capacity (FEV₁/FVC) ratio of .48 and an initial FEV₁ of 66% predicted. He did have a significant response to bronchodilators, with his FEV₁/FVC increasing to .64 and his FEV₁ improving to 78% predicted (12% response).

DISCUSSION

This patient has features of asthma and COPD, as well as a previous tobacco habit and a diagnosis by a physician of asthma. The chest radiograph showing moderate hyperinflation is supportive of either asthma, COPD, or ACO. His PFTs, however, show an FEV₁/FVC ratio <0.7 both pre- and postbronchodilator, and he demonstrates marked reversibility. Due to his previous diagnosis of asthma, current symptoms, and PFTs, a diagnosis of ACO should be considered in this patient.

CLINICAL VIGNETTE 14.2

A 46-year-old male presents to your clinic complaining of increasing shortness of breath and wheezing and increasing frequency of "chest colds" (he describes as increased cough and sputum production). He relates that over the past 10 years, he has noted a steady increase in his wheezing symptoms. He denies any current changes in sputum, weight loss, fevers, or chills. He has a medical history of allergic rhinitis, hyperlipidemia, hypertension, and atrial fibrillation. He is a former cigarette smoker, quitting 2 years ago, but has a 45 pk/yr history. His medications include, albuterol MDI PRN, levothyroxine, apixaban, cetirizine and metoprolol.

On physical exam the patient is afebrile and hemodynamic parameters are normal. Respiratory rate is 22 with a Sa 02 of 94% on RA. Lungs have diffuse scattered expiratory wheezing with a prolonged expiratory phase. Heart was irregularly irregular with no murmurs or gallops. Extremities were free of clubbing, cyanosis, or peripheral edema. PFTs were performed and his FEV_1/FVC ratio was .57, his FEV_1 was 1.92 (72% predicted). There was minimal response to bronchodilators; his FEV_1/FVC ratio increased to .60 and FEV_1 to 2.07. A methacholine challenge was performed, and he had significant (>20%) reduction in his FEV_1 with $</= 4$ mg of methacholine administered.

DISCUSSION

This gentleman presents with increased wheezing, cough and sputum production. Allergic rhinitis is useful to assess as it gives us clues about underling allergies. His PFTs are supportive of COPD, with an FEV_1/FVC ratio <.7 and no significant response to bronchodilator therapy. However, his methacholine challenge test is positive and definitely suggestive of airway hyperresponsiveness (AHR). Due to his increased AHR, it is reasonable to consider a diagnosis of ACO in this patient.

CLINICAL VIGNETTE 14.3

A 45-year-old male presents complaining of increasing cough and shortness of breath. He explains that he is a farmer and has been experiencing intermittent cough, wheezing, and shortness of breath for many years, but it is increasing in frequency and severity. He has no previous history of asthma, but notes he hasn't seen a physician since his last high school sports physical 27 years ago. He takes no medications. He has a 40 pack-year history of cigarette smoking, and continues to smoke, but only half the amount as previously. He denies any blood in his sputum, weight loss, fevers, or chills. He does admit to allergies to cats and pollens, and he further notes he has persistent nasal discharge.

On physical exam, he is afebrile, and his hemodynamic parameters are normal. His respiratory rate is 20 breaths per minute (BPM), and he is maintaining his oxygen saturation >95% on room air. He appears barrel-chested, and lung auscultation reveals mild diffuse wheezing with a prolonged expiratory phase. Pulmonary function testing reveals an FEV_1/FVC of 0.49, FEV_1 of 62%, and a bronchodilator response of 5% (<200 mL). Further studies including a complete blood count (CBC) with differential and Immunoglobulin E (IgE) were obtained, and the patient was found to have elevated eosinophils, and the serum IgE was >2x upper limits of normal.

DISCUSSION

This patient presents with progressive wheezing, cough, and shortness of breath. He has a significant tobacco history, but no history of asthma (although he admittedly doesn't regularly seek healthcare). He does, however, have symptoms consistent with allergic rhinitis. His PFTs are consistent with COPD with an FEV_1/FCV ratio <0.7 and an insignificant bronchodilator response. However, his laboratory studies suggest he may have some atopic inflammation that could be driving some of his respiratory symptoms. Given this mixed picture, it is reasonable to consider the diagnosis of ACO in this patient.

CLINICAL VIGNETTE 14.4

A 52-year-old female presents complaining of chronically uncontrolled wheezing, cough, and shortness of breath. She denies hemoptysis, weight loss, fevers, or chills. She has a medical history significant for COPD, hypothyroidism, overactive bladder, and osteoarthritis of her hands. She currently is prescribed albuterol nebulizers that she uses 4x daily along with an albuterol MDI that she uses 2–4x daily, inhaled ipratropium daily, oxybutynin, and naproxen. She has a 5–7 pack-year history of tobacco use, but quit 30 years ago.

On exam, she is afebrile, and her hemodynamic parameters are normal. Her respiratory rate is 20 BPM, and she is maintaining her oxygen saturation >95% on room air. Lung auscultation reveals diffuse wheezing and prolonged expiratory phase. A CT chest notes moderate emphysematous changes, but otherwise is normal. PFTs show an FEV_1/FVC ratio of 0.48 and FEV_1 of 60%. After bronchodilators, her FEV_1/FVC improved to 0.57. Exhaled nitric oxide testing was performed, and she was found to have a FeNo of 55 PPB. Further, sputum cytology was performed and found an elevated number of eosinophils.

DISCUSSION

This female patient presents with a minimal, remote smoking history and chronically uncontrolled wheezing, cough, and shortness of breath. Her PFTs show obstruction with some, but not significant, bronchodilator response. Her FeNo of 55 PPB is supportive of eosinophilic inflammation, which is also confirmed with sputum studies. Given evidence of eosinophilic inflammation in the setting of obstructive lung disease and partial bronchodilator response, ACO should be considered.

14.1 INTRODUCTION

Asthma-COPD overlap (ACO) is an emerging area of the literature with consensus definitions only recently being proposed. Distinguishing asthma from COPD in older smokers can be difficult, and defining the overlap between these diseases has also proved challenging. Typically, studies examining diagnostic tests focus on either asthma or COPD, with individuals diagnosed with both COPD and asthma excluded from many studies that might better help us classify the diagnosis of this phenotype. When examining the literature regarding diagnostic testing in ACO, careful attention must be paid to the definition of ACO as that definition varies greatly in the literature.

The recent consensus statements by the Global Initiative for Asthma (GINA) and the Global Initiative for Chronic Obstructive Lung Disease (GOLD),[1] as well as the Spanish COPD Guidelines,[2] serve to help clarify the diagnosis of ACO. The GINA/GOLD strategy documents rely heavily on the patient's history and spirometry, while the Spanish criteria assign some value to other measures. We do not propose a specific definition of ACO in this chapter, however, this chapter will discuss diagnostic testing in asthma, COPD, and ACO including spirometry, pulmonary function testing, radiographic studies, serum and sputum markers, exhaled nitric oxide, and genetic modalities of evaluating patients for ACO.

14.2 SPIROMETRY

Spirometry is a fundamental diagnostic test in the evaluation of chronic airway diseases including asthma, COPD,

and ACO. Spirometry should be the first diagnostic step after a thorough history and physical examination that suggests obstructive airway disease.[1] The three main spirometric values that are useful in the diagnosis of asthma, COPD, and ACO are the FEV_1, the FEV_1/FVC ratio, and the postbronchodilator response.

Lung function in asthma may be normal between symptomatic episodes, while ACO and COPD will have persistent airflow obstruction. If spirometry is not performed at the initial encounter, it ought to be performed at a subsequent visit and, if at all possible, prior to initiation of therapy. Also consider that some patients may require repeat testing to make a diagnosis. Furthermore, spirometric values can be influenced by inhaled corticosteroid, as well as long-acting muscarinic or beta-agonist therapy, unless the patient has had a prolonged therapy-free period prior to testing.[1]

14.2.1 FORCED EXPIRATORY VOLUME IN ONE SECOND

In obstructive lung disease, the prebronchodilator FEV_1 is usually low (<70% predicted), but not necessarily so. The GOLD criteria use the FEV_1 in tandem with the FEV_1/FVC ratio as the primary spirometric parameters to diagnose and classify COPD (Table 14.1). Likewise, the FEV_1, and to a lesser extent the FEV_1/FVC ratio, is also used to classify the severity of asthma.[3,4] In addition to being used to classify disease severity, numerous organizations have released a consensus statement suggesting the FEV_1 be used to guide therapy in COPD.[5] Several studies have tried to determine whether FEV_1 is different between asthma, COPD, and ACO groups. Certainly, the FEV_1 in ACO is lower than that in healthy individuals.[6] Interestingly, several have found that ACO also has a significantly lower FEV_1 than asthma.[7,8]

Table 14.1 Pulmonary function testing

	Normal	Asthma	COPD	ACO
FEV_1/FVC	>0.70	<0.70 although may be normal	<0.70	<0.70 is generally agreed upon
FEV_1 (Pre- BD)	>70% Predicted	<70% Predicted although may be normal	<70% Predicted	<70% Predicted
Bronchodilator response		Complete reversibility in most patients	Minimal reversibility	Incomplete to marked reversibility[a]
DLCO	Normal	Normal to increased	Decreased	Normal to decreased[8,10]
Airway-hyper reactivity		Present especially when symptomatic	Usually minimal	Present—and sometimes with less provocation[8]

[a] Marked Reversibility is defined as >12%–15% increase in FEV_1 and 400 mL. (GINA/GOLD. Diagnosis of Diseases of Chronic Airflow Limitation: Asthma, COPD and Asthma COPD Overlap Synrome (ACO); 2015. Available at http://www.ginasthma.org: GINA/GOLD; Cosio BG et al., Chest., 149, 45–52, 2016.)

In other studies, ACO had a lower FEV_1 than both asthma and COPD.[9] Still others have shown no difference in baseline FEV_1 between ACO and COPD.[10] In summary, FEV_1 is decreased in COPD, and can be decreased in asthma and ACO, and therefore cannot be used in isolation to distinguish between them. The FEV_1 in ACO, however, tends to be lower than in asthma and similar to that of COPD.[7–10]

14.2.2 FORCED EXPIRATORY VOLUME IN ONE SECOND/FORCED VITAL CAPACITY (FEV_1/FVC) RATIO

Generally, obstructive lung disease (asthma, COPD, and ACO) is defined by a low FEV_1/FVC ratio. A low FEV_1/FVC ratio can be defined as either <0.70 by the GOLD criteria, or less than the lower limit of normal (adjusted for demographic and physical variations with a reference equation), as defined by the American Thoracic Society (ATS) criteria.[3,11] A reduced FEV_1/FVC ratio is required for the diagnosis of COPD.[3,5,12] Asthma, on the other hand, can have a normal or reduced FEV_1/FVC ratio.[4] After bronchodilator, the FEV_1/FVC ratio in asthma can be normal, but in COPD, and likely in ACO, it will remain less than 0.7.[1,3,4,12] These findings are supported by several population-based studies showing a lower postbronchodilator FEV_1/FVC ratio in COPD and ACO compared to asthma.[8,9] The normalization of the FEV_1/FVC ratio in asthma reflects a greater degree of reversibility with bronchodilators and can also be seen in ACO.

14.2.3 POSTBRONCHODILATOR SPIROMETRY

In obstructive lung disease, spirometry should be repeated after the inhalation of a short-acting beta-agonist, typically albuterol or salbutamol.[3,12] Asthma can show a significant and sometimes complete reversal to normal after bronchodilator therapy, but this can depend on disease severity and control.[1,4] COPD will likely show little to no reversibility, and, by definition, the postbronchodilator FEV_1/FVC

must remain <0.7 or the adjusted lower limit of normal.[1,3,12] Other analysis, however, has revealed a significant number of those with COPD do exhibit bronchodilator response.[13] Individuals with ACO can exhibit incomplete reversibility of airflow obstruction with bronchodilator treatment. Because of these differences, a marked bronchodilator response has been proposed as a defining characteristic of ACO.[1,2] A marked bronchodilator response is defined as a greater than 12%–15% increase in FEV_1 and an increase of 400 mL.[1,10]

14.2.4 FORCED EXPIRATORY FLOW AT 25%–75% OF FVC (FEF_{25-75})/MAXIMAL MIDEXPIRATORY FLOW

The FEF_{25-75} is the fraction of air in midexpiration—or the fraction of air expired from the 25th to the 75th percent of the expiratory limb of the flow volume loop. The intent of measuring this fraction of expired air is to capture the impact of the small airways on PFT. Further, this measurement is considered effort independent.[14] Researchers examining the FEF_{25-75} among those with COPD found that a low FEF_{25-75} is predictive of frequent exacerbations. That same study found that a previous diagnosis of asthma by a physician (among the COPD group) also strongly predicted increased frequency of exacerbations compared to the COPD group that had never had a previous diagnosis of asthma.[15] In patients with asthma, a decreased FEF_{25-75} in the setting of a normal FEV_1 was associated with increased asthma severity, oral steroid use, and asthma exacerbations in a pediatric population.[16] Unfortunately, at this time there are no published data comparing the FEF_{25-75} between asthma, COPD, or ACO groups.

14.3 PULMONARY FUNCTION TESTING

14.3.1 LUNG VOLUMES

Generally, in well-controlled asthmatics, lung volumes are normal.[17] If asthma is poorly controlled, increases in the residual volume (RV) and total lung capacity can be seen.[17] On the other hand, a hallmark of COPD is nonreversible airway obstruction that leads to progressive increases in the RV and total lung capacity (TLC) as a result of air trapping.[18] ACO, like COPD, has significantly higher TLC, RV, and functional residual capacity (FRC) values compared to asthma.[8] Therefore, lung volume measurements can also be useful in evaluating a patient for ACO.

14.3.2 DIFFUSING CAPACITY OF THE LUNGS FOR CARBON MONOXIDE

Diffusing capacity of the lungs for carbon monoxide ($D_L CO$) is measured to determine how easily oxygen travels from the alveoli of the lungs to the bloodstream. In asthma, the $D_L CO$ is generally thought to be normal, but can be increased. In COPD, it is known that the $D_L CO$ is decreased, and this is related to the degree of emphysematous changes.[19] The literature reports that the $D_L CO$ in ACO is both unchanged like in asthma[8] and decreased like in COPD with emphysema.[10] These changes likely depend on whether a significant amount of emphysema is present with ACO.

14.3.3 BRONCHOPROVOCATION AND AIRWAY HYPERRESPONSIVENESS TESTING

Clinically, AHR or bronchial hyperresponsiveness (BHR) is an exaggerated bronchoconstriction response to a variety of both allergic and nonallergic inhaled stimuli including smoke, cold air, pollution, chemical fumes, and specific allergens. This tendency to an exaggerated response can be measured by bronchoprovocation studies. Bronchoprovocation studies are typically performed in patients that have symptoms consistent with asthma, but have normal spirometry. Agents that are used in bronchoprovocation studies include methacholine, mannitol, hypertonic saline, or adenosine. Methacholine is the most widely used clinically, as it is widely available in an FDA-approved preparation and causes bronchoconstriction directly.[20] Mannitol is used by some and as opposed to methacholine, has a secondary bronchoconstriction effect mediated by mast cells.[4]

In bronchoprovocation tests, baseline spirometry is measured, then methacholine (or another agent) is inhaled, and spirometry is measured again. Asthmatics are sensitive to methacholine and generally have a decrease in FEV_1. Conventionally, a methacholine challenge test is considered positive when there is a decline in the FEV_1 of 20% after administration of methacholine. The provocative concentration that is required to cause a positive reaction is termed the PC_{20} and determines the severity of bronchial hyperreactivity.[20] Typically, there is very little change in FEV_1 in response to methacholine in normal patients or patients with COPD. It is reported, however, that in patients with moderate to severe COPD, there is a small decrease in

FEV_1, mainly due to changes in RV.[21] In ACO, increases in AHR are typical.

Patients with ACO appear to have more severe AHR than those with COPD or asthma alone. A group of asthmatics and those with ACO were compared after performance of a methacholine challenge test executed according to the ATS protocol.[8,20] As per convention, the test was considered positive if there was a decrease in FEV_1 of greater than 20% at a cumulative concentration of methacholine of 16 or less (PC_{20} <16 mg/mL).[20] The rates of AHR were similar in asthma and ACO; however, in ACO, the dose of methacholine required to induce a decline in the FEV_1 was much smaller.[8] Another group using a different protocol for the methacholine challenge test followed this study. In this study, airway hyperresponsiveness was defined as a 20% reduction in FEV_1 after a cumulative dose </= 1 mg of methacholine. A significantly higher percentage of the ACO group (92.1%) demonstrated AHR compared to the COPD (14.5%), asthma (66.6%), and healthy (3.5%) groups.[6]

Methacholine testing has limitations of poor specificity. Some propose that agents such as mannitol, hypertonic saline, and adenosine are preferable agents because they do not directly cause airway smooth-muscle contraction, like methacholine.[22] Hypertonic saline inhalation has been used to define AHR in obstructive lung disease as well. Those with ACO had more airway responsiveness than COPD, defined as a decline in the FEV_1 by 15% or more, in response to inhalation of hypertonic saline.[10] Likewise, individuals with ACO demonstrated increased AHR in response to hypertonic saline than those with no underlying obstructive lung disease.[22] Using mannitol as a bronchoprovocation agent, ACO and asthma had similar rates of AHR. However, like methacholine, the concentrations of mannitol required to induce AHR were lower in the ACO group.[8]

14.4 RADIOGRAPHIC STUDIES

High-resolution CT (HRCT) scans are often used to determine the cause of unexplained dyspnea (Table 14.2). In mild to moderate asthma, HRCT scans are typically normal, but air trapping and increased bronchial wall thickening can be seen. In COPD, air trapping and emphysema are frequently

Table 14.2 Imaging findings

	Asthma	COPD	ACO
Emphysema	–	++	+[23,24]
Bronchial wall thickening	+	+	++[24,26]
Air trapping	+ or –	Same as ACO	Same as COPD but with more improvement after bronchodilator[23]

observed. CT scans can be used to quantify emphysema in COPD patients, usually in the context of research protocols. These techniques have been applied to asthma and ACO as well. Perhaps best studied is the emphysema index. The emphysema index measures the areas of low attenuation (<950 HU) and calculates an index value using postprocessing imaging software. There have been several groups that have examined differences in HRCT imaging between normal, asthma, COPD, and ACO groups. When interpreting and discussing their results, it is important to be cognizant of the fact that there was no control for age, tobacco exposure, or duration of disease.

When the HRCTs of patients with ACO and COPD are compared, those diagnosed with COPD have more emphysema than those with ACO at baseline.[23,24] When CT scans are used to try to differentiate between ACO and asthma, those with more emphysema are more likely to have ACO.[25] Thus, these findings suggest that patients with ACO have more emphysematous changes than patients with asthma alone, but less than patients with COPD alone.

Bronchial wall thickness, an approximation of airway inflammation, has also been studied in asthma, COPD, and ACO. Patients with ACO have significantly increased bronchial wall thickening (measured as airway wall area) compared to those with COPD.[26,24] The bronchial wall thickening can be reduced by 12 weeks of budesonide treatment.[26]

Air trapping can be estimated on CT scan as well. In this case, radiographic air trapping is defined as areas <856 HU on an expiratory CT scan. There are no statistically significant differences in air trapping between COPD and ACO.[23,24] After treatment with a bronchodilator, however, those with ACO had more improvement in radiographic air trapping than those with COPD.[23]

14.5 BIOMARKERS

Because an ACO diagnosis can be difficult and may rely on subjective opinion, more definitive markers need to be defined. Objective biomarkers of ACO would be an attractive

addition to the diagnosis of ACO. There have been numerous studies attempting to identify sputum, serum, and other objective markers to assist in the diagnosis of ACO.

14.5.1 SPUTUM

Sputum biomarkers are an attractive target because sputum is easily obtained from patients with obstructive lung disease. It also directly reflects the inflammatory state of the airways. The most widely available sputum analysis is sputum cell count and differential.

Different inflammatory pathways predominate in patients with COPD as compared to those with asthma and ACO (Table 14.3). Generally speaking, inflammation in asthma is eosinophilic and driven by CD4 cells, whereas, inflammation in COPD is typically neutrophilic and driven by CD8 cells.[3,27,28] Noneosinophilic asthma with limited response to inhaled corticosteroids (ICS) is also recognized,[29] as well as COPD with eosinophilic inflammation.[30] There have been several studies recently that focus specifically on sputum cell counts and differentials in the ACO population.

Whether ACO has a predominantly neutrophilic, eosinophilic, or a mixed inflammatory picture is controversial. This is likely due to two underlying cohorts of ACO being studied. First, there is a cohort of asthmatic smokers that developed irreversible airway obstruction. Their sputum tends to show neutrophilic inflammation due to smoking. There is also a cohort of patients that has COPD with eosinophilic inflammation and reversible airway obstruction. A large, cross-sectional study of more than 4000 patients with airway disease, including asthma, COPD, ACO, and chronic cough was performed. In this study, 53% of those with ACO had eosinophilic bronchitis, 19% had neutrophilic bronchitis, and 10% had a mixed inflammatory pattern. Notably, there was a higher proportion of sputum eosinophilia in patients that had stable disease and a relative shift to increased sputum neutrophilia in exacerbated disease states.[31] In another study, with more carefully defined ACO, sputum neutrophils predominated in both the ACO and COPD groups, with eosinophils predominating in asthma.[22] Likewise, a large biological clustering

Table 14.3 Sputum analysis

	Asthma	COPD	ACO
Sputum cytology	Generally eosinophilic	Generally neutrophilic[a]	Eosinophilic Vs. Neutrophilic[b]
Cytokines	IL-5, IL-13[c]	IL-1B, IL-6, IL-8, CCL 13[d]	IL-1B, TNFa, IL-8, IL-10,[e] NGAL, MPO[f]

[a] GOLD. Global Strategy for the Diagnosis, Management, and Prevention of Chronic Obstructive Pulmonary Disease; 2006; National Heart LaBi. Expert Panel Report 2: Guidelines for the Diagnosis and Management of Asthma; 2007; Papi A et al., *Am J Respir Crit Care Med.*, 162, 1772–177, 2000.

[b] Gibson PG and Simpson JL., *Thorax*, 64, 728–735, 2009; D'Silva L et al., *Can Respir J.*, 18, 144–148, 2011.

[c] Manise M et al., *PLOS ONE.*, 8, e58388, 2013.

[d] Gibson PG and Simpson JL., *Thorax*, 64, 728–735, 2009.

[e] IL-1B and TNFa were found to be the best discriminator between asthma, COPD, and ACO (Ghebre MA et al., *J Allergy Clin Immunol.*, 135, 63–72, 2015.)

[f] Iwamoto H et al., *Eur Respir J.*, 43, 421–429, 2014.

analysis supports neutrophilic inflammation in both ACO and COPD, and eosinophilic inflammation in asthma.[32]

14.5.1.1 Cytokines

In addition to examining sputum cytology, sputum cytokine levels have been measured in an attempt to distinguish asthma, COPD, and ACO. In asthma, it is known that eosinophilic cytokines such as IL-5 and IL-13 predominate.[33] In COPD, neutrophilic cytokines predominate, including IL-6, IL-8, and IL-1β.[34]

In a biological clustering analysis, ACO was found to have higher sputum levels of IL-1β, tumor necrosis factor alpha (TNFα), IL-8, and IL-10.[23] COPD had elevated sputum levels of IL-6 and CCL13.[23] In this cohort, the best discriminator between asthma, COPD, and ACO was sputum IL-1β levels greater than 130 pg/mL and TNFα levels greater than 5 pg/mL. These elevated cytokine levels were found only in the ACO subjects. Others measured IL-1β, IL-6, IL-8, IL-10, and TNFα in a cohort of ACO patients before and after treatment with omalizumab, an anti-IgE therapy. There were no differences in these cytokine levels after treatment.[35] This may be because a higher level of bacterial colonization in ACO, rather than allergic inflammation, was driving these cytokines.[32]

Others have compared healthy volunteers, COPD, and ACO. They found that sputum levels of neutrophil gelatinase-associated lipocalin (NGAL) and myeloperoxidase (MPO) were significantly elevated in the ACO group when compared to the other groups.[36]

14.5.2 SERUM AND SPUTUM BIOMARKERS

Serum biomarkers have also been sought to help better delineate asthma, COPD, and ACO (Table 14.4). These biomarkers have focused on inflammatory markers including peripheral eosinophilia, IgE, and other inflammatory cytokines.

14.5.2.1 Peripheral eosinophilia

Along with increases in sputum eosinophilia, peripheral eosinophilia has been reported in ACO. In fact, peripheral eosinophilia of 5% or higher has been used as a minor criteria for ACO.[10] Likewise, when comparing asthma and ACO, those in the asthma group had a higher percentage and absolute number of peripheral eosinophils.[8]

14.5.2.2 IgE levels and allergy testing

IgE has long been known as a serum marker of allergic inflammation and asthma. Because of these correlations, it has been investigated in ACO. An elevated IgE modestly increases the probability of asthma but does not rule out COPD.[1] It is also reported that there is a large subset of COPD patients (35%) with allergic sensitization that have elevated IgE levels.[37] When comparing ACO and asthma, ACO had significantly higher IgE levels (322 U/mL) compared to the asthma group (199 U/mL).[28] When comparing ACO to COPD, those with ACO had higher serum levels of IgE, however, influencing that finding was the fact that serum IgE levels of >100 IU/mL were used as a minor criteria for the diagnosis of ACO.[10]

Table 14.4 Serum analysis

	Asthma	COPD	ACO
Peripheral cytology	Eosinophilic	Neutrophilic	Eosinophilic
IgE levels	+	−[a]	+/−[b]
Serum cytokines			
CRP[c]	−	+	+
TNF[c]	−	+	+
IL-6[d]	−	+	+
IL-8[c]	−	+	+
IL-17[e]	−	+	+
IL-18[e]	−	+	+
sRAGE[f]	−		+
SP-A[f]	−		+
Plasma nitrates[g]	−	+	−

[a] Found to be higher than asthma (Cosio BG et al., *Chest*, 149, 45–52, 2016.)

[b] Up to 35% of individuals with COPD have an elevated IgE (Tamada T et al., *Int J Chron Obstruct Pulmon Dis.*, 10, 2169–2176, 2015.)

[c] CRP, TNFa, IL-8 higher in COPD and ACO than healthy controls (Miravitlles M et al., *Respir Med.*, 107, 1053–1060, 2013; Garcia-Rio F et al., *Respir Res.*, 11, 63, 2010.)

[d] IL-6 increased in ACO compared to asthma and healthy controls. (Fu JJ et al., *Allergy Asthma Immunol Res.*, 6, 316–324, 2014.)

[e] IL-17 and IL-18 higher in ACO and COPD than asthma and healthy controls. (Soodaeva S et al., *Eur Resp J.*, 46, 2015.)

[f] Iwamoto H et al., *Eur Respir J.*, 43, 421–429, 2014.

[g] Miravitlles M et al., *Respir Med.*, 107, 1053–1060, 2013; Garcia-Rio F et al., *Respir Res.*, 11, 63, 2010.

IgE levels to specific aeroallergens have also been studied. In a large population dataset, those with ACO were more likely to have elevated levels of IgE to house dust mite, cat dander, Timothy grass, or *Cladosporium* compared to COPD and healthy controls. The levels of sensitization were similar to those with asthma.[6] Skin-prick testing to common allergens including cat, dog, dust mite, grasses, and fungi were performed in those with ACO and asthma. Overall, there were similar levels of positive skin-prick tests in those with ACO and asthma.[8] Taken as a whole, these data suggest that allergic sensitization may play a role in ACO. However, when interpreting IgE levels, the race, age, and gender of the patient must be taken into account, as the female gender and Hispanic and African American groups have been found to have higher levels of IgE.[38]

14.5.2.3 Inflammatory cytokines

Systemic inflammation plays a prominent role in the pathogenesis of COPD and its comorbidities. C reactive protein (CRP), tumor necrosis factor alpha (TNFα), IL-8, and nitrates all are higher in COPD than healthy controls.[39,40] These inflammatory biomarkers also have been examined in ACO. CRP, TNFα, and IL-8 were all elevated in both COPD and ACO. The only difference was that the plasma nitrates/nitrates were much lower in ACO compared to COPD.[9] Others show that IL-6 is increased in ACO compared to healthy controls, asthmatics[40] and COPD.[30] Serum IL-17 and IL-18 also were higher in ACO and COPD than in asthma and healthy controls.[41]

Other potential novel biomarkers have also been investigated. Plasma-soluble receptor for advanced glycation end products (sRAGE) is shown to be elevated in ACO as compared to asthma patients, and surfactant protein A (SP-A) is postulated to help differentiate overlap from asthma, but not overlap from COPD.[36] Amyloid A also has been evaluated and no differences between COPD, healthy, and ACO groups were found.[7]

14.6 EXHALED NITRIC OXIDE TESTING

Exhaled nitric oxide (NO) has been used in a clinical context since the late 1990s. Papi was the first to associate elevated sputum eosinophilia and increased exhaled NO with reversible airflow obstruction, a disease feature typically associated with asthma.[28] Furthermore, Papi et al. found that exhaled NO concentrations, but not percentage of sputum eosinophilia, correlated with degree of airflow reversibility. More recently, Chou found that in patients with COPD, there are significant correlations between exhaled NO and sputum eosinophilia.[42] As with all tests, there are limitations to exhaled NO concentrations as Barnes notes in a review that reports that current smoking and ICS use reduces exhaled NO concentrations.[43] The role of exhaled NO also has been investigated in the setting of ACO (Table 14.5).

The consensus statement set forth by the scientific committees of GINA/GOLD discusses the role of fractional exhaled NO (FeNO) in the diagnosis of ACO, and suggests that a high level of exhaled NO (>50 ppb) in nonsmokers supports eosinophilic airway inflammation and, therefore, is supportive of ACO. Tamada et al. conducted a study measuring FeNO in patients with COPD in an attempt to be able to classify those with asthma-like atopic features by objective measures. The authors postulate that the FeNO levels in patients are useful to help identify the ACO group.[37] The study was a multicenter cross-sectional study that targeted patients with COPD, and it ultimately enrolled 331 participants. Authors used PFT values to diagnose COPD then added FeNO as a measure of asthma-like inflammation. They report that the average FeNO was 20 ppb and 16.3% of those with COPD had a FeNO level of >35 ppb. The authors propose that an FeNO of >35 ppb combined with PFTs supportive of COPD to be diagnostic of ACO. Overall, Tamada et al. estimate the prevalence rate of ACO is 16.3% in their COPD population based on FENO >35 ppb. This is notable given there is general agreement that among those with COPD, 10%–20% have features of asthma.[44]

14.7 GENETIC TESTING

With an ever-evolving role of genetics used for diagnosis and therapeutics, several authors have investigated the role of genes in the diagnosis of asthma-COPD overlap.

Christenson and colleagues hypothesize that there are partially overlapping airway gene expression changes in asthma and COPD, and that these genetic changes can help identify a COPD subgroup more similar to asthma.[45] To examine this, they compared disease-associated airway epithelial gene expression in asthma and COPD cohorts. The

Table 14.5 Exhaled nitric oxide

	Asthma	COPD	ACO
FeNO[c]	Elevated in most asthmatics	Normal in most with COPD	Normal or elevated: >50PPB[a] >35PPB[b]

[a] GINA/GOLD. Diagnosis of Diseases of Chronic Airflow Limitation: Asthma, COPD and Asthma COPD Overlap Synrome (ACO); 2015. Available at http://www.ginasthma.org: GINA/GOLD.

[b] Barnes PJ et al., *Chest*, 138, 682–692, 2010.

[c] FeNO testing is influenced by current cigarette smoking and use of inhaled corticosteroids.

authors used a T helper type 2-signature expression score and found that this score was highest in a COPD subpopulation that had increased asthma-like features, such as increased response to ICS, bronchodilator reversibility, blood eosinophilia, and airway wall eosinophilia. Interestingly, a higher score also correlates with decreased lung function, but not an asthma history in the COPD cohorts.[45]

Hardin et al. performed genome-wide-association analyses in an attempt to identify specific genes associated with ACO. Study subjects were current or former smoking, non-Hispanic whites or African Americans diagnosed with COPD. The overlap patients were defined as having been diagnosed with asthma and COPD before the age of 40. Their analysis concludes that while no specific genes met genome-wide association study levels of statistical significance, single nucleotide polymorphisms in the genes CSMD1, SOX5, and GPR65 are associated with asthma-COPD overlap.[24]

REFERENCES

1. GINA/GOLD. Diagnosis of Diseases of Chronic Airflow Limitation:Asthma, COPD and Asthma COPD Overlap Syndrome (ACOS); 2015. Available at http://www.ginasthma.org: GINA/GOLD.
2. Miravitlles M, Soler-Cataluna JJ, Calle M et al. Spanish COPD Guidelines (GesEPOC): Pharmacological treatment of stable COPD. *Aten Primaria*. 2012;44(7):425–437.
3. GOLD. Global Strategy for the Diagnosis, Management, and Prevention of Chronic Obstructive Pulmonary Disease; 2006. goldcopd.org, accessed June 16, 2016.
4. National Heart, Lung, and Blood Institute. National Asthma Education and Prevention Program: Expert panel report III: Guidelines for the diagnosis and management of asthma; 2007. https://www.nhlbi.nih.gov/files/docs/guidelines/asthgdln.pdf; accessed June 18, 2016
5. Qaseem AW, Wilt TJ, Weinberger SE et al. Diagnosis and management of stable chronic obstructive pulmonary disease: A clinical practice guideline update from the american college of physicians, american college of chest physicians, american thoracic sociery and european respiratory society. *Ann of Intern Med*. 2011;3(155):179–191.
6. de Marco RM, Rossi A, Anto JM et al. Asthma, COPD and overlap syndrome: Alongitudinal study in young European adults. *Eur Respir J*. 2015;46(3):587–590.
7. Fu JJ, Gibson PG, Simpson JL et al. Longitudinal changes in clinical outcomes in older patients with asthma, COPD and asthma-COPD overlap syndrome. *Respir*. 2014;87(1):63–74.
8. Lee HY, Kang JY, Yoon HK et al. Clinical characteristics of asthma combined with COPD feature. *Yonsei Med J*. 2014;55(4):980–986.
9. Miravitlles M, Soriano JB, Ancochea J et al. Characterisation of the overlap COPD-asthma phenotype. Focus on physical activity and health status. *Respir Med*. 2013;107(7):1053–1060.
10. Cosio BG, Soriano JB, Lopez-Campos JL et al. Defining the asthma-COPD overlap syndrome in a COPD cohort. *Chest*. 2016;149(1):45–52.
11. Pellegrino R, Viegi G, Brusasco V et al. Interpretative strategies for lung function tests. *Eur Respir J*. 2005;26(5):948–968.
12. Celli BR, MacNee W, Agusti A et al. Standards for the diagnosis and treatment of patients with COPD: A summary of the ATS/ERS position paper. *Eur Resp J*. 2004;23(6):932–946.
13. Hanania NA, Celli BR, Donohue JF et al. Bronchodilator reversibility in COPD. *Chest*. 2011;140(4):1055–1063.
14. Grippi MA and Tino G. Pulmonary function testing. In: MA Grippi, JA Elias, JA Fishman et al., eds. *Fishman's Pulmonary Diseases and Disorders*. 5th ed. New York, NY: McGraw-Hill Education; 2015.
15. Wan ES, DeMeo DL, Hersh CP et al. Clinical predictors of frequent exacerbations in subjects with severe chronic obstructive pulmonary disease (COPD). *Respir Med*. 2011;105(4):588–594.
16. Rao DR, Gaffin JM, Baxi SN et al. The utility of forced expiratory flow between 25% and 75% of vital capacity in predicting childhood asthma morbidity and severity. *J Asthma*. 2012;49(6):586–592.
17. Irvin CG and Bates JH. Physiologic dysfunction of the asthmatic lung: What's going on down there, anyway?. *Proc Am Thorac Soc*. 2009;6(3):306–311.
18. Jarenback L, Ankerst J, Bjermer L et al. Flow-volume parameters in COPD related to extended measurements of lung volume, diffusion, and resistance. *Pulm Med*. 2013;2013:782052.
19. McLean A, Warren PM, Gillooly M et al. Microscopic measurments of emphysema: Relation to carbon monoxide gas transfer. *Thorax*. 1992;47(3):144–149.
20. Society AT. Amertican thoracic society guidelines for methacholine and exercise challenge testing 1999. *Am J Respir Crit Care Med*. 2000;161:309–329.
21. Walker PP, Hadcroft J, Costello RW et al. Lung function changes following methacholine inhalation in COPD. *Resp Med*. 2009;103(4):535–541.
22. Gibson PG and Simpson JL. The overlap syndrome of asthma and COPD: What are its features and how important is it?. *Thorax*. 2009;64(8):728–735.
23. Gao Y, Zhai X, Li K et al. Asthma COPD overlap syndrome on CT densitometry: A distinct phenotype from COPD. *COPD*. 2016;13(4):471–476.
24. Hardin M, Cho M, McDonald ML et al. The clinical and genetic features of COPD-asthma overlap syndrome. *Eur Respir J*. 2014;44(2):341–350.

25. Xie M, Wang W, Dou S et al. Quantitative computed tomography measurements of emphysema for diagnosing asthma-chronic obstructive pulmonary disease overlap syndrome. *Int J Chron Obstruct Pulmon Dis.* 2016;11:953–961.

26. Suzuki T, Tada Y, Kawata N et al. Clinical, physiological, and radiological features of asthma-chronic obstructive pulmonary disease overlap syndrome. *Int J Chron Obstruct Pulmon Dis.* 2015;10:947–954.

27. National Heart, Lung, and Blood Institute. Expert Panel Report 2: Guidelines for the Diagnosis and Management of Asthma; 2007. https://www.nhlbi.nih.gov/files/docs/guidelines/asthgdln.pdf; accessed June 18, 2016

28. Papi A, Romagnoli M, Baraldo S et al. Partial reversibility of airflow limitation and increased exhaled NO and sputum eosinophiia in chronic obstructive pulmonary disease. *Am J Respir Crit Care Med.* 2000;162:1772–177.

29. Berry M, Morgan A, Shaw DE et al. Pathological features and inhaled corticosteroid response of eosinophilic and non-eosinophilic asthma. *Thorax.* 2007;62(12):1043–1049.

30. Saha S and Brightling CE. Eosinophilic airway inflammation in COPD. *Int J of Chron Obstruct Pulmon Dis.* 2006;1(1):39–47.

31. D'Silva L, Hassan N, Wang HY et al. Heterogeneity of bronchitis in airway disease in teritary care clinical practice. *Can Respir J.* 2011;18(3):144–148.

32. Ghebre MA, Bafadhel M, Desai D et al. Biological clustering supports both "Dutch" and "British" hypotheses of asthma and chronic obstructive pulmonary disease. *J Allergy Clin Immunol.* 2015;135(1):63–72.

33. Manise M, Holtappels G, Van Crombruggen K et al. Sputum IgE and cytokines in asthma: Relationship with sputum cellular profile. *PLOS ONE.* 2013;8(3):e58388.

34. Barnes PJ. The cytokine network in asthma and chronic obstructive pulmonary disease. *J Clin Invest.* 2008;118(11):3546–3556.

35. Yalcin AD, Celik B, and Yalcin AN. Omalizumab (anti-IgE) therapy in the asthma-COPD overlap syndrome (ACOS) and its effects on circulating cytokine levels. *Immunopharmacol Immunotoxicol.* 2016;38(3):253–256.

36. Iwamoto H, Gao J, Koskela J et al. Differences in plasma and sputum biomarkers between COPD and COPD-asthma overlap. *Eur Respir J.* 2014;43(2):421–429.

37. Tamada T, Sugiura H, Takahashi T et al. Biomarker-based detection of asthma-COPD overlap syndrome in COPD populations. *Int J Chron Obstruct Pulmon Dis.* 2015;10:2169–2176.

38. Gergen PJ, Arbes SJ, Jr., Calatroni A et al. Total IgE levels and asthma prevalence in the US population: Results from the national health and nutrition examination survey 2005-2006. *J Allergy Clin Immunol.* 2009;124(3):447–453.

39. Garcia-Rio F, Miravitlles M, Soriano JB et al. Systemic inflammation in chronic obstructive pulmonary disease: A population-based study. *Respir Res.* 2010;11:63.

40. Fu JJ, McDonald VM, Gibson PG et al. Systemic inflammation in older adults with asthma-COPD overlap syndrome. *Allergy Asthma Immunol Res.* 2014;6(4):316–324.

41. Soodaeva S, Postnikova L, Boldina M et al. Serum IL-17 and IL-18 levels in asthma-COPD overlap syndrome patients. *Eur Resp J.* 2015;46(Suppl. 59) :4886–4887.

42. Chou KT, Su KC, Huant SF et al. Exhaled nitric oxide predicts eosinophilic airway inflammation in COPD. *Lung.* 2014;192(4):499–504.

43. Barnes PJ, Dweik RA, Gelb AF et al. Exhaled nitric oxide in pulmonary diseases: A comprehensive review. *Chest.* 2010;138(3):682–692.

44. Gibson PG and McDonald VM..Asthma-COPD overlap 2015: Now we are six. *Thorax.* 2015;70(7):683–691.

45. Christenson SA, Steiling K, van den Berge M et al. Asthma-COPD overlap. Clinical relevance of genomic signatures of type 2 inflammation in chronic obstructive pulmonary disease. *Am J Respir Crit Care Med.* 2015;191(7):758–766.

Environmental control of asthma, COPD, and asthma-COPD overlap

GENNARO D'AMATO, CAROLINA VITALE, ANTONIO MOLINO, AND MARIA D'AMATO

CLINICAL VIGNETTE 15.1

An increasing body of evidence shows the occurrence of severe asthma epidemics during thunderstorms in the pollen season.

On May 28, 2012, a 36-year-old, 20-weeks-pregnant woman presented to an emergency department (ED) with acute shortness of breath, about 2 hours after being outdoors during a thunderstorm.

She was affected by seasonal asthma and sensitized to *Parietaria* (pellitory of the wall) pollen and was on inhaled corticosteroid and long-acting β_2-agonist combination therapy.

She had already been admitted to the ED for severe dyspnea on two previous occasions.

The first time she experienced near-fatal asthma in concomitance with a thunderstorm was in June 2004, and she was treated in the ED of the Antonio Cardarelli Hospital in Naples, Italy. The second time she experienced near-fatal asthma in concomitance with a thunderstorm, she was admitted to the ED of the same hospital 7 years later, on May 24, 2011, despite appropriate treatment with inhaled corticosteroids and bronchodilators.

Since the first episode, the patient had avoided being outdoors when a thunderstorm was approaching.

In 2012 an unexpected thunderstorm occurred while she was driving her motorbike, and she experienced increasing dyspnea that had to be treated in the ED some hours later. She was admitted to the ED and was unsuccessfully treated with adrenaline, high-dose steroids; then she was intubated and transferred to the intensive-care unit. Despite 4 days of systemic therapy with oxygen, methylprednisolone, and albuterol, her clinical picture dramatically improved only after infusions of magnesium sulfate, with a normalization of arterial blood gas parameters. At day eight, the patient was extubated, steroids were slowly tapered down, magnesium sulfate was infused for two additional days, and fluticasone via aerosol was given. Clinical and ultrasound checks did not show any fetal distress. The patient could then be discharged with inhalers and oral prednisone. The childbirth occurred with caesarean section at week 32, and the baby was in good health with a normal Apgar's index.

As in the previous two episodes, symptoms appeared after a thunderstorm occurred during the Parietaria pollen season (pollen count was 36 grains/m³ air on May 28 and 108 grains/m³ on May 27). Main pollutants levels did not show any significant change in respect to the previous days.

In conclusion, this case report is a dramatic example of how environmental conditions directly caused by thunderstorms can trigger an asthma attack; specifically, it described the first case of relapse of near-fatal thunderstorm-related asthma.[1]

15.1 INTRODUCTION

The massive increase of chemical and biologic pollutants in the atmosphere over the last century has made poor air quality a sentinel environmental issue in many regions of the world. The negative impact of poor air quality on human health is now well recognized. There are numerous well-conducted studies that have confirmed the association between short- and long-term exposure to air pollutants and adverse human health effects.[2–9]

The prevalence of obstructive airway diseases such as asthma and chronic obstructive pulmonary disease (COPD) has increased dramatically to epidemic proportions worldwide. Besides air pollution from industry-derived emissions and motor vehicles, the rising trend can be explained, in large part, by the profound changes in the environments where we live around the planet, in both developed and developing countries. The world economy has been transformed over the last 50 years with developing countries being at the core of these changes. Many of these changes are considered to have negative effects on respiratory health, and they increase the frequency and severity of respiratory diseases such as asthma, COPD, and asthma-COPD overlap (ACO) in the general population. Increased concentrations of greenhouse gases in the atmosphere, especially carbon dioxide (CO_2), have contributed substantially to global warming of the planet, as well as having caused more marked variations in temperature, increased air pollution, more frequent forest fires, prolonged droughts, severe floods, powerful thunderstorms, and more severe and prolonged heat waves, all of which can affect respiratory health.[4]

These changes in climate and air quality, both outdoors and indoors, have a measurable impact not only on the morbidity but also on the mortality of patients with asthma and other obstructive respiratory diseases such as COPD and ACO. There is also considerable evidence that subjects affected by asthma are at an increased risk of exacerbations with continuous exposure to gaseous and particulate components of air pollution.[10]

Global warming is expected to affect the onset, duration, and intensity of the allergenic pollen season as well as the rate of asthma and COPD exacerbations due to air pollution, respiratory infections, and cold-air inhalation. Control of the environment requires attention to exposures that originate from both outdoor and indoor environments. This emphasis leading to reduction of outdoor and indoor air pollution can help improve symptoms of obstructive respiratory diseases and reduce the health burden of these diseases.

Asthma and COPD significantly have a substantial economic burden on our health care system. Asthma and COPD are among the top 10 chronic medical conditions that are associated with significant activity restriction, impaired quality of life, and substantial health care utilization.

Asthma is a chronic inflammatory disorder, characterized by reversible airway obstruction and hyperresponsiveness. In a Global Initiative of Asthma (GINA) report on the burden of asthma, it has been estimated that asthma is one of the most common chronic diseases, affecting 300 million people worldwide.[11] The asthma prevalence rate in the United States is approximately 10.9%, representing 35.5 million individuals.[12] The number of disability-adjusted life years (DALYs) lost due to asthma worldwide has been estimated to be approximately 15 million per year. The economic costs associated with asthma account for 1%–2% of total healthcare budgets for developed countries. In the United States, the total cost of asthma in 2004 was estimated at $16.1 billion, with $11.5 billion the result of direct costs (71.4%) and $4.6 billion secondary to indirect costs (28.6%).[13] The ERS white book, published in 2003, estimated the total costs of asthma in Europe at approximately 17.7 billion Euros per annuum.[14] An estimate of the costs of asthma in children in 25 European Union countries in 2005 was estimated to be 3 billion Euros. The use of wheeze as the definition for asthma leads to a considerably higher cost of 5.2 billion Euros. However, it should be noted that the annual costs for childhood asthma per country varies widely.[15]

According to the World Health Organization (WHO), COPD "is a lung disease characterized by chronic obstruction of lung airflow that interferes with normal breathing and is not fully reversible." The pathophysiologic spectrum of COPD includes chronic bronchitis and emphysema. COPD carries a high mortality burden; it is the fourth-leading cause of death in the United States, yet it may be largely underdiagnosed.[16] COPD is associated with significant economic burden. In the European Union, COPD accounts for 56% (38.6 billion Euros) of the cost of respiratory disease. In the United States, the estimated direct costs of COPD are $32 billion and the indirect costs are $20.4 billlion.[16]

A significant proportion of patients who present with chronic respiratory symptoms, particularly older patients, have diagnoses or features of both asthma and COPD, and are found to have chronic airflow limitation (that is not completely reversible after bronchodilatation). Although there is no general agreement to define these patients, the term ACO has been proposed by the Science Committees of both GINA and GOLD.[11,16]

ACO patients experience frequent exacerbations, have poor quality of life, experience a more rapid decline in lung function, and have high mortality rates, and consume a disproportionate amount of health-care resources than asthma or COPD alone.[11,16]

In this chapter, opportunities for intervention to control environmental determinants of asthma, COPD, and ACO are discussed.

15.2 COMPONENTS OF OUTDOOR AIR POLLUTION IN URBAN AREAS

Several studies[17–25] confirmed the negative effect of urban air pollution on human health and on respiratory diseases.

Air pollutants exert their detrimental effects on the lung and airways by several mechanisms, such as

1. Attenuation of ciliary activity of airway epithelial cells
2. Increase in permeability of airway epithelium
3. Inflammatory changes in cells of airways and lung parenchyma
4. Modulation of cell cycle and death of cells of respiratory system

Air pollutants exhibit their proinflammatory effects on airways by causing direct cellular injury or by inducing intracellular signaling pathways and transcription factors that are known to be sensitive to the oxidative stress.

Epidemiologic studies have demonstrated that urbanization, high levels of vehicle emissions, and westernized lifestyle are correlated to an increase in the frequency of obstructive respiratory diseases prevalent in people who live in urban areas compared with those who live in rural areas.[17–28]

Reduction in exposure to air pollutants to prevent asthma episodes can be approached at a policy level through changes in indoor and outdoor air pollution and by modifying the lifestyle of asthma patients.

The most abundant components of air pollution in urban areas are nitrogen dioxide (NO_2), ozone (O_3), and particulate matter (PM).

1. Nitrogen dioxide (NO_2) is a precursor of photochemical smog found in urban and industrial regions, and is most often generated by vehicle exhaust and power plants. In conjunction with sunlight and hydrocarbons, NO_2 results in the production of O_3. Similar to O_3, NO_2 is an oxidizing pollutant, but has a lower chemical reactivity. NO_2 exposure is associated with increased ED visits, wheezing, and medication use among children with asthma. Controlled exposure studies on asthmatic patients have shown that NO_2 can enhance the allergic response to inhaled allergens. Furthermore, NO_2 concentrations in ambient air have also been associated with cough, wheezing, and shortness of breath in atopic patients.[24–27]

2. As mentioned, ozone (O_3) is generated at ground level by photochemical reactions involving NO_2, hydrocarbons, and ultraviolet (UV) radiation. Inhalation of O_3 induces epithelial damage and consequent inflammatory responses in the upper and lower airways manifested as increased levels of inflammatory cells and mediators in nasal and bronchoalveolar lavage.[24] Exposure to increased atmospheric levels of O_3 induces a reduction of lung function and an increase in airway hyperreactivity induced by bronchoconstrictor agents.[26,27] Epidemiologic studies have provided strong evidence that high ambient concentrations of O_3 are associated with an increased rate of asthma exacerbations, increased hospital admissions, and/or ED visits for all respiratory diseases, including asthma. Furthermore, several studies[26–31] suggest that O_3 increases asthma morbidity by enhancing airway inflammation and epithelial permeability. It has been speculated that O_3 and other pollutants may render allergic-atopic patients more susceptible to the antigen they are sensitized.[29,30] Beck et al.[29] observed that high environmental O_3 levels enhance allergenicity of birch pollen with clinical relevance for susceptible individuals. The acute health effects of exposure to ambient O_3 have been examined in many geographical regions. O_3 exposure has both a priming effect on allergen-induced responses and an intrinsic proinflammatory action in the airways of allergic-atopic asthmatic patients. In the long term, continuous exposure to high O_3 levels impairs respiratory function, and causes or exacerbates airway inflammation in healthy patients and in asthma patients. At the population level, long-term exposure to O_3 may reduce lung function in schoolchildren and adults, and increase the prevalence of asthma and asthmatic symptoms. In addition, studies have shown that asthma can be exacerbated by O_3, as measured by increased visits to EDs on days with higher levels of O_3 and other pollutants. Recently Malig et al.[31] explored ozone's connection to asthma and total respiratory ED visits. A multisite, time-stratified, case-crossover study of O_3 exposures for approximately 3.7 million respiratory ED visits from 2005 through 2008 was conducted among California residents living within 12 miles of an O_3 monitor.[31] The result was that short-term O_3 exposures among California residents living near an O_3 monitor were positively associated with ED visits for asthma, acute respiratory infections, pneumonia, chronic obstructive pulmonary disease, and upper respiratory tract inflammation from 2005 through 2008. Those associations were typically larger and more consistent during the warm season.

3. PM is a mixture of organic and inorganic solid and liquid particles of different origins, size, and composition. Ultrafine particulate matter (UFPM), with diameters of 0.1 mm or less, is a major byproduct of vehicle emissions. These particles accumulate into larger fine PM with a diameter of 2.5 mm ($PM_{2.5}$, PM with a diameter of 2.5 mm or less) within short distances from the point

of release. PM_{10} consists of $PM_{2.5}$ and larger particles of mainly crustal or biological origin, including many aero-allergens. Based on epidemiological and laboratory studies[32-34] $PM_{2.5}$ appears to be a more potent agent for the development of respiratory and cardiovascular disease compared with PM_{10}. PM_{10} can penetrate the lower airways, and $PM_{2.5}$ is thought to constitute a notable health risk because it can be inhaled more deeply into the lungs at the alveoli level. Although human lung parenchyma retains $PM_{2.5}$, particles larger than 5 mm and smaller than 10 mm reach the proximal airways only, wherein they are eliminated by mucociliary clearance if the airway mucosa is intact. A large portion of urban PM originates from diesel engines, as diesel exhaust particles (DEP), which include other components, such as polycyclic aromatic hydrocarbons (PAH).

4. DEPs account for up to 90% of airborne PM in the world's largest cities and are composed of fine (2.5–0.1 mm) and ultrafine (0.1 mm) particles, which can also coalesce to form aggregates of varying sizes. PM_{10} levels have been associated with early respiratory exacerbations in children with persistent asthma and with higher prevalence rates even after having considered the dispersion of the particles. Although there is compelling evidence that ambient air pollution exacerbates existing asthma, the link with the development of asthma syndrome is still less well established, as few studies provide extensive exposure data. Researchers have elucidated the mechanisms whereby fine particles induce adverse effects; they appear to affect the balance between antioxidant pathways and airway inflammation. Gene olymorphisms involved in antioxidant pathways can modify responses to air pollution exposure. Acute exposure to diesel exhaust causes specific effects like irritation of nose and eyes, headache, lung function abnormalities, respiratory changes, fatigue, and nausea, whereas chronic exposure is associated with cough, sputum production, and diminished lung function. Studies[33-36] have demonstrated inflammation in the airways of healthy individuals after exposure to diesel exhaust and DEP, and elevated expression and concentrations of inflammatory mediators have similarly been observed in the respiratory tract after diesel exhaust and DEP exposure. Recently, Carlsten et al.[21] observed that inhalation of diesel exhaust at environmentally relevant concentrations augments allergen-induced allergic inflammation in the lower airways of atopic individuals. Particularly, diesel exhaust not only augmented the allergen-induced increase in airway eosinophils, interleukin-5 (IL-5), and eosinophil cationic protein (ECP), but also augmented markers of nonallergic inflammation and monocyte chemotactic protein (MCP)-1, and suppressed activity of macrophages and myeloid dendritic cells.[21]

In the context of outdoor air pollution, we also need to consider that open biomass burning plays an important role in atmospheric pollution and in climate change.

15.3 POLLUTANTS OF THE INDOOR ENVIRONMENT

15.3.1 INDOOR POLLUTANTS

Indoor pollution sources that release gases or particles into the air are the primary cause of indoor air quality (IAQ) problems in homes and some people feel better as soon as they remove the source of the pollution. There are many sources of indoor air pollution in any home. These include combustion sources such as oil, gas, kerosene, coal, wood, and tobacco products; building materials and furnishings including deteriorated, asbestos-containing insulation, wet or damp carpet, and cabinetry or furniture made of certain pressed wood products; products for household cleaning and maintenance, personal care, or hobbies; central heating and cooling systems; humidification devices; and outdoor sources that seep inside, such as radon, pesticides, and outdoor air pollution.

Some sources, such as building materials, furnishings, and household products like air fresheners, release pollutants more or less continuously. Other sources, related to activities carried out in the home, release pollutants intermittently. These include smoking; the use of unvented or malfunctioning stoves, furnaces, or space heaters; the use of solvents in cleaning and hobby activities; the use of paint strippers in refinishing activities; and the use of cleaning products and pesticides in housekeeping. High pollutant concentrations can remain in the air for long periods after some of these activities. Volatile organic compounds (VOC) are emitted as gases from certain solids or liquids. VOCs include a variety of chemicals, some of which may have short- and long-term adverse health effects. Concentrations of many VOCs are consistently higher indoors (up to ten times higher) than outdoors. VOCs are emitted by a wide array of products numbering in the thousands. Microbial volatile organic compounds (MVOC) are a variety of compounds formed in the metabolism of fungi and bacteria. MVOCs are affected by different factors including, but not restricted to, the substrate, moisture content of the material, and temperature.[37] MVOCs can be used as a tracer of suspected or hidden microbial contamination, as well as in detection of moisture problems, risk of fungal development, and sources of odors in buildings.[38] The most obvious health effect of MVOC exposure is eye and upper-airway irritation. However, symptoms of irritation have appeared at MVOC concentrations several orders of magnitude higher than those measured indoors (single MVOC levels in indoor environments have ranged from a few ng/m^3 up to 1 mg/m^3).[39] Organic chemicals are widely used as ingredients in household products. Paints, varnishes, and wax all contain organic solvents, as do many cleaning, disinfecting, cosmetic, degreasing, and hobby products. Fuels are made up of organic chemicals. All of these products can release organic compounds while being used and, to some extent, when stored. Poor ventilation can increase indoor pollutant levels as a result of inadequate outdoor air exchange, which is necessary to dilute indoor sources of emissions and to allow the escape of indoor air pollutants from the home. Elevated temperature and humidity levels can also increase concentrations of some pollutants. IAQ refers to the air quality within and around buildings and structures, especially as it relates to the health and comfort of building occupants. Understanding and controlling common pollutants indoors can help reduce an inhabitant's risk of indoor health problems.

With respect to indoor pollution, few studies have associated levels of air pollutants other than environmental tobacco smoke with increase asthma and COPD prevalence or symptoms. Environmental tobacco smoke is one of the most significant risks for respiratory symptoms and diseases worldwide. Consistent results support short-term (aggravation) and, less commonly, long-term (prevalence augmentation) effects on asthma related to poor indoor air.

The data available are also reliable for indoor nitrogen dioxide and PM, which have been associated with asthma and COPD. Whereas formaldehyde and VOC seem to be the main pollutants in indoor settings, relevant studies on asthma are still lacking.[4]

15.3.2 INDOOR ALLERGENS

The most common indoor allergens are dust mites, furry pets, cockroaches, and molds.[40-47]

15.3.2.1 Dust mites

The major dust mite allergens are Der f 1 and Der p 1 from the two most common house dust mite species, *Dermatophagoides farinae* and *Dermatophagoides pteronyssinus*. Several different approaches to dust mite allergen exposure reduction have been studied, and they focus on source removal (i.e., killing the dust mites) and/or removal of the allergen. As the major dust mite allergens are carried on larger particles (>10 microns), they quickly settle to dependent surfaces after disturbance of the reservoir. The primary avoidance measure approaches include interventions that target the bed. These include frequent washing of all bed linens in hot water and use of allergen impermeable mattress. It is also effective to pull up carpet and apply acaricides or allergen-denaturing agents. Application of acaricides and allergen-denaturing agents is cumbersome, but one Cochrane review suggests that acaricides may be beneficial.[41] However, further studies are needed to offer a definitive recommendation. Home or room dehumidification, with a goal of reducing relative humidity less than 45% can reduce dust mite populations. Sustained reduction of indoor relative humidity is difficult to achieve, and carpet removal is expensive and of unclear benefit. First-line approaches to reduce dust mite allergen exposure include washing of bed linens and use of allergen-impermeable mattress and pillow encasements, as these measures are highly effective in reducing dust mite allergens in the bed. In studies with carefully selected patients who are very likely to have dust mite–driven asthma, dust mite interventions that result in a substantial reduction in dust mite allergen levels showed a clinical benefit.[40]

15.3.2.2 Furry pets

The most common furry pets are cats and dogs. Cat and dog allergens can be found in virtually all homes, but, not surprisingly, homes with pets contain much higher levels of the allergens than homes without pets. The major dog allergen is Can f 1 and the major cat allergen is Fel d 1. These allergens, in contrast to dust mite and cockroach allergens, are predominantly carried on smaller particles (<10–20 microns) so remain airborne for long periods and are readily detectable in air samples from homes. A recent study addressed the question of whether certain dog breeds are "hypoallergenic" by measuring dog allergen levels in dust and air samples collected from homes with a variety of dog breeds, including ones considered hypoallergenic. The investigators found that homes with hypoallergenic dogs had similar levels of dog allergen as homes with nonhypoallergenic dogs. Almost all studies support the notion that significant reductions in animal allergen levels require source removal (relocating the pet). Even after removing the pet from the home, it can take several months before significant reductions in allergen levels are observed. However, there is no evidence supporting the hypothesis that sustained animal allergen exposure leads to tolerance and is therefore better or equivalent to pet removal from the home in asthma management, so this cannot be a recommended approach for pet-allergic asthmatics.[40] However, given the unconditional love provided by pets to their owners, complete avoidance is often not practical, and therefore interventions such as removing the pet from the bedroom and main activity room; frequent vacuuming; HEPA filtration in the bedroom and main activity room; cheese cloth or vent filters over outflow vents into the bedroom; protective encasements for pillows, mattresses, and box springs; and frequent washing of bedding may help significantly reduce the patient's total allergen burden. Furthermore, allergen immunotherapy may be very effective at mitigating symptoms allowing patients to keep their pets.[42]

15.3.2.3 Cockroaches

The most common cockroaches in U.S. inner cities are the German and American cockroaches, and the major German cockroach allergens, Bla g 1 and Bla g 2, are the best studied in terms of health effects. Cockroach allergen exposure among sensitized inner-city children with asthma was first linked to asthma morbidity by the National Cooperative Inner-City Asthma Study (NCICAS) in 1997. Since then, the link with asthma morbidity has been replicated, and highly effective methods based on integrated pest management principles to reduce cockroach allergen levels have been identified. Moreover, in a successful multifaceted environmental intervention in inner-city children with asthma, the degree of reduction in cockroach allergen was correlated with the degree of improvement in asthma symptoms, providing strong support for recommending cockroach allergen environmental control measures as an integral part of asthma management in cockroach-sensitized children with asthma.[40]

15.3.2.4 Molds

There are a very large number of mold species, but very few have been well studied with respect to their effects on asthma. Molds can be found in both indoor and outdoor environments. Aspergillus and Penicillium species are among the most common indoor molds, and Alternaria can be found in both indoor and outdoor environments but is considered the outdoor mold causing the most clinical symptoms in mold-sensitized individuals.

Sensitization to molds has been associated with increased asthma severity and death, hospital admission and intensive care admissions in adults, and increased bronchial reactivity in children.[43-48] In a retrospective study of 11 asthmatic patients who had a respiratory arrest, 10 out of 11 were skin-test-positive for *Alternaria alternata*.[46]

Black et al. reported that 20 of 37 patients (54%) admitted to the ICU for asthma had a positive skin test for one or more fungal allergens.[47] Targonsky et al. reported that, during the pollen season, mean concentrations of mold spores, but not tree, grass, or ragweed pollen, were significantly higher on the days when there were deaths related to asthma compared to days when no asthma deaths were recorded.[48]

The pathogenetic mechanisms by which certain mold allergens induce more severe airway disease compared to other common allergens remain to be elucidated. A possible explanation is that fungi, compared to other allergens, have the additional ability to actively germinate and infect the host skin or attempt to colonize the respiratory tract. It was suggested that mold allergens acting in concert with other nonallergen proteins or toxins produce an enhanced host response. For example, mold release mVOC, which manifest as the mildew odors associated with mold contaminated areas. These mVOCs have been reported to cause a spectrum of irritant upper and respiratory symptoms in exposed individuals with or without rhinitis and asthma.[49] Because molds prefer warm, moist environments, mold growth can be decreased by interventions that reduce moisture and humidity, such as dehumidification, air conditioning, and increased ventilation.

Humidifiers and vaporizers increase indoor humidity, and can become colonized with mold, so they should not be used in homes of people with asthma. If small amounts of molds are already present, thorough cleaning with fungicides is recommended using personal protective equipment (e.g., a NIOSH N95 rated respirator). If cleaning is not possible, the item should be eliminated. Keeping windows closed to reduce exposure to outdoor molds and running the air conditioner, which acts as a natural dehumidifier, will help prevent indoor mold growth. However, it is important to avoid perfrigeration or frosting, which can occur when the indoor temperature is lower than 75–77°F. A HEPA room air filter may also help, but this intervention has not been extensively studied.[50] Water leaks can contribute to the growth of indoor molds, so it is important to prevent and eliminate water intrusion wherever possible. When outdoors, patients should avoid heavy exposure to moldy vegetation and use a properly fitting particulate mask when working with moldy material, such as mulching. Although there have been no randomized trials of mold abatement in persons with asthma, there is adequate evidence to recommend these basic interventions to reduce exposure for mold-sensitized patients with asthma. Furthermore, the NAEPP and Joint Task Force Practice Parameter guidelines recommend considering measures to control indoor dampness and molds.[51]

15.4 EFFECTS OF CLIMATE CHANGE ON AIR POLLUTION AND ALLERGENIC POLLEN

Climate change may affect air pollutant levels in several ways: regional weather (e.g., changes of wind patterns, amount and intensity of precipitation, and increase of temperature), the severity and frequency of air pollution episodes, and on anthropogenic emissions. For example, an increase of energy demand for space heating or cooling can lead to enhancement of the urban heat island effect, which may increase some secondary pollutants (i.e., ozone) and indirectly lead to increased natural sources of air pollutant emissions, such as decomposition of vegetation, soil erosion, and wildfires.[2-4]

Tropospheric ozone (O_3) is formed in the presence of bright sunshine and elevated temperatures by the reaction between VOC and nitrogen oxides (NO), both emitted from natural and anthropogenic sources. An association between tropospheric ozone concentrations and temperature has been demonstrated from measurements in outdoor smog chambers and from measurements in ambient air, even if it does not occur when the ratio of VOC to NO is low. Tropospheric ozone concentrations are increasing in most regions, and this trend is expected to continue over the next 50 years.

Pollen from birch trees that have been exposed to higher ozone levels induce larger wheal and flare responses in skin-prick tests compared to lower ozone-exposed pollen, suggesting that ozone increases allergenicity of pollen.[2-4] Changes in temperature and precipitation may also increase frequency and severity of forest fires, which can have significant public health consequences. Changes in wind patterns may increase episodes of long-distance anemophilous spread of pollutants and pollen grains, thereby making large-scale circulation patterns as important as regional exposures.[2-4]

Climate change appears to induce an increased concentration of all health-related air pollutants. Climate change influences not only the levels and the type of air pollution but also allergenic pollens. Global warming affects the onset, duration, and intensity of the pollen season as well as the allergenicity of the pollen. Studies on plant responses to elevated atmospheric levels of CO_2 indicate that plants exhibit enhanced photosynthesis and reproductive effects and produce more pollen. Moreover, the plants flower earlier in urban areas than in corresponding rural areas, with earlier pollination of about 2–4 days. Over the last few decades, many studies have shown changes in production, dispersion, and allergen content of pollen and spores, and the nature of the changes may vary in different regions and between species. Current knowledge on the worldwide effects of climate change on respiratory allergic diseases is provided by several studies on the relationship between asthma and environmental factors, such as meteorological variables, airborne allergens, and air pollution. Published data suggest an increasing effect of aeroallergens on allergic patients, leading to a greater likelihood for development of an allergic respiratory disorder in sensitized patients and aggravation of symptoms in patients already diagnosed with these conditions.[2–10]

15.4.1 THUNDERSTORM ASTHMA AND REDUCTION OF THE RISK OF ASTHMA CRISES

According to current climate change scenarios, there will be an increase in intensity and frequency of heavy rainfall episodes, including thunderstorms explained by the fact that warmer air carries more moisture, leading to heavier rainfalls. Thunderstorm asthma is a term used to describe an observed increase in acute bronchospasm cases following the occurrence of thunderstorms in the local vicinity.[52,53] Associations between thunderstorms and asthma morbidity have been identified in multiple locations around the world, predominantly in Europe and in Australia, during the pollen season, and it is now recognized that thunderstorms are a risk factor for asthma attacks in patients suffering from pollen allergy (Table 15.1 and 15.2).[52,53]

Thunderstorms can concentrate pollen grains at ground level, which may release allergenic particles of respirable size into the atmosphere after they rupture by osmotic shock. Therefore, during the first 20–30 minutes of a thunderstorm, patients suffering from pollen allergy may inhale a high concentration of the allergenic material that is dispersed into the atmosphere.[54–63] On 21st November 2016, there was a very unusual weather occurrence with wind and torrential rain combined with a high pollen count, sending high quantity of pollen allergens across the city in Melbourne, Australia. Hospitals were swamped with emergency patients affected by a thunderstorm-related severe asthma attacks (more than 8,500 patients in Emergency Departments and 8 died).[63]

15.5 MEASURES TO IMPROVE OUTDOOR AIR QUALITY

A significant amount of research still needs to be conducted to better understand the health impact of air pollution. Future investigations should use a multidisciplinary

Table 15.1 Thunderstorm-associated asthma outbreaks worldwide[57–63]

Year/Country/Observations

- 1983 U.K.: 26 sudden cases of asthma attacks in relation to thunderstorms
- 1992 Australia: Late-spring thunderstorms in Melbourne were observed to trigger epidemics of asthma attacks (5 to 10-fold rise).
- 1997 U.K.: Asthma or other airways disease hospital visits were noted to increase; 640 cases visited the ED during a 30-hour period in June 1994, nearly 10 times the expected number.
- 1992–2000 Canada: 18,970 hospital ED asthma visits among children 2–15 years of age were noted. Summer thunderstorm activity was associated with an OR of 1.35 (95% CI 1.02–1.77) relative to summer periods with no thunderstorm activity.
- 1993–2004 U.S.: 215,832 asthma ED visits were observed, of which 24,350 of these visits occurred on days following thunderstorms. A significant association was found between daily counts of asthma ED visits and thunderstorm occurrence. Asthma visits were 3% higher on days following thunderstorms.
- 2000 Australia: Asthma visits during thunderstorms increased. History of hay fever and allergy to ryegrass were strong predictors for asthma exacerbation during thunderstorms in the spring.
- 2001 Australia: The incidence of excess hospital attendances for asthma during late spring and summer was strongly linked to the occurrence of thunderstorm outflow.
- 2002 U.K.: A case–control study of 26 patients presenting to Cambridge University Hospital with asthma after a thunderstorm found that *Alternaria alternata* sensitivity was a compelling predictor of this asthma epidemic in patients with seasonal asthma; grass pollen allergy was also found to be an important factor in thunderstorm-related asthma.
- 2004 Italy: Six cases of thunderstorm-related asthma because of pollen (Paretaria) were reported.
- 2010 Italy: Twenty cases of thunderstorm-related asthma because of pollen (olive tree) were reported.
- 2010 Australia: Epidemics of thunderstorm asthma that occurred in Melbourne during the spring found that the spring season in conjunction with heavy winter rainfall in and around Melbourne predicted a severe pollen season and raised the risk of allergic rhinitis and asthma in pollen-sensitive individuals.
- 2016 Australia: More than 8,500 people were affected by severe asthma attacks and nine died.

Table 15.2 Characteristics of thunderstorm-associated asthma epidemics

1. The occurrence of epidemics is closely linked to thunderstorms.
2. The thunderstorm-related epidemics are limited to late spring and summer, when there are high levels of airborne pollen grains.
3. There is a close temporal association between the arrival of a thunderstorm, a major rise in the concentration of pollen grains, and the onset of epidemics.
4. Patients with pollen allergy, who stay indoors with the windows closed during a thunderstorm, are not affected.
5. There are no high levels of gaseous and particulate components of air pollution.
6. There is a major risk for patients who are not under adequate asthma treatment.
7. Patients with allergic rhinitis and without previous asthma can experience severe bronchoconstriction.

approach incorporating biologic, genetic, epidemiologic, and clinical methods. However, public health approaches to decrease the general public's exposure to air pollution should take into consideration the following goals:

- Reduce the use of fossil fuels and control vehicle emissions
- Reduce private traffic in towns and improve public transportation, which also favors pedestrian traffic
- Plant nonallergenic trees in cities[4]

As for the last point, it is important to consider that unfortunately each year, hectares of forests are destroyed by large fires, frequently due to criminal intent. Moreover, although there is no general agreement, increasing the antioxidant defenses of the human airways by eating antioxidant foods should be encouraged. Governments and international organizations such as WHO and European Union are facing a growing problem related to the respiratory effects induced by gaseous and particulate pollutants arising from motor vehicle emissions. The last release of the Intergovernmental Panel on Climate Change (IPCC) stated that climate change is very likely due to human activity. This statement is supported by an impressive amount of data published in the last several years, which have had an impact on policymakers who are now advocating implementation of preventive measures (such as the Kyoto Protocol) and alternative energy sources. The desired positive effects of these measures will hopefully be observable in the next decade, but, in the short term, global temperature will continue to increase despite these aggressive air-quality improvement measures.

The detrimental effects of ambient air pollution can be reduced by decreasing the time spent on outdoor activities, and the level of activity when the air quality index (AQI) is higher than a specified level. The AQI is a number used by government agencies to communicate to the public the current degree of air pollution or how polluted it is forecasted to become. It is calculated from four major air pollutants: ground level O_3, particle pollution, CO, and SO_2.

The AQI tells people how clean or unhealthy the air is and what associated health effects might be a concern. The AQI can be found on government websites; in the local media, such as newspapers and television; and through mobile phones applications. When the AQI reaches a certain high level, people should reduce the time outdoors and avoid exercising in polluted air. AQI values can vary from one season to another and in different places even in the same city, and at different times of day. In urban areas, CO may be high in the central area during rush hours because of large numbers of vehicles and usually poor airflow. O_3 level is often higher in warmer months and peaks in the afternoon to early evening. Particle pollution is often elevated near busy roadways, especially during morning or evening rush hours.

Subjects with chronic respiratory disease, such as COPD and asthma, should adapt their daily activity according to the local AQI report.[64]

Wearing personal protective equipment (N95 mask or equivalent) might be useful for avoiding detrimental effect of ambient air pollutants. Masks have been proven useful in reducing respiratory virus transmission during a pandemic. Using a nose mask during haze environment can help people to prevent adverse effects from vehicular pollution.[64]

Masks can be divided into at least two categories. One type works by mechanical filtration that reduces the PM and the other by absorbing gaseous chemicals through the activated carbon inside. Surgical facemasks and plain facemasks are designed for preventing and avoiding the spread of spillage droplets, and filtering out large particulate materials usually hundreds of micrometers in size. But they are not of any use in preventing inhalation of fine articles like $PM_{2.5}$. N95 and R95 facemasks are efficient filter masks that can absorb as high as 95% of airborne particles in the inhaled air.[64] The later type is more efficient and is recommended as an efficient protective measure in minimizing exposure to gas emissions. But the disadvantage of these kinds of masks are obvious: they are not comfortable due to their high-respiratory resistance and cannot be worn for a long time. The efficiency of air filtration and chemical absorption will be lowered when used for a certain time, and frequent replacement would result in a high financial burden. To date, there is no recommended guidance for masks in preventing the effects of air pollution.

15.5.1 THE FARM ENVIRONMENT IS ABLE TO REDUCE THE RISK OF ASTHMA

The relationship between exposure to a farming environment and the reduced risk of asthma has been investigated in several studies, however there is still much to understand. Exposure to a farming environment seems to protect individuals from respiratory allergy. The timing and duration of exposure seem to play critical roles. The largest reduction in risk of developing respiratory allergies is seen among those who are exposed prenatally and continuously thereafter. Von Mutius et al. carried out a study analyzing the impact of different environmental and social conditions on the development of allergies in two genetically homogeneous populations. The prevalence of asthma and allergic disorders was assessed in reunified Germany (in the former East Germany and in the former West Germany). The results showed that hay fever, skin-test reactivity to common aeroallergens, and asthma were considerably more prevalent in western Germany, where air quality was lower due to traffic-related air pollutants and NO_2 exposure as compared to eastern Germany.[65]

The Amish and Hutterites are U.S. agricultural populations whose lifestyles are remarkably similar in many respects but whose farming practices, in particular, are distinct; the former follow traditional farming practices whereas the latter use industrialized farming practices. The populations also show striking disparities in the prevalence of asthma, and little is known about the immune responses underlying these disparities. Stein et al.[66] studied environmental exposures, genetic ancestry, and immune profiles among 60 Amish and Hutterite children, measuring levels of allergens and endotoxins, and assessing the microbiome composition of indoor dust samples. Despite the similar genetic ancestries and lifestyles of Amish and Hutterite children, the prevalence of asthma and allergic sensitization was four and six times as low in the Amish, whereas median endotoxin levels in Amish house dust was 6.8 times as high. Profound differences in the proportions, phenotypes, and functions of innate immune cells were also found between the two groups of children. In a mouse model of experimental allergic asthma, the intranasal instillation of dust extracts from Amish but not Hutterite homes significantly inhibited airway hyperreactivity and eosinophilia. The results of the study by Stein et al. in humans and mice indicate that the Amish environment induces protection against asthma by engaging and shaping the innate immune response.[66]

15.6 MEASURES TO IMPROVE INDOOR AIR QUALITY

Air filtration is frequently recommended as a component of environmental control measures for patients with allergic respiratory disease. The association between preventive asthma care and comprehensive environmental control practices was examined in a review of 3,727 adults with asthma using data from the Four-State National Asthma Survey.[67] Comprehensive management was defined as the implementation of combinations of at least five of eight measures. Air filtration was found to be the fourth (27.4 %) most commonly implemented strategy, preceded only by no smoking (80%), no pets (53.9 %), and washing sheets in hot water (43.2 %), and followed by pillow covers (23.7 %), mattress covers (23.4 %), no carpets (14.5 %), and use of a dehumidifier (13.8 %).

Residential air filtration can be provided by whole house filtration (WHF) via the home's heating, ventilation, or air conditioning system (HVAC); by portable room air cleaners

(PRACs); or a combination of the two. Use of high-efficiency particulate air (HEPA) filters reduce airborne allergens in the indoor environment and may provide clinical benefits for patients with respiratory allergies.[68] The role of air filtration in disease prevention has been studied for a long time but it continues to be debated. Several investigations have demonstrated that indoor air cleaning devices can reduce concentrations of asthma triggers in indoor air. Recently, Brown et al. evaluated the performance of different grades of filters in a modeling, identifying filters to be effective at reducing airborne asthma triggers by at least 50%. Several studies examined the efficacy of air filtration in reducing airborne pet allergen levels and improving asthma in sensitized patients.[67–70] Overall, these studies have found that this approach only modestly reduces airborne allergen levels and is not effective to improve symptoms of asthma.

Of course, it is important to abolish indoor smoking to reduce the risk for asthma worsening/exacerbations in asthmatic subjects.

CONCLUSIONS AND KEY POINTS

A body of evidence suggests that major changes induced by human activity to our planet are occurring and involve air quality and global warming.

In this chapter we have tried to focus on the following points based on scientific evidence:

- Currently, it is primarily the pollution generated by vehicles that degrades the quality of air in the cities of industrialized countries, whereas industrial pollution still constitutes the largest source of air pollution in countries undergoing progressive industrialization.
- Climate change affects the social and environmental determinants of health—clean air, safe drinking water, sufficient food, and secure shelter. The direct health costs estimated by the WHO will be between $2 and $4 billion per year by the year 2030.
- Exposure to air pollution has been linked to many signs of allergic respiratory diseases, including asthma and COPD exacerbations, increased bronchial hyperresponsiveness, increased medication use, visits to EDs, and hospital admissions.
- Asthma and COPD are heterogeneous diseases that are strongly influenced by environmental factors. Many of these factors are influenced by meteorological events and climate change that vary in type and intensity across the world.
- Respiratory and primary health professionals are key to ensuring that awareness of the importance of clean air is raised, that patients are getting the right advice with regards to both short- and long-term exposure.
- Air pollution is associated with mortality and morbidity from respiratory and cardiovascular disease.
- PM and O_3 are aggravating factors of asthma and increase the effects of airborne allergens through various mechanisms.

- Living near heavy traffic roads is associated with impaired respiratory health and lung development.
- Subjects living in urban areas tend to be more affected by plant-derived respiratory disorders than those living in rural areas.
- Global warming effects the onset, duration, and intensity of pollen season (longer and more intense).
- Subjects affected by pollen allergy should be alerted to the danger of being outdoors during a thunderstorm during the pollen season.

Since strategies to reduce climate change and air pollution are political in nature, citizens and health professionals must voice their strong support for clean policies on both the national and international level.[71]

REFERENCES

1. D'Amato G, Corrado A, Cecchi L et al. A relapse of near-fatal thunderstorm-asthma in pregnancy. *Eur Ann Allergy Clin Immunol.* May 2013;45(3):116–117.
2. IPCC AR4 WG1. *Climate change 2007: The physical science basis. Contribution of Working Group I to the Fourth Assessment Report of the Intergovernmental Panel on Climate Change.* S Solomon, D Qin, M Manning et al., eds. Cambridge University Press; 2007.
3. Intergovernmental Panel on Climate Change. 2014 IPCC fifth assessment report: Climate change. Available at http://ar5-syr.ipcc.ch/. Accessed February 1, 2016.
4. D'Amato G, Holgate ST, Pawankar R et al. Meteorological conditions, climate change, new emerging factors, and asthma and related allergic disorders. A statement of the world allergy organization. *World Allergy Organ J.* 2015;8:25.
5. Crowley RA. Climate change and health: A position paper of the American college of physicians. *Ann Intern Med.* 2016;164:608–610.
6. Ayres JG, Forberg B, Annesi-Maesano I et al. Climate change and respiratory disease. European respiratory society position statement on behalf of the environment & human health committee. *Eur Respir J.* 2009;34:295–302.
7. D'Amato G, Vitale C, De Martino A et al. Effects on asthma and respiratory allergy of climate change and air pollution. *Multidiscip Respir Med.* 2015;10:39.
8. D'Amato G and Cecchi L. Effects of climate change on environmental factors in respiratory allergic diseases. *Clin Exp Allergy.* 2008;38:1264–1274.
9. Zhang Y, Bielory L, Mi Z et al. Allergenic pollen season variations in the past two decades under changing climate in the United States. *Glob Chang Biol.* 2015;21:1581–1589.
10. To T, Zhu J, Larsen K et al. Progression from asthma to chronic obstructive pulmonary disease. Is air pollution a risk factor? Canadian Respiratory Research Network. *Am J Respir Crit Care Med.* August 15, 2016;194(4):429–438.
11. GINA Report. 2017. Global Strategy for asthma management and prevention. GINA Committee Report. Available at www.ginasthma.org.
12. Masoli, M, Fabian, D, Holt, S et al. The global burden of asthma: Executive summary of the GINA dissemination committee report. *Allergy.* 2004;59:469–478.
13. National Heart, Lung, and Blood Institute. Morbidity and mortality: 2004 chartbook on cardiovascular, lung, and blood diseases. Washington, DC: US Department of Health and Human Services; 2004.
14. European Respiratory Society. European lung white book. *Huddersfield European Respiratory Society Journals Ltd 2003.*
15. Van derAkker-van Marie ME, Brull J, and Detmar SB. Evaluationof cost of disease: Assessing the burden to society of asthma in children in the European Union. *Allergy.* 2005;60:140–149.
16. GOLD 2017. Global strategy for the diagnosis, management and prevention of COPD. Available at www.GOLDCOPD.org.
17. Powell P, Brunekreef B, and Grigg J. How do you explain the risk of air pollution to your patients? *Breathe* 2016;1:201–203.
18. D'Amato G. Outdoor air pollution, climate and allergic respiratory diseases: Evidence of a link. *Clin Exp Allergy.* 2002;32:1391–1393.
19. Biagioni BJ, Tam S, Chen YR et al. Effect of controlled human exposure to diesel exhaust and allergen on airway surfactant protein D, myeloperoxidase, and club (Clara) cell secretory protein 16. *Clin Exp Allergy.* 2016;doi:10.1111/cea.12732.
20. Bra back L and Forsberg B. Does traffic exhaust contribute to the development of asthma and allergic sensitization in children: Findings from recent cohort studies. *Environ Health.* 2009;8:17.
21. Carlsten C, Blomberg A, Pui M et al. Diesel exhaust augments allergen induced lower airway inflammation in allergic individuals: A controlled human exposure study. *Thorax.* 2016;71:35–44.
22. Jung DY, Leem JH, Kim HC et al. Effect of traffic-related air pollution on allergic disease: Results of the children's health and environmental research. *Allergy Asthma Immunol Res.* 2015;7:359–366.
23. Chung HY, Hsieh CJ, Tseng CC et al. Association between the first occurrence of allergic rhinitis in preschool children and air pollution in Taiwan. *Int J Environ Res Public Health.* 2016;13:268.
24. Gauderman WJ, Avol E, Lurmann F et al. Childhood asthma and exposure to traffic and nitrogen dioxide. *Epidemiology.* 2005;16:737–743.
25. D'Amato G and Holgate ST. The impact of air pollution on Respiratory Health. *Eur Res Mono.* 2002;21.
26. Bernstein JA, Alexis N, Barnes C et al. Health effects of air pollution. *J Allergy Clin Immunol.* 2004;114:1116–1123.

27. McConnell R, Berhane K, Gilliland F et al. Asthma in exercising children exposed to ozone: A cohort study. *Lancet.* 2002;359:386–391.

28. McDonnell WF, Abbey DE, Nishino N et al. Longterm ambient ozone concentration and the incidence of asthma in nonsmoking adults: The AHSMOG study. *Environ Res.* 1999;80:110–121.

29. Beck I, Jochner S, Gilles S et al. High environmental ozone levels lead to enhanced allergenicity of birch pollen. *PLOS ONE.* 2013;8:e80147.

30. Peden DB, The epidemiology and genetics of asthma risk associated with air pollution. *J Allergy Clin Immunol.* February 2005;115(2):213–219; quiz 220.

31. Malig BJ, Pearson DL, Chang YB et al. A time-stratified case-crossover study of ambient ozone exposure and emergency department visits for specific respiratory diagnoses in California (2005–2008). *Environ Health Perspect.* 2016;124:745–753.

32. Sacks JD, Stanek LW, Luben TJ et al. Particulate matter-induced health effects: Who is susceptible? *Environ Health Perspect.* 2011;119:446–454.

33. Ristovski ZD, Miljevic B, Surawski NC et al. Respiratory health effects of diesel particulate matter. *Respirology.* 2012;17:201–212.

34. Oftedal B, Brunekreef B, Nystad W et al. Residential outdoor air pollution and allergen sensitization in schoolchildren in Oslo, Norway. *Clin Exp Allergy.* 2007;37:1632–1640.

35. Riedl M and Diaz Sanchez D. Biology of diesel exhaust effects on respiratory function. *J Allergy Clin Immunol.* 2005;115:221–228.

36. Laumbach RJ and Kipen HM. Respiratory health effects of air pollution: Update on biomass smoke and traffic pollution. *J Allergy Clin Immunol.* 2012;129:3–11.

37. Sunesson A, Vaes W, Nilsson C et al. Identification of volatile metabolites from five fungal species cultivated on two media. *Appl Environ Microbiol.* August 1995;61(8):2911–2918.

38. Schleibinger H, Laussmann D, Bornehag CG et al. Microbial volatile organic compounds in the air of moldy and mold-free indoor environments. *Indoor Air.* April 2008;18(2):113–124.

39. Korpi A, Järnberg J, and Pasanen AL. Microbial volatile organic compounds. *Crit Rev Toxicol.* 2009;39(2):139–193.

40. Matsui EC, Environmental control for asthma: Recent evidence. *Curr Opin Allergy Clin Immunol.* August 2013;13(4):417–425.

41. Nurmatov U, van Schayck CP, Hurwitz B et al. House dust mite avoidance measures for perennial allergic rhinitis: An updated cochrane systematic review. *Allergy.* February 2012;67(2):158–165.

42. Portnoy J, Kennedy K, Sublett J et al. Environmental assessment and exposure control: A practice parameter--furry animals. *Ann Allergy Asthma Immunol.* April 2012;108(4):223.e1–e15. doi: 10.1016/j.

anai.2012.02.015. No abstract available. Erratum in: Ann Allergy Asthma Immunol. September 2012;109(3):229.

43. D'Amato G, Vitale C, Lanza M et al. Near fatal asthma: Treatment and prevention. *Eur Ann Allergy Clin Immunol.* 2016;48:116–122.

44. Zureik M, Neukirch C, Leynaert B et al. Sensitisation to airborne moulds and severity of asthma: Cross sectional study from European community respiratory health survey. *BMJ.* 2002;325:1–7.

45. Denning D.W, O'Driscoll B.R, Hogaboam C.M. et al. The link between fungi and severe asthma: A summary of the evidence. *Eur Respir J.* 2006;27:615–626.

46. O'Hollaren MT, Yunginger JW, Offord KP et al. Exposure to an aeroallergen as a possible precipitating factor in respiratory arrest in young patients with asthma. *N Engl J Med.* February 7, 1991;324(6):359–363.

47. Black PN, Udy AA, Brodie SM. Sensitivity to fungal allergens is a risk factor for life-threatening asthma. *Allergy.* May 2000;55(5):501–504.

48. Targonski PV, Persky VW, and Ramekrishnan V. Effect of environmental molds on risk of death from asthma during the pollen season. *J Allergy Clin Immunol.* 1995;95:955–961.

49. Bobbitt RC Jr1, Crandall MS, Venkataraman A et al. Characterization of a population presenting with suspected mold-related health effects. *Ann Allergy Asthma Immunol.* January 2005;94(1):39–44.

50. Bernstein JA, Levin L, Crandall MS et al. A pilot study to investigate the effects of combined dehumidification and HEPA filtration on dew point and airborne mold spore counts in day care centers. *Indoor Air.* December 2005;15(6):402–407.

51. Barnes CS, Horner WE, Kennedy K et al. Environmental allergens workgroup.home assessment and remediation. *J Allergy Clin Immunol Pract.* May–June 2016;4(3):423–431.e15.

52. D'Amato G, Vitale C, D'Amato M et al. Thunderstorm-related asthma: What happens and why. *Clin Exp Allergy.* 2016;46:390–396.

53. D'Amato G, Cecchi L, and Annesi-Maesano I. A transdisciplinary overview of case reports of thunderstorm-related asthma outbreaks and relapse. *Eur Respir Rev.* June 1 2012;21(124):82–87.

54. Taylor PE, Hagan R, Valenta R et al. Release of allergens in respirable aerosols: A link between grass pollen and asthma. *J Allergy Clin Immunol.* 2002;109:51–56.

55. D'Amato G, Vitale C, Lanza M et al. Climate change, air pollution, and allergic respiratory diseases: An update. *Curr Opin Allergy Clin Immunol.* October 2016;16(5):434–440.

56. D'Amato G, Liccardi G, and Frenguelli G. Thunderstorm-asthma and pollen allergy. *Allergy.* 2007; 62: 11–16. doi:10.1111/j.1398-9995.2006.01271.x.

57. Venables KM, Allitt U, Collier CG et al. Thunderstorm-related asthma – epidemic 24/25 June 1994. *Clin Exp Allergy*. 1997;27:725–36.

58. Packe GE, Ayres JG. Asthma outbreak during a thunderstorm. *Lancet*. 1985;2:199–204.

59. Bellomo R, Gigliotti P, Treloar A et al. Two consecutive thunderstorm associated epidemic of asthma in Melbourne. *Med J Aust*. 1992;156:834–837.

60. Girgis ST, Marks GB, Downs SH et al. Thunderstorm-associated asthma in an inland town in south-eastern Australia who is at risk? *Eur Respir J*. 2000;16:3–8.

61. Villeneuve PJ, Leech J, and Bourque D. Frequency of emergency room visits for childhood asthma in Ottawa, Canada: The role of weather. *Int J Biometeorol*. 2005;50:48–56.

62. Grundstein A, Sarnat SE, Klein M et al. Thunderstorm associated asthma in Atlanta, Georgia. *Thorax*. 2008;63:659–660.

63. D'Amato G, Annesi-Maesano I, Molino A, VitaleC et al. *Thunderstorm related asthma attacks*, JACI in press.

64. Xu-Qin Jiang, Xiao-Dong Mei, Air pollution and chronic airway diseases: What should people know and do? *J Thorac Dis*. January 2016;8(1):E31–E40.

65. von Mutius E, Martinez FD, Fritzsch C et al. Thiemann HH.Prevalence of asthma and atopy in two areas of West and East Germany. *Am J Respir Crit Care Med*. February 1994;149(21):358–364.

66. Stein MM, Hrusch CL, Gozdz J et al. Innate Immunity and Asthma Risk in Amish and Hutterite Farm Children. *N Engl J Med*. 2016;375(5):411–421.

67. Roy A and Wisnivesky JP. Comprehensive use of environmental control practices among adults with asthma. *Allergy Asthma Proc*. 2010;31:72–77.

68. Sublett JL, Seltzer J, Burkhead R et al. American academy of allergy, asthma & immunology indoor allergen committee. Air filters and air cleaners: Rostrum by the American academy of allergy, asthma & immunology indoor allergen committee. *J Allergy Clin Immunol*. 2010;125:32–38.

69. Du L, Batterman S, Parker E, Godwin C et al. Particle concentrations and effectiveness of free-standing air filters in bedrooms of children with asthma in Detroit, Michigan. *Build Environ*. 2011;46:2303–2313.

70. Lanphear BP, Hornung RW, Khoury J et al. Effects of HEPA air cleaners on unscheduled asthma visits and asthma symptoms for children exposed to secondhand tobacco smoke. *Pediatrics*. 2011;127:93–101.

71. Bergoglio JM. *Encyclical letter 'Laudato si' of the Holy Father Francis on Care for Our Common Home*. Vatican Press; 2015.

Medications for asthma, COPD, and asthma-COPD overlap

ROBERT LEDFORD, MAX FELDMAN, AND THOMAS CASALE

16.1 INTRODUCTION

The number of people affected by obstructive lung diseases worldwide represents a significant global health problem. The appropriate management of these patients is essential to reducing symptom burden and, as a corollary, maintaining and, when possible, improving, lung function. However, the treatments available for obstructive lung disease management are numerous and cover the spectrum from highly familiar inhalants to newer biologic agents. Further complicating the matter, the two primary obstructive lung diseases—asthma and chronic obstructive lung disease (COPD)—are not treated identically. There are important differences in the recommended therapeutic algorithms for these diseases. Patients affected by asthma and COPD present with similar complaints related to lung function deterioration and airflow obstruction. Many of the therapies available have been approved and utilized for both conditions. However, the approach is fundamentally not the same for several critical reasons. Physicians treating patients with asthma and COPD must be capable of differentiating diseases with similar presentations and determining the most appropriate approach to pharmacologic therapy. The simultaneous difficulty and significance of this differentiation should not be understated. Using tables, summaries of best practices, and clinical vignettes, we will highlight the key differentiating points between the management of asthma and COPD, as well as discuss the overlap syndrome between the two that is increasingly being recognized as a related but distinct clinical entity. The goal of this chapter is to provide physicians with a useful tool to help them deliver high-quality care that is tailored to the correct patient population of those burdened by obstructive lung disease.

16.1.1 CLINICAL VIGNETTES

CLINICAL VIGNETTE 16.1

A 35-year-old woman with no known past medical history comes to her primary care physician to discuss her shortness of breath. She noticed increasing dyspnea with exertion over the last several weeks of insidious onset. She typically takes a brisk walk in the morning for several miles without any shortness of breath. However, over the last several weeks, she has been progressively limited in the duration and pace of her exercise. She notes that this is accompanied by cough on most mornings as well. She denies any fever, chills, nasal congestion, rhinorrhea, chest pain, or leg swelling. When questioned further, she notes that the cough is present at other times of the day as well. She coughs when she laughs, intermittently when talking on the phone, and at nighttime when she lays down to sleep. She denies

any reflux, difficulty swallowing, dyspepsia, or other nocturnal symptoms. She works as an accountant, does not smoke, and denies sensitivity to any airborne particles. Her family history is as follows: father died at age 65 from myocardial infarction, mother is still alive at age 65 and has type 2 diabetes and hypertension, and her son at age 7 has eczema. On exam, the patient has a clear oropharynx, nasal mucosa is normal, there is no cervical lymphadenopathy or jugular venous distention, cardiac exam is normal and without S3, lungs are clear but there is a prolonged expiratory phase as well as wheeze on forced exhalation, the abdominal exam is normal, and there is no pedal edema.

What would be the next best test to determine the cause of the woman's symptoms?

Spirometry is performed and demonstrates a FEV_1/FVC ratio that is 0.65 and FEV_1 that is 70% of predicted and reversible by 330 mL to 90% of predicted with inhalation of bronchodilator.

What diagnosis is suggested?

The patient likely has asthma. She has an obstructive lung disease with reversibility, a family history of atopy, and symptoms commensurate with asthma. The robustness of reversibility argues against COPD as do her lack of exposure to a triggering etiologic agent for COPD and the episodic nature of her symptoms. Other causes, such as upper airway cough syndrome, are not as likely without associated symptoms.

What is the suggested first line of therapy for this patient?

This patient's clinical scenario suggests newly diagnosed asthma with currently poorly controlled symptoms. She should be started on inhaled corticosteroid (ICS) therapy at a medium dose concentration or low-dose concentration/long-acting β_2-agonists (LABA) combination. She should also be given a rescue/reliever inhaler in the form of short-acting β_2-agonist (SABA).

What is a key step to help increase likelihood of success for the regimen above?

It is critical that clinicians demonstrate correct inhaler techniques and then ensure patient understanding by demonstration. Patient should also be provided with an asthma action plan to understand what to do if she is not improving and a follow-up appointment be scheduled to reassess her condition in 4–6 weeks or sooner if she is not improving.

CLINICAL VIGNETTE 16.2

A 22-year-old man with a history of intermittent asthma presents to his primary care physician due to worsening breathing. He notes that he recently cleaned his garage and then began having increased wheezing and shortness of breath with activities. Additionally, he feels tightness in his chest when he leaves the house for work in the morning and notes that his eyes are itchy, and he has been sneezing more when outside. He feels that these symptoms are due to the pollen he has seen on his car. He recently moved to the area and denies known aeroallergen sensitivity but states there were no oak trees where he lived previously. His current medications include as-needed albuterol along with two puffs twice daily of 180 mcg/actuation inhaled budesonide (low dose). He has been using his albuterol multiple times every day. On exam, his ocular conjunctiva is injected with cobblestone appearance noted. There is boggy, pale nasal mucosa. There is no cervical lymphadenopathy. Lungs have wheeze bilaterally with diminished air movement. Cardiac exam is normal with mild tachycardia. Abdominal exam is normal. Spirometry revealed and FEV_1/FVC ratio of 0.65, and an FEV_1 of 75% of predicted.

What is the likely cause of the patient's worsening symptoms?

The tree pollen seems to have triggered allergic disease burden in this patient and subsequently worsened his asthma control.

What is the next best step in management of the patient?

Paramount, the patient requires improved asthma control. Control of allergic symptoms should also be undertaken, and this will likely improve his asthma over time as well; but priority should be made for decreased lower respiratory symptoms and improved lung function. There are options available to step-up therapy. Addition of LABA to his scheduled ICS is a very appropriate next step. The physician could also consider addition of LTRA to his current ICS dose, especially given his allergic symptom burden. Alternatively, the physician could increase the dose of the ICS.

What is an important next step after the medication change?

It is critical that a close follow-up appointment be made to reassess the patient's clinical symptoms and consider addition of further controllers as needed.

The patient returns in 2 weeks and is feeling much improved. He notes that as the pollen has diminished and he has been using his new ICS/LABA, he has required his rescue SABA only rarely.

Should the regimen be changed?

At this point, it would be prudent to maintain the patient on his current controller regimen. Reassess the patient again in another 3 months to determine if he remains well controlled. If so, the physician and patient could discuss step-down to ICS monotherapy (or lowering of dose based on previous option selected) and further management of allergic disease with allergy testing and consideration of referral to an asthma/allergy specialist.

CLINICAL VIGNETTE 16.3

A 44-year-old woman with a history of asthma returns to follow up with her primary care physician. She first noticed increased effort breathing and dyspnea on exertion 4 months ago, and was limiting her physical activities as a result. This shortness of breath was associated with frequent coughing. She was already using a combination fluticasone/salmeterol inhaler at low dose (45 mcg/actuation of fluticasone) with two puffs twice daily. At that time, her physician stepped up her controller regimen by increasing the ICS component of her combination inhaler to 115 mcg/actuation. The patient noticed improvement of her limitations and dyspnea with exertion gradually over the last 4 months and now feels back to her previous baseline. She has not been having cough either at night or during the day, she denies any awakening from sleep due to cough or shortness of breath, and has resumed her previous physical activities. She denies any thrush, hoarseness, dry mouth, or cough with use of her inhaler. She can't remember when the last time she needed her rescue inhaler. She is a nonsmoker. On exam, her lungs are clear with mildly prolonged expiratory phase on forced exhalation. The remainder of the physical exam is normal. Spirometry revealed an FEV_1/FVC ratio of 0.75, and FEV_1 of 95% of predicted.

What is the next best step in management?

This patient had an asthma exacerbation that was treated with step-up therapy to level 4. She now has improved symptoms, and her exam is at baseline. Given that she has been controlled for a reasonable length of time, it would be prudent to examine the possibility of step-down therapy. She does not have any modifiable risk factors. The next best step is to reduce the ICS component of her inhaler by approximately 50% or to the next available strength. Change of her controller inhaler to the low-dose ICS/LABA strength and carefully monitoring her for symptom change is recommended.

What is a key component of her new management plan?

The patient needs to understand her updated asthma action plan and have close follow up to ensure stability during de-escalation of therapy (see Chapter 21 on asthma exacerbation management). The physician should emphasize the importance of appropriate vaccinations (e.g., influenza, pertussis) to help minimize risk of further exacerbation.

CLINICAL VIGNETTE 16.4

A 66-year-old man with a 50 pack-year tobacco smoking history presents to his primary care physician. He has been dealing with chronic cough that is mildly productive over the last several months. He first believed that he had a "chest cold," but the failure of the cough to improve and chronic mucus production has caused him to seek his physician's guidance. Upon further questioning, he notes that he has been less capable of playing with his grandson in the yard over the last several weeks with insidious progression of this limitation. He denies any chest pain, palpitations, weight gain, orthopnea, fevers, chills, or recent travel or immobility. He takes a baby aspirin daily for heart protection but is otherwise on no medications. He quit smoking 7 years ago when his grandson was born. On exam, he has normal nasal and ocular mucosa, there is no cervical lymphadenopathy, there is no jugular venous distention, cardiac exam is regular and without displacement of point of maximal impulse or presence of S3 gallop, lungs have bronchial breath sounds in the periphery bilaterally with wheeze on forced exhalation but no dullness to percussion or egophony noted, the abdominal exam is normal, and there is no pedal edema. The primary care physician orders a complete blood count, a chest radiograph, and complete lung functions with DLCO. There is no leukocytosis and the differential on the white blood cell count is normal. The chest radiograph demonstrates hyperinflation but no bullous changes. Complete lung functions reveal a $FEV_1/FVC < 0.6$, FEV_1 predicted of 60%, FEV_1 reversibility of 10%, and a diminished diffusion capacity.

What is the likely diagnosis?

The patient is presenting with symptoms suggestive of chronic airflow limitation and cough that have been persistent over the last several months. He does not describe significant variability. He has endured significant exposure to tobacco smoke. Lung function testing demonstrates an obstructive lung disease with mild reversibility and impaired diffusion. In totality, the most likely diagnosis is COPD with chronic bronchitis phenotype.

What is the next best step in management?

The patient has significant symptoms and limitation of activities and thus controller therapy, and not simply rescue or symptomatic therapy, should be initiated. The recommended medication would be long-acting bronchodilator, either in the form of β_2-agonist or anticholinergic. If either does not control his symptoms, then a combination of a LABA/long-acting muscarinic antagonist (LAMA) can be considered.

CLINICAL VIGNETTE 16.5

A 51-year-old woman with a history of COPD presents to her primary care physician for routine follow up. She has been on controller therapy for several years

in the form of combination fluticasone/salmeterol at the 250/50 mcg dosing twice a day. Unfortunately, she still experiences a chronic productive cough, breathlessness with limited activities on most days, decreased ambulatory distances, and has been hospitalized twice in the last 12 months for COPD exacerbation. She continues to smoke cigarettes though she has been able to cut back to half a pack daily with the use of nicotine replacement. She is reticent to use any alternative smoking cessation pharmacotherapies and is not sure she can fully quit smoking. On exam, she has a normal oropharyngeal exam, cardiac exam is normal, lungs have poor air movement bilaterally with bronchial breath sounds and faint wheeze appreciated on force exhalation, abdominal exam is normal, and there is no pedal edema.

In addition to continuing efforts to help with smoking cessation, what would be the next best step in management?

Given that patient has significant symptom burden and associated exacerbation history, there are clear signs of poor control of her COPD. She is on medium-dose ICS/LABA combination at present. She would now be categorized level D in the GOLD guidelines. Step-up therapy is indicated. The best choice would be to add long-acting anticholinergic to her regimen. Alternatively, roflumilast addition could be considered, given the patient's chronic bronchitis phenotype. Theophylline would be another consideration.

What other measures would be important for her physician to consider?

Patients with this level of disease burden should be referred for pulmonary rehabilitation. Also, it is paramount that she receive a pneumococcal vaccine (unless she has received this already) and a yearly influenza vaccination.

CLINICAL VIGNETTE 16.6

A 61-year-old woman presents to her primary care physician to discuss her difficulty breathing. She has been having progressive difficulty with exercise tolerance for the last year but has been largely ignoring it. When she spent time with family members recently for a reunion, they commented on her exercise limitations which prompted this visit. She endorses chronic cough that is occasionally productive during that time period as well. Her symptoms of shortness of breath and cough are present daily though she notes that some days are better than others. She denies any weight gain, orthopnea, leg swelling, reflux, weight loss, fevers, or chills. She has a history of asthma diagnosed as an adolescent that during her lifetime would occasionally flare requiring use of her rescue inhaler. She still had an albuterol inhaler from a previous visit to a walk-in clinic and has been using this with some relief when her dyspneic symptoms are more prominent. She is a former smoker with a 20 pack-year history but quit when she was 40 years of age. On exam, there is a clear oropharynx, there is no jugular venous distention or cervical lymphadenopathy, the cardiac exam is normal and without S3 or displaced point of maximal impulse, the lungs have diminished breath sounds bilaterally with wheeze noted in the end of the expiratory phase, there is no clubbing, the abdominal exam is normal, and there is no pedal edema. A chest radiograph demonstrates hyperinflation of the lungs bilaterally with apical bullous changes but no lymphadenopathy or mass. A complete blood count is normal and without eosinophilia on the leukocyte differential. Lung functions are obtained and show $FEV_1/FVC < 0.6$, FEV_1 of 65% predicted, mildly diminished diffusion capacity, normal lung capacity, and a bronchodilator response with an increase of FEV_1 by 14% and 240 mL.

What diagnosis is suspected?

This patient has chronic symptoms of airflow limitation and cough that do not demonstrate significant variability. Chest radiograph demonstrates hyperinflation and bullous changes consistent with emphysema. However, there is marked reversibility of her lung obstruction that is uncharacteristic of COPD. Furthermore, she has a personal history of asthma earlier in life. The most likely diagnosis is asthma-COPD overlap syndrome (ACO).

What is the next best step in management?

Given the likelihood of ACO in this patient, the next step in management should be to start a combination ICS/LABA therapy. She should be carefully monitored for symptom improvement and therapy escalated as indicated based on her response. Additionally, this patient should be screened for alpha-1-antitrypsin deficiency given bullous changes on her chest radiograph.

16.2 MEDICATION CLASSES

16.2.1 SHORT-ACTING β₂-AGONISTS

16.2.1.1 Mechanism

SABAs bind to $β_2$ adrenergic receptors on bronchial smooth muscle and other cells, activating the adenylyl cyclase enzyme, which increases intracellular levels of cyclic AMP. This results in bronchial smooth-muscle relaxation, increased mucociliary clearance, and inhibition of mast cell mediator release.[1]

16.2.1.2 Medications

Albuterol is a 50:50 racemic mixture of the R-albuterol and S-albuterol isomers. R-albuterol is responsible for the majority of the bronchodilator effect, which led to the development of levalbuterol, a single enantiomer formulation of R-albuterol. Despite its theoretical superiority, there does not appear to be a clinical benefit over albuterol, although some patients report fewer adrenergic side effects with levalbuterol.[2] Onset of action of both medications is within minutes of administration and lasts for 4–6 hours. When proper technique is used, albuterol administered by metered-dose inhaler (MDI) provides the same amount of bronchodilation when compared to delivery of medication by nebulizer at comparable doses. However, a nebulizer or MDI with spacer may be preferred when factors such as age, poor coordination, or respiratory distress preclude proper MDI technique.

16.2.1.3 Side effects

An exaggerated physiologic tremor is commonly seen with SABA use that is temporary and self-limited. Sinus tachycardia and other more serious cardiac arrhythmias can be seen in susceptible patients by activation of $β_1$ receptors on cardiac tissue, however this is uncommon due to the selectivity of albuterol and levalbuterol for $β_2$ receptors. Hypokalemia can also occur especially with overuse of a SABA.[3]

16.2.1.4 Use in asthma

SABAs are among the most potent bronchodilators approved for use in asthma and are highly effective for the quick relief of asthma symptoms. Their use as monotherapy should be reserved for those with mild, intermittent asthma only, and clinicians should regularly inquire about the frequency of SABA use as a gauge for asthma control. Frequent use of SABA is a risk factor for asthma exacerbations and asthma related death, which is likely due to poor underlying control; however, the development of tolerance due to downregulation of beta receptors in bronchial tissue may be a contributing factor.[4] SABAs are the drug of choice for prophylaxis against exercise-induced bronchospasm.

16.2.1.5 Use in COPD

Similar to asthma, SABAs are used for the quick relief of symptoms and exacerbations in COPD. SABAs can be used alone or in combination with a short-acting muscarinic antagonist (SAMA). The combination of both SABA and SAMA provide more bronchodilation and, therefore, may be preferred in patients with stable COPD and daily symptoms.[5]

16.2.2 LONG-ACTING β₂-AGONISTS

16.2.2.1 Mechanism

Mechanisms for LABA is different than SABA as it stays anchored to the beta 2 receptor for 12 hours.

16.2.2.2 Medications

The two inhaled LABAs approved for use in asthma are salmeterol and formoterol. They both have an effect that lasts for 10–12 hours, however formoterol has a quicker onset of action within five minutes whereas salmeterol takes 20–30 minutes to take effect.[6] Formoterol is a full β₂-agonist and has higher intrinsic activity compared to salmeterol.[6]

A subclass called Ultra-LABAs has emerged, named for their long duration of action allowing for once-daily dosing. Medications in this class are currently only approved in the United States for the treatment of COPD and include indacaterol, olodaterol, and vilanterol.

16.2.2.3 Side effects

Recently, the FDA has removed the boxed warning for asthma related deaths pertaining to LABA when used with ICS based on post-marketing surveillance studies that does not show more serious asthma related side effects than using ICS's alone. There remains a boxed warning for increased asthma related deaths for LABAs when used without ICSs.

16.2.2.4 Use in asthma

LABAs are long-term controller medications used in moderate to severe persistent asthma when symptoms are not adequately controlled with ICS. In adults with uncontrolled asthma on low-dose ICS, the addition of a LABA as step-up therapy was shown to be more effective in achieving control than increasing the dose of ICS.[7] The rapid-acting formoterol can be effectively used as a reliever medication in addition to maintenance regular therapy (not PRN); however, it should not be used without the coadministration of ICS.

There is uncertainty surrounding the use of LABAs in asthma after this class was questioned to increase the frequency of severe exacerbations and asthma-related mortality. The Salmeterol Multicenter Asthma Research Trial (SMART) showed a small but statistically significant increase of respiratory-related and asthma-related deaths when salmeterol was added to usual asthma care.[8] This outcome was most common in African Americans and in those not concurrently using ICS. In response to this data, the FDA issued a black box warning on all LABAs cautioning about increased risk of asthma-related death and requested large prospective trials to be undertaken to assess LABA safety. Two of these trials were recently published that showed no increased risk of serious asthma-related

events in patients using ICS and LABA versus ICS monotherapy.[9,10] This data suggests that while one should avoid LABA monotherapy in asthma, LABAs when combined with ICS are probably safe.

16.2.2.5 Use in COPD

Bronchodilators are the cornerstone of maintenance therapy in COPD, and LABAs can be used as monotherapy or as an add on to LAMAs for maintenance therapy. LABAs have been shown to improve FEV₁, dyspnea, health-related quality of life, and exacerbation rate.[11] No maintenance medications have been shown to improve mortality or rate of decline of lung function in COPD.[11]

16.2.3 INHALED CORTICOSTEROIDS

16.2.3.1 Mechanism

ICSs exert their clinical effect on the airways by multiple different mechanisms. Glucocorticoids have a potent anti-inflammatory effect by increasing transcription of anti-inflammatory cytokines and NF-kB, and by decreasing transcription of inflammatory cytokines, chemokines, and adhesion molecules. At the cellular level this results in a decrease in the number of eosinophils, T-lymphocytes, mast cells, and dendritic cells in the airway. ICSs also increase the expression of beta receptors in the airway augmenting the effect of β₂-agonists and protecting against the downregulation of β receptors typically seen with chronic β₂-agonist use.[12]

16.2.3.2 Medications

The relative clinical comparability of the various ICS treatments for asthma are summarized in Table 16.1. Factors such as particle size/formulation, cost, and delivery method should be considered when selecting therapy.

16.2.3.3 Side effects

Dysphonia, cough, and oral thrush are local side effects of ICS and occur due to the direct deposition of the corticosteroid onto the surface of the mouth, oropharynx, and larynx. These side effects are dose dependent and common with close to 2/3 of patients reporting at least one.[13] Oral thrush is a direct effect of oropharyngeal exposure and can be minimized with improving good inhaler technique, using a spacer device and routine rinsing of the mouth after inhaler use. These measures however do not reduce dysphonia or cough as these are caused by corticosteroid deposition in the larynx.[13] Dysphonia due to vocal cord weakening is often more problematic in individuals who speak a lot for work or in general.

ICSs can enter the systemic circulation either by direct absorption from the lung or after they are deposited in the mouth, swallowed, and absorbed by the GI tract where they

Table 16.1 Low-, medium-, and high-dose inhaled corticosteroids for asthma in patient ≥ 12 years of age

Inhaled corticosteroid	Total daily dose (mcg)		
	Low	Medium	High
Beclometasone diproppionate (CFC)	200–500	> 500–1000	> 1000
Beclometasone diproppionate (HFA)	100–200	> 200–400	> 400
Budesonide (DPI)	200–400	> 400–800	> 800
Ciclesonide (HFA)	80–160	> 160–320	> 320
Flunisolide (CFC)	500–1000	> 1000–2000	> 2000
Flunisolide (HFA)	320	> 320–640	> 640
Fluticasone furoate (DPI)		100	200
Fluticasone propionate (DPI or HFA)	100–250	> 250–500	> 500
Mometasone furoate	110–220	> 220–440	> 440
Triamcinolone acetonide	400–1000	> 1000–2000	> 2000

Source: Adapted from Global Initiative for Asthma. Global Strategy for Asthma Management and Prevention, 2016. Available at www .ginasthma.org.

are subject to first-pass metabolism.[14] The amount of systemic absorption and risk of systemic side effects depends on the ICS, dose, particle size, and the delivery system used. In addition, the concomitant use of intranasal corticosteroids might add to this risk.

Adrenal Insufficiency: There is some degree of measurable suppression of the hypothalamic-pituitary-adrenal axis with medium-dose ICS, however clinically significant consequences are very uncommon, and if they do occur, are almost always observed in patients treated with high-dose ICS for long periods of time.[15]

Osteoporosis: There is a small but increased risk of osteoporosis in patient's taking high-dose ICS for long periods of time, and it would be reasonable to screen these patients periodically with a bone-density examination, especially for those at increased risk because of race, body habitus, and age.[15] Patient's taking low- or medium-dose ICS do not appear to be at elevated risk.

Reduced Growth Velocity in Children: Treatment of children with low- to medium-dose ICS appears to initially reduce growth velocity resulting in approximately 1 cm difference of height after one year. However, after the first year, growth velocity returns to baseline.[16] For those children who are on a normal growth curve and then begin to fall below this curve, closer monitoring is recommended and if persistent, then evaluation by an endocrinologist may be necessary.

Ophthalmologic: ICS use is a risk factor for the development of both cataracts and glaucoma.[17,18] The risk is highest in those using high-dose ICS for long periods of time and in those with a family history of glaucoma. It is important to determine whether the cataracts are posterior versus anterior as posterior cataracts are more typical of corticosteroid usage.

16.2.3.4 Use in asthma

ICSs are the preferred controller therapy for persistent asthma. They have been shown to reduce asthma symptoms, decrease the need for rescue inhaler use, decrease the frequency and severity of exacerbations, reduce hospitalizations, and reduce asthma-related mortality.[19] While regular use of ICS has been shown to increase FEV_1 and decrease asthma severity, these medications ultimately do not cure the disease.[20] Clinical response is dose dependent, however the majority of clinical benefit is achieved at low doses. It is always important to reassess asthma patients on ICS for control and to step down to a lower concentration if feasible.

16.2.3.5 Use in COPD

The role of ICS in stable COPD is controversial, and their benefit is likely limited to a select group of patients with more severe disease. Benefits including improvement in symptoms and decreased frequency of exacerbations have been observed primarily in patients with $FEV_1 < 60\%$ predicted.[12] However, ICS can be used as an adjunctive treatment when symptoms are poorly controlled on bronchodilators alone. No controller medications have been shown to reduce mortality from COPD or to modify the long-term decline in lung function. There is a small increased risk of pneumonia in patients with COPD treated with ICS, therefore the decision to use this class of agents in these patients should be individualized after a discussion of risks and benefits.[21]

16.2.4 LEUKOTRIENE RECEPTOR MODIFYING AGENTS

16.2.4.1 Mechanism

Leukotrienes are byproducts of the 5-lipoxygenase pathway in arachidonic acid metabolism. They have multiple effects that are important to the pathogenesis of asthma, including eosinophil and mast cell recruitment, stimulation of mucus secretion, increased contractility and proliferation of bronchial smooth-muscle cells, and increased vascular permeability of endothelial cells.[22] These mechanisms make leukotrienes an attractive target for the treatment of asthma.

16.2.4.2 Medications

Montelukast and zafirlukast block leukotriene receptors, while zileuton inhibits the formation of leukotrienes by inhibiting 5-lipoxygenase. While there have been no head-to-head trials comparing these agents, the favorable side-effect profile and once daily dosing of montelukast has made it the preferred treatment in this class.

16.2.4.3 Side effects

Post-marketing surveillance has raised concern for an increased risk of suicide in young adults using montelukast. However, subsequent trials have found no association. Cases of severe liver toxicity are associated with zileuton, and liver function should be monitored regularly in patients treated with this medication.

16.2.4.4 Use in asthma

Leukotriene modifying agents (LTMAs) are indicated for the treatment of persistent asthma. They have been shown to reduce asthma symptoms, reduce the frequency of asthma exacerbations, reduce required ICS doses, and provide a small bronchodilator effect.[1] However, these agents are generally less effective than ICS as monotherapy and less effective than LABAs as add-on therapy.[1,23] Adherence to once-daily montelukast is superior to that of ICS, which makes it a good option for patients with a history of inhaler noncompliance. Patients that are likely to have the most benefit from LTMA treatment are those who have concurrent allergic rhinitis or aspirin-sensitive asthma where the underlying mechanism is thought to be leukotriene overproduction. In addition, LTMAs can be used for prophylaxis in patients with exercise-induced bronchospasm (although less effective than SABA), and unlike SABAs, there is no development of tolerance with chronic use.

16.2.4.5 Use in COPD

Currently there is no established role for LTMAs in the treatment of COPD.

16.2.5 ANTI-IgE

16.2.5.1 Mechanism

IgE is a major mediator of immediate hypersensitivity reactions making it a key player in the pathogenesis of asthma and other atopic conditions. This has made IgE an attractive target for the treatment of asthma. Omalizumab is a humanized monoclonal IgG1 antibody that inhibits the binding of IgE to the IgE receptor on the surface of mast cells and basophils. Omalizumab also works by reducing FcεR1 expression on the mast cell, basophil cell, and the antigen presenting dendritic cell surface.

16.2.5.2 Medications

Omalizumab is the only anti-IgE therapy approved for the treatment of asthma. It is administered as a subcutaneous injection every 2–4 weeks. The starting dose and frequency are determined by patient weight and total IgE level.

16.2.5.3 Side effects

Anaphylactic reactions such as bronchospasm, hypotension, urticaria, and angioedema have been reported with use of omalizumab in approximately 0.2% of patients. This is most likely to happen during the first three doses; however, it has also been reported late in the treatment course. Most reactions occur within two hours of administration, therefore patients should be monitored for an appropriate period of time in a health-care setting prepared to handle anaphylaxis. The most commonly reported side effects are arthralgia, fatigue, and dizziness.

16.2.5.4 Use in asthma

Candidates for treatment with omalizumab are those with moderate to severe persistent asthma who are 12 years or older and not adequately controlled on ICS or ICS with LABA therapy. These patients must demonstrate positive reactivity to a perennial aeroallergen and have serum IgE levels between 30–700 IU/mL. The addition of omalizumab to this population reduces the frequency of asthma exacerbations, decreases rescue inhaler use, and improves asthma symptoms.[24] Patient response to omalizumab is variable, and peripheral eosinophil count > 300/mcL may be a predictor of favorable response.[25] Patients should be continued on omalizumab for at least 16 weeks before treatment is said to have failed. While the cost of omalizumab can be upward of $10,000 per year, it has been shown to be cost effective for patients with greater than 20 hospital days per year due to asthma if effective.[1]

16.2.5.5 Use in COPD

Currently there is no established role for omalizumab in the treatment of COPD.

16.2.6 ANTI-IL-5

16.2.6.1 Mechanism

Eosinophils play an important role in the pathogenesis of asthma. The recruitment, differentiation, and survival of eosinophils is promoted by IL-5.[26]

16.2.6.2 Medications

Mepolizumab (administered as a SQ injection every 4 weeks) and reslizumab (administered as an IV infusion every 4 weeks) are the two anti-IL-5 monoclonal antibodies currently approved by the FDA for the treatment of eosinophilic asthma. Pivotal studies of reslizumab required higher peripheral eosinophil counts than did mepolizumab to show consistent therapeutic effects.[27,28] Benralizumab is an anti-IL-5 receptor alpha antibody that not only blocks eosinophils promoted by IL-5, but also causes antibody-dependent cellular apoptosis of eosinophils and basophils. Clinical trials to date indicate that it too may be an effective option for the treatment of severe eosinophilic asthma.[29,30]

16.2.6.3 Side effects

Anaphylactic reactions have been reported in association with both medications. Anaphylaxis with reslizumab was observed within 20 minutes of administration, whereas mepolizumab has the potential to cause delayed anaphylaxis after a few days. Both medications should only be given in a health-care setting that is equipped to handle anaphylaxis. There is a possible increased incidence of herpes zoster with mepolizumab, and patients over the age of 50 should receive the Zostavax before starting therapy if there are no other contraindications. There is increased incidence of malignancies (diverse types) observed in patients treated with reslizumab compared to placebo.

16.2.6.4 Use in asthma

Mepolizumab is FDA approved for add-on maintenance treatment of severe asthma in patients 12 and older with an eosinophilic phenotype (this term is not formally defined, however a reasonable definition would be peripheral eosinophil count >150 cells/mcL based on trial inclusion criteria). In patients with severe eosinophilic asthma, the addition of mepolizumab resulted in decreased rate of exacerbations, decreased ED visits and hospital admissions for asthma, and reduced oral corticosteroid doses.[28,31] In patients with higher eosinophil levels (>500 cells/mcL), a significant increase in FEV_1 was observed.

Reslizumab is FDA approved for add-on maintenance treatment of patients with severe asthma aged 18 years and older with an eosinophilic phenotype. In patients with severe asthma and peripheral eosinophils > 400 cells/mcL, reslizumab was shown to decrease the frequency of exacerbations and improve FEV_1.[27]

16.2.6.5 Use in COPD

Currently there is no established role for these agents in the treatment of COPD.

16.2.7 ALLERGY IMMUNOTHERAPY

16.2.7.1 Mechanism

Subcutaneous immunotherapy (SCIT) involves the administration of increasingly larger doses of a clinically relevant allergen into the skin to induce tolerance; whereas sublingual immunotherapy (SLIT) involves oral administration and does not require dose escalation. Allergen immunotherapy alters the allergic immune response that causes symptoms through various mechanisms including upregulation of T-regulatory cells, reduction of allergen-specific IgE, and decrease in tissue infiltration by eosinophils and mast cells.[20]

16.2.7.2 Side effects

Subcutaneous immunotherapy has the potential to induce anaphylaxis and therefore must be administered in a health-care setting that is equipped to treat anaphylaxis. Patients must be monitored for anaphylaxis for at least 30 minutes following therapy. Risk of anaphylaxis is higher in patients with moderate to severe asthma, and in those with poorly controlled asthma. The risk is increased when FEV_1 is less than 70% of predicted.[18,20] The most common side effect is a local injection site reaction.

The most common side effects of SLIT are localized to the oropharynx, including pruritus and throat irritation; this uncommonly can progress to potentially life-threating laryngeal edema. These side effects tend to lessen in severity and frequency after one week of therapy. While SLIT has a much lower risk of anaphylaxis compared to SCIT, it is still recommended that patients be prescribed an epinephrine auto-injector and instructed on its use.

16.2.7.3 Use in asthma

Subcutaneous immunotherapy is approved for the treatment of asthma for which there is a clinically important allergic trigger. Patients should be considered for immunotherapy if they have symptoms refractory to environmental control and pharmacologic therapy, have adverse effects from pharmacologic therapy, or wish to avoid or decreased long-term pharmacotherapy. In patients with allergic asthma, SCIT has been shown to improve asthma symptoms, reduce SABA use, and decrease allergen-specific and nonspecific airway hyperresponsiveness.[18] Similar results have been demonstrated with SLIT[32]; however in the USA, SLIT is not approved for asthma. Patients should be aware that a typical course of allergen immunotherapy is 3–5 years and requires at least monthly visits for administration of SCIT. Potential side effects, cost, and required frequency of visits should all be discussed before therapy is initiated. Whereas SCIT can be administered for multiple sensitizing allergens, SLIT is only available for grass and ragweed in the United States. In general, SCIT has a more robust effect on inducing tolerance compared to SLIT.

16.2.7.4 Use in COPD

Currently there is no established role for SCIT or SLIT in the treatment of COPD.

16.2.8 LONG-ACTING MUSCARINIC ANTAGONIST

16.2.8.1 Mechanism

Muscarinic antagonists block the effect of acetylcholine on muscarinic receptors in the bronchial tree, attenuating parasympathetic input that causes bronchoconstriction and mucus secretion. Their mechanism of bronchodilation is unique to and synergistic with that of beta agonists. They also may have an anti-inflammatory effect by altering the attraction and survival of neutrophils and other inflammatory cells.[33] LAMAs have a longer residence time on M3 muscarinic receptors, which are primarily responsible for cholinergic-induced bronchoconstriction.

16.2.8.2 Medications

Tiotropium 1.25 ug per actuation is the only LAMA approved for asthma in the United States. Tioptropium, umcclidinium, and aclidiniumare LAMAs are approved for COPD in the United States. Once-daily glycopyrronium is also available in Europe. The bronchodilator effect of tiotropium and umeclidinium lasts more than 24 hours, allowing for the convenience of once-daily dosing.

16.2.8.3 Side effects

Systemic absorption of muscarinic antagonists from the lungs and GI tract are minimal, which make them very well tolerated. The most common reported side effect is dry mouth, a result of direct deposition of the medication on the oropharynx.[33] Uncommonly patients report a bitter or metallic taste. A recent meta-analysis raised concern about increased cardiovascular events in patients with COPD treated with inhaled anticholinergics; however, a subsequent randomized trial did not confirm this finding. In general, clinical experience and studies suggest these agents result in fewer cardiac side effects compared to LABA.[34–36]

16.2.8.4 Use in asthma

Tiotropium was recently approved by the FDA for add-on therapy in persistent asthma. Tiotropium has been shown to improve lung function in patients with poor control despite ICS and LABAs; however, there does not appear to be any significant effects on asthma symptoms.[37] Data comparing LABA versus LAMA as first line step-up therapy is limited, but comparable effects have been noted.[38] LABAs should remain the preferred step-up therapy given the abundance of data demonstrating their benefit, whereas LAMAs should be reserved for those with a contraindication to LABAs or

when LABAs are ineffective until asthma guidelines are updated.

16.2.8.5 Use in COPD

Bronchodilators are the cornerstone of maintenance therapy in COPD. In a head-to-head trial, maintenance therapy with tiotropium was found to be superior to salmeterol in preventing exacerbations in COPD patients.[39] Although tiotropium reduces exacerbations and improves symptoms in COPD patients, there are no controller medications that have been shown to reduce the rate of lung function decline or mortality.[12] LABA/LAMA and LABA/LAMA/ICS combinations are in development for obstructive airways diseases. Anoro is the first once-daily LAMA/LABA product to be cleared as a maintenance treatment for COPD in the United States, and is a combination of vilanterol with umeclidinium bromide.

16.2.9 SHORT-ACTING MUSCARINIC ANTAGONIST

16.2.9.1 Mechanism

SAMA are not muscarinic receptor specific and therefore bind to all 3 M receptors in the airways (See Section 16.2.8.1).

16.2.9.2 Medications

Ipratropium is the only SAMA currently available in the United States and can be administered by MDI or nebulizer. Its bronchodilator effects last for approximately eight hours.[12]

16.2.9.3 Side effects

The side-effect profile of SAMAs are similar to LAMAs discussed in an earlier section.

16.2.9.4 Use in asthma

Ipratropium is less effective as a reliever medication than albuterol. The combination of albuterol and ipratropium during an acute exacerbation produces a small improvement in lung function and decreases hospital admission rates compared to albuterol monotherapy.[1] The role of ipratropium in the long-term management of asthma is limited to those who have intolerable side effects to SABAs.

16.2.9.5 Use in COPD

Ipratropium is used as a reliever medication in COPD. The bronchodilator effect of ipratropium is more potent and lasts longer than most SABAs, and, therefore, it is the preferred reliever monotherapy.[40] The greatest benefit in lung function is derived when SAMAs are used in combination with SABAs, and, therefore, this combination should be the preferred treatment for COPD exacerbations.[6]

16.2.10 ORAL CORTICOSTEROIDS

16.2.10.1 Mechanism

Oral corticosteroids exhibit the same mechanism of action as described for ICS previously.

16.2.10.2 Side Effects

Short-term use of oral corticosteroids can result in hyperglycemia, increased appetite, fluid retention, weight gain, mood alteration, insomnia, peptic ulcer disease, and rarely, avascular necrosis. Most of these side effects are reversible.

Long-term use (>2 weeks) of oral corticosteroids include osteoporosis, osteopenia, hypertension, diabetes, suppression of HPA axis, obesity, cataracts, glaucoma, skin thinning, myopathy (including risk of respiratory muscle myopathy), dysphoria, sleep disturbance, and agitation. Every attempt should be made to use alternative therapies, control environmental triggers, treat comorbid conditions that could exacerbate respiratory disorders, and use appropriate adjuncts to control respiratory symptoms before starting oral corticosteroids.

16.2.10.3 Use in asthma

Oral corticosteroids can be used as either short-term "burst" therapy to gain control of an exacerbation or as long-term controller therapy in severe, persistent asthma. Its use in acute exacerbations reduces the need for referral to the emergency room, reduces hospital admissions, and prevents early relapse after treatment in the ER.[1] The usual treatment course is for 5–14 days at 0.5 to 1 mg/kg, which is considered high-dose therapy. Oral corticosteroids can be stopped once symptoms have subsided and lung function has returned to normal, however, some patients clinically benefit from a slower taper. In hospitalized patients, oral glucocorticoids are as effective as IV glucocorticoids.[41] The use of oral corticosteroids for maintenance therapy should be considered only in patients with severe, persistent asthma that do not respond to or have contraindications to other therapies. The benefits of long-term oral corticosteroid therapy must always be weighed against the risk of side effects and when used should be maintained at the minimal effective daily or alternating daily dose necessary for achieving asthma control. Patients treated with prolonged corticosteroids should undergo a slow taper before discontinuing.

16.2.10.4 Use in COPD

The short-term use of oral corticosteroids is well established for the treatment of COPD exacerbations, however,

in contrast to asthma, its role as a chronic controller therapy is less clear.[12] Its use in treating acute exacerbations has been shown to improve symptoms, lung function, shorten length of hospital stay, and reduce 30-day readmission rates due to recurrent exacerbations.[12] Treatment duration ranges from 5–14 days and should be tailored to the severity of exacerbation and rate of response. In hospitalized patients, oral glucocorticoids are noninferior to IV glucocorticoids.[42] The role of oral corticosteroids for chronic maintenance therapy in COPD is unclear with little data supporting their efficacy. The use of chronic corticosteroids should be weighed strongly against their numerous side effects.

16.2.11 THEOPHYLLINE

16.2.11.1 Mechanism

Theophylline causes nonspecific inhibition of phosphodiesterase isoenzymes and antagonizes adenosine receptors. The inhibition of phosphodiesterase III and IV causes bronchial smooth-muscle relaxation resulting in a small degree of bronchodilation; however, the majority of its clinical effect is likely due to its immunomodulatory, anti-inflammatory, and bronchoprotective effects on the airway.[43] Theophylline has also been shown to increase mucociliary clearance, increase systemic venous return and cardiac output, increase diaphragmatic contractility, and increase respiratory drive.

16.2.11.2 Side effects

Theophylline has a narrow therapeutic index and wide interpatient variation in metabolism. This requires careful and individualized dose titration and education of both the patient and providers on physiologic states, tobacco use, and medications that may alter theophylline metabolism. When theophylline levels are maintained at nontoxic levels (between 8–13 ug/mL), it is a very well-tolerated medication with very few noticeable side effects. Potentially fatal toxicity results from antagonism of adenosine receptors, which can cause metabolic abnormalities, tremor, vomiting, seizures, hypotension, and ventricular arrhythmias. Chronic toxicity may have a more insidious onset and may not correlate to serum levels.

16.2.11.3 Use in asthma

The risk of side effects and the emergence of novel therapies has caused theophylline to fall out of favor for the treatment of asthma. Theophylline has been shown to improve pulmonary function and symptoms when asthma is not adequately controlled on ICS and, therefore, may have a role as additive maintenance therapy when other alternatives are unacceptable.[44] Theophylline may also have a role as primary maintenance therapy in patients that require or prefer an oral medication when monteleukast is not sufficient; however, this should only be considered after the risks and benefits have been thoroughly discussed.

16.2.11.4 Use in COPD

Theophylline has been shown to improve FEV_1, dyspnea, and PaO^2 when used as additive maintenance therapy in stable COPD.[45] Given its risk of toxicity and need for monitoring, it is generally not preferred over LABAs or LAMAs.

16.2.12 ROFLUMILAST

16.2.12.1 Mechanism

Roflumilast is an oral phosphodiesterase IV inhibitor approved for the treatment of COPD. While the specific mechanism by which roflumilast exerts its therapeutic effect on patients with COPD is not well defined, it is likely similar to that of theophylline.

16.2.12.2 Side effects

Roflumilast has been associated with psychiatric side effects including worsening depression and suicidality and should be used cautiously in a patient with a history of depression after discussion of its risks and benefits. Roflumilast has also been reported to cause severe weight loss. Most commonly reported side effects were mild and included nausea and headache.

16.2.12.3 Use in asthma

Currently there is no established role for the use of roflumilast in the treatment of asthma.

16.2.12.4 Use in COPD

Roflumilast reduces the risk of COPD exacerbation in patients with a history of frequent COPD exacerbations (at least two per year) compared to placebo.[46] While roflumilast is not a bronchodilator, it has been shown to provide modest improvements in FEV_1.[46] Its use is typically reserved for patients that have frequent exacerbations despite maximal inhaler therapy.

16.3 DISCUSSION

16.3.1 ASTHMA MANAGEMENT

The guidelines from the Global Initiative for Asthma (GINA) have been updated annually since 2002. The workgroup is comprised of international experts in the care of asthma who review relevant literature and data where it exists to provide best practices recommendations. Asthma is a heterogeneous disease and the options for treatment are myriad; navigating this landscape can be daunting for the primary care physician and nonasthma specialist. As any physician who cares for patients burdened by this disease can attest, control is paramount to quality of life. However, due to cost, side effects, and encumbrance of medication routines, when feasible after patients are well controlled, efforts should be made to reduce the therapeutic regimen. As a result, physicians who are on the forefront of asthma care need to be capable of assessing risk factors for asthma worsening, determining appropriate initial controller and rescue therapy, ensuring patient understanding and demonstration of the skill set needed to use medications, regularly reviewing response to treatments, and considering escalating or deescalating therapy as appropriate. A summary of the most recent consensus guidelines from the GINA guidelines and literature review is provided in Tables 16.2–16.6.[1,47] These tables highlight the assessment of risk factors for asthma/lung function worsening, useful questions to determine symptom control for patients, recommended regimens for control and relief of symptoms based on patient risk/symptom profile, as well as a framework for escalation and de-escalation of therapy. There are innumerable subtleties/nuances involved in the sophisticated care of complex genetic and environmentally affected diseases such as asthma. These guidelines and tables are an effort to simplify this practice to improve management of chronic asthma for the general practicing physician. As such, they cannot replace expert-level knowledge, and, therefore, more complex select asthma cases should be referred to an asthma specialist for additional testing and management guidance. In general, the principles of asthma management are to (1) strongly consider use of ICS as a controller therapy in patients with asthma symptoms or risk factors for asthma,

Table 16.2 Risk factors for exacerbations/worsening lung function in asthma

- Poor symptom control
- Ineffective ICS due to adherence or technique
- $FEV_1 < 60\%$
- Ongoing exposures: tobacco smoke, occupational irritants, food, or aeroallergens, if documented sensitivity
- Obesity
- Poorly controlled GERD
- Chronic rhinitis and rhinosinusitis
- Eosinophilia in blood or sputum
- Pregnancy
- History of intubation or ICU admission for asthma
- Any severe exacerbation in last 12 months (e.g., oral steroid or hospitalization needed)

Source: Adapted from Global Initiative for Asthma. Global Strategy for Asthma Management and Prevention, 2016. Available at www.ginasthma.org.

Table 16.3 Assessment of asthma symptom control

In the past 4 weeks has the patient experienced:
- Daytime symptoms more than twice per week
- Need to use rescue inhaler more than twice per week
- Any limitation of activities due to asthma
- Any nocturnal waking due to asthma

If none of these are present, then the patient is well controlled.

If 1–2 of these are present, then the patient is partly controlled.

If 3–4 of these are present, then the patient is uncontrolled/poorly controlled.

Source: Adapted from Global Initiative for Asthma. Global Strategy for Asthma Management and Prevention, 2016. Available at www.ginasthma.org.

(2) escalate therapy until symptoms are well controlled and lung function is stable, (3) consider adjunct therapy as needed and personalize asthma care plans based on patient-specific characteristics, (4) frequently reassess patients who are requiring either step-up or step-down therapy, (5) maintain a combination of ICS/LABA treatment when stepping down from higher to a lower dose of ICS component, and (6) refer patients to asthma specialists when traditional therapy does not yield the desired results.

16.3.2 COPD MANAGEMENT

The guidelines from the Global Initiative for Chronic Obstructive Lung Disease (GOLD) workgroup are updated regularly to reflect the literature and best-practices recommendations from experts in the field. The management of COPD focuses on symptoms as well as lung function, and in that way mirrors the two-pronged approach to the management of asthma. Accompanying Tables 16.7–16.9[48] highlight key areas of management consideration, notably (1) the categorization of patients based on their spirometry, exacerbations, and symptoms; (2) the recommended first-line therapies with listed alternatives for each category; and (3) summary of key management points. Although asthma and COPD share similar presenting symptoms (cough, shortness of breath, limitation of activity due to symptoms) and can be difficult to distinguish from each other in certain instances, there are several key factors that differ in their management (Table 16.10).[49] Briefly, the key management differences center on the preferred first-line agents, the additional risk of ICS in the COPD patient population, and the approach to the stable patient. It cannot be overemphasized that ICS are the mainstay treatment for asthma and in most patients should remain the core element of their controller regimen. Alternatively, in COPD, the addition of ICS should be reserved for patients with severe disease and those not responsive to isolated bronchodilator or in the presence of peripheral eosinophilia. Furthermore, with regards to COPD, there exists an additional significant risk

of pneumonia when compared to COPD patients not managed with ICS.[50] This increased risk abates when the ICS is withdrawn. There is considerable emphasis in the literature to follow the GOLD guidelines, which clearly reserve ICS use as an adjunct in more severe patients (i.e., those with frequent or severe exacerbations and those with $FEV_1 \leq 60\%$ predicted). Much work has been done to emphasize the risk of ICS due to their overuse in patients with COPD categorized as having less severe disease. However, it should be noted that ICS have proven benficial as an adjunct therapy for COPD to reduce exacerbations, improve all-cause mortality, and improve lung function.[51] Therefore, physicians must be cognizant that the long-term effects of these pneumonia episodes, the lack of known data to suggest clinical deterioration as a result, and the known benefit of adjunctive ICS must be considered on balance in each patient scenario. Importantly, the approach to the stable/improved patient with COPD also differs fundamentally from the approach to those with asthma. While step-down therapy is a cornerstone of asthma management, there is no consensus about step-down therapy with COPD. It is likely reasonable to cautiously withdraw ICS from combination therapy with long-acting bronchodilators in patients with well-controlled symptom burden and no exacerbations on current therapy. Since there has been a link to decline in lung function despite good symptom control in these patients,[52] this observation diminished the enthusiasm for step-down approaches in the management of COPD.

16.3.3 ACO MANAGEMENT

The ACO is increasingly recognized as a distinct clinical entity encountered in the adult population. Large segments of the global population are exposed during their lifetime to inhaled particles (e.g., tobacco smoke, indoor and outdoor air pollutants, noxious occupational inhalants) that are known to confer increased risk of COPD. It is inevitable that many of these patients also have preexisting asthma phenotypes with associated intermittent respiratory symptoms, sensitivity to respiratory infections and aeroallergens, and personal and familial history of atopy. The end result of this sequence is that patients can have features of both asthma and COPD. Furthermore, an epidemiologic study links poorly controlled asthma in children to the development of fixed airway obstruction earlier in adulthood.[53] This subset of patients is not a homogenous group and the relative burden of each symptom domain is variable.[54] Despite the ambiguity involved in the assessment of such patients and particular symptom profile they exhibit, it is critical that they be accurately identified. Cohorts of patients that have been found to have poor reversibility and chronic symptoms (i.e., suggestive of COPD) with a self-reported history of asthma have been shown to have increased frequency of exacerbations regardless of GOLD category, increased health-care utilization, and a more rapid decline in lung function.[55] There is, as of yet, not a specific definition of ACO. However, clinical features that

Table 16.4 Stepwise approach for asthma according to GINA guidelines

Therapy level	Step 1	Step 2	Step 3	Step 4	Step 5
Presentation	No risk factors for exacerbation and symptoms are well controlled	Risk factor(s) for exacerbation present or symptoms only partly controlled	Uncontrolled symptoms	Uncontrolled symptoms and poor response to prior step therapy	Severe symptoms and/or poor response to prior step therapy
Preferred controller	None	Low-dose ICS	• If age > 11: low-dose ICS/LABA • If age < 11: medium-dose ICS	• If age > 11: – Low- dose ICS/formoterol as controller and rescue[d] – Or medium/high-dose ICS/LABA • If age < 11: – referral to specialist	Referral to specialist for further assessment and adjunct treatment
Alternatives for control	Consider low-dose ICS if FEV$_1$ < 80% of predicted	• LTRA[a] • If age > 11: consider theophylline	• Medium/high-dose ICS[b] • Low-dose ICS + LTRA • If age > 11: low-dose ICS + theophylline	• If age > 18: add tiotroprium to regimen • High-dose ICS + LTRA • If age > 11: high-dose ICS + theophylline	• If age > 18: add tiotroprium to regimen • Add oral corticosteroids to regimen • Consider biologic therapy (Anti-IL-5 or Anti-IgE)
Rescue/reliever	PRN SABA	PRN SABA	• If controller is low-dose ICS/formoterol, then use as PRN rescue as well[c] • If not, then PRN SABA	• If controller is low-dose ICS/formoterol, then use as PRN rescue as well • If not, then PRN SABA	• If controller is low-dose ICS/formoterol, then use as PRN rescue as well • If not, then PRN SABA

Source: Adapted from Global Initiative for Asthma. Global Strategy for Asthma Management and Prevention, 2016. Available at www.ginasthma.org.

[a] LTRA are less effective than ICS for asthma control but may be considered for patients unable to use inhalers, having side effects from ICS, or with concomitant allergic rhinosinusitis disease.

[b] Medium/high-dose ICS is less effective than addition of LABA in patients > 11 years of age.

[c] Use of low-dose ICS/formoterol combination as both controller and rescue has shown to significantly reduce exacerbations and yield equally effective symptom control. It should be noted that this therapy is not FDA approved, but is being used in Europe.

[d] If patient is already on combination low-dose ICS/formoterol from step 3, then dose can be increased for maintenance therapy, though not FDA approved in the United States.

are suggestive have been proposed to help establish a clinical definition that serves to improve the identification and subsequent study of these patients. The GINA/GOLD ACO guidelines suggest that ACO is characterized by persistent, though variable, airflow limitation symptoms and features of both the COPD as well as asthma phenotype. Thus, ACO is defined by patients that share features of both diseases rather than by differences from either (Table 16.11). Patients with ACO exhibit chronic symptoms, a typical COPD feature, with variability in symptom burden, a frequent asthma feature. Patients with ACO have a reduced FEV$_1$/FVC ratio that typically remains less than 0.7 after bronchodilator, a COPD feature. However, they may exhibit a pronounced response to bronchodilator therapy with increase > 12% in FEV$_1$ or of > 400 mL, an asthma feature. Therapy for ACO is focused on the importance of ICS use in patients with features of asthma, regardless of their existence in isolation or in the context of an overlap syndrome. Patients diagnosed with ACO should be treated with ICS as the cornerstone of therapy, similar to asthma. Long-acting bronchodilators as adjunctive therapies should be added as needed, typically with early initiation as symptoms dictate. As in asthma, the current recommendations would be to add therapeutics with alternative mechanisms of action (e.g., LABA or LAMA) before the escalation of ICS dose. Single-agent LABA should be avoided in patients with ACO, which is similar to what is recommended in the management of asthma.

Table 16.5 Step-down approach for asthma according to GINA guidelines

Current step	Current medication	Step down recommended
Step 5[a]	High-dose ICS/LABA + oral corticosteroid	Reduce dose of oral corticosteroid or replace with additional high-dose ICS
Step 4	Medium- to high-dose ICS/LABA[b]	Reduce ICS component of ICS/LABA combination by 50%
	Medium-dose ICS/formoterol as controller and rescue	Reduce to low-dose ICS/formoterol as controller and rescue
	High-dose ICS + alternative agent	Reduce ICS by 50% and continue alternative agent
Step 3'	Low-dose ICS/LABA	Change to once daily use of low-dose ICS/LABA
	Low-dose ICS/formoterol as controller and rescue	Change to once daily use of low-dose ICS/formoterol as controller and continue PRN use as rescue
	Medium-dose ICS	Reduce ICS by 50%
Step 2	Low-dose ICS[c]	Change to once daily use of low-dose ICS
	LTRA	Consider stopping controller if no symptoms for 6 months and no risk factors for worsening lung function present, but this is rare

Source: Adapted from Global Initiative for Asthma. Global Strategy for Asthma Management and Prevention, 2016. Available at www .ginasthma.org.
[a] Strongly consider referral to asthma specialist for any Step 5 patients for step-down management
[b] When using a combination ICS/LABA and step-down therapy, focus on reduction of ICS dose but avoid elimination of LABA component, as this has been shown to worsen asthma symptoms (Brozek JL).
[c] Patients receiving ICS should not be taken off them completely.

Table 16.6 Key points for asthma management

- Low threshold to initiate controller ICS for patients with symptom burden, poor lung function by spirometry, or risk factors for exacerbations
- ICS is the fundamental management tool in asthma
- LABA should not be used in isolation
- Deliberate caution in the step-down process should be used to ensure continued control of symptoms and stable lung function
- When using step-down therapy, reduce ICS component of ICS/LABA rather than eliminating LABA
- If step-up therapy is not successful, low threshold for referral to specialist in asthma

Table 16.7 GOLD classification of COPD

Patient category	Patient characteristics	Risk classification[a,b]	CAT score for symptom burden	mMRC score for breathlessness
A	Low risk, less symptoms	GOLD 1 or 2 and < 2 exacerbations and no hospitalizations	< 10	< 2
B	Low risk, more symptoms	GOLD 1 or 2 and < 2 exacerbations and no hospitalizations	≥ 10	≥ 2
C	High risk, less symptoms	GOLD 3 or 4 or ≥ 2 exacerbations or any hospitalizations	< 10	< 2
D	High risk, more symptoms	GOLD 3 or 4 or ≥ 2 exacerbations or any hospitalizations	≥ 10	≥ 2

Source: Adapted from the Global Strategy for the Diagnosis MaPoC, Global Initiative for Chronic Obstructive Lung Disease (GOLD) 2016.
[a] GOLD classification is based on spirometry and FEV_1 postbronchodilator.
- GOLD 1: $FEV_1 \geq 80\%$ predicted
- GOLD 2: $50\% \leq FEV_1 < 80\%$ predicted
- GOLD 3: $30\% \leq FEV_1 < 50\%$ predicted
- GOLD 4: $FEV_1 < 30\%$ predicted
[b] Risk classification is based on either spirometry or clinical history of exacerbations in preceding 12 months and should err on the side of whichever factor confers higher risk.

Table 16.8 Step-up therapy for COPD according to GOLD guidelines

Patient category	Recommended therapy	Alternatives to consider
A	PRN short-acting bronchodilator[a]	• Combination of SABA/SAMA[b] • LABA[b] • LAMA[b]
B	Long-acting bronchodilator	• Combination of LABA/LAMA[c] • Short-acting bronchodilator + theophylline[d]
C	LAMA or ICS/LABA	• Combination of LABA/LAMA[c] • Combination of ICS/LAMA • Long-acting bronchodilator + roflumilast[e] • Short-acting bronchodilator + theophylline[d]
D	ICS/long-acting bronchodilator	• Combination ICS/LABA/LAMA • ICS/long-acting bronchodilator + roflumilast[e] • Short-acting bronchodilator + theophylline[d]

Source: Adapted from the Global Strategy for the Diagnosis MaPoC, Global Initiative for Chronic Obstructive Lung Disease (GOLD) 2016. It is not clear whether increasing the dose of ICS component in COPD improves either symptoms or disease modification.
[a] Either short-acting β_2-agonist (SABA) or short-acting muscarinic-antagonist (SAMA) is acceptable, though SAMA may be preferred.
[b] There is no convincing evidence to use multiple or long-acting agents for this patient population.
[c] Newer data suggest there may be superiority of LAMA/LABA over ICS/LABA (Wedzicha JA).
[d] Theophylline may be useful in situations where cost or access is prohibitive for long-acting bronchodilators.
[e] Roflumilast, a phosphodiesterase-4 inhibitor, can be considered as add-on therapy if patient has chronic bronchitis phenotype.

Table 16.9 Key points for medication management of COPD

- Long-acting bronchodilators are preferred over short-acting for maintenance therapy.
- Combination of beta-agonists and anti-muscarinic is reasonable if needed for symptom control.
- Theophylline is not recommended unless other therapies are unavailable or have failed.
- ICS are recommended for patients with severe COPD not well controlled with long-acting bronchodilators.
- ICS as monotherapy is not recommended.
- Consideration should be given for ICS taper/withdrawal in patients on combination therapy with reduced risk (i.e., improved FEV_1, limited/no exacerbations).
- There is an increased risk of pneumonia without associated increase in mortality in COPD patients on ICS.

Table 16.10 Distinguishing characteristics between asthma and COPD

Discrepancy issue	Asthma	COPD
ICS	The principle controller medication for care	Should only be used as adjunct therapy in patients with more severe symptoms or higher risk
ICS risk	• There are risks associated, especially with high-dose formulations, but benefits substantially outweigh risks in most instances • No increased pneumonia risk seen[a]	• Significant increased risk in pneumonia without accompanying mortality risk • Careful consideration of continued use[b]
Long-acting bronchodilators	Useful as adjunct therapy in step-up management	The principle recommended therapy for patients who have more than trivial symptom burden
Step-down approach	Well validated and a key part of asthma management	Not well established as part of COPD management and must weigh risks of medications with benefits of symptom control

[a] Studies have failed to show an increased risk of pneumonia in asthma patients treated with ICS (Bansal V).
[b] Physicians must discuss the proven benefits of ICS with patients who have severe COPD and significant FEV_1 decline versus the risk of pneumonia, as well as bone mineral density loss and other potential side effects.

Table 16.11 Characteristics of asthma, COPD, and asthma-COPD overlap (ACO)

Domain	Asthma	ACO	COPD
Symptoms	Highly variable with time of day and season	Persistent and chronic but with variability	Chronic with little variability except during exacerbations
FEV_1 bronchodilator response	12% and often > 400 mL	Variable but often > 12% and > 400 mL	May be > or < 12% but not likely > 400 mL
Cornerstone of therapy	ICS	ICS (+/– long-acting bronchodilator)	Long-acting bronchodilator
Primary adjuvant therapy	Long-acting bronchodilator	Long-acting bronchodilator	Alternative long-acting bronchodilator and/or ICS
Step-down approach	Fundamental and often possible when control is achieved	Not well defined	May be feasible though concern for worsening lung function despite symptoms control

16.4 CONCLUSION

Asthma, COPD, and ACO are diseases that share many similar presenting features and have significant overlap of therapeutic options for management. However, there are key differences in first-line therapies, approach to the poorly controlled patient, and recommendations for potential de-escalation of therapy when control or stability is achieved. These variances are not merely academic; they are critical to the best care of patients by maintaining or improving lung function and minimizing side effects and adverse events associated with pharmacologic therapy. Despite the seemingly daunting task of manipulating theses subtleties, physicians on the front line of patient care can make a tremendous impact on patient outcomes and health. Using cornerstone guidelines, such as GINA and GOLD, and reference tables such as those we have included in this section, physicians can correctly determine the most appropriate therapy for these patients as well as constructing a plan for further care as dictated by response to treatment. Referral to specialists will clearly be necessary at times, but all physicians need to have a fundamental working knowledge of obstructive lung disease management to improve the care of the millions of individuals affected worldwide.

REFERENCES

1. Johnson M. Beta2-adrenoceptors: Mechanisms of action of beta2-agonists. *Paediatr Respir Rev.* 2001;2(1):57–62.
2. Ahrens R. and Weinberger M. Levalbuterol and racemic albuterol: Are there therapeutic differences? *J Allergy Clin Immunol.* 2001;108(5):681–684.
3. Guhan AR, Cooper S, Oborne J et al. Systemic effects of formoterol and salmeterol: A dose-response comparison in healthy subjects. *Thorax.* 2000;55(8):650–656.
4. Haselkorn T, Fish JE, Zeiger RS et al. Consistently very poorly controlled asthma, as defined by the impairment domain of the expert panel report 3 guidelines, increases risk for future severe asthma exacerbations in the epidemiology and natural history of asthma: Outcomes and treatment regimens (TENOR) study. *J Allergy Clin Immunol.* 2009;124(5):895–902. e1–e4.
5. In chronic obstructive pulmonary disease, a combination of ipratropium and albuterol is more effective than either agent alone. An 85-day multicenter trial. COMBIVENT inhalation aerosol study group. *Chest.* 1994;105(5):1411–1419.
6. Lotvall J. Pharmacological similarities and differences between beta2-agonists. *Respir med.* 2001;95(Suppl. B):S7–S11.
7. Ducharme FM, Ni Chroinin M, Greenstone I et al. Addition of long-acting beta2-agonists to inhaled steroids versus higher dose inhaled steroids in adults and children with persistent asthma. *Cochrane Database syst Rev.* 2010(4):CD005533.
8. Nelson HS, Weiss ST, Bleecker ER et al. The salmeterol multicenter asthma research trial: A comparison of usual pharmacotherapy for asthma or usual pharmacotherapy plus salmeterol. *Chest.* 2006;129(1):15–26.
9. Peters SP, Bleecker ER, Canonica GW et al. Serious asthma events with budesonide plus formoterol vs. Budesonide alone. *N Engl J Med.* 2016;375(9):850–860.
10. Stempel DA, Raphiou IH, Kral KM et al. Serious asthma events with fluticasone plus salmeterol versus fluticasone alone. *N Engl J Med.* 2016;374(19):1822–1830.
11. From the Global Strategy for the Diagnosis, Management and Prevention of COPD, Global Initiative for Chronic Obstructive Lung Disease (GOLD) 2016. Available from: http://goldcopd.org. Accessed 5/31/2016.

12. Barnes PJ. Inhaled corticosteroids. *Pharmaceuticals.* 2010;3(3):514–540.

13. Williamson IJ, Matusiewicz SP, Brown PH et al. Frequency of voice problems and cough in patients using pressurized aerosol inhaled steroid preparations. *Eur Respir J.* 1995;8(4):590–592.

14. Derendorf H, Nave R, Drollmann A et al. Relevance of pharmacokinetics and pharmacodynamics of inhaled corticosteroids to asthma. *Eur Respir J.* 2006;28(5):1042–1050.

15. Kelly HW and Nelson HS. Potential adverse effects of the inhaled corticosteroids. *J Allergy Clin Immunol.* 2003;112(3):469–478; quiz 79.

16. The Childhood Asthma Management Program (CAMP): Design, rationale, and methods. Childhood asthma management program research group. *Control Clin Trials.* 1999;20(1):91–120.

17. Mitchell P, Cumming RG, and Mackey DA. Inhaled corticosteroids, family history, and risk of glaucoma. *Ophthalmol.* 1999;106(12):2301–2306.

18. Garbe E, Suissa S, and LeLorier J. Association of inhaled corticosteroid use with cataract extraction in elderly patients. *JAMA.* 1998;280(6):539–543.

19. Global Initiative for Asthma. Global Strategy for Asthma Management and Prevention, 2016. Available at www.ginasthma.org. Accessed 5/31/2016.

20. National Asthma E and Prevention P. Expert Panel Report 3 (EPR-3): Guidelines for the diagnosis and management of asthma-summary report 2007. *J Allergy Clin Immunol.* 2007;120(5 Suppl):S94–138.

21. Singh S, Amin AV, and Loke YK. Long-term use of inhaled corticosteroids and the risk of pneumonia in chronic obstructive pulmonary disease: A meta-analysis. *Arch Intern Med.* 2009;169(3):219–229.

22. Peters-Golden M, Henderson WR and Jr. Leukotrienes. *N Engl J Med.* 2007;357(18):1841–1854.

23. Chauhan BF and Ducharme FM. Anti-leukotriene agents compared to inhaled corticosteroids in the management of recurrent and/or chronic asthma in adults and children. *Cochrane Database Syst Rev.* 2012;5:Cd002314.

24. Hanania NA, Alpan O, Hamilos DL et al. Omalizumab in severe allergic asthma inadequately controlled with standard therapy: A randomized trial. *Ann Intern Med.* 2011;154(9):573–582.

25. Busse W, Spector S, Rosen K et al. High eosinophil count: A potential biomarker for assessing successful omalizumab treatment effects. *J Allergy Clin Immunol.* 2013;132(2):485–486.e11.

26. Garcia G, Taille C, Laveneziana P et al. Anti-interleukin-5 therapy in severe asthma. *Eur Respir Rev.* 2013;22(129):251–257.

27. Castro M, Zangrilli J, Wechsler ME et al. Reslizumab for inadequately controlled asthma with elevated blood eosinophil counts: Results from two multicentre, parallel, double-blind, randomised, placebo-controlled, phase 3 trials. *Lancet Respir Med.* 2015;3(5):355–366.

28. Ortega HG, Liu MC, Pavord ID et al. Mepolizumab treatment in patients with severe eosinophilic asthma. *N Engl J Med.* 2014;371(13):1198–1207.

29. Bleecker ER, FitzGerald JM, Chanez P et al. Efficacy and safety of benralizumab for patients with severe asthma uncontrolled with high-dosage inhaled corticosteroids and long-acting beta2-agonists (SIROCCO): A randomised, multi-centre, placebo-controlled phase 3 trial. *Lancet.* 2016;388(10056):2115–2127.

30. FitzGerald JM, Bleecker ER, Nair P et al. Benralizumab, an anti-interleukin-5 receptor alpha monoclonal antibody, as add-on treatment for patients with severe, uncontrolled, eosinophilic asthma (CALIMA): A randomised, double-blind, placebo-controlled phase 3 trial. *Lancet.* 2016;388(10056):2128–2141.

31. Bel EH, Wenzel SE, Thompson PJ et al. Oral glucocorticoid-sparing effect of mepolizumab in eosinophilic asthma. *N Engl J Med.* 2014;371 (13):1189–1197.

32. Virchow JC, Backer V, Kuna P et al. Efficacy of a house dust mite sublingual allergen immunotherapy tablet in adults with allergic asthma: A randomized clinical trial. *JAMA.* 2016;315(16):1715–1725.

33. Alagha K, Palot A, Sofalvi T et al. Long-acting muscarinic receptor antagonists for the treatment of chronic airway diseases. *Ther Adv Chronic Dis.* 2014;5(2):85–98.

34. Celli B, Decramer M, Leimer I et al. Cardiovascular safety of tiotropium in patients with COPD. *Chest.* 2010;137(1):20–30.

35. Singh S, Loke YK, and Furberg CD. Inhaled anticholinergics and risk of major adverse cardiovascular events in patients with chronic obstructive pulmonary disease: A systematic review and meta-analysis. *JAMA.* 2008;300(12):1439–1450.

36. Tashkin DP, Celli B, Senn S et al. A 4-year trial of tiotropium in chronic obstructive pulmonary disease. *N Engl J Med.* 2008;359(15):1543–1554.

37. Kerstjens HA, Disse B, Schroder-Babo W et al. Tiotropium improves lung function in patients with severe uncontrolled asthma: A randomized controlled trial. *J Allergy ClinI Immunol.* 2011;128(2):308–314.

38. Peters SP, Kunselman SJ, Icitovic N et al. Tiotropium bromide step-up therapy for adults with uncontrolled asthma. *N Engl J Med.* 2010;363(18):1715–1726.

39. Vogelmeier C, Hederer B, Glaab T et al. Tiotropium versus salmeterol for the prevention of exacerbations of COPD. *N Engl J Med.* 2011;364(12):1093–1103.

40. Chervinsky P. Concomitant bronchodilator therapy and ipratropium bromide. A clinical review. *Am J Med.* 1986;81(5A):67–73.

41. Dembla G, Mundle RP, Salkar HR et al. Oral versus intravenous steroids in acute exacerbation of asthma—randomized controlled study. *J Assoc Physicians India*. 2011;59:621–623.

42. Tashkin DP. Oral vs IV corticosteroids for in-hospital treatment of COPD exacerbations. *Chest*. 2007;132(6):1728–1729.

43. Barnes PJ. Theophylline. *Am J Respir Crit Care Med*. 2013;188(8):901–906.

44. Evans DJ, Taylor DA, Zetterstrom O et al. A comparison of low-dose inhaled budesonide plus theophylline and high-dose inhaled budesonide for moderate asthma. *N Engl J Med*. 1997;337(20):1412–1418.

45. Ram FS, Jones PW, Castro AA et al. Oral theophylline for chronic obstructive pulmonary disease. *Cochrane Database Syst Rev*. 2002(4):CD003902.

46. Chong J, Poole P, Leung B et al. Phosphodiesterase 4 inhibitors for chronic obstructive pulmonary disease. *Cochrane Database Syst Rev*. 2011(5):CD002309.

47. Brozek JL, Kraft M, Krishnan JA et al. Long-acting beta2-agonist step-off in patients with controlled asthma. *Arch Intern Med*. 2012;172(18):1365–1375.

48. Wedzicha, J. A. et al. Indacaterol-glycopyrronium versus salmeterol-fluticasone for COPD. *N Engl J Med*. 2016;374(23):2222–2234.

49. Bansal V, Mangi MA, Johnson MM, Festic E. Inhaled corticosteroids and incident pneumonia in patients with asthma: Systematic review and meta-analysis. *Acta Medica Academica*. 2015;44(2):135–158.

50. Kew KM and Seniukovich A. Inhaled steroids and risk of pneumonia for chronic obstructive pulmonary disease. *Cochrane Database Syst Rev*. 2014(3):CD010115.

51. Festic E and Scanlon PD. Incident pneumonia and mortality in patients with chronic obstructive pulmonary disease. A double effect of inhaled corticosteroids? *Am J Respir Crit Care Med*. 2015;191(2):141–148.

52. Magnussen H, Disse B, Rodriguez-Roisin R et al. Withdrawal of inhaled glucocorticoids and exacerbations of COPD. *N Engl J Med*. 2014;371 (14):1285–1294.

53. McGeachie MJ, Yates KP, Zhou X et al. Patterns of growth and decline in lung function in persistent childhood asthma. *N Engl J Med*. 2016;374(19):1842–1852.

54. Hardin M, Silverman EK, Barr RG et al. The clinical features of the overlap between COPD and asthma. *Respir Res*. 2011;12:127.

55. Hardin M, Cho M, McDonald ML et al. The clinical and genetic features of COPD-asthma overlap syndrome. *Eur Respir J*. 2014;44(2):341–350.

Biologics and emerging therapies for asthma, COPD, and asthma-COPD overlap

ANGIRA DASGUPTA, AMBER J. OBERLE, AND PARAMESWARAN NAIR

CLINICAL VIGNETTE 17.1

A 42-year-old woman; never-smoker; with allergies to grass, cats, and ragweed; rhinosinusitis and nasal polyposis; and a recently identified aspirin sensitivity, who was on treatment with 1,000 mcg equivalent of an inhaled corticosteroid (ICS) and a long-acting β_2-agonist (LABA), a long-acting muscarinic antagonist (LAMA), and a leukotriene receptor antagonist (LTRA), had three exacerbations in the previous year that required treatment with short courses of prednisone. Her specialist decides to maintain her on a low dose of prednisone (7.5 mg daily) to avoid the frequent courses of prednisone. Her forced expiratory volume in one second (FEV_1) and vital capacity (VC) prebronchodilator are 1.6 L (62% predicted) and 3.2 L (78% predicted) respectively, with a ratio of 50%. The FEV_1 and VC improve to 1.9 L and 3.4 L after inhaling 200 μg of salbutamol. Her high-resolution thoracic CT scan does not show emphysema or bronchiectasis. Her total serum IgE is 480 IU/L. Other measurements include blood eosinophil count of 0.6/μL, sputum eosinophil count of 8% with moderate free granules, and an exhaled nitric oxide (NO) of 48 ppb.

CLINICAL VIGNETTE 17.2

A 63-year-old man, with a 40 pack-year history of cigarette smoking and allergies to grass pollen and possibly to isocyanate exposure at work, is referred for recurrent symptoms of wheezing, shortness of breath, and purulent sputum. He is also known to have stable coronary artery disease and is on baby aspirin, a beta-blocker, and a low-dose daily diuretic. He was on treatment with a combination of ICS and LABA as well as a LAMA. His FEV_1 and VC prebronchodilator are 1.4 L (60% predicted) and 2.7 L (72% predicted) with an FEV_1/VC ratio of 52%. The FEV_1 improved modestly to 1.5 L after inhaling 200 μg of salbutamol. A high-resolution thoracic CT scan shows paraseptal and centrilobular emphysema and mild cylindrical bronchiectasis of the lingula. His total serum IgE is 140 IU/L. Other measurements at the time of a previous asthma exacerbation revealed a peripheral blood eosinophil count of 0.5/μL, sputum eosinophil count of 7% with moderate free granules associated with a neutrophil count of 85%, and a total cell count of 43 million cells/g.

17.1 INTRODUCTION

Guideline-based management of asthma, COPD, or their overlap (asthma-COPD overlap or ACO) is similar for all three of these conditions in many ways.[1,2] It entails the use of inhaled bronchodilators (short- and long-acting antimuscarinic or β_2-agonists), ICS and oral corticosteroids, leukotriene modifying agents (LTMAs), phosphodiesterase 4 inhibitors (roflumilast), and other medications using symptoms, lung function, and patient-related outcome scores to titrate doses of these agents to achieve asthma control. However, there are a subset of patients who, despite standard guideline-based care, are difficult to control, and experience more frequent exacerbations, worsening of lung function, and poorer quality of life. These patients often display characteristics of both asthma and COPD.[3,4] Accumulating evidence shows that these patients have more complex mechanisms driving their disease, necessitating tailored treatment based upon individual patient characteristics.[5,6]

"Overlap syndrome" is a not a new concept. It is an extension of the "Dutch hypothesis," whereby chronic airflow limitation may arise as a result of chronic asthma or the association of bronchodilator reversibility and airway hyperresponsiveness in patients with smoking-related airway diseases or exposure to other environmental determinants.[7] Underlying shared biological similarities are reinforced by recent unbiased cluster analytical techniques of cytokines involved in the pathobiology of these diseases.[8] Intuitively, it would make more sense to direct therapies with a clear understanding of the components (i.e., airflow obstruction, airway hyperresponsiveness [AHR], and airway inflammation) associated with these diseases rather than based on the "disease label."[9] Identifying airway inflammation through various biomarkers has proven to be a useful and exciting method for more targeted therapy, especially if the use of biologics is contemplated.[5] The strategy is to optimize airway inflammation guided by its specific nature (e.g., eosinophilic, neutrophilic, mixed, and paucigranulocytic) and is best achieved by using sputum quantitative assays to measure airway inflammation.[10] Indeed, this strategy has been shown to be superior to standard therapy in asthma as well as COPD.[11,12] It is intuitive that this will also be applicable in patients with ACO. Some of these patients require long-term high doses of corticosteroids, which predispose them to serious complications, including cataracts, glaucoma, osteoporosis, avascular bone necrosis, diabetes, and others. Biologics are helpful in such situations, as oral corticosteroid sparing agents or as add-on medications to standard therapy.[1,13]

The clinical endotype of patients requiring biologics is usually one of the following: (a) allergic or nonallergic patients with uncontrolled eosinophilic inflammation despite high doses of inhaled or oral corticosteroids, and (b) uncontrolled neutrophilic inflammation with or without associated airway eosinophilia. A third endotype of paucigranulocytic bronchitis (i.e., normal sputum cell counts) associated with hyperresponsive airways is currently not amenable to therapy with currently available biologics or small molecule antagonists. Procedures, such as bronchial thermoplasty, that attenuate airway smooth-muscle mass may be the best strategy to treat their symptoms. It is worth considering that these cellular endotypes correspond with the endotypes defined by more sophisticated "omics platform based characterization," such as the "Th2-high," "Th2-low," or the "Th2-low and Th-17 low" immune endotypes.[14,15]

Current clinical evidence of the efficacy and safety of biologicals and small molecule antagonists to treat these endotypes is limited to patients with asthma. However, there is emerging evidence for their efficacy in COPD, and clinical trials are currently underway. This chapter will illustrate a therapeutic approach to each of these unique, but not mutually exclusive, clinical endotypes for both asthma and COPD, and discuss the use of currently approved biologics using a case-based approach. However, these endotypes are not static, but rather dynamic, and might change over time in an individual. Therefore, it is important to reassess quantitative sputum counts whenever the patients are symptomatic to identify persistence of a particular endotype, which would then increase the likelihood of response to therapy targeted at a specific inflammatory mediator. This is not an exhaustive account of all the biological agents that are currently being evaluated for airway diseases. The potential targets and drugs have been reviewed in detail elsewhere.[16–18]

17.1.1 DISCUSSION OF CLINICAL VIGNETTE 1

This patient has severe atopic asthma with partially reversible airflow obstruction, and thus has asthma and associated chronic airflow limitation with persistent eosinophilic bronchitis and peripheral blood eosinophilia despite being on high doses of inhaled and oral corticosteroids. This illustrates a typical "eosinophil or high Th2 phenotype." The most widely available biomarker for this phenotype is peripheral blood eosinophilia, and when elevated, is usually associated with a response to corticosteroids. However, it is a poor marker of airway eosinophilia and has a lower diagnostic accuracy for the detection of airway eosinophilia especially when asthma becomes severe.[19] A possible explanation for this discrepancy is the local production of eosinophilopoietic cytokines, such as IL-5 and IL-13, by innate lymphoid cells-type 2 (ILC-2) residing in the airways.[20,21] Other biomarkers of the Th2 phenotype such as fraction of exhaled nitric oxide (FeNO) and serum periostin have certain disadvantages. FeNO has a wide normal range and is not specific for eosinophilic inflammation in patients who are on high doses of corticosteroids, while serum periostin estimation is currently not available for routine use in clinical practice.[22] Thus, sputum analysis affords a more comprehensive and accurate phenotype of patients with airway eosinophilia. In the absence of sputum analysis, blood eosinophil count is likely an acceptable surrogate[19,23] and when combined with other biomarkers like FeNO, may improve the diagnostic accuracy for the detection of airway eosinophilia.[24] An absolute eosinophil count greater than 150–400/μL, or a sputum eosinophil count greater than 3%, seem to be the best predictors of exacerbations and response to anti-IL5 agents.[19]

All the biologics that are currently being developed (Table 17.1) are directed against cytokines that either directly or indirectly recruit eosinophils into the airway (Figure 17.1). Omalizumab, a humanized IgG anti-IgE monoclonal antibody, was the first biologic to be approved by the Food and

Drug Administration (FDA) in the United States and to be recommended by international guidelines for the treatment of asthma.[1] Although it is indicated in patients with moderate to severe allergic asthma with serum IgE levels between 30 and 700 IU/mL experiencing frequent exacerbations and persistent airflow limitation, its effect in patients who are oral-corticosteroid dependent is less well established.[25] Nevertheless, it would be reasonable to consider a trial of omalizumab as

Table 17.1 Biologics for asthma and their clinical efficacies

Monoclonal	Isotype	Target	Effect on FEV$_1$	Effect on exacerbation	Prednisone-sparing effect
Omalizumab	IgG1	IgE	++	++	Being evaluated
Mepolizumab	IgG1	IL5	+	+++	++
Reslizumab	IgG4	IL5	++	+++	Not evaluated
Benralizumab	IgG1	IL5Rα	++	++	+++
Lebrikizumab	IgG4	IL13	+	+	Not evaluated
Tralokinumab	IgG4	IL13Rα1 and 2	+	+	Being evaluated
Dupilumab	IgG4	IL4Rα/13	++	++	Being evaluated

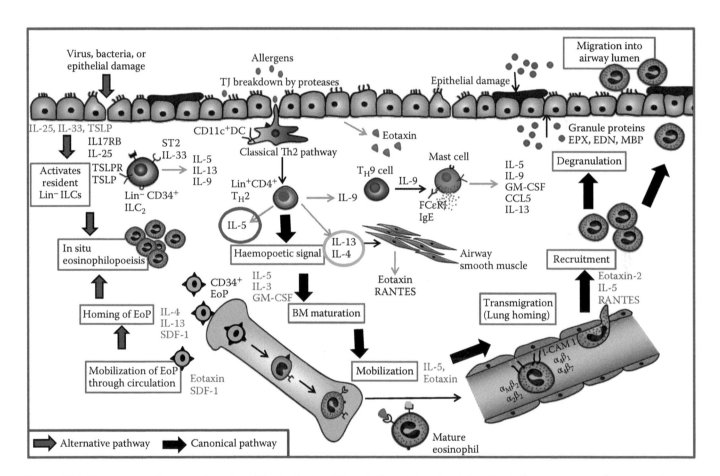

Figure 17.1 Tissue recruitment of eosinophils. In the traditional allergic (or atopic) patient, the exposure of an aeroallergen to the epithelial cells of the airway lumen stimulates the Th2 mediated allergic cascade leading to IgE class switching in the B cell. Upon re-exposure, the allergen binds to the high affinity IgE receptor on the mast cell stimulating degranulation and release of mediators implicated in symptoms of asthma such as bronchoconstriction, mucous production, and edema. The T helper cell also releases the cytokine IL-5, a potent stimulator for the production, recruitment, maturation, and survival of eosinophils within the airway lumen.

In the non-allergic (or non-classical pathway), an exposure (e.g., virus, bacteria, pollutants, allergens) may trigger the release of alarmins (IL-25, IL-33, and TSLP) from the airway epithelium that could lead to the recruitment of eosinophils into the airway. The activation of the innate type 2 lymphoid cells and release of cytokines like IL-5 and IL-13 may also contribute to in-situ eosinophil differentiation in the airway tissues.

Novel anti-eosinophilic biologics and their targets are discussed further in Table 17.1.

Mepolizumab, Reslizumab, and Benralizumab target IL-5. Dupilumab target IL4 and IL13.

the first line of monoclonal therapy in this patient before considering biologics directed against the other Th2 cytokines implicated in severe asthma, as the patient has a history of significant clinical allergies.

The most extensively studied biologic specifically directed against the eosinophil is anti-IL-5. Mepolizumab, reslizumab (both effective in phase 3 clinical trials and approved for clinical use by the FDA and the European Medical Agency), and benralizumab are effective in reducing exacerbations in patients with increased blood or sputum eosinophil counts when high-dose ICSs or oral corticosteroids are ineffective.[26-29] The relative risk reduction in exacerbations for the two approved biologics are comparable (Table 17.1), and they may be effective in patients with eosinophilic asthma[30] independent of the patient's atopic status.[31] Mepolizumab, in an observational study, has also been reported to be effective in patients who have previously been exposed but who have not necessarily failed to improve on omalizumab.[32] Thus, either reslizumab or mepolizumab may be a reasonable choice for this patient if there is inadequate response to therapy with omalizumab. The dose and route of administration of these two biologics may be relevant in patients with severe eosinophilic asthma who are on daily high doses of prednisone. As previously reported, the prednisone-sparing effect of 100 mg subcutaneous (s/c) mepolizumab is less than that of 750 mg intravenous (i/v) mepolizumab, and this may be due to inadequate suppression of local eosinophilopoietic processes.[20,21] However, a direct comparison of s/c, i/v, or body-weight-adjusted versus a fixed dose of monoclonal antibodies may be necessary to resolve this observation in prednisone-dependent patients. It would appear reasonable to start with an s/c-dosing strategy and to switch to i/v dosing if there is insufficient clinical response. The magnitude of improvement reported for FEV_1 seems to be greater with reslizumab, but this is likely to be dependent on how critical eosinophils are to the cause of airflow obstruction rather than the biology of the molecule.[17]

Although there is no direct head-to-head comparative data available, the prednisone-sparing effect of benralizumab seems to be more impressive than that of the other biologics.[33] Despite a 75% reduction in prednisone dose (compared to 25% for placebo), the annualized reduction in rate of asthma exacerbation was 70% for every 8 weeks dosing of 30 mg s/c compared to 32% for every 4 weeks dosing of mepolizumab 100 mg s/c in a similar patient population.[13] The reductions in exacerbation rate of benralizumab in patients with less severe asthma (on lower maintenance doses of corticosteroids) have been less impressive.[34-36] This may have been related to nuances related to patient selection, countries from where patients were recruited, or simply that blood eosinophils (based on which the patients were recruited) in these milder patients may not truly reflect the key effector role of eosinophils in these patients.

Both benralizumab[37] and mepolizumab[38] have also been evaluated in patients with asthma and associated COPD with sputum and blood eosinophilia. Although both drugs were effective in reducing sputum and blood eosinophil count, the effect on FEV_1, and exacerbations were modest compared to previous reports in patients without associated COPD. Thus, it remains to be resolved if anti-IL5 therapies will have the same effect in patients with asthma and COPD (smoker-related bronchitis or emphysema) as those without smoking-related bronchitis. Phase 3 studies of mepolizumab in this patient population have just been completed and have reported modest effect sizes (~14%–18% risk reduction in exacerbations). Further information should be forthcoming.

Other investigational antieosinophil biologics which have reached phase 3 clinical trials but not yet approved by the FDA are anti-IL13 (tralokinumab), anti-IL4R (dupilumab), antithymic stromal lymphopoietin (TSLP), anti-CRTh2,[39,40] in addition to several others, including anti-IL9.[41-43] Nasal polyposis is largely driven by eosinophilic infiltration, and reslizumab has been reported to be more efficacious in those patients with associated sinus disease.[44] Dupilumab is the only biologic that has been specifically evaluated and shown to improve sinus disease outcomes.[45] CRTh2 antagonists also have the potential to be effective in these patients. Another reason for persistent eosinophilia despite treatment with corticosteroid is corticosteroid resistance or insensitivity. Several mechanisms have been suggested to explain this process.[46] The two most examined ones are (a) phosphorylation of the glucocorticoid receptor (GR), which reduces its translocation into the nucleus and therefore impairs corticosteroid responsiveness, and (b) reduction in histone deacetylase 2 (HDAC2) activity resulting in increased acetylation of the GR, which prevents it from inhibiting NF-κB–driven inflammation.[47,48] Several kinases might be involved in the phosphorylation mechanism, such as p38 MAPK-alpha, p38 MAPK-gamma, and JNK1; inhibition of these kinases (e.g., p38 MAPK inhibitor) increases corticosteroid responsiveness.[49] There are several drugs which can increase HDAC2 activity, notably low-dose theophylline, nortriptyline, and macrolides, as well as novel therapies such as inhaled PI3Kd or p38 MAPK inhibitors, which are currently being investigated.[50,51]

In summary, a reasonable treatment strategy for this patient would be to ensure compliance and adequate inhaler therapy,[52] initiate therapy with either omalizumab or one of the anti-IL5 therapies (mepolizumab or reslizumab). Then begin therapy with omalizumab, and if there is inadequate response within 6 months, switch to 100 mg s/c mepolizumab. If this is not effective, switch to three mg/kg i/v reslizumab. However, it is also reasonable based on this patient's clinical presentation to begin treatment with either of these anti-IL5 agents. Benralizumab may be another alternative, when it is approved for clinical use.

17.1.2 DISCUSSION OF CLINICAL VIGNETTE 2

In contrast to the first case scenario, this patient has a history of asthma and associated chronic airflow limitation due to smoker's bronchitis and emphysema. He also has a pleotropic bronchitis manifesting as mixed eosinophilic and neutrophilic bronchitis. In addition, the increase in his total cell count indicates that neutrophilic bronchitis is likely due to an infective etiology.[53] It is important to recognize that peripheral blood examination is not helpful to identify this pleiotropic bronchitis. The role of neutrophils in airway diseases is still not fully understood. It is possible that they release reactive oxygen species and proteases, which have the potential to cause exacerbations and are poorly responsive to corticosteroids. The problem with targeting neutrophils is that they are important cells in combating infection due to their protective role in our innate immune defense system. A common practice for recurrent neutrophilic bronchitis is to use add-on macrolides, which has been found to reduce exacerbation rates[54] and improve quality of life.[55] A recent large study reported impressive results with the use of azithromycin in an unselected group of patients with moderate to severe asthma independent of the type of bronchitis.[56] The mechanism of benefit is still unclear.

More specific antineutrophil-directed therapies such as brodalumab, a human anti-IL17 receptor monoclonal antibody, in initial clinical trials did not demonstrate a significant clinical benefit in patients with moderate to severe asthma.[57] Airway neutrophilia can be reduced by blocking neutrophil attractant chemokines such as CXCL1 (GRO-a), CXCL5 (ENA-78), and CXCL8 (IL8), which are increased in patients with COPD and with severe asthma, especially in patients who smoke. Orally active small molecule antagonists against CXCR2,[58] while effective in reducing circulating and sputum neutrophil counts, do not appear to offer significant clinical benefits in asthma[59,60] or in COPD.[61] The dominant cytokine in patients with pleiotropic bronchitis seems to be IL6.[62] However, it remains to be seen whether antagonism of the IL6-signaling pathway would be beneficial in these patients.

In summary, a reasonable treatment strategy for this patient would be to ensure compliance and adequate inhaler therapy, which may include a LABA and LAMA,[63] in addition to administer empiric therapy with macrolide antibiotics. The patient may be considered for anti-IL5 therapies. If there is inadequate response after 4–6 months, it should be discontinued.

17.2 CONCLUSION

Anti-IL5 therapies are effective in patients with an eosinophilic phenotype, independent of their atopic status, although anti-IgE therapy seems to be the reasonable first option for patients whose airway disease is critically driven by an IgE-mediated allergic pathway. Their role in patients with asthma and associated COPD related to smoking is less well established. In patients with associated sinus disease, anti-IL4R–directed therapy may be a suitable alternative. A prednisone-sparing effect has currently been demonstrated only for mepolizumab. New biologics targeting epithelial alarmins (e.g., IL33, TSLP) and chemokines such as CRTh2 are currently being evaluated. The optimum dose and route of administration of anti-IL5 therapies need further evaluation. There is currently no effective biologic for patients with noneosinophilic asthma, however, IL6- and IL23-directed therapies are likely to be beneficial and merit evaluation in this endotype.

Several antieosinophilic biologic agents are being developed for the treatment of poorly controlled asthma. This list compares the currently available and investigational novel biologic targets based on their efficacy on lung-function improvement, exacerbation reduction, and prednisone-sparing effect. While thus far there are only three FDA-approved agents (omalizumab, mepolizumab, and reslizumab), it is expected that more will be ready for clinical use in the coming years.

ACKNOWLEDGMENT

We thank Dr. Manali Mukherjee for Figure 17.1.

REFERENCES

1. Global Initiative for Asthma Report, Global Strategy for Asthma Management and Prevention 2017. www.ginaasthma.org, accessed 16 Jan 2017.
2. Global Initiative for COPD 2017. www.goldcopd.org, accessed 16 Jan 2017.
3. Barrecheguren M, Esquinas C, and Miravitlles M. The asthma-chronic obstructive pulmonary disease overlap syndrome (ACOS): Opportunities and challenges. *Current Opin Pulm Med.* 2015;21(1):74–79.
4. Gibson PG and Simpson JL. The overlap syndrome of asthma and COPD: What are its features and how important is it? *Thorax.* 2009;64(8):728–735.
5. Dasgupta A, Neighbour H, and Nair P. Targeted therapy of bronchitis in obstructive airway diseases. *Pharmacol Ther.* 2013;140(3):213–222.
6. Postma DS and Rabe KF. The Asthma-COPD overlap syndrome. *N Eng J Med.* 2015;373(13):1241–1249.
7. de V, Tammeling GJ, and Orie NG. Hyperreactivity of the bronchi in bronchial asthma and chronic bronchitis. *Ned Tijdschr Geneeskd.* 1962;106:2295–2296.
8. Ghebre MA, Bafadhel M, Desai D et al. Biological clustering supports both "Dutch" and "British" hypotheses of asthma and chronic obstructive pulmonary disease. *J Allergy Clin Immunol.* 2015;135(1):63–72.
9. Hargreave FE and Parameswaran K. Asthma, COPD and bronchitis are just components of airway disease. *Eur Respir J.* 2006;28(2):264–267.
10. Pizzichini E, Pizzichini MM, Efthimiadis A et al. Measurement of inflammatory indices in induced sputum: Effects of selection of sputum to minimize salivary contamination. *Eur Respir J.* 1996;9(6):1174–1180.

11. Jayaram L, Pizzichini MM, Cook RJ et al. Determining asthma treatment by monitoring sputum cell counts: Effect on exacerbations. *Eur Respir J.* 2006;27(3):483–494.

12. McDonald VM, Higgins I, Wood LG et al. Multidimensional assessment and tailored interventions for COPD: Respiratory utopia or common sense? *Thorax.* 2013;68(7):691–694.

13. Bel EH, Wenzel SE, Thompson PJ et al. Oral glucocorticoid-sparing effect of mepolizumab in eosinophilic asthma. *N Eng J Med.* 2014;371(13):1189–1197.

14. Brasier AR, Victor S, Boetticher G et al. Molecular phenotyping of severe asthma using pattern recognition of bronchoalveolar lavage-derived cytokines. *J Allergy Clin Immunol.* 2008;121(1):30–37.e6.

15. Choy DF, Hart KM, Borthwick LA et al. TH2 and TH17 inflammatory pathways are reciprocally regulated in asthma. *Sci Transl Med.* 2015;7(301):301ra129.

16. Darveau ME, Jacques E, Rouabhia M et al. Increased T-cell survival by structural bronchial cells derived from asthmatic subjects cultured in an engineered human mucosa. *J Allergy clin Immunol.* 2008;121(3):692–699.

17. Hambly N and Nair P. Monoclonal antibodies for the treatment of refractory asthma. *Curr Opin Pulm Med.* 2014;20(1):87–94.

18. Ray A, Raundhal M, Oriss TB et al Current concepts of severe asthma. *J Clin Invest.* 2016;126(7):2394–2403.

19. Mukherjee M and Nair P. Blood or sputum eosinophils to guide asthma therapy? *Lancet Respir Med.* 2015;3(11):824–825.

20. Sehmi R, Smith SG, Kjarsgaard M et al. Role of local eosinophilopoietic processes in the development of airway eosinophilia in prednisone-dependent severe asthma. *Clin Exp Allergy.* 2016;46(6):793–802.

21. Smith SG, Chen R, Kjarsgaard M et al. Increased numbers of activated group 2 innate lymphoid cells in the airways of patients with severe asthma and persistent airway eosinophilia. *J Allergy Clin Immunol.* 2016;137(1):75–86.e8.

22. Nair P and Kraft M. Serum periostin as a marker of T(H)2-dependent eosinophilic airway inflammation. *J Allergy Clin Immunol.* 2012;130(3):655–656.

23. Nair P and O'Byrne PM. Blood eosinophils to guide asthma therapy. *Chest.* 2016;150:485–487.

24. Korevaar DA, Westerhof GA, Wang J et al. Diagnostic accuracy of minimally invasive markers for detection of airway eosinophilia in asthma: A systematic review and meta-analysis. *Lancet Respir Med.* 2015;3(4):290–300.

25. Normansell R, Walker S, Milan SJ et al. Omalizumab for asthma in adults and children. *Cochrane Database Syst Rev.* 2014(1):Cd003559.

26. Castro M, Zangrilli J, Wechsler ME et al. Reslizumab for inadequately controlled asthma with elevated blood eosinophil counts: Results from two multicentre, parallel, double-blind, randomised, placebo-controlled, phase 3 trials. *Lancet Respir Med.* 2015;3(5):355–366.

27. Haldar P, Brightling CE, Hargadon B et al. Mepolizumab and exacerbations of refractory eosinophilic asthma. *N Eng J Med.* 2009;360(10):973–984.

28. Nair P, Pizzichini MM, Kjarsgaard M et al. Mepolizumab for prednisone-dependent asthma with sputum eosinophilia. *N Eng J Med.* 2009;360(10):985–993.

29. Ortega HG, Liu MC, Pavord ID et al. Mepolizumab treatment in patients with severe eosinophilic asthma. *N Eng J Med.* 2014;371(13):1198–1207.

30. Aleman F, Lim H, and Nair P. Eosinophilic endotype of asthma. *Immunol Allergy Clin North Am.* 2016;36:559–568.

31. Ortega H, Chupp G, Bardin P et al. The role of mepolizumab in atopic and nonatopic severe asthma with persistent eosinophilia. *Eur Respir J.* 2014;44(1):239–241.

32. Magnan A, Bourdin A, Prazma CM et al. Treatment response with mepolizumab in severe eosinophilic asthma patients with previous omalizumab treatment. *Allergy.* 2016;71:1335–1344.

33. Nair P, Wenzel S, Rabe KF et al. Oral Glucocorticoid-Sparing effect of benralizumab in severe asthma. *N Engl J Med.* 2017;376:2448–2458.

34. Ferguson GT, FitzGerald JM, Bleecker ER et al. Benralizumab for patients with mild to moderate, persistent asthma (BISE): A randomised, double-blind, placebo-controlled, phase 3 trial. *Lancet Respir Med.* 2017;5:568–576.

35. FitzGerald JM, Bleecker ER, Nair P et al. Benralizumab, an anti-interleukin-5 receptor α monoclonal antibody, as add-on treatment for patients with severe, uncontrolled, eosinophilic asthma (CALIMA): A randomised, double-blind, placebo-controlled phase 3 trial. *Lancet.* 2016;388:2128–2141.

36. Bleecker ER, FitzGerald JM, Chanez P et al. Efficacy and safety of benralizumab for patients with severe asthma uncontrolled with high-dosage inhaled corticosteroids and long-acting β-agonists (SIROCCO): A randomised, multicentre, placebo-controlled phase 3 trial. *Lancet.* 2016;388:2115–2127.

37. Brightling CE, Bleecker ER, Panettieri RA Jr et al. Benralizumab for chronic obstructive pulmonary disease and sputum eosinophilia: A randomised, double-blind, placebo-controlled, phase 2a study. *Lancet Respir Med.* 2014;2(11):891–901.

38. Dasgupta A, Kjaragaard M, Capaldi D et al. A pilot randomized clinical trial of mepolizumab in COPD with eosinophilic bronchitis. *Eur Respir J* 2017; 49(3): pii:1602486.

39. Barnes N, Pavord I, Chuchalin A et al. A randomized, double-blind, placebo-controlled study of the CRTH2 antagonist OC000459 in moderate persistent asthma. *Clin Exp Allergy.* 2012;42(1):38–48.

40. George L and Brightling CE. Eosinophilic airway inflammation: Role in asthma and chronic obstructive pulmonary disease. *Ther Adv Chronic Dis.* 2016;7(1):34–51.

41. Corren J, Lemanske RF, Hanania NA et al. Lebrikizumab treatment in adults with asthma. *N Eng J Med.* 2011;365(12):1088–1098.

42. Gauvreau GM, O'Byrne PM, Boulet LP et al. Effects of an anti-TSLP antibody on allergen-induced asthmatic responses. *N Eng J Med.* 2014;370(22):2102–2110.

43. Wenzel S, Ford L, Pearlman D et al. Dupilumab in persistent asthma with elevated eosinophil levels. *N Eng J Med.* 2013;368(26):2455–2466.

44. Castro M, Mathur S, Hargreave F et al. Reslizumab for poorly controlled, eosinophilic asthma: A randomized, placebo-controlled study. *Am J Respir Crit Care Med.* 2011;184(10):1125–1132.

45. Bachert C, Mannent L, Naclerio RM et al. Effect of subcutaneous dupilumab on nasal polyp burden in patients with chronic sinusitis and nasal polyposis: A randomized clinical trial. *JAMA.* 2016;315(5):469–479.

46. Barnes PJ. Corticosteroid resistance in patients with asthma and chronic obstructive pulmonary disease. *J Allergy Clin Immunol.* 2013;131(3):636–645.

47. Irusen E, Matthews JG, Takahashi A et al. p38 Mitogen-activated protein kinase-induced glucocorticoid receptor phosphorylation reduces its activity: Role in steroid-insensitive asthma. *J Allergy Clin Immunol.* 2002;109(4):649–657.

48. Matthews JG, Ito K, Barnes PJ et al. Defective glucocorticoid receptor nuclear translocation and altered histone acetylation patterns in glucocorticoid-resistant patients. *J Allergy Clin Immunol.* 2004;113(6):1100–1108.

49. Mercado N, Hakim A, Kobayashi Y et al. Restoration of corticosteroid sensitivity by p38 mitogen activated protein kinase inhibition in peripheral blood mononuclear cells from severe asthma. *PLOS ONE.* 2012;7(7):e41582.

50. Ito K, Lim S, Caramori G et al. A molecular mechanism of action of theophylline: Induction of histone deacetylase activity to decrease inflammatory gene expression. *Proc Natl Acad Sci U S A.* 2002;99(13):8921–8926.

51. Mercado N, To Y, Ito K et al. Nortriptyline reverses corticosteroid insensitivity by inhibition of phosphoinositide-3-kinase-delta. *J Pharmacol Exp Ther.* 2011;337(2):465–470.

52. Nair P. Anti-interleukin-5 monoclonal antibody to treat severe eosinophilic asthma. *N Eng J Med.* 2014;371(13):1249–1251.

53. Nair P, Aziz-Ur-Rehman A, and Radford K. Therapeutic implications of 'neutrophilic asthma'. *Curr Opin Pulm Med.* 2015;21(1):33–38.

54. Brusselle GG, Vanderstichele C, Jordens P et al. Azithromycin for prevention of exacerbations in severe asthma (AZISAST): A multicentre randomised double-blind placebo-controlled trial. *Thorax.* 2013;68(4):322–329.

55. Reiter J, Demirel N, Mendy A et al. Macrolides for the long-term management of asthma–a meta-analysis of randomized clinical trials. *Allergy.* 2013;68(8):1040–1049.

56. Gibson PG, Yang IA, Upham JW et al. Effect of azithromycin on asthma exacerbations and quality of life in adults with persistent uncontrolled asthma (AMAZES): A randomised, double-blind, placebo-controlled trial. *Lancet.* 2017;390:659–668.

57. Busse WW, Holgate S, Kerwin E et al. Randomized, double-blind, placebo-controlled study of brodalumab, a human anti-IL-17 receptor monoclonal antibody, in moderate to severe asthma. *Am J Respir Crit Care Med.* 2013;188(11):1294–1302.

58. Donnelly L and Barnes PJ. Chemokine receptor CXCR2 antagonism to prevent airway inflammation. *Drug Fut.* 2011;36:465–472.

59. Nair P, Gaga M, Zervas E et al. Safety and efficacy of a CXCR2 antagonist in patients with severe asthma and sputum neutrophils: A randomized, placebo-controlled clinical trial. *Clin Exp Allergy.* 2012;42(7):1097–1103.

60. O'Byrne PM, Metev H, Puu M et al. Efficacy and safety of a CXCR2 antagonist, AZD5069 in patients with uncontrolled asthma: A randomised trial. *Lancet Respir Medicine.* 2016;4:797–806.

61. Rennard SI, Dale DC, Donohue JF et al. CXCR2 antagonist MK-7123. A phase 2 Proof-of-Concept trial for chronic obstructive pulmonary disease. *Am J Respir Crit Care Med.* 2015;191(9):1001–1011.

62. Chu DK, Al-Garawi A, Llop-Guevara A et al. Therapeutic potential of anti-IL-6 therapies for granulocytic airway inflammation in asthma. *Allergy Asthma Clin Immuno.* 2015;11(1):14.

63. Wedzicha JA, Banerji D, Chapman KR et al. Indacaterol-Glycopyrronium versus Salmeterol-Fluticasone for COPD. *N Engl J Med.* 2016;374:2222–2234.

Endoscopic and surgical treatment for asthma, COPD, and asthma-COPD overlap

DIANE TISSIER-DUCAMP, A. BOURDIN, ALAIN PALOT, CÉLINE TUMMINO, LAURIE PAHUS, AND PASCAL CHANEZ

Despite recent improvements in the pharmacological arsenal for asthma and chronic obstructive pulmonary disease (COPD), including new long-acting muscarinic antagonists (LAMA) long-acting β_2-agonists (LABA) combinations for COPD and biologics for severe asthma, many patients remain uncontrolled, causing a major burden both for the patient and for the health-care system.[1] However, in addition to current medical therapies, novel endoscopic and surgical treatments have been developed and are emerging as important therapies for many of these challenging patients.

One example of these newer treatments is bronchial thermoplasty (BT), which has been developed and became available in the last decade. BT has been shown to improve quality of life and control of asthma in some patients.[2] On the other hand, endoscopic lung reduction using coil placement may bring some relief in exercise-induced breathlessness, and subsequently improve exercise tolerance and quality of life in COPD patients with high levels of static hyperinflation (residual volume [RV] > 220%).[3] If asthma-COPD overlap (ACO) represents a real overlap between asthma and COPD,[4] one can question the potential for these interventions to help those patients with residual symptoms and disability despite current treatments.

In this chapter, we provide three vignettes of patients: one with COPD, one with asthma, and a third one descriptive of a more complex clinical situation. The patient with COPD was treated with coil insertion, and the other two received bronchial thermoplasty. For the last vignette, we evaluate the potential for coils in a patient described initially as suffering from severe asthma.

18.1 COPD

18.1.1 INTRODUCTION

COPD is defined by permanent and progressive airways obstruction.[5] Pulmonary emphysema may decrease the elastic retraction forces and induce exaggerated expiratory bronchiolar collapse involved in thoracic distension.[6] Dyspnea in COPD is considered to be a consequence of such distension, which initially appears during intense exercise but could become disabling and dramatically impair quality of life.

Currently, very few treatments effectively decrease pulmonary distension and improve symptoms during exercise: pharmacological treatments face a maximal plateau effect[7] and surgical lung volume reduction only gets utilized in highly selected patients with major distension and heterogeneous emphysema. The risk of morbidity and mortality of such a surgery remains substantial, and this technique is now progressively being abandoned worldwide.[8] Accordingly, less-invasive techniques have been developed. At this time, unidirectional valves and coils are the most advanced devices in their clinical development. Unidirectional valves are devices that are inserted during bronchoscopy. Because of their shape, they are opening only during expiration, whereas they remain closed during inspiration leading to progressive deflation of the treated lobe. The main issue with this technique is related to the frequent existence of collateral ventilation usually seen in patients with incomplete scissors likely implicated in reinflation of the treated lobe—and, in the end, in the absence of clinical benefit. This issue can be addressed through a barometer device (called Chartis) used during bronchoscopy, which can determine whether important collateral ventilation will preclude success. These devices are developed in emphysematous lungs, and they improved forced expiratory volume in one second (FEV_1) and forced vital capacity (FVC) by respectively 140 (95% CI: 55–225) and 370 mL (95% CI: 107–588 mL) in the Dutch randomized controlled trial, whereas six-minute walking test distance gained 76 m (47–100) over the control group. Safety issues are a real cause for concern since some death, pneumothorax, device migration, or a requirement for replacement or removal occurred in the treated groups.[9–11]

Insertion of shaped-memory coils during bronchoscopy is more dedicated to increase lung elastic recoil forces through increased tensing of the upper lobes. One French and one American randomized controlled trial demonstrated clinical benefits of uncertain magnitude as a greater improvement in the six-minute walking test distance in the treated arms vs. control was respectively by +21 m (95% CI −4 to infinite) and +14.6 m (97.5% CI 0.4 to infinite).[3,12] Because many other endobronchial techniques are currently developed, a meta-analysis aimed at giving pooled results, but, as expected, heterogeneity precludes clarity of the conclusion.[13,14]

18.1.2 DISCUSSION

Endoscopic lung volume reduction is a promising technique that provides hope to patients and physicians. Patients suffering from COPD, particularly severe emphysema, have impaired quality of life due to disabling dyspnea during exercise related to pulmonary distension. Very few available conventional treatments are highly effective and safe for severe COPD. The endobronchial lung volume reduction with coils seems to be hopeful as an appropriate procedure for the most severe patients. However, benefits obtained from this treatment are inconsistent from one study to another, and, as described previously, discrepancies exist between United States and European Union experiences.[3,12] Mandatory improvements are required to predict a positive treatment response but also to define its mechanisms of action. Real life cost-effectiveness is another issue that requires further assessment. Although short-term adverse effects are now well described, long-term issues need to be assessed, and this will require the development of rigorously organized registries.

Currently, bronchodilator reversibility, a feature of asthma, has been considered an exclusion criteria for participating in clinical trials on lung volume reduction. Indeed, variability of airway obstruction is a mandatory

CLINICAL VIGNETTE 18.1

A 72-year-old COPD patient with severe emphysematous lung changes but no exacerbations presents for further evaluation. He had no relevant medical history except for a smoking history of 30 pack years; he stopped smoking 5 years earlier. The patient describes major impairment of his quality of life related to daily disabling dyspnea with the slightest effort. Clinical examination showed a distended lung with a barrel chest, pursed-lips breathing indicating a high level of intrinsic positive expiratory pressure consistent with his excessive distal airway collapsibility, and chest distention. Chest X-ray showed hyperinflation consistent with COPD (see Figure 18.1). Pulmonary function testing revealed severe nonreversible obstructive impairment: FEV_1/FVC: 0.50, FEV_1 = 0.70 L (28% predicted value) associated with major chest distention; functional residual capacity (FRC): 6.77 L (198% predicted value); residual volume (RV): 6,53 L (259%); arterial blood gas at rest while breathing room air showed pH of 7.42, PaO_2 of 70 mmHg, and $PaCO_2$ of 38 mmHg. The six-minute walking test demonstrated exercise-induced oxygen desaturation (from 90% to 84%) while covering 441 m. Borg dyspnea scale changed from 5/10 at baseline to 10/10 at the end of the effort.

Management was optimized in this weaned-from-smoking patient and included a pharmacological treatment combining a long-acting β_2-agonist and a long-acting muscarinic antagonist agent in conjunction with a long-term rehabilitation program. Because of his major quality of life alteration closely related to symptoms during exercise and because he was too old for a lung transplant, he was enrolled in the REVOLENS clinical trial, which compared the efficacy and safety of coils with pharmacological treatment compared to pharmacological treatment alone on exercise-induced symptoms. The patient met the eligibility criteria: severe bilateral symptomatic emphysema, FEV_1 < 50%, RV > 220% postbronchodilators, and currently enrolled in a respiratory rehabilitation program. The patient underwent a first bronchoscopy procedure for placement of nine coils in the left lobe without incident during the procedure, and 6 weeks later, the patient underwent a second bronchoscopy with contralateral placement of nine coils inserted in the right upper lobe without incident short or long term. Anterior-posterior chest X-ray (Figure 18.2) shows correct placement of the coils in both lower lobes.

Several months later, the patient reported a reduction of symptoms during exercise and an improvement in quality of life. Pulmonary function testing before and after the endoscopic procedure (Table 18.1) showed no significant improvement: FEV_1/FVC = 46%, FEV_1 = 0.71 L (28%), decreased pulmonary distension (FRC: = 6.29 [183%], RV = 5.39 [214%]), and the six-minute walking test remained unchanged. The chest and computed tomography (CT) scan (Figure 18.3) showed the spirals in the two upper lobes.

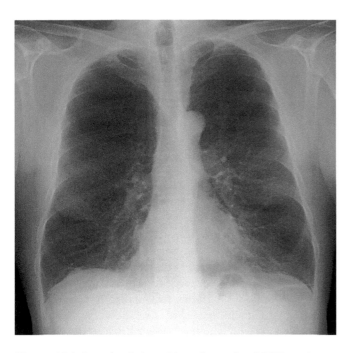

Figure 18.1 Standard chest X-ray from the COPD patient before intervention distention and destruction of the lung parenchyma.

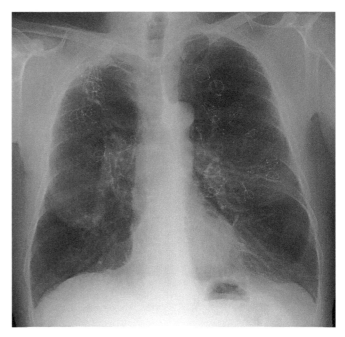

Figure 18.2 Standard chest X-ray from the COPD patient after intervention showing the spirals in the 2 upper lobes.

Table 18.1 Pulmonary function assessment before and after endoscopic treatment

	Dyspnea	PBD FEV$_1$	FEV/VC	CRF	RV	TM6 d	TM6 desat
Before	At rest	28%	46%	198%	259%	441 m	84%
12 m	At rest	28%	47%	168%	190%	401 m	87%
24 m	At rest	29%	57%	185%	238%	378 m	88%

PBD FEV$_1$: Post bronchodilator FEV$_1$
CRF: Residual functional capacity
RV: Residual volume
TM6 d: Walked distance in 6 minutes
TM6 desat: Maximal *desaturation* during 6 min walk test

criterion to confirm asthma diagnosis, as stated in the last Global Initiative for Asthma (GINA) update,[4] although it is commonly observed to be difficult to demonstrate in the most severe cases. Even though asthma per se is not a good indication for coils, clinical situations in which distension and static hyperinflation can be documented as predominantly relying on emphysematous changes of the lung and decreased elastic recoil forces—and not only as a consequence of airways obstruction—may potentially overcome this feeling.

Alternatives such as lung volume reduction surgery (LVRS) and lung transplantation are worth discussing with such patients. Now a robust experience of LVRS is available, and more than 1600 patients could be pooled in the last meta-analysis.[15] Improved selection criteria and greater experience in expert centers are key points likely to explain how it could go over the negative results of the National Emphysema Treatment Trial (NETT).[16] Safety concerns are still to be addressed especially in nonexpert centers, as this technique is rarely performed.

COPD is a more frequent indication for lung transplantation, probably because other conditions benefited from medical improvements. Comorbidities and age (and this was an issue for the present patient) are important hurdles in this area, and long-term survival benefits are debated.[8,17]

18.2 ASTHMA

18.2.1 INTRODUCTION

Severe asthma continues to represent a major challenge for clinicians. New treatment strategies and approaches are urgently needed for these patients. Appropriate patient selection is paramount when considering any new treatment modality, be it pharmacological or device-based. Bronchial thermoplasty (BT), is a nonpharmacological, device-based therapy that delivers controlled thermal energy to the

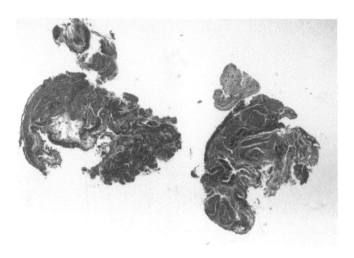

Figure 18.3 Endobronchial biopsies obtained from the severe asthma patient before bronchial thermoplasty displaying the important contribution of bronchial smooth muscle bundlles in the submucosa.

airway walls through a series of three bronchoscopic procedures.[18] It was approved in 2010 by the U.S. Food and Drug Administration (FDA) for the treatment of severe persistent asthma in patients 18 years and older whose asthma is not well controlled with inhaled corticosteroids (ICS) and long-acting β_2-agonists (LABAs), and it has been European Medicines Agency (EMA)–approved in Europe since 2011. The clinical-development program consisted of five main clinical trials, four in subjects with asthma, and three were randomized. The largest sham-controlled, device-based clinical trial in severe asthma, the Asthma Intervention Research 2 (AIR2) Trial,[2,19,20] has recently published five-year efficacy and safety data. Several studies demonstrated its potential mechanisms of action and the relationships between clinical efficacy and structural changes.[21-23] Indeed, even though the debate is still open, decreased smooth muscle layer thickness and, more unexpectedly, decreased neuroendocrine cell contingency within the airway epithelium were shown as the most obvious structural changes explaining how it works.[22,24-26] The short- and long-term safety have been investigated with no severe adverse events despite more than 1000 patients having been treated in clinical trials and real life at present. Few cases of hemoptysis and pneumothoraces have been reported and were managed without major persistent harm or negative outcomes for the patients.

CLINICAL VIGNETTE 18.2

A sea carpenter born in 1964 began to suffer from asthma in 2004. His asthma was uncontrolled from the time of diagnosis, leading to numerous hospitalizations and emergency room visits. He had no significant past medical history, family history, or comorbid conditions. He was a past smoker with a cumulative smoking history of less than 10 pack years. He was not able to work any longer due to his severe asthma. His main complaint was an intractable cough resistant to all treatments and leading to rib fractures. In 2014 he was on maximal treatment, receiving 2000 μg ICS: Fluticasone, 200 μg Salmétérol, and 44 μg glycopyrronium, 48 μg LABA/LAMA, and 40 mg oral prednisone daily. He was dyspneic after brief exercise and had 12 emergency room visits during the last year. He was wheezy at rest, and the asthma-control questionnaire score was always higher than two at each outpatient visit. Despite several therapeutic trials with drugs including methotrexate, cyclosporine, and omalizumab, his asthma remained uncontrolled. His condition deteriorated despite high daily doses of oral corticosteroids, leading to bilateral cataracts and severe osteoporosis. His lung function demonstrated persistent airflow obstruction, with an FEV_1 of 25% (0.850 liter) (6% postbronchodilator reversibility) with an $FEV_1/FVC < 0.7$, a normal diffusing capacity of the lungs for carbon monoxide (D_LCO), and an RV at 120% of predicted value. A six-minute walking test was not associated with oxygen desaturation despite marked dyspnea. Imaging of the airways by CT scan displayed only thickening of the airway walls without emphysema, and there was no evidence of significant bronchiectasis or interstitial lung disease. No relevant triggers for his symptoms were identified. Fiberoptic bronchoscopy showed some features of bronchomalacia, and endobronchial biopsies showed minimal inflammatory cell infiltrates but increased bronchial smooth muscle mass > 15% of the submucosal area on 10 biopsies (Figure 18.3). Despite long-term azithromycin treatment (at a similar regimen than in the azithromycin for prevention of exacerbations in severe asthma [AZISAST] study)[27] and continuous positive airway pressure (CPAP) during the night, because a moderate, obstructive sleep apnea syndrome was documented (Apnea-Hypopnea Index [AHI] of 17 hours, mostly related to hypopnea, without any central event), his asthma remained uncontrolled. The patient was considered eligible for BT. Three sessions were administered, without any adverse event. One year after the last session, his asthma was improved but still uncontrolled with an ACQ = 1.5; OCS requirement was decreased to 20 mg a day, and he experienced only one exacerbation during the follow-up without ER requirement. His quality of life improved mainly due to the disappearance of his intractable cough, and his FEV_1 improved to 65% (2.21 L, +1.150 L compared to previous assessment) (Table 18.2). This benefit on this outcome was sustained at 24 months, even though he still required OCS and ICS/LABA combination therapy, as unacceptable symptoms relapsed with OCS tapering. A follow-up CT scan of the chest revealed no significant changes before and 12 months after bronchial thermoplasty (Figure 18.4).

Table 18.2 Clinical symptoms and lung function evaluations before and after bronchial thermoplasty

| | Control | | | CS mg median | | | |
	ACQ	ER/Hosp	EXA	dose	PBD FEV$_1$	Cough	TM6
Before	2.5	12	14	40	40%	+++	400 m
12 m	2	0	6	30	60%	+	NA
24 m	2	0	3	20	65%	±	420 m

ACQ: Composite score of control: Asthma control questionnaire
ER/Hospitalizations: Emergency/hospitalization visits and stays
EXA: Exacerbations requiring increase in systemic corticosteroids
CS: Systemic corticosteroids
PBD: Post bronchodilator FEV$_1$
TM6: Distance walked during 6 minutes

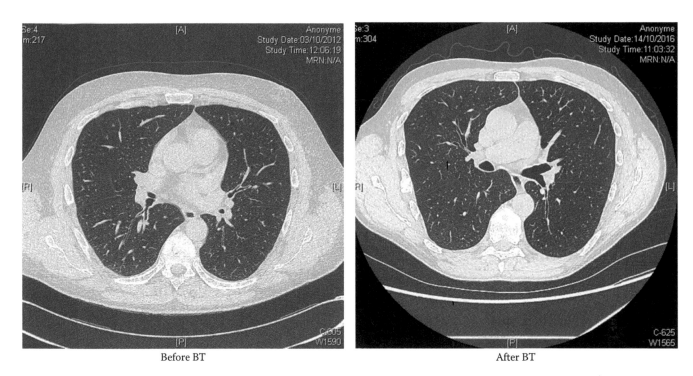

Before BT   After BT

Figure 18.4 Chest CT scan slides obtained from the severe asthma patient showing some increase in the airway wall before and 12 months after bronchial thermoplasty without any major change.

18.2.2 DISCUSSION

In severe asthma, the armamentarium of potential new treatments is increasing. However, first, it is important to secure the diagnosis of asthma, assess adherence to the prescribed medications, and investigate and treat potential environmental triggers, as well as comorbid conditions, according to current guidelines. This initial assessment often takes 6 to 12 months as reported in the 2014 European Respiratory Society (ERS)/American Thoracic Society (ATS) Task Force.[28] While novel biologics targeting interleukin 5 have been recently approved, BT has also been approved for potential use in uncontrolled severe asthmatics.[29] The mechanisms underlying its efficacy have been recently studied. BT in severe asthmatics reduces airway smooth muscle (ASM) area, but also mucosal and ASM-associated nerve endings, neuroendocrine epithelial cells, and, to a lesser extent, bronchial smooth muscle thickening.[22,30,31] These effects correlate with asthma control with fewer exacerbations, hospitalizations, and intensive care unit (ICU) admissions for asthma, decreased Asthma Control Test and Asthma-Related Quality of Life Questionnaire scores, and reduced requirement of OCS. In most of the studies, BT failed to reduce airway obstruction. The present severe asthma vignette is a good illustration of the potential success of this new approach. The short- and long-term safety aspects have been reported with minimal tolerance problems.[2] Despite its effect on airway structure, particularly on the bronchial smooth muscle, the absence of effect on lung function is surprising and worth discussion. First, the causality and correlation between structural changes and lung function are not clearly established. Second, the benefit on asthma control and exacerbations is perhaps dissociated, with no functional improvement, possibly reflecting a decreased in airway responsiveness, as reported by Cox[32] in mild to moderate asthma. It can be hypothesized that decreased airway smooth muscle mass will reduce the extent of exaggerated bronchoconstriction and also limit severity of airflow obstruction, in the case of an exacerbation; it can also help in daily living activities. In other terms, ASM reduction is likely related to an increased PD20. Unfortunately, the permanent airway obstruction observed in severe asthma patients with low baseline FEV_1 values, and sometimes the impossibility to withdraw bronchodilators for adequate duration may preclude the assessment of airway hyperresponsiveness in these severe asthma patients with greatly impaired airflow. Third, as shown in some imaging reports,[21] a diffusion of the thermal effect seems to occur in bronchi distal to the treated segments, as evidenced by ground-glass hyperdensities, visible in the untreated middle lobe or any treated lobe or segment. The measurement of parameters linked to distal airways may represent a potential outcome to assess BT efficacy.[33] The last question with BT is its place in the treatment algorithm of severe asthma, as several biologics are also available to treat this condition. In our experience, which is similar to the patient in the vignette, most of these patients with severe asthma have been previously exposed to one or two biologics directed against a T2-related phenotype. Treatment failure after 4–6 months may require consideration of a new biologic or shifting to BT. Lastly, non T2 or noneosinophilic severe asthma represents a major challenge for specialists who manage asthma, and, therefore, a patient with this phenotype represents a potential target for BT. However, more mechanistic research is needed to identify the optimal patients most suitable for BT, as that will save time, reduce false hopes, and save money for patients and society.

18.3 ASTHMA-COPD OVERLAP (ACO)

18.3.1 INTRODUCTION

Chronic airway diseases have been recognized to be heterogeneous for a long time. Most chest physicians have reported cases of smoking asthmatics with a full recovery of their lung function after a short course of corticosteroids. On the other hand, some patients with asthma may display a fixed component of airway obstruction even though they were

CLINICAL VIGNETTE 18.3

This patient suffered from asthma at the age of 20 when finishing his university curriculum to become an engineer. Asthma was mainly related to the presence of a cat where he lived with several fellow students. He was born prematurely and had a cardiac abnormality (aortic coarctation), which was corrected at age 5. This last intervention was complicated by a transient pneumothorax with a full recovery. No specific respiratory disease was found in his family. His childhood and adolescence was free of health concerns, and he was able to ski and enjoy his family life. He never smoked and did not drink. After graduating as an engineer, he worked in an alpine resort. He was able to exercise normally and received an ICS/LABA prescription treatment for asthma from his chest physician between 2006 and 2011. His best FEV_1 during this period was 70% of predicted value. After a flu episode in the winter of 2011, his condition deteriorated, and his asthma became uncontrolled despite treatment. After this episode, he experienced twice-yearly exacerbations requiring systemic corticosteroids. Despite the addition of a LAMA, azithromycin, and omalizumab, his best FEV_1 values remained below 40%. The investigation found no major trigger or comorbid conditions, and his adherence to treatment was estimated to be excellent. His RV was 180%, and he was able to complete exercise on a bicycle in the laboratory. FEV_1 values varied between 25% and 40% during or after exacerbations. His blood eosinophil count was below 300 eosinophils/µl, and total IgE count was less than 120 KIU/L. There were no criteria for allergic bronchopulmonary aspergillosis (ABPA) or vasculitis. No macroscopic abnormality was found at endoscopy, and the pathological report of bronchial biopsies described pauci-inflammatory wall infiltration with increased smooth muscle mass (Figure 18.5). The patient was deemed eligible for a BT trial. Three sessions were applied during a 3-month period, with hemoptysis as a serious adverse event leading to a hospitalization after one of the procedures. One year after the last session, his asthma was better controlled, and the patient reported only one exacerbation during the follow-up without ER requirement. Improvement in quality of life was mainly attributed to the exacerbation-rate reduction, whereas FEV_1 was still severely impaired, measured at 35% of predicted value (Table 18.3). At 24 months the patient reported two exacerbations, and his maximal achievable FEV_1 was 28%, but his exercise capacity remained reduced. The RV was 220% at maximal bronchodilation. Chest CT scan was reassessed, and several cysts and centrilobular emphysema lesions were described, resulting in a possible diagnosis of Langerhans cell histiocytosis being finally confirmed (Figure 18.6). At this stage, endoscopic lung volume reduction was evaluated as a therapeutic option for this patient who previously received BT. BT in this patient did not lead to a major improvement in quality of life but did result in a reduction in exacerbation. On the other hand, the increased RV and the CT scan aspect suggested the potential benefit for endoscopic reduction of emphysema. The history and follow-up of this patient supports the coexistence of features of both asthma and COPD.

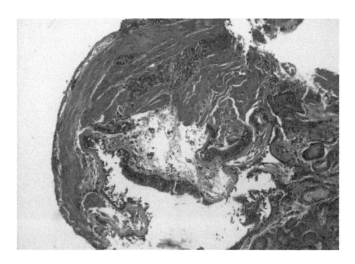

Figure 18.5 Endobronchial biopsies obtained from ACO phenotype asthma patient before bronchial thermoplasty displaying the important contribution of bronchial smooth muscle bundles in the submucosa.

never smokers. The combination of clinical and functional features of asthma and COPD has led to the concept of ACO.[34] The origin of the condition is still controversial. GINA and GOLD guidelines acknowledged this, and promoted the acronym of ACO instead of ACOS—because the association is evident, whereas "syndrome" suggested that a new entity should be distinguished. Furthermore, current case definitions may confuse the understanding of this syndrome by general practitioners who manage asthma and COPD.

18.3.2 DISCUSSION

Postma and Rabe underlined the need for better defining and characterizing ACO, as illustrated by the variability of definitions used in available studies.[34] The main concern is related to the need to establish a consensus definition for ACO in the field of chronic disorders. One may question the heterogeneity of these diseases and the need to add another

Table 18.3 Clinical and pulmonary function testing before and after bronchial thermoplasty in an ACO patient

	Control ACQ	ER/Hosp	EXA	CS mg median dose	PBD FEV$_1$	Cough	TM6
Before	1.5	0	4	0	30%	0	NA
12 m	1	0	2	0	34%	0	NA
24 m	1	0	2	0	37%	0	NA

ACQ: Composite score of control: Asthma Control Questionnaire
ER/Hospitalizations: Emergency/hospitalization visits and stays
EXA: Exacerbations requiring increase in systemic corticosteroids
CS: Systemic corticosteroids
PBD: Post bronchodilator FEV$_1$
TM6: Distance walked during 6 minutes

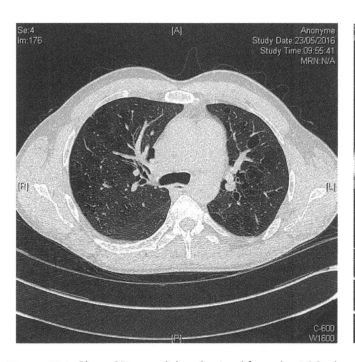
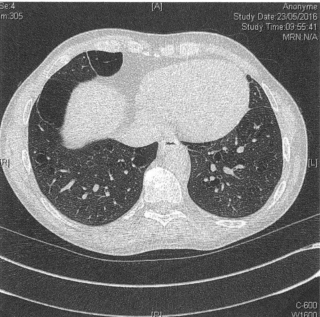

Figure 18.6 Chest CT scan slides obtained from the ACO phenotype asthma patient after bronchial thermoplasty showing some emphysema lesions; the initial imaging was identical.

entity, with the potential to reduce confusion among specialists, primary care physicians, and patients. Regarding these diseases, it is important to better understand their underlying mechanisms and design treatments that address the main mechanism(s) responsible for daily symptoms and future negative risks. In the case of our patient, the history suggests a diagnosis of asthma with both variable but reversible symptoms and significant FEV_1 improvement after inhaling a bronchodilator, even though it did not return to normal. BT was an option when omalizumab failed and the endobronchial biopsies displayed an increase in smooth muscle mass. We can argue that the morphological changes on CT scan and the persistent airflow obstruction with increased RV may warrant endoscopic treatment of emphysema. Whether patients with ACO exhibit worse outcomes than those with COPD only is an area of debate. There are no real options than to follow cohorts of well-characterized patients and to integrate new outcomes, such as imaging and inflammatory markers to assess and understand the natural history of these patients. We are just beginning to consider the role of early events during lung development and early life on the overall picture of the patient with a chronic airway disorder.

18.4 CONCLUSION

Chronic airway disorders are clearly heterogeneous respiratory diseases. As we try to integrate more rapidly into current care the most recent knowledge acquired from research on respiratory disease mechanisms in order to choose the best treatment options, we are facing new challenges. First, precise and multiscale phenotyping criteria are now obtainable in routine practice, and this increases the likelihood of finding overlapping features. In fact, we don't perfectly know how to weigh different traits and which thresholds should drive treatment choices. Second, the availability of many different therapeutic options highlights the need for more complex and frequently updated treatment algorithms. In our experience, endoscopic treatments for bronchial diseases should be performed in specialized centers with a progressive approach and while integrating research and innovative treatment options. This is the only way to better understand the efficacy/tolerance ratio of new therapies and to provide them to the right patient at the right time.

REFERENCES

1. Demoly P, Annunziata K, Gubba E et al. Repeated cross-sectional survey of patient-reported asthma control in Europe in the past 5 years. *Eur Respir Rev Off J Eur Respir Soc.* Mar 1, 2012;21(123):66–74.

2. Wechsler ME, Laviolette M, Rubin AS et al. Bronchial thermoplasty: Long-term safety and effectiveness in patients with severe persistent asthma. *J Allergy Clin Immunol.* December 2013;132(6):1295–302.

3. Deslée G, Mal H, Dutau H et al. Lung volume reduction coil treatment vs Usual care in patients with severe emphysema: The REVOLENS randomized clinical trial. *JAMA.* January 12, 2016;315(2):175–184.

4. Global Strategy for Asthma Management and Prevention, Global Initiative for Asthma (GINA;last updated April 2015. Available at: http://www.ginasthma.org. [Internet]. Available at http://www.ginasthma.org

5. GOLD - the Global initiative for chronic Obstructive Lung Disease [Internet]. [cited April 4, 2016]. Available at http://www.goldcopd.org/guidelines-global-strategy-for-diagnosis-management.html

6. McDonough JE, Yuan R, Suzuki M et al. Small-airway obstruction and emphysema in chronic obstructive pulmonary disease. *N Engl J Med.* October 27, 2011;365(17):1567–1575.

7. Wedzicha JA, Banerji D, Chapman KR et al. Indacaterol-Glycopyrronium versus Salmeterol-Fluticasone for COPD. *N Engl J Med.* June 9, 2016;374(23):2222–2234.

8. Marchetti N and Criner GJ. Surgical approaches to treating emphysema: Lung volume reduction surgery, bullectomy, and lung transplantation. *Semin Respir Crit Care Med.* August 2015;36(4):592–608.

9. Klooster K, ten Hacken NHT, Hartman JE et al. Endobronchial valves for emphysema without interlobar collateral ventilation. *N Engl J Med.* December 10, 2015;373(24):2325–2335.

10. Davey C, Zoumot Z, Jordan S et al. Bronchoscopic lung volume reduction with endobronchial valves for patients with heterogeneous emphysema and intact interlobar fissures (the BeLieVeR-HIFi study): A randomised controlled trial. *Lancet Lond Engl.* September 12, 2015;386(9998):1066–1073.

11. Herth FJF, Eberhardt R, Gompelmann D et al. Radiological and clinical outcomes of using Chartis™ to plan endobronchial valve treatment. *Eur Respir J.* February 2013;41(2):302–308.

12. Sciurba FC, Criner GJ, Strange C et al. Effect of endobronchial coils vs Usual care on exercise tolerance in patients with severe emphysema: The RENEW randomized clinical trial. *JAMA.* May 24, 2016;315(20):2178–2189.

13. Van Agteren JE, Hnin K, Grosser D et al. Bronchoscopic lung volume reduction procedures for chronic obstructive pulmonary disease. *Cochrane Database Syst Rev.* 23, 2017;2:CD012158.

14. Shah PL, Herth FJ, van Geffen WH et al. Lung volume reduction for emphysema. *Lancet Respir Med.* February 2017;5(2):147–156.

15. Van Agteren JE, Carson KV, Tiong LU et al. Lung volume reduction surgery for diffuse emphysema. *Cochrane Database Syst Rev*. October 14, 2016;10:CD001001.

16. Fishman A, Martinez F, Naunheim K et al. A randomized trial comparing lung-volume-reduction surgery with medical therapy for severe emphysema. *N Engl J Med*. May 22, 2003;348(21):2059–2073.

17. ISHLT: The International Society for Heart & Lung Transplantation [Internet]. [cited June 10, 2017]. Available at http://www.ishlt.org/registries/slides.asp?slides=heartLungRegistry

18. Trivedi A, Pavord ID, Castro M. Bronchial thermoplasty and biological therapy as targeted treatments for severe uncontrolled asthma. *Lancet Respir Med*. July 2016;4(7):585–592.

19. Cox G, Thomson NC, Rubin AS et al. Asthma control during the year after bronchial thermoplasty. *N Engl J Med*. March 29, 2007;356(13):1327–1337.

20. Thomson NC, Rubin AS, Niven RM et al. Long-term (5 year) safety of bronchial thermoplasty: Asthma Intervention Research (AIR) trial. *BMC Pulm Med*. Feb 11, 2011;11:8.

21. Debray M-P, Dombret M-C, Pretolani M et al. Early computed tomography modifications following bronchial thermoplasty in patients with severe asthma. *Eur Respir J*. March 2017;49:1601565.

22. Pretolani M, Bergqvist A, Thabut G et al. Effectiveness of bronchial thermoplasty in patients with severe refractory asthma: Clinical and histopathologic correlations. *J Allergy Clin Immunol*. April 2017;139(4):1176–1185.

23. Boulet L-P, Laviolette M. Acute effects of bronchial thermoplasty: A matter of concern or an indicator of possible benefit to small airways? *Eur Respir J*. March 2017;49:1700029. DOI: 10.1183/13993003.00029-2017.

24. Pretolani M, Dombret M-C, Thabut G et al. Reduction of airway smooth muscle mass by bronchial thermoplasty in patients with severe asthma. *Am J Respir Crit Care Med*. Dec 15, 2014;190(12):1452–1454.

25. Bonta PI, d' Hooghe J, Sterk PJ et al. Reduction of airway smooth muscle mass after bronchial thermoplasty: Are we there yet? *Am J Respir Crit Care Med*. May 15, 2015;191(10):1207–1208.

26. Kirby M, Ohtani K, Lisbona RML et al. Bronchial thermoplasty in asthma: 2-year follow-up using optical coherence tomography. *Eur Respir J*. September 1, 2015;46(3):859–862.

27. Brusselle GG, Vanderstichele C, Jordens P et al. Azithromycin for prevention of exacerbations in severe asthma (AZISAST): A multicentre randomised double-blind placebo-controlled trial. *Thorax*. April 2013;68(4):322–329.

28. Chung KF, Wenzel SE, Brozek JL et al. International ERS/ATS guidelines on definition, evaluation and treatment of severe asthma. *Eur Respir J*. February 2014;43(2):343–373.

29. Dombret M-C, Alagha K, Boulet LP, Brillet PY, Joos G, Laviolette M, et al. Bronchial thermoplasty: A new therapeutic option for the treatment of severe, uncontrolled asthma in adults. *Eur Respir Rev Off J Eur Respir Soc*. December 2014;23(134):510–518.

30. Chakir J, Haj-Salem I, Gras D et al. Effects of Bronchial Thermoplasty on Airway Smooth Muscle and Collagen Deposition in Asthma. *Ann Am Thorac Soc*. November 2015;12(11):1612–1618.

31. Salem IH, Boulet L-P, Biardel S et al. Long-Term Effects of Bronchial Thermoplasty on Airway Smooth Muscle and Reticular Basement Membrane Thickness in Severe Asthma. *Ann Am Thorac Soc*. August 2016;13(8):1426–1428.

32. Cox G, Miller JD, McWilliams A et al. Bronchial thermoplasty for asthma. *Am J Respir Crit Care Med*. May 1, 2006;173(9):965–969.

33. Bommart S, Marin G, Molinari N et al. Club cell secretory protein serum concentration is a surrogate marker of small-airway involvement in asthmatic patients. *J Allergy Clin Immunol*. January17, 2017;140(2):581–584.

34. Postma DS and Rabe KF. The Asthma-COPD Overlap Syndrome. *N Engl J Med*. Septembre 24, 2015;373(13):1241–1249.

19

Supplemental oxygen and pulmonary rehabilitation for chronic obstructive pulmonary disease (COPD), asthma, and asthma-COPD overlap

RALPH J. PANOS

19.1 INTRODUCTION

The asthma-chronic obstructive pulmonary disease (COPD)-overlap (ACO) is a recently described clinical phenotype for individuals with features of both asthma and COPD.[1] Although both disorders are characterized by airway inflammation and eosinophils, type 2 helper T lymphocytes predominate in asthma, whereas neutrophils and CD8 lymphocytes prevail in COPD.[1] Despite these pathophysiologic differences, the clinical manifestations of asthma and COPD are very similar, with multiple overlapping/intersecting respiratory symptoms and physiologic derangements, including breathlessness, wheezing, airflow obstruction with bronchodilator responsivity, and bronchial hyperresponsiveness. Because

these clinical manifestations and pulmonary physiologic abnormalities overlap, it is often difficult or impossible to determine the underlying process. Furthermore, pharmacologic management of asthma and COPD utilizes the same medications, albeit in very different sequences: both use short-acting β_2-agonists for urgent relief, but the initial mainstay of asthma management is inhaled corticosteroids whereas, in COPD, utilization of anticholinergics and long-acting β_2-agonists precedes the use of corticosteroids. The pharmacologic treatment of ACO is discussed in Chapter 16. In this chapter, we will discuss the use of supplemental oxygen and pulmonary rehabilitation. Because of the lack of prospective, randomized trials of these interventions in ACO, general principles and the use of supplemental oxygen and pulmonary rehabilitation in asthma and COPD are discussed.

CLINICAL VIGNETTE 19.1: SUPPLEMENTAL OXYGEN AND COPD

A 59-year-old man transferred his care from the private sector to the Veterans Health Administration (VHA) in the United States. He had been diagnosed several years ago with COPD after smoking up to three packs per day and stopping 1 year ago. He experiences shortness of breath when walking up one flight of steps, 1/3 mile on level ground, and with activities of daily life, such as bathing and dressing. He has intermittent wheezing and a cough productive of white to gray phlegm with no blood. He had pneumonia about 8–10 years ago and has frequent episodes of bronchitis treated with antibiotics and oral corticosteroids. He was hospitalized approximately 3–4 months ago for respiratory distress after breathing cooking fumes. He worked as a boiler technician in military service, where he was exposed to asbestos, and has also worked as an auto mechanic and commercial/residential/industrial electrician. He snores at night, and his former wife noted apneic events. He awakens at night with shortness of breath and gasping. Although he does not have a morning headache, he frequently awakens feeling tired and drowsy. He feels fatigued throughout the day and falls asleep watching TV or talking with someone but not with driving. Other medical disorders include cardiac disease with placement of coronary artery stents, hypertension, hyperlipidemia, diabetes, and chronic kidney disease. His medications include aspirin, 81 mg daily; carvedilol, 12.5 mg twice daily; glipizide, 5 mg daily; lisinopril, 5 mg daily; omeprazole, 20 mg daily; pravastatin, 40 mg daily; nebulized albuterol/ipratropium, 3–4 times daily; and budesonide 160/formoterol 4.5 mcg, 2 puffs twice daily.

His height is 66 inches and weight is 219 pounds. Vital signs are blood pressure of 107/75 mmHg, pulse of 73 beats/minute, respiratory rate at 18 breaths per minute, and SpO_2 of 86% while breathing room air. Head, ears, nose, and throat exams are normal and the Mallampati Score is class 4. Chest is hyperresonant to percussion. Breath sounds are diminished throughout with poor air movement, and there are no wheezes, rales, or rhonchi. Auscultation of the chest reveals normal heart sounds and no murmurs or gallops. His abdomen is soft and nontender, with normally active bowel sounds. Extremities show a well-healed surgical scar on the right arm but no clubbing, cyanosis, or edema. Neurological examination is normal.

Pulmonary function tests are shown in Table 19.1. Chest radiographs reveal hyperinflation, increased retrosternal airspace, flattened diaphragms, and parenchymal hyperlucency (Figure 19.1).

Table 19.1   Clinical vignette 19.1: Pulmonary function tests

Spirometry	Prebronchodilator			Postbronchodilator	
	Actual	Predicted	% Predicted	Actual	% Predicted
FVC (l)	3.2	3.61	90	3.58	99
FEV$_1$(l)	0.89	2.91	31	1.11	38
FEV$_1$/FVC (%)	27			31	
Lung volumes					
TLC (l)	6.97	6.18	113		
RV (l)	3.72	2.07	180		
Diffusing capacity					
DLCO (mL/min/mmHg)	6.70	30.03	22		

Abbreviations: DLCO, diffusing capacity; FVC, forced vital capacity; FEV$_1$, forced expiratory volume in 1 second; l, liters; RV, residual volume; TLC, total lung capacity.

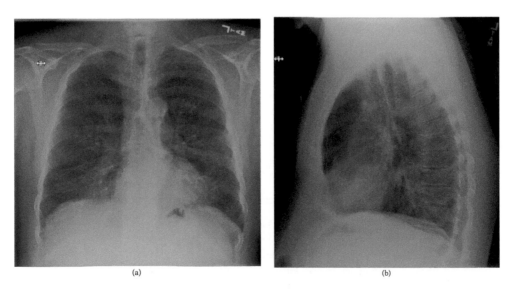

(a)   (b)

Figure 19.1 **(a)** Anteroposterior chest radiograph, **(b)** Lateral chest radiograph. Chest radiographs reveal hyperinflation, increased retrosternal airspace, flattened diaphragms, and parenchymal hyperlucency.

Supplemental oxygen was titrated to 3 liters per minute (l pm) to maintain a resting SpO_2 at 93% and prevent exertional desaturations. A polysomnography study revealed obstructive sleep apnea with a respiratory disturbance index (RDI) of 26.6 events per hour but no central apneas. The SpO_2 dropped to a nadir of 80% while breathing room air. There were no periodic limb movements. He was started on bilevel noninvasive ventilation, IPAP 14 cm H_2O and EPAP 8 cm H_2O with 3 lpm supplemental oxygen, which prevented nocturnal desaturations during sleep and reduced the RDI to three events per hour.

CLINICAL VIGNETTE 19.2: SUPPLEMENTAL OXYGEN AND ASTHMA

A 22-year-old man with a history of asthma since early childhood presents to the emergency room (ER) with increasing respiratory distress that started early in the day after exposure to charcoal smoke at a barbeque. He has used at least 10 puffs of his albuterol rescue inhaler with no relief. His asthma had been well controlled with budesonide/formoterol, which he uses twice daily, plus normally less than 2–4 puffs of his albuterol weekly. He sleeps through the night and has been able to exercise regularly with no respiratory limitations. He has not been to the ED or hospitalized for his asthma. Previously, he was diagnosed with hay fever and has seasonal oculorhinitis, which he treats with over-the-counter medications. He is taking no other medications and has had no other medical disorders.

He is in respiratory distress with audible wheezes. Heart rate is 132, respiratory rate is 28, blood pressure is 155/90, and SpO_2 is 88%. He is using accessory muscles to breathe. Chest auscultation reveals diffuse wheezing but poor air movement and tachycardia. Peak flow cannot be performed reliably. A portable chest radiograph reveals hyperinflation and no parenchymal opacification, and an arterial blood gas demonstrates pH of 7.39, PCO_2 of 35, and PO_2 of 53. Due to the impending respiratory failure suggested by ineffectual ventilation evidenced by a near normal PCO_2 despite a respiratory rate of 28, bilevel noninvasive ventilation with IPAP 12 and EPAP 6 cm H_2O with 4 LPM supplemental oxygen is initiated with concurrent intravenous corticosteroids and albuterol nebulized treatments. Within 6 hours, his respiratory distress is gone, and he is breathing comfortably with no further wheezing. The bilevel noninvasive ventilation is discontinued and supplemental oxygen is titrated to maintain his $SpO_2 >$ 92%. After 12 hours, his supplemental oxygen is titrated down to room air and he is discharged home with an oral corticosteroid taper.

CLINICAL VIGNETTE 19.3: PULMONARY REHABILITATION AND COPD

A 68-year-old man is experiencing exertional breathlessness after walking less than 50 yards. The shortness of breath causes him to limit his exertion and his travel outside of the home. Very occasionally, he notes a whistling sensation in his chest. He also has a chronic cough productive of small amounts of white phlegm with no hemoptysis. He has had several episodes of bronchitis treated with antibiotics and corticosteroids over the past 2 years but has not been seen in the ER or hospitalized for respiratory reasons. He never had pneumonia, tuberculosis, or known tuberculosis exposure. He smoked two to three packs per day for nearly 45 years, and he quit smoking 8 years ago. He was diagnosed with COPD nearly 10 years ago. Other medical diagnoses include hypertension, hyperlipidemia, diabetes with peripheral neuropathy and microalbuminuria, atrial flutter treated with ablation, and gout. Supplemental oxygen was started 4 years ago for resting hypoxemia. He is currently using 3 LPM continuously. Other medications include albuterol, 2 puffs as needed (he rarely uses his albuterol); budesonide 160/formoterol 4.5 mcg, 2 puffs twice daily; cholecalciferol, 1000 units daily; diltiazem, 240 mg daily; gabapentin, 400 mg thrice daily; glipizide, 15/20 mg morning/night; lisinopril, 10 mg daily; pravastatin, 80 mg daily; saxagliptin, 5 mg daily; allopurinol 150 mg daily; and tiotropium, 18 mcg daily.

His height is 72 inches, and weight is 260 pounds. Vital signs are blood pressure of 145/77 mmHg, pulse at 93 beats/minute, respiratory rate at 16 breaths per minute, and SpO_2 of 93% breathing 3 LPM oxygen. Head, ears, nose, and throat exam is normal. Chest is barrel-shaped and resonant to percussion. Breath sounds are diminished throughout, and there are no wheezes, rales, or rhonchi. Auscultation of the chest reveals normal heart sounds and no murmurs or gallops. Abdomen is soft and not tender with normally active bowel sounds. There is no clubbing, cyanosis, or edema. Sensation is diminished in the lower extremities.

Chest radiograph is shown in Figure 19.2 and shows hyperinflation with increased anterior-posterior diameter, paucity of lung markings in the apices, and mild linear opacifications in the bases. A chest CT scan showing apical centrilobular emphysema is shown in Figure 19.3. Pulmonary function test results are presented in Table 19.2.

Based on his persistent respiratory symptoms despite maximal pharmacologic treatment and supplemental oxygen, he was referred to pulmonary rehabilitation and completed a 12-week program of exercise and education. Pulmonary rehabilitation metrics, pre-, post-, 6 months, and 12 months after the program are shown in Table 19.3. During the course of pulmonary rehabilitation, his exercise capacity increased and his daily activity level at home also improved. With diabetes, diet, and exercise education, his fasting blood glucose dropped from more than 300 to 170–195.

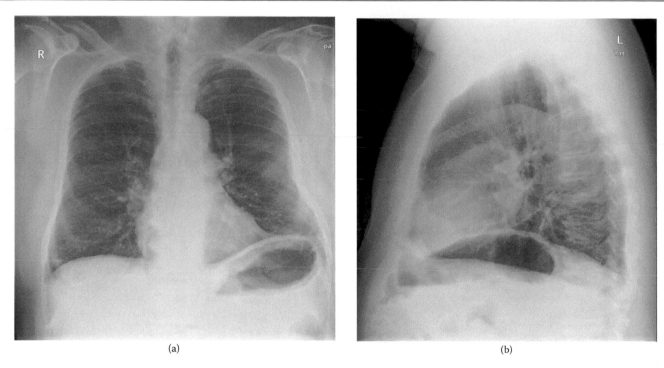

(a) (b)

Figure 19.2 **(a)** Anteroposterior chest radiograph, **(b)** Lateral chest radiograph. Chest radiographs shows hyperinflation with increased anterior-posterior diameter, paucity of lung markings in the apices, and mild linear opacifications in the bases.

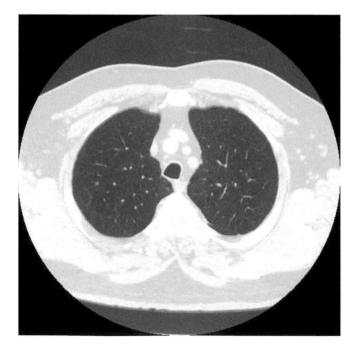

Figure 19.3 Chest computed tomography (CT) scan. CT scan shows apical centrilobular emphysema.

Table 19.2   Clinical vignette 19.3: Pulmonary function tests

Spirometry	Prebronchodilator				Postbronchodilator	
	Actual	Predicted	% Predicted	LLN	Actual	% Predicted
FVC (l)	3.27	4.83	68	3.86	3.41	71
FEV$_1$(l)	1.63	3.59	45	2.77	1.94	54
FEV$_1$/FVC (%)	50	74	67	64	57	77
Lung volumes						
TLC (l)	6.92	7.43	93	6.03		
ERV (l)	0.80	1.15	70			
RV (l)	3.53	2.60	136	1.78		
Diffusing capacity						
DLCO (mL/min/mmHg)	12.87	25.43	51	15.75		

Abbreviations: DLCO, diffusing capacity; ERV, expiratory reserve volume; FVC, forced vital capacity; FEV$_1$, forced expiratory volume in 1 second; l, liters; LLN, lower limit of normal; RV, residual volume; TLC, total lung capacity.

Table 19.3   Clinical characteristics before and after pulmonary rehabilitation

Metric	Pre-PR	Post-PR immediate	Post-PR 6 months	Post-PR 12 months
SABA use (puffs/week)	0	7	0	0
Respiratory hospitalization	0	0	0	0
Respiratory ER visits	0	0	0	0
Questionnaires				
UCSD SOB	50	35	38	7
HADS anxiety	7	6	6	4
HADS depression	12	11	8	3
PHQ-9	8	6	0	16
SGRQ	65	55	44	34
Dartmouth COOP	19	23	21	25
CAT	21	16	15	15
Pulmonary Knowledge Test	80	95	70	95
MMRC	3	2	2	2
BODE	5	3	3	3
Weight	259	248	250	238
Waist circumference	51	49.5	50	49.25
BMI	35.1	33.6	33.9	32.3
6MWD				
Distance	590	932	945	1000
Minimal SpO$_2$	88%	91%	89%	89%
Maximal HR	126	96	117	84

Abbreviations: BMI, body mass index; BODE, BODE Index (body mass index, airflow obstruction, dyspnea, exercise); CAT, Chronic Obstructive Pulmonary Disease Activity Test; Dartmouth COOP, Dartmouth Cooperative Functional Assessment Charts; ER, emergency room; HADS, Hospital Anxiety and Depression Scale; HR, heart rate; 6MWD, 6 minute walk distance; MMRC, Modified Medical Research Council Dyspnea Scale; PHQ-9, Patient Health Questionnaire 9; PR, pulmonary rehabilitation; SABA, short acting β_2-agonist; SGRQ, Saint George's Respiratory Questionnaire; SpO$_2$, peripheral capillary oxygen saturation; UCSD SOB, University of California San Diego Shortness of Breath Questionnaire.

CLINICAL VIGNETTE 19.4: PULMONARY REHABILITATION AND ASTHMA

A 31-year-old woman with a history of lifelong asthma presents to her primary care physician after starting an exercise program for weight reduction but not being able to exercise for more than 5 or 10 minutes before developing mild chest tightness and wheezing relieved with 2 puffs of albuterol. Her asthma has been well controlled with low-dose inhaled corticosteroids, and she normally only uses her albuterol once or twice monthly. She last presented to the ER with asthma symptoms at age 14, and she was hospitalized once at age 8 but never required intensive care or intubation. Her usual exacerbating factors are mold, mildew, and fragrant odors, which she avoids. Her blood pressure is slightly elevated at 148/90, and her weight has been increasing to a BMI of 29, due mainly to inactivity.

Pulmonary rehabilitation is prescribed, and she begins a graduated-exercise program. Prior to exercising, she uses two puffs of albuterol and acclimates to the exercise environment for 5 minutes with a brisk walk. With this pre-exercise regimen, she is able to progress through the 12-week pulmonary rehabilitation program, increasing her exercise capacity to 30 minutes walking on a treadmill with no wheezing or respiratory limitation. Upon completion of the rehabilitation program, she continues the pre-exercise conditioning regimen, and expands and intensifies her workout routine. After 6 months, she is able to reduce her BMI to 24 and is now able to exercise rigorously for an hour or more.

19.2 SUPPLEMENTAL OXYGEN AND COPD

More than 1 million patients with COPD in the United States use Medicare-reimbursed long-term supplemental oxygen therapy at an annual cost of $2 billion.[2] Supplemental oxygen improves survival in patients with hypoxemia at rest ($PaO_2 < 55$ torr or $SpO_2 < 88\%$; or $PaO_2 < 60$ and > 55 torr with evidence of cor pulmonale).[3,4] The mechanisms by which supplemental oxygen improve mortality are not known.[5] Oxygenation should be measured on room air at rest, with exertion, and during sleep, after the administration of supplemental oxygen to insure that desaturation is prevented. Although Medicare and many insurance plans reimburse for supplemental oxygen during exercise or at night with evidence of exercise or nocturnal desaturation, there is no substantive evidence that supplemental oxygen during exercise or at night is beneficial in individuals with stable COPD (Table 19.4).

19.3 RESTING HYPOXEMIA

Supplemental oxygen was the first therapy demonstrated to prolong survival in individuals with COPD and resting hypoxemia. This evidence was generated in two landmark, randomized, controlled trials performed in the 1970s, the Nocturnal Oxygen Treatment Trial (NOTT)[3] and the Medical Research Council (MRC) study.[4]

Table 19.4 U.S. medicare oxygen reimbursement guidelines

Patient condition	PaO$_2$	SpO$_2$
Awake, at rest	≤ 55 mm Hg or 56–59 mm Hg and dependent edema or cor pulmonale or pulmonary hypertension by right heart catheterization or echocardiogram or P pulmonale on ECG (P wave > 3 mm in leads II, III, or AVF) or erythrocythemia (HCT > 56%)	≤ 88% or = 89% and dependent edema or cor pulmonale or pulmonary hypertension by right heart catheterization or echocardiogram or P pulmonale on ECG (P wave > 3 mm in leads II, III, or AVF) or erythrocythemia (HCT > 56%)
Exercise	≤ 55 mm Hg and documentation that use of supplemental oxygen ameliorates the decline in oxygen levels (Duration of desaturation and type/level of exertion are not specified.)	≤ 88% mm Hg and documentation that use of supplemental oxygen ameliorates the decline in oxygen levels (Duration of desaturation and type/level of exertion are not specified.)
Sleep	≤ 55 mm Hg or PaO$_2$ declines > 10 mm Hg from awake, resting level and dependent edema or cor pulmonale or pulmonary hypertension by right heart catheterization or echocardiogram or P pulmonale on ECG (P wave > 3 mm in leads II, III, or AVF) or erythrocythemia (HCT > 56%) (Duration of desaturation and type/level of exertion are not specified.)	≤ 88% or SpO$_2$ declines > 5% from awake, resting level and dependent edema or cor pulmonale or pulmonary hypertension by right heart catheterization or echocardiogram or P pulmonale on ECG (P wave > 3 mm in leads II, III, or AVF) or erythrocythemia (HCT > 56%) (Duration of desaturation and type/level of exertion are not specified.)

Source: Modified from Panos, R.J., *Management of Stable Chronic Obstructive Pulmonary Disease.* RJ Panos and WL Eschenbacher, eds. COPD Primer. DeGruyter; February, 2016. http://www.degruyter.com/view/product/468864.

The MRC study examined whether supplemental oxygen for 15 or more hours daily (including overnight use) compared with no oxygen for at least 3 years affected the survival of 87 subjects (66 men and 21 women) who were < 70 years old with airflow obstruction (FEV_1 < 1.2 L) and a room air resting PaO_2 of 40–60 mm Hg.[4] Oxygen was delivered by nasal cannula, usually at 2 L/minute (or higher if needed to achieve a PaO_2 > 60 mm Hg). Study participants had severe COPD with mean FEV_1 of 0.76 L (men) and 0.58 L (women), PaO_2 of 49–52 torr, PCO_2 of 56–59 torr, mild pulmonary hypertension, and mean pulmonary artery pressure of 33–35 mmHg. Supplemental oxygen improved longevity, 55% survival in the oxygen group compared with 33% survival in the control group. The survival advantage was evident from the start of the study in women, but only became evident in men after about 500 days. For men, the risk of death after 500 days appeared to be constant, 12% annually in participants receiving oxygen and 29% annually in the control group, whereas, for women, the risk of death from study enrollment was 5.7% annually in subjects receiving oxygen and 36.5% in controls. Most patients died suddenly at home during the night of presumed respiratory failure. The mean pulmonary artery pressure and red cell mass declined slightly in men surviving for > 500 days and receiving supplemental oxygen compared with the control group. Supplemental oxygen did not appear to alter the decline in other physiologic variables, work time, or exacerbations.[4]

NOTT[3] compared continuous supplemental oxygen with nocturnal oxygen treatment in 203 subjects with optimally treated COPD, resting hypoxemia (PaO_2 ≤ 55 torr or ≤ 59 torr), and at least one of edema, hematocrit ≥55%, or electrocardiographic evidence of P pulmonale (3 mm P waves in leads II, III, aVf). Resting oxygen measurements were obtained twice over a three-week, exacerbation-free observation period. Individuals who had received oxygen therapy in the previous 2 months for 30 days or more were excluded. Only about 20% (203 of 1043) of screened subjects were eligible for participation in the study; interestingly, 21% of the excluded individuals experienced an elevation in arterial PaO_2 with optimal treatment during the observation period, which increased their oxygen to a level that prevented enrollment. The two groups had similar physiologic characteristics with severe airflow obstruction, hypoxemia, and minimal hypercarbia and pulmonary hypertension. The nocturnal treatment group averaged 12.0 h/d of oxygen use and the continuous treatment group used supplemental oxygen for an average of 17.7 h/d. Over the average 19.3 months of study participation, the relative risk of death for the nocturnal oxygen treatment group was 1.94 (95% confidence limits, 1.17, 3.24). The 12- and 24-month mortality rates were 20.6 ± 4.0% versus 11.9 ± 3.2%, and 40.8 ± 5.5% versus 22.4 ± 4.6%, continuous versus nocturnal treatment, respectively. Significant decreases in hematocrit and pulmonary vascular resistance but not in other physiologic variables occurred in the continuously treated group compared with the nocturnal group.[3]

19.4 MILD RESTING OR NOCTURNAL HYPOXEMIA

Other studies of supplemental oxygen therapy in individuals with COPD and mild resting hypoxemia or nocturnal desaturation have not demonstrated improvements in survival. Gorecka and colleagues[6] studied 135 individuals with severe airflow obstruction (mean FEV_1 of 0.83L), mild resting hypoxemia PaO_2 of 56–65 torr randomized to treatment with supplemental oxygen to increase the PaO_2 to at least 65 torr for at least 17 hours daily, or no treatment. The cumulative survival rate was 88% at one year, 77% at 2 years, and 66% at 3 years, and there were no differences in survival between the two groups over the mean observation period of 40.9 months. Additionally, longer oxygen use (>15 hours daily) did not improve survival[6].

The recently completed Long-Term Oxygen Treatment Trial (LOTT) was a large prospective study enrolling 738 patients with COPD and either moderate resting hypoxemia (SpO_2 of 89%–93%) or moderate exercise desaturation (SpO_2 < 90% for ≥ 10 seconds and ≥ 80% for ≥ 5 minutes while walking) randomized to supplemental oxygen (long-term oxygen treatment [LTOT]) or conventional room air.[7] Patients with resting desaturation randomized to LTOT were prescribed 24-hour oxygen; patients with only exercise desaturation randomized to LTOT were prescribed oxygen during exercise and sleep. Participants were followed for at least one year and up to 6 years. There was no difference in the principal outcome, time to death, or first hospitalization (hazard ratio = 0.94, 95% confidence interval [CI] [0.79, 1.12], P = 0.52) and no difference in rates of all hospitalizations (rate ratio = 1.02, 95% CI [0.92, 1.14]), COPD exacerbations (rate ratio = 1.09, 95% CI [0.99, 1.20]), and COPD-related hospitalizations (rate ratio = 0.99, 95% CI [0.84, 1.18]). There were no consistent differences in measures of quality of life, lung function, or six-minute walking test. This study found that in patients with stable COPD and moderate resting hypoxemia or exertional desaturation, supplemental oxygen did not improve survival or any other measured outcome and, thus, raises the question whether supplemental oxygen treatment benefits these individuals.[7]

Chaouat and coworkers[8] studied the effect of nocturnal supplemental oxygen in 76 individuals with moderate to severe airflow obstruction, mild to moderate daytime hypoxemia (PaO_2, 56–69 torr), and nocturnal desaturation (defined as SpO_2 < 90% for ≥ 30% of sleep time). All subjects underwent polysomnography studies to exclude obstructive sleep apnea. During the mean follow-up period of 35.1

± 14.3 months, the mortality rate was similar in the two groups, 22% (9 of 41) of subjects receiving nocturnal oxygen and 20% (7 of 35) of control subjects. The same proportion of subjects required institution of continuous supplemental oxygen, 12 (29%) in the nocturnal oxygen group and 10 (29%) in the control group. Further, there were no differences in pulmonary vascular hemodynamics between the two groups. Based on these results, the investigators concluded that nocturnal oxygen therapy in isolation should not be prescribed for individuals with COPD and nocturnal desaturation.[8]

19.5 EXERTIONAL DESATURATION

There is no uniform definition of exertional desaturation or standardized exercise protocol to elicit decreases in oxygen levels in individuals with COPD. The most widely used clinical threshold for exertional hypoxemia in individuals with chronic stable COPD is defined by the Centers for Medicare and Medicaid Services (CMS) as a $PaO_2 \leq 55$ mmHg or an arterial oxygen saturation $\leq 88\%$ measured during exercise.[9] In studies of supplemental oxygen in exertional desaturation, investigators have used different absolute values or relative decrements for varying durations in either oxygen tension or saturation to define exertional desaturation. Examples of various definitions include $PaO_2 \leq 55$ mmHg or ≤ 8–8.5 kPa (1 kPa = 7.5 mmHg), $SpO_2 \leq 88\%$–90%, and relative declines in $SpO_2 > 2\%$–5%. Measurements beyond these absolute thresholds or relative declines are considered significant. Oxygenation is dynamic and not constant during exertion, and, therefore, some studies require a desaturation below a threshold value be maintained for a specified duration to be considered significant. Finally, the type and intensity of activity, activities of daily living, six-minute walking test, treadmill walk, step test or shuttle exercise, and incremental maximal or steady-state cycle ergometry may affect exertional desaturation.[5]

A retrospective analysis of 7700 patients with COPD who were prescribed supplemental oxygen revealed that 1425 (18.5%) had a resting $PaO_2 > 8$ kPa (60 mmHg) and, therefore, were assumed to have either nocturnal or exercise-related desaturation as the indication for prescribed supplemental oxygen treatment.[10] These patients had a similar longevity to patients with COPD and resting hypoxemia, PaO_2 between 6.7–8 kPa (50–60 mmHg), who were also treated with supplemental oxygen but a lower survival rate compared with a gender- and age-matched general population. The eight-year survival of 471 participants in the National Emphysema Treatment Trial with resting normoxemia and exertional desaturation ($SpO_2 < 90\%$ during a seven-minute treadmill walk) who received medical management was similar among individuals treated with continuous, intermittent, or no oxygen.[11]

Exercise performance in individuals with COPD who are normoxemic at rest but who desaturate with exertion may be improved with supplemental oxygen.[12,13] Breathlessness declined and distance walked increased with supplemental oxygen compared with room air during the six-minute walking test in 11 patients with COPD (mean FEV_1 of 0.9 l, a resting SaO_2 of 94.7%, and a mean minimal exertional SaO_2 of 84.8%).[13] Further, the training work rate increased more rapidly, and the maximal workload achieved and level of endurance were greater in 29 patients with COPD and resting normoxemia treated with supplemental oxygen compared with compressed air during 7 weeks of high-intensity cycle ergometer exercise.[14] Supplemental oxygen in concentrations up to 50% reduces respiratory rate and dynamic hyperinflation during exercise in patients with COPD and mild hypoxemia.[15] However, other studies have not demonstrated significant improvements in the exercise capacity of patients with exertional desaturation treated with supplemental oxygen.[16–18] A meta-analysis of supplemental oxygen use during exercise training in patients with COPD concluded that oxygen did not increase exercise training benefits and recommended any exercise program, with or without oxygen supplementation.[19]

Supplemental oxygen improves health-related quality of life in individuals with COPD and exertional desaturation.[20] 28 of 50 (68%) patients with COPD (mean FEV_1 % predicted of 25.9 ± 8.0, resting PaO_2 of 9.2 ± 1.0 kPa, and SpO_2 after six-minute walking test of 82 ± 5.4%) increased their distance in the six-minute walking test (≥ 54 m) or decreased their Borg dyspnea scale (≥ 1) during a 12-week double-blind, randomized, crossover trial.[20] Health-related quality of life measured by the Chronic Respiratory Questionnaire; levels of anxiety and depression determined by the Hospital Anxiety and Depression Scale; and general health, physical, and emotional states measured by the Short Form (36) Health Survey also improved. However, despite these benefits, nearly half (41%) of the responders preferred not to continue supplemental oxygen after the study. Supplemental oxygen may alleviate cerebral desaturation during exertion and maintain cognitive function.[21]

19.6 SHORT-BURST OXYGEN

In the United Kingdom, short-burst oxygen (intermittent use of oxygen for short periods before or immediately after exertion) is frequently used to ameliorate dyspnea.[22–27] Although earlier studies suggested that short-burst oxygen alleviated breathlessness and potentially increased the distance walked in 6 minutes[28–30] more recent studies show that short-burst oxygen prior to or immediately after exertion does not reduce dyspnea or increase the distance walked in 6 minutes.[31–34] A meta-analysis showed that short-burst oxygen therapy does not decrease dyspnea, and its effect on other parameters, such as exercise capacity, oxygen saturation, and other ventilatory parameters is not consistent.[26]

19.7 ADVERSE EFFECT OF SUPPLEMENTAL OXYGEN

Although usually considered benign, supplemental oxygen may have untoward effects. Fires may be started by lighters, cigarettes, stoves, or even cell phones.[35-38] A review of 3673 admissions to a burn center showed that 27 (0.74%) were related to supplemental oxygen[39] and 34 of 38 (89%) of deaths associated with fires related to supplemental oxygen occurred in individuals who were smoking while using supplemental oxygen.[40] There is also preliminary evidence that oxygen treatment may increase lower airway oxidative stress and inflammation.[41]

Supplemental oxygen does not improve survival in patients with COPD and mild resting hypoxemia and does not appear to reduce the mortality of patients with exertional desaturation. Use of oxygen in individuals with COPD and exertional desaturation has variable and inconsistent effects on exercise capacity, dyspnea, and health-related quality of life.[42]

19.8 OXYGEN AND ASTHMA

Because asthma is principally a disorder of the airways, alveolar gas exchange capacity is limited only during asthma exacerbations that significantly perturb airflow and cause ventilatory limitations to oxygenation and possibly perfusion due to hypoxemic vasoconstriction. Derangements in ventilation and perfusion during severe asthma exacerbations may cause hypoxemia and hypercarbia. Chronic supplemental oxygen is rarely, if ever, required in the management of asthma. During acute exacerbations, oxygenation should be monitored by pulse oximetry and supplemental oxygen instituted to maintain the SpO_2 greater than 90%. Hypercarbia leading to respiratory acidosis requires measurement of the arterial PCO_2 and pH with an arterial blood gas. Elevated PCO_2 or reduced pH (signifying respiratory academia) suggest severe disease and potential impending respiratory failure. Oxygen should be administered to maintain the $SpO_2 > 90\%$ regardless of the PCO_2 or pH. End tidal CO_2 monitoring may be beneficial to detect CO_2 retention and worsening respiratory failure that might require intubation and mechanical ventilation.[43,44]

Heliox, a mixture of helium and oxygen, usually at a ratio of 20:80 or 30:70, may be used in nebulizer treatments during severe asthma exacerbations.[45] The lower density of Heliox compared to air/oxygen mixtures causes less turbulent flow in the larger airways therby reducing resistance and potentially improving ventilation for better medication and oxygen delivery. Heliox reduces the sensation of breathlessness and hospitalization rates while increasing peak expiratory flow rates, and it may decrease the work of breathing, but it has not been shown to diminish intubation rates during asthma exacerbations.[46,47]

19.9 PULMONARY REHABILITATION

Pulmonary rehabilitation is a multidisciplinary program of education and exercise that teaches patients with respiratory disorders about their disease, its management including pharmacological and nonpharmacological therapies, and mechanisms to cope with respiratory symptoms and their effects on daily activities, as well as an exercise and conditioning program. Individuals with COPD and other respiratory disorders tend to decrease their physical activity over time; this reduction in activity leads to loss of both muscle mass and tone, reducing the capacity for exercise and daily activities.[48,49] This process leads to a gradual downward spiral of "the less one does, the less one is capable of doing" that culminates in being housebound and socially estranged from family and friends.

The American Thoracic Society/European Respiratory Society Task Force on Pulmonary Rehabilitation defined pulmonary rehabilitation as "a comprehensive intervention based on a thorough patient assessment followed by patient-tailored therapies, which include, but are not limited to, exercise training, education, and behavior change, designed to improve the physical and psychological condition of people with chronic respiratory disease and to promote the long-term adherence of health-enhancing behaviors."[50,51] Pulmonary rehabilitation is a multimodality intervention that may include exercise, education, motivational interviewing, instruction about the underlying respiratory disorder and its treatment, nutritional counseling, and advanced-care planning delivered by an interdisciplinary team that may include physicians, nurses, physical therapists, respiratory therapists, occupational therapists, nutritionists, and social workers. These programs are usually developed for individuals with COPD but may include nearly all respiratory disorders, and can be utilized at nearly any point in the course of disease with salubrious, beneficial effects on respiratory symptoms, overall well-being and quality of life, improved exercise capacity, and reduced healthcare utilization (Table 19.5).[50-52]

Pulmonary rehabilitation has the best effects when it is integrated into a comprehensive management program that encourages behavior change and a shift from provider-initiated to patient-initiated care. For those with COPD, pulmonary rehabilitation improves respiratory symptoms.[53,54] In addition to improving respiratory symptoms, pulmonary rehabilitation decreases health-care utilization and may improve survival.[55] Patients with COPD who maintain physical activity have less breathlessness with exertion, better health-related quality of life, improved long-term function and independence, and better psychological and physiological function. Physical inactivity is associated with worse survival, increased risk of respiratory-related hospitalization, lower self-reported health status, and greater systemic inflammation.[56] Home-based pulmonary rehabilitation programs have the same benefits as hospital-based programs.[57,58]

Table 19.5 Potential benefits of pulmonary rehabilitation

Diminished respiratory symptoms, especially
breathlessness

Enhanced exercise capacity and endurance

Increased activity and function

Improved understanding of the underlying respiratory
disorder and its management

Boost in overall well-being and quality of life

Enhanced self-efficacy and sense of control over disease
and destiny

Less depression and anxiety

Reduction in health-care utilization

Better survival, especially after hospitalization for a
COPD exacerbation

Source: Adapted from Nici L and ZuWallack R., *Semin. Respir. Crit. Care Med.*, 36(4), 567–574, 2015.

19.10 PULMONARY REHABILITATION AND COPD

A large 2015 Cochrane analysis of 65 randomized controlled trials of pulmonary rehabilitation in individuals with COPD concluded that, based on its beneficial effects on respiratory symptoms and health-related quality of life, further comparison studies of pulmonary rehabilitation and conventional management are no longer warranted.[53,54] Instead, the authors suggested that future pulmonary rehabilitation studies should concentrate on the determination of the critical elements of pulmonary rehabilitation programs that confer these benefits; the optimal program length, location, intensity, and level of supervision required; and the duration of benefits and best use of maintenance or reprisal of program participation. This analysis showed that pulmonary rehabilitation improved all four quality of life domains measured by the Chronic Respiratory Questionnaire—dyspnea, fatigue, emotional function, and mastery—and these effects all exceeded the minimal clinically important difference (dyspnea 0.79 [0.56, 1.03], fatigue 0.68 [0.45,0.92], emotional function 0.56 [0.34,0.78], mastery 0.71 [0.47,0.95], and mean difference [95% confidence interval]) (McCarthy 2015). The improvement in the overall St. George's Respiratory Questionnaire, −6.89 (−9.26, −4.52) and all of its individual domains exceeded the minimal clinically important difference (−4). Pulmonary rehabilitation improved both maximal and functional exertional capacity.

Exercise capacity does not necessarily equate with physical activity.[59] Exercise is "a subset of physical activity that is planned, structured, repetitive, and purposeful,"[60] whereas physical daily activity is defined as "the totality of voluntary movement produced by skeletal muscles during every day functioning."[61,62] Reduced physical activity is a universal finding in individuals with COPD. This inactivity occurs in individuals with mild airflow obstruction as well as those

with more severe physiologic impairments, and decreased activity may proceed the diagnosis of COPD.[63,64] Most individuals with COPD have lower levels of physical activity measured by both walking duration and intensity when compared with analogous individuals who do not have COPD.[65–68] Studies evaluating the effect of pulmonary rehabilitation on physical activity show inconsistent effects.[59]

The optimal time in the course of COPD when pulmonary rehabilitation should be offered remains unclear. Most guidelines recommend pulmonary rehabilitation for patients with more advanced disease, frequently those with a modified Medical Research Council (mMRC) dyspnea scale score ≥ 2.[50,51,69,70] Review of four randomized controlled trials of patients with COPD and mMRC dyspnea scale scores ≥ 1 revealed short-term improvement in health-related quality of life measured by the St. George's Respiratory Questionnaire, mean difference −4.2 (95% CI, −4.51, −3.89), nonclinically important improvement in the distance walked in 6 minutes, and no difference in mortality. Maximal exercise capacity and muscle strength could not be assessed.[71] When compared with conventional care, pulmonary rehabilitation initiated after a COPD exacerbation reduces hospital readmissions (pooled odds ratio 0.22 [95% CI 0.08–0.58], number needed to treat [NNT] 4 [95% CI 3–8], over 25 weeks) and mortality (OR 0.28, 95% CI 0.10 to 0.84, NNT 6 [95% CI 5–30] over 107 weeks). Health-related quality of life measured by all domains of the Chronic Respiratory Questionnaire and exercise capacity measured by the six-minute walking test and shuttle walk tests also improved.[72] These promising results have been questioned by recent studies with less beneficial effects on hospital readmissions, necessitating more careful analysis with specific attention to participation, program setting, timing, and content.[73]

An analysis of randomized controlled trials of postdischarge patient self-management programs after hospitalization for COPD exacerbations showed improvements in the St. George's Respiratory Questionnaire, mean difference −3.84 (95% CI −1.29, −6.40) that are less than the minimal clinically important difference and no effect on all-cause mortality or hospital readmission rates.[74,75]

Pulmonary rehabilitation also reduces COPD exacerbations.[76,77] In a review of 170 veterans referred to pulmonary rehabilitation, Major and colleagues[76] showed that respiratory-related emergency room visits declined by 38%, and hospitalizations decreased by 44% in the year after completing rehabilitation. In addition, when compared with patients who were referred to pulmonary rehabilitation but did not participate, those completing pulmonary rehabilitation had 44% fewer emergency room visits and 61% fewer hospitalizations.[76] Regular physical activity is associated with a reduced risk of hospitalization due to COPD exacerbations.[62–78,79]

Other benefits of pulmonary rehabilitation in patients with COPD include reduction in anxiety and depression.[80,81] Although anxiety and depression are associated with failure to complete pulmonary rehabilitation, increased respiratory symptoms, and reduced functional status, some patients with these symptoms may have greater improvement in exercise capacity.[82–86]

Pulmonary rehabilitation is usually provided as a hospital- or clinic-based outpatient service, but there is increasing evidence that home- or community-based programs are also beneficial.[58,87] In a meta-analysis, nonhospital-based pulmonary rehabilitation improved distance walked in 6 minutes and health-related quality of life measured by all domains of the Chronic Respiratory Questionnaire compared with usual treatment and these benefits were not different from the improvements achieved by outpatient programs.[87]

19.11 PULMONARY REHABILITATION AND ASTHMA

Individuals with asthma may limit or eliminate exercise or physical exertion due to acute and subacute exacerbations of respiratory symptoms. Lower levels of asthma control are associated with increasing functional impairment, as well as effects on work, regular life activities,[88] greater psychological distress, and poorer quality of life.[89] Physical activity may precipitate wheezing or other respiratory symptoms in individuals with exercise-induced asthma.[90] An estimated 10%–50% of elite athletes may have exercise-induced asthma.[91] Adults with asthma may have a reduced overall level of physical fitness compared with peers who do not have asthma.[92–94] Several studies have demonstrated an association between increasing levels of physical exercise and a reduced risk of asthma-related respiratory symptoms or exacerbations,[95–97] whereas other investigations have not revealed an association between exercise- and asthma-related respiratory symptoms.[98–100] Trevor and colleagues[101] showed that individuals with asthma who completed pulmonary rehabilitation had improved physical function and emotional well-being measured by the Beck Depression Inventory and Short Form (36) Health Survey.

At least two controlled trials have evaluated the effects of exercise training in patients with asthma.[102,103] Mendes and colleagues[102] assigned adults with asthma to either a control program (education and breathing exercises) or a training program (education, breathing exercises, and aerobic training). After 3 months, the training group experienced improvements in physical limitations, symptom frequency, psychological score, and anxiety and depression levels, and had more days with no asthma symptoms. Individuals with worse baseline psychological scores had better improvement. Turner and coworkers[103] evaluated 35 individuals with fixed-airway obstructive asthma who were randomized to either supervised-exercise training or usual care for 6 weeks. The exercise training group experienced improvements in symptoms and activity levels measured by the Asthma Quality of Life Questionnaire, and were able to

walk farther in 6 minutes immediately and 3 months after completing the intervention.

Two Cochrane analyses have reviewed breathing exercises and physical training in asthma.[104,105] Review of breathing exercise (such as Papworth method, Buteyko breathing technique, or yoga) studies revealed that, although individual trials demonstrated benefits, the Cochrane analysis could neither support nor refute the effectiveness of breathing exercises in adults with asthma.[104] Physical training improved cardiopulmonary fitness measured by an increase in maximal oxygen uptake, but there were no changes in lung function.[105] There also appeared to be a benefit in health-related quality of life but differences in assessment methods prevented the pooling of data. Most importantly, no adverse effects were reported for physical training.

In a review of 17 studies including 599 subjects with asthma, Eichenberger and colleagues (106) showed that exercise training increased days without asthma-related respiratory symptoms, FEV_1, exercise capacity, and suggested improvement in quality of life, bronchial hyperresponsiveness, and exercise-induced bronchoconstriction. Multiple linear regression analysis demonstrated that the improvements in quality of life were due to changes in airway hyperreactivity and lung function, and better exercise capacity was related to changes in airway hyperreactivity.[106]

Because exercise is considered important in the management of asthma,[107] individuals with asthma should be taught how to prevent exercise-induced symptoms (Table 19.6).[108] Most guidelines recommend excellent baseline control of respiratory symptoms prior to initiating an exercise program.[90,108] Use of inhaled corticosteroids for at least 4 weeks prior to exercise testing reduces exercise-induced bronchoconstriction.[109] Respiratory symptoms may be minimized with careful and thorough pre-exercise warm-up.[110] Short-acting β_2-agonists, mast cell stabilizing medications (cromolyn sodium, nedocromil) and anticholinergics effectively reduce exercise-induced bronchospasm with a relative efficacy: short-acting β_2-agonist > mast cell

Table 19.6 Management of exercise-induced bronchoconstriction in individuals with asthma

Baseline
- Optimal baseline control of respiratory symptoms
- Use of inhaled corticosteroids for at least 4 weeks

Prophylactic treatments
- Use of short-acting bronchodilators prior to exercise: Relative efficacy: short-acting β_2-agonist > mast cell stabilizers > anticholinergics

Preventative measures
- Thorough pre-exercise warm-up
- Avoid environmental triggers such as pollen, mold, fungus, cold, or air pollution

stabilizers > anticholinergics.[111] Prophylactic single-dose treatment with both short- and long-acting β_2-agonist bronchodilators effectively and safely prevents exercise-induced asthma; however, current guidelines do not recommend the use of long-acting β_2-agonist bronchodilators without concurrent inhaled corticosteroids.[112] Avoidance of potential environmental triggers, such as pollen, mold, fungus, cold, or air pollution is also key to the prevention of respiratory symptoms during exercise.

Additionally, asthma self-management education varies with the age of asthma onset.[113] Overall, approximately three quarters (76.4%) of adults with active asthma have been taught what to do during an asthma attack, but only 28.7% have an asthma action plan. Patient-reported asthma self-management education declines as the age of asthma onset increases.[113]

19.12 CONCLUSION

Supplemental oxygen is a long-standing treatment for patients with stable COPD and resting hypoxemia, and it was one of the first therapies to improve survival in COPD. Despite its current use, there is no substantive evidence that supplemental oxygen during exercise or at night is beneficial in individuals with stable COPD. Because asthma is a disorder of the airways, the lung parenchyma and gas exchange function is well preserved maintaining normal oxygenation. However, during asthma exacerbations, ventilation/perfusion mismatching may lead to hypoxemia, and although supplemental oxygen is frequently utilized, there are no prospective, randomized trials supporting this practice. Supplemental oxygen treatment in ACO has not been prospectively studied, and resting hypoxemia is not usually described in this syndrome.[1] During ACO exacerbations, supplemental oxygen treatment may be used to maintain normal oxygen levels, but, similar to asthma or even COPD exacerbations, there is a lack of evidence to support these practices.

Pulmonary rehabilitation has significant salubrious benefits for individuals with COPD and asthma but has not been studied in ACO. Because of its potential comprehensive advantageous effects, pulmonary rehabilitation in conjunction with optimal pharmacological treatment warrants evaluation in individuals with ACO.

REFERENCES

1. Postma DS and Rabe KF. The asthma-COPD overlap syndrome. *N Engl J Med.* 2015;373(13):1241–1249.
2. Croxton TL and Bailey WC. Long-term oxygen treatment in chronic obstructive pulmonary disease: Recommendations for future research: An NHLBI workshop report. *Am J Respir Crit Care Med.* 2006;174(4):373–378.
3. Nocturnal oxygen therapy trial group. Continuous or nocturnal oxygen therapy in hypoxemic chronic obstructive lung disease: A clinical trial. *AnnalInter Med.* 1980;93:391–398.
4. Medical research council working party. Long-term domicilliary oxygen therapy in chronic hypoxic cor pulmonale complicating chronic bronchitis and emphysema. *Lancet.* 1981;1:681–686.
5. Panos RJ and W Eschenbacher. Exertional desaturation in patients with chronic obstructive pulmonary disease. *COPD* 2009;6(6):478–487.
6. Gorecka D, Gorzelak K, Sliwinski P et al. Effect of long-term oxygen therapy on survival in patients with chronic obstructive pulmonary disease with moderate hypoxaemia. *Thorax.* 1997;52:674–679.
7. Long-Term Oxygen Treatment Trial Research Group., Albert RK, Au DH, Blackford AL et al. A randomized trial of long-term oxygen for COPD with moderate desaturation. *N Engl J Med.* October 27, 2016;375(17):1617–1627.
8. Chaouat A, Weitzenblum E, Kessler R et al. A randomized trial of nocturnal oxygen therapy in chronic obstructive pulmonary disease patients. *Eur Respir J.* November 1999;14(5):1002–1008.
9. Centers for Medicare and Medicaid Services, National coverage Determinations Manual, Chapter 1, Part 4, Section 240.2. Home Use of Oxygen.
10. Veale D, Chailleux E, Taytard A et al. Characteristics and survival of patients prescribed long-term oxygen therapy outside of prescription guidelines. *Eur Respir J.* 1998;12:780–784.
11. Drummond MB, Blackford AL, Benditt JO et al. Continuous oxygen use in nonhypoxemic emphysema patients identifies a high-risk subset of patients: Retrospective analysis of the national emphysema treatment trial. *Chest.* 2008;134(3):497–506.
12. Stein DA, Bradley BL, Miller WC et al. Mechanisms of oxygen effects on exercise in patients with chronic obstructive pulmonary disease. *Chest.* 1982;81:6–10.
13. Jolly EC, Di Boscio V, Aguirre L et al. Effects of supplemental oxygen during activity in patients with advanced COPD without severe resting hypoxemia. *Chest.* 2001;120:437–443.
14. Emtner M, Porszasz J, Burns M et al. Benefits of supplemental oxygen in exercise training in nonhypoxemic chronic obstructive pulmonary disease patients. *Am J Respir Crit Care Med.* 2003;168:1034–1042.
15. Somfay A, Porszasz J, Lee SM et al. Dose-response effect of oxygen on hyperinflation and exercise endurance in nonhypoxemic COPD patients. *Eur Respir J.* 2001;18:77–84.
16. Wadell K, Henriksson-Larsén K, and Lundgren R. Physical training with and without oxygen in patients with chronic obstructive pulmonary disease and exercise-induced hypoxaemia. *J Rehab Med.* 2001;33:200–205.

17. Rooyackers JM, Dekhuijzen PNR, Van Herwaarden CLA et al. Training with supplemental oxygen in patients with COPD and hypoxaemia at peak exercise. *Eur Respir J.* 1997;10:1278–1284.

18. Garrod R, Paul EA, and Wedzicha JA. Supplemental oxygen during pulmonary rehabilitation in patients with COPD with exercise hypoxaemia. *Thorax.* 2000;55:539–543.

19. Nonoyama ML, Brooks D, Lacasse Y et al. Oxygen therapy during exercise training in chronic obstructive pulmonary disease. *Cochr Data Syst Rev.* 200718;(2)CD005372.

20. Eaton T, Garrett JE, Young P et al. Ambulatory oxygen improves quality of life of COPD patients: A randomized controlled study. *Eur Respir J.* 2002;20:306–312.

21. Jensen G, Nielsen HB, Ide K et al. Cerebral oxygenation during exercise in patients with terminal lung disease. *Chest.* 2002;122:445–450.

22. Wedzicha JA. Domiciliary oxygen therapy services: Clinical guidelines and advice for prescribers. Summary of a report of the royal college of physicians. *J R Coll Physicians Lond.* 1999;33:445–447.

23. Okubadejo AA, Paul EA, and Wedzicha JA. Domiciliary oxygen cylinders: Indications, prescription and usage. *Respir Med.* 1994;88:777–785.

24. Roberts CM. Short burst oxygen therapy for relief of breathlessness in COPD. *Thorax.* 2004;59:638–640.

25. O'Neill B, Bradley JM, Heaney L et al. Short burst oxygen therapy in chronic obstructive pulmonary disease: A patient survey and cost analysis. *Int J Clin Pract.* 2005;59:751–753.

26. O'Neill B, MacMahon J, and Bradley J. Short-burst oxygen therapy in chronic obstructive pulmonary disease. *Respir Med.* 2006;100:1129–1138.

27. Stevenson NJ and Calverley PMA. Effect of oxygen on recovery from maximal exercise in patients with chronic obstructive obstructive pulmonary disease. *Thorax.* 2004;59:668–672.

28. Woodcock AA, Gross ER, and Geddes DM. Oxygen relieves breathlessness in "pink puffers". *Lancet.* 1981;1:907–909.

29. Evans TW, Waterhouse JC, Carter A et al. Short burst oxygen treatment for breathlessness in chronic obstructive airways disease. *Thorax.* 1986;41:611–615.

30. Killen JW and Corris PA. A pragmatic assessment of the placement of oxygen when given for exercise induced dyspnoea. *Thorax.* 2000;55:544–546.

31. McKeon JL, Murree-Allen K, and Saunders NA. Effects of breathing supplemental oxygen before progressive exercise in patients with chronic obstructive pulmonary disease. *Thorax.* 1988;43:53–56.

32. Rhind CB, Prince KL, Scott W et al. Symptomatic oxygen therapy in hypoxic chronic bronchitis (abstract). *Thorax.* 1986;42:245.

33. Nandi K, Smith AA, Crawford A, MacRae KD et al. Oxygen supplementation before or after submaximal exercise in patients with chronic obstructive pulmonary disease. *Thorax.* 2003;58:670–673.

34. Lewis CA, Eaton TE, Young P et al. Short-burst oxygen immediately before and after exercise is ineffective in nonhypoxic COPD patients. *Eur Respir J.* 2003;22:584–588.

35. Baruchin O, Yoffe B, and Baruchin AM. Burns in inpatients by simultaneous use of cigarettes and oxygen therapy. *Burns.* 2004;8:836–838.

36. Chang TT, Lipinski CA, and Sherman HF. A hazard of home oxygen therapy. *J Burn Care Rehabil.* 2001;22:71–74.

37. Lacasse Y, LaForge J, and Maltais F. Got a match? Home oxygen therapy in current smokers. *Thorax.* 2006;61:374–375.

38. Tamir G, Issa M, and Yaron HS. Mobil phone-triggered thermal burns in the presence of supplemental oxygen. *J Burn Care Res.* 2007;28:348–350.

39. Robb BW, Hungness ES, Hershko DD et al. Home oxygen therapy: Adjunct or risk factor. *J Burn Care Rehabil.* 2003;24:403–406.

40. Wendling, T and Pelletier A. Fatal fires associated with smoking during long-term oxygen therapy—Maine, Massachusetts, New Hampshire, and Oklahoma—2000-2007. *MMWR.* 2008;57:852–854.

41. Carpagnano GE, Kharitonov SA, Foschino-Barbaro MP et al. Supplementary oxygen in healthy subjects and those with COPD increases oxidative stress and airway inflammation. *Thorax.* 2004;59:1016–1019.

42. Panos RJ., *Management of Stable Chronic Obstructive Pulmonary Disease.* RJ Panos and WL Eschenbacher, eds. COPD Primer. DeGruyter; February, 2016. Available at http://www.degruyter.com/view/product/468864.

43. Adams JY, Sutter ME, and Albertson TE. The patient with asthma in the emergency department. *Clin Rev Allergy Immunol.* 2012;43(1–2):14–29.

44. Urso DL. Treatment for acute asthma in the emergency department: Practical aspects. *Eur Rev Med Pharmacol Sci.* March 2010;14(3):209–214. Review. PubMed PMID: 20391960.

45. Expert Panel Report 3 (EPR-3) (2007) Guidelines for the diagnosis and management of asthma—Summary report 2007. *J Allergy Clin Immunol* 120(5 Suppl):S94–S138.

46. Rodrigo GJ and Castro-Rodriguez JA. Heliox-driven β2-agonists nebulization for children and adults with acute asthma: A systematic review with meta-analysis. *Ann Allergy Asthma Immunol.* 2014;112(1):29–34.

47. Colebourn CL, Barber V, and Young JD. Use of helium-oxygen mixture in adult patients presenting with exacerbations of asthma and chronic obstructive pulmonary disease: A systematic review. *Anaesthesia.* January 2007;62(1):34–42.

48. Vaes AW, Garcia-Aymerich J, Marott JL et al. Changes in physical activity and all-cause mortality in COPD. *Eur Respir J.* 2014;44:1199–1209.

49. Waschki B, Kirsten AM, Holz O et al. Disease progression and changes in physical activity in patients with COPD. *Am J Respir Crit Care Med.* 2015;192:295–306.

50. Spruit MA, Singh SJ, Garvey C et al. An official American Thoracic Society/European Respiratory Society statement: Key concepts and advances in pulmonary rehabilitation. *Am J Respir Crit Care Med.* October 15, 2013;188(8):e13–64. doi:10.1164/rccm.201309-1634ST.

51. Spruit MA, Singh SJ, Garvey C et al. An official American thoracic society/european respiratory society statement: Key concepts and advances in pulmonary rehabilitation. *Am J Respir Crit Care Med.* 2013;188(8):e13–e64.

52. Nici L and ZuWallack R. chronic obstructive pulmonary disease-evolving concepts in treatment: Advances in pulmonary rehabilitation. *Semin Respir Crit Care Med.* August 2015;36(4):567–574.

53. Lacasse Y, Goldstein R, Lasserson TJ et al. Pulmonary rehabilitation for chronic obstructive pulmonary disease. *Cochrane Database Syst Rev.* October 18, 2006;(4):CD003793.

54. McCarthy B, Casey D, Devane D et al. Pulmonary rehabilitation for chronic obstructive pulmonary disease. *Cochrane Database Syst Rev.* February 23, 2015;(2):CD003793.

55. Ries AL. Pulmonary rehabilitation: Summary of an evidence-based guideline. *Respir Care.* September 2008;53(9):1203–1207.

56. Watz H, Pitta F, Rochester CL et al. An official European respiratory society statement on physical activity in COPD. *Eur Respir J.* 2014;44:1521–1537.

57. Vieira DS, Maltais F, and Bourbeau J. Home-based pulmonary rehabilitation in chronic obstructive pulmonary disease patients. *Curr Opin Pulm Med.* March 2010;16(2):134–143.

58. Maltais F, Bourbeau J, Shapiro S et al. Effects of home-based pulmonary rehabilitation in patients with chronic obstructive pulmonary disease: A randomized trial. *Ann Intern Med.* December 16, 2008;149(12):869–878.

59. Spruit MA, Pitta F, McAuley E et al. Pulmonary rehabilitation and physical activity in patients with chronic obstructive pulmonary disease. *Am J Respir Crit Care Med.* October 15, 2015;192(8):924–933.

60. Caspersen CJ, Powell KE, and Christenson GM. Physical activity, exercise, and physical fitness: Definitions and distinctions for health-related research. *Public Health Rep.* 1985;100:126–131.

61. Steele BG, Belza B, Cain K et al. Bodies in motion: Monitoring daily activity and exercise with motion sensors in people with chronic pulmonary disease. *J Rehabil Res Dev.* 2003;40(5 Suppl 2):45–58.

62. Pitta F, Troosters T, Probst VS et al. Quantifying physical activity in daily life with questionnaires and motion sensors in COPD. *Eur Respir J.* 2006;27:1040–1055.

63. Van Remoortel H, Hornikx M, Demeyer H et al. Daily physical activity in subjects with newly diagnosed COPD. *Thor ax* 2013;68:962–963.

64. Gouzi F, Préfaut C, Abdel laoui A et al. Evidence of an early physical activity reduction in chronic obstructive pulmonary disease patients. *Arch Phys Med Rehabil.* 2011;92:1611–1617.e2.

65. Watz H, Waschki B, Meyer T et al. Physical activity in patients with COPD. *Eur Respir J.* 2009;33:262–272.

66. Schoenhofer B, Ardes P, Geibel M et al. Evaluation of a movement detector to measure daily activity in patients with chronic lung disease. *Eur Respir J.* 1997;10:2814–2819.

67. Hernandes NA, Teixeira Dde C, Probst VS et al. Profile of the level of physical activity in the daily lives of patients with COPD in Brazil. *J Bras Pneumol.* 2009;35:949–956.

68. Singh S and Morgan MD. Activity monitors can detect brisk walking in patients with chronic obstructive pulmonary disease. *J Cardiopulm Rehabil.* 2001;21:143–148.

69. Bolton CE, Bevan-Smith EF, Blakey JD et al. British Thoracic society guideline on pulmonary rehabilitation in adults. *Thorax.* 2013;68(Suppl 2):21–230.

70. Marciniuk DD, Brooks D, Butcher S et al. Optimizing pulmonary rehabilitation in chronic obstructive pulmonary disease – practical issues: A Canadian thoracic society clinical practice guideline. *Can Respir J.* 2010;17(4):159–168.

71. Rugbjerg M, Iepsen UW, Jørgensen KJ et al. Effectiveness of pulmonary rehabilitation in COPD with mild symptoms: A systematic review with meta-analyses. *Int J Chron Obstruct Pulmon Dis.* April 17, 2015;10:791–801.

72. Puhan MA, Gimeno-Santos E, Scharplatz M et al. Pulmonary rehabilitation following exacerbations of chronic obstructive pulmonary disease. *Cochrane Database Syst Rev.* October 5, 2011;(10):CD005305.

73. Maddocks M, Kon SS, Singh SJ et al. Rehabilitation following hospitalization in patients with COPD: Can it reduce readmissions? *Respirology.* April 2015;20(3):395–404. doi:10.1111/resp.12454. Epub December 22, 2014.

74. Majothi S, Jolly K, Heneghan NR et al. Supported self-management for patients with COPD who have recently been discharged from hospital: A systematic review and meta-analysis. *Int J Chron Obstruct Pulmon Dis.* April 29, 2015;10:853–867.

75. Jordan RE, Majothi S, Heneghan NR et al. Supported self-management for patients with moderate to

severe chronic obstructive pulmonary disease (COPD): An evidence synthesis and economic analysis. *Health Technol Assess.* May 2015;19(36):1–516.

76. Major S, Moreno M, Shelton J et al. Veterans with chronic obstructive pulmonary disease achieve clinically relevant improvements in respiratory health after pulmonary rehabilitation. *J Cardiopulm Rehabil Prev.* November–December 2014;34(6):420–429.

77. Sahin H, Varol Y, Naz I et al. The effect of pulmonary rehabilitation on COPD exacerbation frequency per year. *Clin Respir J.* 2018 Jan;12(1):165-174

78. Garcia-Aymerich J, Farrero E, Felez MA et al. Risk factors of readmission to hospital for a COPD exacerbation: A prospective study. *Thorax.* 2003;58:100–105.

79. Garcia-Aymerich J, Lange P, Benet M et al. Regular physical activity reduces hospital admission and mortality in chronic obstructive pulmonary disease: A population-based cohort study. *Thorax.* 2006;61:772–778.

80. Paz-Díaz H, Montes de Oca M, López JM et al. Pulmonary rehabilitation improves depression, anxiety, dyspnea and health status in patients with COPD. *Am J Phys Med Rehabil.* 2007;86:30–36.

81. Griffiths TL, Burr ML, Campbell IA et al. Results at 1 year of outpatient multidisciplinary pulmonary rehabilitation: A randomised controlled trial. *Lancet.* 2000;355:362–368.

82. Bhandari NJ, Jain T, Marolda C et al. Comprehensive pulmonary rehabilitation results in clinically meaningful improvements in anxiety and depression in patients with chronic obstructive pulmonary disease. *J Cardiopul Rehabilita Preven.* 2013;33:123–127.

83. Janssen DJ, Spruit MA, Leue C et al. Symptoms of anxiety and depression in COPD patients entering pulmonary rehabilitation. *Chronic Resp Disease.* 2010; 7:147–157.

84. von Leupoldt A, Taube K, Lehmann K et al. The impact of anxiety and depression on outcomes of pulmonary rehabilitation in patients with COPD. *Chest.* 2011;140:730–736.

85. Harris D, Hayter M, and Allender S. Improving the uptake of pulmonary rehabilitation in patients with COPD: Qualitative study of experiences and attitudes. *Br J Gen Pract.* 2008;58:703–710.

86. Withers NJ, Rudkin ST, and White RJ. Anxiety and depression in severe chronic obstructive pulmonary disease: The effects of pulmonary rehabilitation. *J Cardiopulm Rehabil.* 1999;19:362–365.

87. Neves LF, Reis MH, and Gonçalves TR. Home or community-based pulmonary rehabilitation for individuals with chronic obstructive pulmonary disease: A systematic review and meta-analysis. *Cad Saude Publica.* June 20, 2016;32(6): S0102-311X2016000602001.

88. Wertz DA, Pollack M, Rodgers K et al. Impact of asthma control on sleep, attendance at work, normal activities, and disease burden. *Ann Allergy Asthma Immunol.* 2010;105:118–123.

89. Adams RJ, Wilson DH, Taylor AW et al. Psychological factors and asthma quality of life: A population based study. *Thorax.* 2004;59:930–935.

90. Smoliga JM, Weiss P, and Rundell KW. Exercise induced bronchoconstriction in adults: Evidence based diagnosis and management. *BMJ.* January 13, 2016;352:h6951.

91. Parsons JP and Mastronarde JG. Exercise-induced bronchoconstriction in athletes. *Chest.* 2005;128:3966–3974.

92. Clark CJ and Cochrane LM. Assessment of work performance in asthma for determination of cardiorespiratory fitness and training capacity. *Thorax.* 1988;43:745–749.

93. Garfinkel SK, Kesten S, Chapman KR et al. Physiologic and nonphysiologic determinants of aerobic fitness in mild to moderate asthma. *Am Rev Respir Dis.* 1992;145:741–745.

94. Malkia E and Impivaara O. Intensity of physical activity and respiratory function in subjects with and without bronchial asthma. *Scand J Med Sci Sports.* 1998;8:27–32.

95. Garcia-Aymerich J, Varraso R, Antó JM et al. Prospective study of physical activity and risk of asthma exacerbations in older women. *Am J Respir Crit Care Med.* 2009;179:999–1003.

96. Ford ES, Heath GW, Mannino DM et al. Leisure-time physical activity patterns among US adults with asthma. *Chest.* 2003;124:432–437.

97. Kilpelainen M, Terho EO, Helenius H et al. Body mass index and physical activity in relation to asthma and atopic diseases in young adults. *Respir Med.* 2006;100:1518–1525.

98. Chen Y, Dales R, and Krewski D. Leisure-time energy expenditure in asthmatics and non-asthmatics. *Respir Med.* 2001;95:13–18.

99. Eijkemans M, Mommers M, de Vries SI et al. Asthmatic symptoms, physical activity, and overweight in young children: A cohort study. *Pediatrics.* 2008;121:e666–e672.

100. Corbo GM, Forastiere F De Sario M et al. Wheeze and asthma in children: Associations with body mass index, sports, television viewing, and diet. *Epidemiology.* 2008;19:747–755.

101. Trevor JL, Bhatt SP, Wells JM et al. Benefits of completing pulmonary rehabilitation in patients with asthma. *J Asthma.* 2015;52(9):969–973.

102. Mendes FA, Gonçalves RC, Nunes MP et al. Effects of aerobic training on psychosocial morbidity and symptoms in patients with asthma: A randomized clinical trial. *Chest.* 2010;138:331–337.

103. Turner S, Eastwood P, Cook A et al. Improvements in symptoms and quality of life following exercise training in older adults with moderate/severe persistent asthma. *Respiration.* 2011;81(4):302–310.

104. Freitas DA, Holloway EA, Bruno SS et al. Breathing exercises for adults with asthma. *Coc Database Syst Rev.* 2013;(10):CD001277.

105. Carson KV, Chandratilleke MG, Picot J et al. Physical training for asthma. *Cochrane Data Syst Rev.* 2013;(9):CD001116.

106. Eichenberger PA, Diener SN, Kofmehl R et al. Effects of exercise training on airway hyperreactivity in asthma: A systematic review and meta-analysis. *Sports Med.* 2013;43:1157–1170.

107. Ram FS, Robinson RM, Black PN. Effects of physical training in asthma: A systematic review. *Br J Sports Med.* 2000;34:162–167.

108. Pedersen BK and Saltin B. Exercise as medicine—Evidence for prescribing exercise as therapy in 26 different chronic diseases. *Scand J Med Sci Sports.* December 2015;25(Suppl 3):1–72.

109. Koh MS, Tee A, Lasserson TJ et al. Inhaled corticosteroids compared to placebo for prevention of exercise induced bronchoconstriction. *Coch Data Syst Rev.* 2007;(3):CD002739.

110. Stickland MK, Rowe BH, Spooner CH et al. Effect of warm-up exercise on exercise-induced bronchoconstriction. *Med Sci Sports Exerc.* 2012;44:383391.

111. Spooner C, Spooner GR, and Rowe BH. Mast-cell stabilising agentsto prevent exercise-induced bronchoconstriction. *Coch Data Syst Rev.* 2003;(4):CD002307.

112. Bonini M, Di Mambro C, Calderon MA et al. Beta2-agonists for exercise-induced asthma. *Coch Data Syst Rev.* 2013;(10):CD003564.

113. Mirabelli MC, Beavers SF, Shepler SH et al. Age at asthma onset and asthma self-management education among adults in the United States. *J Asthma.* 2015;52(9):974–80.

Smoking cessation for asthma, COPD, and asthma-COPD overlap

ADRIENNE L. JOHNSON, ALISON C. MCLEISH, AND TALYA ALSAID-HABIA

20.1 OVERVIEW

Despite the known compromising effects of smoking on lung function and health, cigarette smoking is more common among individuals with asthma and chronic obstructive pulmonary disease (COPD) compared to those without.[1,2] Indeed, individuals with asthma are 1.36 times more likely and individuals with COPD more than twice as likely to be cigarette smokers than individuals without these diseases.[2-4] Moreover, smokers with asthma are more likely to be heavier and more nicotine-dependent smokers than those without asthma.[5,6] Given that smoking is the leading risk factor for COPD,[2] these high rates of smoking are not entirely surprising. The findings for asthma, however, are even more striking when taking into consideration that for at least half of all smokers with asthma, their asthma diagnosis preceded smoking onset.[5]

Cigarette smoking is a significant contributor to the increased rates of morbidity and mortality associated with asthma and COPD. For example, smoking results in increased frequency and severity of respiratory symptoms, poorer asthma control, and decreased lung function.[1,7-10] Indeed, patients with poorly controlled asthma are more likely to be current or former smokers than those with well-controlled asthma, and smoking status has been found to have the greatest influence on whether or not patients achieve asthma control.[8] Smokers with asthma and COPD also report greater interference with daily activities compared to their nonsmoking counterparts, as well as greater health-care utilization.[11,12] Unfortunately, smoking also significantly decreases the effectiveness of inhaled corticosteroids used to treat these conditions.[13]

Given these high prevalence rates and associated negative outcomes, quitting smoking is a critically important goal for patients with asthma and COPD. Quitting smoking decreases the risk of developing smoking-related health problems and may increase the survival time among those persons who have already developed medical problems.[14] In terms of asthma and COPD, specifically, quitting smoking results in significant improvements in lung function, reductions in asthma medication use, and improved quality of life.[15,16]

20.2 CURRENT SMOKING CESSATION GUIDELINES

The majority of all smokers are interested in quitting smoking, and this motivation to quit is typically even higher among smokers with asthma or COPD.[6,16] Notably, provider advice to quit smoking has been cited by smokers as one of the strongest motivators for quitting.[17] As a result, current smoking cessation guidelines recommend that providers not only assess smoking status, but also provide at least a brief intervention to every smoker at each office visit.[17] These brief interventions require 3 minutes or less to implement, yet have been shown to be highly effective.

Table 20.1 The "5 A's" model for smoking cessation[a]

ASK	Ask about and document smoking status for every patient at every visit.
ADVISE	In a clear, strong, and personalized manner, urge every tobacco user to quit.
ASSESS	Is the tobacco user willing to make a quit attempt at this time?
ASSIST	*For patients willing to make a quit attempt*: offer medication and provide or refer for counseling or additional treatment to help the patient quit.
	For patients unwilling to make a quit attempt at this time: provide interventions designed to increase motivation for future quit attempts.
ARRANGE	*For patients willing to make a quit attempt*: arrange for follow-up contacts, beginning within the first week after the quit date.
	For patients unwilling to make a quit attempt at this time: address tobacco dependence and willingness to quit at next clinic visit.

[a] (Fiore MC et al., *Treating Tobacco Use and Dependence: 2008 Update*, U.S. Dept. of Health and Human Services, Public Health Service, Rockville, 2008.)

Providers are encouraged to follow the 5 A's model of smoking cessation intervention (see Table 20.1). For all patients, clinicians need to ask the patient if he or she is a smoker. For those who endorse current cigarette smoking, they then need to advise the patient to quit smoking in a clear, strong, and personalized manner and assess the patient's willingness to make a quit attempt at this time. Below is an example of how to implement the first three of the 5 A's:

> ## CLINICAL VIGNETTE 20.1: INTERACTION BETWEEN PROVIDER AND PATIENT ADDRESSING QUITTING
>
> Provider: Before we get started with your exam, I want to go over the paperwork you filled out. It says here that you are a cigarette smoker. Is that correct?
>
> Patient: Yes, but I just smoke a few cigarettes a day.
>
> Provider: Even light smoking is still dangerous to your health. As your clinician, I need you to know that one of the most important things you can do for your current and future health is to quit smoking. In fact, smoking can make your medications for asthma less effective, and quitting smoking can help us manage your asthma better and may even reduce the number of asthma attacks you have.
>
> Patient: I know smoking is bad for me, but I've been under a lot of stress lately.
>
> Provider: Yes, a lot of people believe that smoking helps you deal with stress, but research has shown us that, in the long run, smoking actually leads to more stress and puts you at risk of developing an anxiety disorder. So quitting smoking will not only improve your physical health, but your emotional health as well. Are you willing to try to quit smoking?

20.2.1 FOR PATIENTS WILLING TO QUIT

For patients who endorse a willingness to quit smoking at this time, providers should then provide practical assistance for quitting. Current smoking cessation guidelines highlight two primary approaches for smoking cessation: counseling and pharmacotherapy.[17]

20.2.1.1 Counseling

Providers can be effective in providing brief counseling interventions during the office visit (see Table 20.2). First, they should assist patients in developing a quit plan that involves the following components: (1) setting a quit date within 2 weeks; (2) informing family, friends, and coworkers about the quit date and soliciting social support; (3) identifying smoking triggers and developing a plan for managing them; and (4) removing tobacco products from places where patients spend a lot of time (e.g., home, work, car). The majority of the discussion should focus on having patients identify their triggers for smoking and helping them develop strategies to manage these triggers. For certain triggers, such as alcohol, avoiding them altogether is the best strategy. For other triggers, patients can try to alter the situation slightly (e.g., drink a different flavor of coffee if coffee is a strong smoking trigger) or use behavioral substitution (e.g., replacing smoking with gum or brushing their teeth). It is also helpful to help patients learn from previous quit attempts by identifying what was and was not helpful. Below is an example of how to develop such a plan.

Table 20.2 Guidelines for developing a quit plan

1. Set quit date within 2 weeks of appointment.
2. Enlist social support by informing family, friends, and coworkers of quit date.
3. Identify smoking triggers and create a plan to deal with them.
4. Remove tobacco products from personal environment (e.g., home, work, car) prior to quit date.

CLINICAL VIGNETTE 20.2: INTERACTION BETWEEN PROVIDER AND PATIENT COUNSELING A PATIENT WHO HAS DECIDED TO QUIT

Provider: I'm glad you are ready to take this important step toward improving your health. Let's go ahead and create a plan for quitting. The first step is to set a quit date, ideally sometime in the next 2 weeks.

Patient: Okay. How about next Monday?

Provider: That sounds perfect, you can start off the week fresh! This means on Sunday night you will want to make sure you remove all cigarettes, lighters, ashtrays, and any other smoking materials from your house and car. Be sure to find and destroy all of those emergency cigarettes you have hidden around. I usually tell people to break all of their remaining cigarettes in half, get them wet, and then throw them away. That way you won't be tempted later when you have a really strong craving.

Patient: That makes sense. That's how I started smoking again after I quit the last time—after finding an old pack of cigarettes in a purse I hadn't used in a long time.

Provider: Yes, that happens a lot. So definitely try to go through old bags, purses, clothes, and things like that before Monday. Now that you've set your quit date, the next step is to let your family and other important people in your life, like friends and coworkers, know you are quitting, so they can provide you support. Who do you think you should tell?

Patient: Definitely my husband and kids. They have been nagging me to quit for years.

Provider: Wonderful! It might be helpful if you let them know how they can be the most supportive. For example, if you were having a really strong craving to smoke, what would you want them to do? Help distract you? Or would you prefer if they left you alone?

Patient: I think I would want them to let me deal with the cravings on my own. In the past when I've tried to quit, I've been really cranky, and I don't want to snap at them.

Provider: So you can let them know that you tend to get irritable when you quit smoking, and that the best thing they can do to support you is be understanding if you snap at them. And you can tell them that you may ask them to leave you alone if you are having a particularly rough time. This plan is really coming along. The last thing we need to do is to figure out what your smoking triggers are and develop a plan for how to deal with them.

Patient: My biggest smoking trigger is driving. I can't smoke at work, so I usually smoke a lot on my way to and from work.

Provider: Smoking and driving seem to go hand-in-hand for a lot of people. One thing I would suggest is trying to give your car a good cleaning before your quit day to get rid of the smell of smoke as much as possible. Something that has worked for people in the past is to change the route they drive to work, maybe find one that doesn't go by many places where you could buy cigarettes. Another trick that works well for people is to substitute another behavior for smoking. So instead of smoking you could chew a piece of sugar-free gum, have a piece of hard candy, or drink a glass of cold water.

Patient: Those sound like great ideas! I'm feeling a lot more confident about quitting smoking now.

Provider: Wonderful. I will also have my nurse give you some more information about quitting as well as some referrals for local quitlines and smoking-cessation programs before you leave today. The last thing we need to talk about is medications that can help you quit smoking. . . .

Although brief interventions are effective, research indicates that more intensive treatments are associated with the highest abstinence rates. Specifically, those with four or more sessions of at least 10 minutes in duration have been shown to be most effective.[17] These intensive programs are appropriate for any smoker and are typically delivered by clinicians who specialize in smoking cessation. They are conducted either in an individual or group-based format, although telephone counseling is also effective. The two primary treatment components of these intensive programs are practical counseling and social support. Practical counseling includes problem solving and skills training (e.g., identifying situations that will likely lead to relapse, psychoeducation on the quitting process and withdrawal symptoms, cognitive restructuring, and other strategies to cope with smoking triggers).[17] Social support as part of the counseling process may include things such as encouragement for the upcoming quit day and open communication about the patient's concerns about quitting.[17]

In addition to these in-person interventions, there are a number of online tools that provide resources for quitting smoking (e.g., website cessation programs, mobile phone apps), as well as national hotlines that provide telephone-based counseling for smoking cessation (see Table 20.3). It may also be useful for providers to develop a list of local resources (e.g., local quitline numbers, information about local treatment programs) and have smoking cessation guides on hand (e.g., *Clearing the Air* [https://smokefree.gov/sites/default/files/pdf/clearing-the-air-accessible.pdf]) to give to patients who are current smokers.

20.2.1.2 Pharmacotherapy

There are seven first-line, FDA-approved medications for smoking cessation.[17] These include nicotine replacement therapies (NRTs [patch, gum, lozenge, nasal spray, and inhaler]), as well as two nonnicotine medications, buproprion SR (Wellbutrin®) and varenicline (Chantix®). Table 20.4 provides a summary of dosing guidelines for these medications. Providers are also strongly encouraged to

Table 20.3 Resources for smoking cessation

American Cancer Society	http://www.cancer.org/healthy/stayawayfromtobacco/index
American Lung Association	http://www.lung.org/stop-smoking/i-want-to-quit/
American Heart Association	http://www.heart.org/quitsmoking
National Cancer Institute	http://www.SmokeFree.gov Toll-free hotline: 1-877-44U-QUIT
National Network of Tobacco Cessation Quitlines	Toll-free hotline: 1-800-QUITNOW TTY: 1-800-332-8615 En Español: 1-855-DÉJELO-YA
U.S. Department of Health and Human Services	http://betobaccofree.hhs.gov/quit-now/index.html

Table 20.4 Dosing recommendations for smoking cessation medications[a]

Medication	Dosage
Over the Counter	
Nicotine patch	If smoking > 10 cigarettes per day: 21 mg patch daily for 4 weeks, then 14 mg patch daily for 2 weeks, then 7 mg patch daily for 2 weeks If smoking < 10 cigarettes per day: 14 mg patch daily for 4 weeks, then 7 mg patch daily for 4 weeks
Nicotine gum	Use 4 mg if smoking > 25 cigarettes per day and 2 mg if smoking < 25 cigarettes per day Use at least 1 piece every 1–2 hours for first 6 weeks, but no more than 24 pieces per day. Use for up to 12 weeks.
Nicotine lozenge	Use 4 mg for patients who smoke their first cigarette within 30 minutes of waking, and 2 mg for those who smoke their first cigarette more than 30 minutes after waking. Use 1 lozenge every 1–2 hours for the first 6 weeks, using a minimum of 9 lozenges per day, but no more than 20. Decrease lozenge use to 1 every 2–4 hours during weeks 7–9 and then to 1 every 4–8 hours during weeks 10–12.
Prescription	
Nicotine nasal spray	A dose of nicotine nasal spray consists of one 0.5-mg dose delivered to each nostril. Initial dosing should be 1–2 doses per hour, increasing as needed for symptom relief. Minimum recommended treatment is 8 doses/day, with a maximum limit of 40 doses/day (5 doses/hour). Recommended duration of therapy is 3–6 months.
Nicotine inhaler	A dose from the nicotine inhaler consists of a puff or inhalation. Each cartridge delivers a total of 4 mg of nicotine over 80 inhalations. Recommended dosage is 6–16 cartridges/day. Recommended duration of therapy is up to 6 months, but patient should taper dosage during the final 3 months of treatment.
Buproprion SR	Start 1–2 weeks prior to quitting. 150 mg every morning for 3 days, then increase to 150 mg twice daily. Dosage should not exceed 300 mg per day. Dosing at 150 mg twice daily should continue for 7–12 weeks. Can be used for up to 6 months postquit.
Varenicline	Start 1 week prior to quit at 0.5 mg once daily for 3 days, followed by 0.5 mg twice daily for 4 days. Starting on quit day (day 8), patient should take 1 mg twice daily for 3 months. Can be used for up to 6 months.

[a] (Adapted from Fiore MC et al., *Treating Tobacco Use and Dependence: 2008 Update*, U.S. Department of Health and Human Services, Public Health Service, Rockville, 2008.)

refer to the FDA package inserts for more complete information on these medications. Both buproprion SR and varenicline must be started prior to quit day. Patients using NRT should ensure they are using the proper dose and, for all versions of NRT except the patch, taking enough doses throughout the day. Of note, patients should be instructed on proper chewing technique for nicotine gum. Specifically, the gum should be chewed slowly until a flavored or peppery taste emerges, then "parked" between the cheek and gum. The gum should be "chewed and parked" slowly and intermittently for about 30 minutes or until the taste disappears. Moreover, acidic drinks (e.g., coffee, juice, soft drinks) interfere with the absorption of the nicotine gum and should be avoided for 15 minutes before chewing and during chewing.

20.2.1.3 Summary

Although both medication and counseling are effective individually, they are nearly twice as effective when combined.[17] Thus, the clinical guidelines state that practitioners should encourage all smokers making a quit attempt to use this combined approach.[17] As such, it is critical that providers are aware of the counseling-based smoking cessation programs in their area. State tobacco quitlines are often a good referral source as they can provide telephone-based counseling as well as assist with obtaining NRT. Further, it should be noted that repeated interventions and quit attempts are often needed before a patient is successful in maintaining abstinence in the long term. Therefore, it is recommended that providers arrange for follow-up with patients making a quit attempt (the last of the 5 A's) whether in person, by phone, or electronically. Moreover, providers should continue to check in regarding smoking cessation at future appointments until long-term abstinence (i.e., at least 12 months) has been attained, as it may be necessary to provide additional brief interventions to help patients remain abstinent after a lapse or make another quit attempt after a full relapse to smoking. Here it will be important to help patients reframe their unsuccessful quit attempt as a learning experience and make a new quit plan that addresses the barriers or triggers encountered in the unsuccessful quit attempt.

20.2.2 FOR PATIENTS UNWILLING TO QUIT

For patients who are not willing to make a quit attempt, the most effective treatment is to increase motivation to quit, which can be accomplished through brief motivational enhancement interventions. Such interventions are based on motivational interviewing (MI), a directive, patient-centered approach that can be successfully implemented in brief office visits and has demonstrated efficacy in enhancing motivation to quit smoking and increasing the likelihood of making a future quit attempt.[17,18] The goal of MI

for smoking cessation is to have the patient examine their beliefs and values about smoking in order to highlight areas of ambivalence, which, once identified, can be used to elicit "change talk" (e.g., reasons for quitting smoking) and a commitment to change. MI consists of four main principles. The first is expressing empathy, which involves asking open-ended questions and using reflective listening to better understand the patient's reasons both for smoking and quitting smoking, as well as normalizing the patient's concerns about quitting while respecting their current level of preparedness to make a change. The second principle, developing discrepancy, involves highlighting the discrepancy between the patient's behaviors (i.e., smoking) and their values, goals, and priorities. The third principle is rolling with resistance, which highlights the need to avoid directly challenging the patient when they express resistance to change. Providers, instead, are encouraged to express empathy for the patient's concerns and ask permission to provide information. The final MI principle, supporting self-efficacy, involves helping the patient identify previous successful quit attempts. The following example illustrates a provider discussing quitting smoking with a patient who is unwilling to make a quit attempt, first using a non-MI approach and then an MI approach.

20.2.2.1 Non-MI approach

CLINICAL VIGNETTE 20.3: INTERACTION BETWEEN PROVIDER AND PATIENT DEMONSTRATING NONMOTIVATIONAL APPROACH

Provider: So you aren't willing to quit smoking?

Patient: I know I should quit, but it's just a really difficult time right now with the stress from work.

Provider: Well, we all have difficult times, but you really need to quit smoking or your asthma is going to get much worse. Don't you want to improve your health?

Patient: Well, yes, but I'm just not sure I can do it.

Provider: Lot's of people feel that way. The truth is, you never know if you can do something until you try. So, I think you should go ahead and just do it.

As is evident in the example, the provider expressed minimal empathy when the patient expressed concerns about being able to quit smoking successfully. Moreover, the provider continued to challenge and push the patient to commit to quitting smoking without highlighting the patient's change talk or the discrepancy between the patient's smoking despite stating a desire to quit. Below is an example of the same interaction using an MI approach.

20.2.2.2 MI approach

CLINICAL VIGNETTE 20.4:
INTERACTION BETWEEN PROVIDER
AND PATIENT DEMONSTRATING
MOTIVATIONAL APPROACH

Patient: I know I should quit, but it's just a really difficult time right now with the stress from work.

Provider: Yes, it can be really daunting to make big changes when you are under a lot of stress. What kinds of things are you doing to help manage your stress?

Patient: I don't know. I guess I try to do nice things for myself every once in a while—like getting a massage or giving myself time to relax on the weekends.

Provider: That's great that you are focused on self-care. That can be an effective way to manage stress. And doing things like coming to your doctors' appointments is another way you are taking care of yourself.

Patient: Yes, I guess that's true. I have a tendency to get sick when I am stressed, so I try really hard to keep that from happening.

Provider: It sounds like your health is really important to you.

Patient: Yes, it is.

Provider: Can I make an observation?

Patient: Sure.

Provider: Well, I'm hearing that you care a lot about your health, and are doing things to try to decrease your stress and stay healthy. I'm wondering how that desire to stay healthy fits with smoking.

Patient: Hah! Good point. I guess it doesn't.

Provider: I guess not.

Patient: I mean, I've thought about quitting before. But then I worry about whether I could do it. And I don't think I could deal with all of the stress in my life without smoking.

Provider: It sounds like you would really like to quit, but are worried you won't be successful, in part, because you aren't sure how you would handle stress without smoking.

Patient: Exactly!

Provider: Can I offer a piece of information?

Patient: Sure.

Provider: Well, like you, a lot of smokers smoke to reduce their stress. But what researchers have found is that smoking actually ends up making you more, rather than less, stressed in the long term.

Patient: Wow. I didn't know that. I keep saying I need to be less stressed and that I want to quit smoking. I guess maybe it's time to think about making a change.

Provider: So you're ready to consider changing your smoking behavior. My staff and I are here to help with that.

In the above example, rather than trying to push the client to quit smoking, the provider expressed empathy with the patient's struggles and tried to highlight the discrepancy between the patient's smoking and the patient's goal of being healthy and less stressed. The provider never directly challenged the client when the client expressed resistance, but rather expressed empathy with the patient's concerns about managing stress and provided information about the nature of stress and smoking. Lastly, the provider identified and reinforced change talk, while not making assumptions about what that change would be (i.e., not jumping to the conclusion that the change would mean quitting smoking). Although seemingly straightforward, MI can be difficult to implement successfully; therefore, it can be helpful to obtain specialized training in MI. As MI can be used to address a number of patient behaviors (e.g., medication adherence), the time spent receiving this training is typically worthwhile. As with patients who are willing to quit, it is also important to follow all of the 5 A's and arrange for follow-up to re-evaluate the patient's motivation to quit smoking.

20.3 SPECIAL CONSIDERATIONS FOR SMOKING CESSATION FOR PATIENTS WITH ASTHMA AND COPD

Although following the recommendations described in this chapter should help improve smoking cessation rates, there are several issues specific to patients with asthma and COPD that warrant consideration.

20.3.1 MANAGING WITHDRAWAL SYMPTOMS

Recent research has shown that there may be few differences between smokers with and without asthma and COPD in terms of abstinence rates during a quit attempt.[19–21] However, at least one study has found that, compared to smokers without asthma, smokers with asthma demonstrated a slower decline in withdrawal symptoms and craving during a quit attempt.[19] Accordingly, smokers with asthma may benefit more from using NRT, possibly for an extended period of time, as well as specialized psychosocial treatments to prepare them for these slower declines in withdrawal symptoms and cravings.

20.3.2 COMORBID PSYCHOPATHOLOGY

Rates of mood and anxiety disorders are elevated among cigarette smokers, as well as individuals with asthma and COPD.[22-24] Thus, it is likely that many smokers with asthma or COPD also have a comorbid mood or anxiety disorder. Unfortunately, comorbid mood and anxiety psychopathologies are associated with greater motivation to smoke, poorer smoking cessation outcomes, greater withdrawal symptoms, and a lack of response to smoking cessation pharmacotherapy.[25-27] Moreover, patients and providers alike are often unaware of this connection between psychopathology and cigarette smoking. Therefore, these patients, in particular, should be referred to mental health providers trained in combined approaches to smoking cessation that incorporate medication with intensive psychosocial smoking cessation interventions. Several specialized smoking cessation interventions have been developed that target anxiety and depression in the context of smoking cessation.[28,29] Additionally, bupropion SR may be a beneficial pharmacotherapy for smokers with comorbid depression, as it has been shown to also be an effective antidepressant.[30]

20.3.3 SYMPTOM MANAGEMENT

Patients with asthma who are able to successfully quit smoking may report a temporary increase in their asthma symptoms upon quitting. These increased symptoms are likely related to the clearing of the mucus that has built up in lungs and esophagus immediately following quitting smoking.[31] It will likely be useful to let patients know to expect this slight exacerbation in symptoms and to reassure them that these symptoms are only temporary, and quitting smoking will ultimately result in improved lung functioning, fewer respiratory symptoms, and improved quality of life.[15,32] Further, as smoking decreases the effectiveness of inhaled corticosteroids and quitting smoking results in improved lung function, patients should be evaluated after quitting to determine the appropriate medication regimen.

20.3.4 SMOKING CESSATION MEDICATIONS

Providers should take caution when prescribing certain smoking cessation medications to patients with asthma who want to quit smoking. First, providers should avoid prescribing the nicotine nasal spray, as it can exacerbate asthma symptoms.[33] Second, providers should use caution when prescribing varenicline, as there can be harmful drug interactions with certain asthma medications (i.e., theophylline).[17,34]

20.4 SUMMARY

- Smoking is more common among individuals with asthma, COPD and asthma COPD overlap, and it is associated with increased rates of morbidity and mortality in both diseases.
- Smoking cessation results improved lung functioning, reduced asthma medication use, and improved quality of life.
- Providers are encouraged to follow the 5 A's model of smoking cessation intervention: Ask, Advise, Assess, Assist, and Arrange (see Table 20.1).
- For smokers unwilling to quit, MI techniques should be used to increase motivation for quitting.
- For smokers willing to quit, a combination of pharmacotherapy and smoking cessation counseling is the most effective treatment.
- Specialized intensive psychosocial smoking cessation interventions may be useful for smokers with asthma or COPD and comorbid mood and anxiety disorders.
- Patients with asthma should be warned of slight, temporary increases in their asthma symptoms upon quitting and reassured that these symptoms are only temporary.
- For smokers with asthma and COPD, providers should take caution before prescribing nicotine nasal spray and varenicline, and reassess respiratory medication dosages after quitting.
- Strategies for smoking cessation applied to asthma and COPD should also apply to ACO.

REFERENCES

1. McLeish AC and Zvolensky MJ. Asthma and cigarette smoking: A review of the empirical literature. *J Asthma*. May 2010;47(4):345–361.
2. Centers for Disease Control and Prevention. Chronic obstructive pulmonary disease [Internet]. Atlanta (GA): U.S Department of Health and Human Services; Available at https://www.cdc.gov/copd/index.html. 2017.
3. Gwynn RC. Risk factors for asthma in US adults: Results from the 2000 behavioral risk factor surveillance system. *J Asthma*. February 2004;41(1):91–98.
4. Percentage of People with Asthma Who Smoke [Internet]. Centers for disease control and prevention. U.S Department of Health and Human Services; Available at https://www.cdc.gov/asthma/asthma_stats/people_who_smoke.htm. 2013. Accessed January 20, 2018.
5. McLeish AC, Cougle JR, and Zvolensky MJ. Asthma and cigarette smoking in a representative sample of adults. *J Health Psychol*. May 2011;16(4):643–652.
6. Precht DH, Keiding L, and Madsen M. Smoking patterns among adolescents with asthma attending upper secondary schools: A Community-Based study. *Pediatrics*. May 2003;111(5):562.

7. Schatz M, Zeiger RS, Vollmer WM et al. Determinants of future long-term asthma control. *J Allergy Clin Immunol*. November 2006;118(5):1048–1053.

8. Pedersen SE, Bateman ED, Bousquet J et al. Determinants of response to fluticasone propionate and salmeterol/fluticasone propionate combination in the gaining optimal asthma control study. *J Allergy Clin Immunol*. November 2007;120(5):1036–1042.

9. Mannino DM, Buist AS, Petty TL et al. Lung function and mortality in the United States: Data from the first national health and nutrition examination survey follow up study. *Thorax*. May 2003;58(5):388–393.

10. Pauwels RA and Rabe KF. Burden and clinical features of chronic obstructive pulmonary disease (COPD). *Lancet*. August 14, 2004;364(9434):613–620.

11. Boulet L, FitzGerald JM, McIvor RA et al. Influence of current or former smoking on asthma management and control. *Can Respir J*. July 20, 2008;15(5):275–279.

12. Eisner MD and Iribarren C. The influence of cigarette smoking on adult asthma outcomes. *Nicotine Tob Res*. January 2007;9(1):53–56.

13. Lazarus SC, Chinchilli VM, Rollings NJ et al. Smoking affects response to inhaled corticosteroids or leukotriene receptor antagonists in asthma. *Am J Respir Crit Care Med*. March 15, 2007;175(8):783–790.

14. Samet JM. Health benefits of smoking cessation. *Clin Chest Med*. December 1991;12(4):669–679.

15. Tønnesen P, Pisinger C, Hvidberg S et al. Effects of smoking cessation and reduction in asthmatics. *Nicotine Tob Res*. February 2005;7(1):139–148.

16. Avallone KM, McLeish AC, Zvolensky MJ et al. Asthma and its relation to smoking behavior and cessation motives among adult daily smokers. *J Health Psychol*. June 2013;18(6):788–799.

17. Fiore MC, Jaén CR, Baker TB et al. *Treating Tobacco Use and Dependence: 2008 Update*. Rockville, MD: U.S. Dept. of Health and Human Services, Public Health Service; 2008.

18. Miller, WR and Rollnick S. *Motivational Interviewing: Helping people change*. 3rd ed. New York, NY: Guilford Press; 2012.

19. McLeish AC, Farris SG, Johnson AL et al. Evaluation of smokers with and without asthma in terms of smoking cessation outcome, nicotine withdrawal symptoms, and craving: Findings from a self-guided quit attempt. *Addict Behav*. 2016;63:149–154.

20. Tashkin DP and Murray RP. Smoking cessation in chronic obstructive pulmonary disease. *Respir Med*. July 2009;103(7):963–974.

21. Gratziou C, Florou A, Ischaki E et al. Smoking cessation effectiveness in smokers with COPD and asthma under real life conditions. *Respir Med*. April 2014;108(4):577–583.

22. Brenes GA. Anxiety and chronic obstructive pulmonary disease: Prevalence, impact, and treatment. *Psychosom Med*. November 2003;65(6):963–970.

23. Goodwin RD, Jacobi F, and Thefeld W. Mental disorders and asthma in the community. *Arch Gen Psychiatry*. November 2003;60(11):1125–1130.

24. van Manen JG, Bindels PJE, Dekker FW et al. Risk of depression in patients with chronic obstructive pulmonary disease and its determinants. *Thorax*. May 2002;57(5):412–416.

25. Japuntich SJ, Smith SS, Jorenby DE et al. Depression predicts smoking early but not late in a quit attempt. *Nicotine Tob Res*. June 2007;9(6):677–686.

26. Piper ME, Cook JW, Schlam TR et al. Gender, race, and education differences in abstinence rates among participants in two randomized smoking cessation trials. *Nicotine Tob Res*. June 2010;12(6):647–657.

27. Piper ME, Smith SS, Schlam TR et al. Psychiatric disorders in smokers seeking treatment for tobacco dependence: Relations with tobacco dependence and cessation. *J Consult Clin Psychol*. February 2010;78(1):13–23.

28. Zvolensky MJ, Yartz AR, Gregor K et al. Interoceptive Exposure-Based cessation intervention for smokers high in anxiety sensitivity: A case series. *J Cognit Psychother*. Winter 2008;22(4):346–365.

29. Brown RA, Kahler CW, Zvolensky MJ et al. Anxiety sensitivity: Relationship to negative affect smoking and smoking cessation in smokers with past major depressive disorder. *Addict Behav*. November 2001;26(6):887–899.

30. Jefferson JW. Bupropion extended-release for depressive disorders. *Expert Rev Neurother*. May 2008;8(5):715–722.

31. Willemse BWM, Postma DS, Timens W et al. The impact of smoking cessation on respiratory symptoms, lung function, airway hyperresponsiveness and inflammation. *Eur Respir J*. March 2004;23(3):464–476.

32. Chaudhuri R, Livingston E, McMahon AD et al. Effects of smoking cessation on lung function and airway inflammation in smokers with asthma. *Am J Respir Crit Care Med*. July 15, 2006;174(2):127–133.

33. Roth MT and Westman EC. Asthma exacerbation after administration of nicotine nasal spray for smoking cessation. *Pharmacotherapy*. June 2002;22(6):779–782.

34. Marotta F, DiPaolo A, and Adib R. Chantix (Varenicline). *J Asthma Allergy Educ*. 2013;4(2):85–86.

Management of acute asthma, COPD, and asthma-COPD overlap

CRISTINA VILLA-ROEL AND BRIAN H. ROWE

21.1 DEFINITION AND ECONOMIC BURDEN

Asthma and chronic obstructive pulmonary disease (COPD) exacerbations are both acute events characterized by a progressive increase in respiratory symptoms often in response to external precipitants.[1,2] Patients with features of both asthma and COPD (asthma-COPD overlap [ACO]) also experience exacerbations.[3] These acute events result in visits to health professionals, school and work absenteeism, impairment of quality of life (QoL), emergency room (ER) visits, hospital admissions, and significant costs to the health-care system throughout the developed world.[4-6]

Asthma and COPD exacerbations represent a considerable number of the ER visits in North America.[7,8] Most adults presenting to the ER with asthma exacerbations are treated and subsequently discharged; only 6%–12% are admitted.[9] In contrast, COPD exacerbations resulting in ER visits often lead to hospitalization (50%–60%).[10] ACO exacerbations are three times more common than COPD exacerbations and have shown to be associated with more frequent hospitalizations and greater mortality rates.[11] Despite this, the evidence in ACO is just emerging, and little is known about this entity.

In the United States, asthma-related health-care costs are significantly higher in individuals experiencing exacerbations when compared to individuals not experiencing them.[4] In Canada, it has been estimated that 7% of the direct costs in asthma could be the result of acute asthma care.[12] Exacerbations with hospitalization are the main cost drivers for both COPD and ACO. In the United States in 2000, there were 8 million outpatient visits for COPD, 1.5 million ER visits, and 673,000 hospital admissions.[13] Resource utilization and costs attributable to ACO exacerbations are significantly higher than those derived from asthma and COPD alone.[11]

21.2 DIAGNOSIS

While patients presenting with acute wheezing episodes may suffer from a variety of cardiorespiratory conditions and mimics of asthma (i.e., gastroesophageal reflux, rhinitis/rhinosinusitis, vocal cord dysfunction), COPD and ACO must be ruled out. The diagnosis of asthma, COPD, or ACO exacerbations usually rely on a comprehensive, albeit focused, history and physical examination (Table 21.1). For example, young patients who wheeze and deny cigarette smoking, endorse allergies/family history of atopy, and respond to short-acting β_2-agonists (SABA), likely have acute asthma. Conversely, those over 55 years of age who have $>$20–30 pack-year histories of smoking, who have never had asthma or atopy, who have had a gradual

Table 21.1 Factors that can assist in the differentiation of asthma, COPD, and ACO exacerbations

Factors		Asthma	ACO	COPD
Pathophysiology	Inflammation	+++	+++	+++
	Infection		+/−	+++
Age of onset	Early	+++		
	Late (age > 40)		+++	+++
Sex	Female > male	+++		
	Male > female		+++	+++
Family history		+++		
Allergic conditions		+++		
Previous diagnosis of asthma		+++	+/−	
History of cigarette smoke exposure			+/−	+++
Comorbidities		+/−	+++	+++
Symptoms	Wheeze	+++	+/−	+/−
	Dyspnea	+++	+++	+++
	Cough	+/−	+/−	+++
	Sputum production		+/−	+++
Course	Intermittent exacerbations	+++		
	Chronic progressive		+/−	+++
Response to treatment	Response to bronchodilators	+++	+/−	+/−
	Response to corticosteroids	+++	+/−	+/−
Post-bronchodilator flow measurement	FEV_1/FVC ratio > 0.7	+++		
	FEV_1/FVC ratio < 0.7		+++	+++
Recovery after exacerbation		+++	+/−	+/−

Note: ACO = asthma-COPD overlap; COPD = chronic obstructive pulmonary disease; FVC = forced vital capacity; FEV_1 = forced expiratory volume in one second

onset of symptoms, and often have other comorbidities (e.g., diabetes, hypertension, etc.), likely have acute COPD. Finally, older patients (>40 years of age) with a previous medical diagnosis of asthma and no smoking history who reveal incomplete reversibility of airflow obstruction in the pre-/postbronchodilator flow measurement likely have ACO.

Objective measures of lung function are most commonly designed to establish a diagnosis, stratify, and manage chronic stable respiratory diseases. During exacerbations, they can be helpful in asthma and ACO with *asthma dominant* profile; however, they are generally not recommended for the assessment of COPD (and ACO with *COPD dominant* profile). If the diagnosis has not been confirmed previously, however, they may be useful in some cases, to suggest a diagnosis of asthma/ACO instead of COPD. Forced expiratory volume in 1 second (FEV_1) and, as a second choice, peak expiratory flow (PEF), help confirm the diagnosis, evaluate the exacerbation severity, and monitor the response to treatment. On the other hand, they are difficult to perform, often do not change with treatment, and are not accurate during COPD exacerbations. The diagnosis of COPD exacerbations relies mainly on the clinical presentation, which commonly reflects a sustained worsening of

symptoms leading to an increase in maintenance medications. Severe exacerbations are potentially life-threatening, thus factors that increase the risk of asthma- or COPD-related death should be identified and evidence-based care promptly provided (Table 21.2).[1,2]

21.3 MANAGEMENT

21.3.1 ROLE OF PATIENTS AND PRIMARY CARE PROVIDERS IN THE MANAGEMENT OF ASTHMA, COPD, AND ACO EXACERBATIONS

The goals of the management of asthma exacerbations are to control symptoms, improve QoL, and prevent relapses and subsequent exacerbations.[1] The goals of the management of COPD exacerbations are to relieve bronchospasm and treat infection/inflammation while maintaining adequate oxygenation.[2]

Depending on the severity of the exacerbation/underlying disease, the external resources and the clinical expertise,

Table 21.2 Factors that increase the risk of asthma- and COPD-related death

Asthma	COPD[a]
History of near-fatal asthma requiring intubation and mechanical ventilation	Older age
ER visits or hospitalizations for asthma in the previous year	Severity of illness
Current or recent use of OCS	Dyspnea (measured with a validated survey instrument)
Unopposed SABA use/no current ICS use	PaO_2/F_iO_2 ratio
Frequent use of SABAs, especially the use of more than a canister of salbutamol in the previous month	APACHE II score at admission
History of mental health or psychosocial issues	Low serum albumin
Poor adherence to asthma medications or poor adherence to (or lack of) a written asthma action plan	Presence of cor-pulmonale/end-stage disease.
Food allergy	Poor exercise capacity
	Long-term use of OCS
	Cardiac disease/comorbidities

Source: The Global Strategy for Asthma Management and Prevention, Global Initiative for Asthma (GINA); 2015. Available at http://www.ginasthma.org/; Global Initiative for Chronic Obstructive Lung Disease (GOLD). Global Strategy for Diagnosis, Management and Prevention of COPD; 2016. Available at http://www.goldcopd.org/.

Note: ER = Emergency Room; OCS = oral corticosteroids; ICS = inhaled corticosteroids; SABA = short-acting β_2 agonist; PaO_2/F_iO_2 = ratio of arterial oxygen partial pressure to fractional inspired oxygen; APACHE = Acute Physiology and Chronic Health Status Evaluation.

[a] Risk factors for in-hospital mortality.

patients and primary care providers (PCPs) can contribute to the achievement of these goals. For example, the use of written asthma action plans (AAPs) adapted to patients' level of asthma control and improving health literacy from patient education can be the first self-management strategy to prevent asthma exacerbations. The assessment of patient severity and medication adjustments (e.g., increasing reliever medications, *stepping up* the dose of existing controller medication, and starting patients on systemic corticosteroids) by a PCP can be the second strategy for the management of mild or moderate asthma exacerbations not adequately controlled with the instructions provided in the written AAP.[1] This stepwise approach would allow acute-care facilities (e.g., ERs or equivalent settings) to focus on the provision of urgent care to severe episodes, and those that were not controlled with the previous two strategies (Table 21.3).

Patient self-management programs should be carefully selected during COPD exacerbations to avoid harm.[14] While some episodes can be managed in an ambulatory basis (including guided adjustment or change to medication), their association with significant mortality often justifies hospital assessment and admission, especially in patients with older age, insufficient home support, history of frequent exacerbations, severe underlying COPD with low FEV_1, serious comorbidities (e.g., heart failure or newly occurring arrhythmias), onset of new physical signs (e.g., cyanosis, peripheral -edema), marked increase in symptoms (e.g., sudden resting dyspnea), and no response to initial medical management (Table 21.4).[2,15]

Individuals with ACO have shown an increased risk of undesired outcomes (e.g., more respiratory symptoms, worse lung function, lower perception of general health status, and higher use of medication, hospitalizations, and exacerbations).[16] This increased risk justifies hospital assessment for all but the most minor exacerbations. The role that patients and PCPs can play in the management of ACO exacerbations has not yet been identified; this will not be possible until its phenotypes and clinical progression are better characterized.[17]

21.3.2 ROLE OF ACUTE-CARE FACILITIES IN THE MANAGEMENT OF ASTHMA, COPD, AND ACO EXACERBATIONS

CLINICAL VIGNETTE 21.1

A 25-year-old female university student nurse presents to the ER with a two-day history of progressive shortness of breath, cough, and wheezing associated with symptoms of a viral upper respiratory infection (e.g., sore throat, myalgia, coryza). The patient has a life-long history of asthma and has recently been experiencing increased fibromyalgia symptoms of pain and fatigue. She denied fever or chest pain, and had been using her salbutamol puffer up to 16 times in the past 24-hour period. She stated that she usually used inhaled salbutamol (1–2 puffs as needed) and inhaled budesonide (two 200 mg inhalations, twice daily), when she remembers and can afford the

Table 21.3 Management options for patients and providers when dealing with an exacerbation of asthma in adults

ASTHMA

Patient
Self-management with a written action plan[a]

Early worsening of symptoms or mild symptoms:

- Increase reliever medication
- Increase controller medication
- Review response[b]

Late worsening of symptoms, PEF or FEV_1 < 60% best or not improving in 48 hours:

- Continue reliever medication
- Continue controller medication
- Add short-course OCS (Prednisone 40–50 mg/day)
- Contact doctor[b]

Primary care provider

Patient assessment based on:

Medical history and focused physical examination

Severity of the exacerbation (e.g., vital signs and pulmonary function tests)

Risk factors for asthma-related death (Table 21.2)

Mild or moderate signs and symptoms:
- Talks in phrases
- Prefers sitting to lying down
- Not agitated
- Minimal use of accessory muscles
- ⇑ Respiratory rate
- ⇑ Pulse rate
- O_2 saturation (on room air) 90%–95%
- PEF > 50% predicted or best

Severe signs and symptoms:
- Talks in words only
- Tripod positioning
- Slightly agitated
- Use of accessory muscles
- ⇑ Respiratory rate
- ⇑ Pulse rate
- O_2 saturation (on room air) < 90%
- PEF ≤ 50% predicted or best

Life-threatening:
- Converses using single words
- Agitated
- Confused or decreased level of consciousness
- Silent chest
- Unable to perform PEF
- Transfer to a monitored setting

Start treatment:
- SABA 4–10 puffs by MDI with spacer every 20 min for 1 hour
- Prednisone 50 mg (oral)
- Controlled oxygen (if available) to reach O_2 saturation (on air) 93%–95%
- Review response in 1 hour[c]

Start treatment and transfer to an acute care facility:
- SABA nebulized (5 mg) or MDI (4–8 puffs) and spacer
- Ipratropium bromide nebulized (500 µg) or MDI (4–6 puffs) and spacer
- Systemic corticosteroids (intravenous if vomiting or too dyspneic to swallow)
- Controlled oxygen (if available)

Source: The Global Strategy for Asthma Management and Prevention, Global Initiative for Asthma (GINA); 2015. Available at http://www.ginasthma.org/.

Note: PEF = peak expiratory flow; FEV_1 = forced expiratory volume in one second; OCS = oral corticosteroids; SABA = short-acting β_2-agonist; O_2 = oxygen; MDI = metered-dose inhalers

[a] Requires self-monitoring of symptoms and/or lung function, use of a written action plan, and regular medical review. These self-management strategies are targeting short-term periods (1–2 weeks) and should be followed by medical review.

[b] Presentation to an acute-care facility should be considered if there is no improvement or rapid deterioration in symptoms occurs despite following the written action plan. If there is improvement in the presenting signs/symptoms, increased dose of controller medication should be advised for the next 2–4 weeks and short-term medical follow-up (within 2–7 days) scheduled for monitoring patient level of asthma control, treatment response, individual risk factors, and engagement in self-management.

[c] Presentation to an acute care facility should be considered if there is no improvement or rapid deterioration in symptoms occurs.

Table 21.4 Management options for patients and providers when dealing with an exacerbation of COPD

COPD	
Patient **Self-management with a written action plan^a**	**Primary care provider**
Early worsening of symptoms or mild symptoms: • Increase SABA, SAAC, or SABA/SAAC combination therapy • Increase oxygen flow • Review response Late worsening of symptoms or not improving in 48 hours: • Contact doctor 	Patient assessment based on: Medical history and focused physical examination (Anthonisen criteria) Severity of the exacerbation (e.g., vital signs, severity of symptoms, disability, and pulmonary function tests) Risk factors for COPD-related death (Table 21.2) Moderate or severe COPD exacerbation: • Shortness of breath from COPD causing the patient to stop after walking ~100 m (or after a few minutes) on the same level (MRC 3 to 4) • 50% ≤ FEV_1 < 80% predicted • Shortness of breath from COPD resulting in the patient being too breathless to leave the house, breathless with activities of daily living (e.g., dressing), or the presence of chronic respiratory failure or clinical signs of right heart failure (MRC 5) • 30% ≤ FEV_1 < 50% predicted • Life-threatening (Table 21.2) • Transfer to a monitored setting Start treatment (if possible): • SAAC or SABA/SAAC combination therapy 4–8 puffs by MDI with spacer every 20 min for one hour or nebulized inhalation (5 mg) • Prednisone 50 mgs PO × 1 dose or IV methylprednisolone (80–125 mg) • Oral of IV antibiotics if ≥ 2 of the following^b: increased dyspnea, increased sputum volume, and increased sputum purulence • Controlled oxygen (if available) to reach O_2 saturation (on air) 88%–92% • Transfer *immediately* to a monitored setting

Mild COPD exacerbation:
• Shortness of breath from COPD when hurrying on the same level or walking up a slight hill (MRC 2).
• FEV_1 ≥ 80% predicted

Start treatment:
• SAAC or SABA/SAAC combination therapy 2–8 puffs by MDI with spacer every 20 min for 1 hour
• Prednisone 50 mgs PO × 1 dose
• Oral antibiotics if ≥ 2 of the following:^b
• increased dyspnea, increased sputum volume and increased sputum purulence
• Controlled oxygen (if available) to reach O_2 saturation (on air) 88%–92%
• Review response in 1 hour^c

Source: O'Donnell DE et al., *Can Respir J.*, 15, 1A–8A, 2008.
Note: COPD = chronic obstructive pulmonary disease; SABA = short-acting β_2-agonist; SAAC = short-acting anticholinergics; MRC = Medical Research Council dyspnea scale; FEV_1 = forced expiratory volume in one second; O_2 = oxygen; MDI = metered-dose inhalers.
a Requires self-monitoring of symptoms and signs, use of a written action plan, and regular medical review. These self-management strategies are targeting short-term periods (2 days) and should be followed by medical review. Contact your doctor if there is no improvement or rapid deterioration in symptoms occurs despite following the action plan.
b Consider recent use and local bacterial resistance pattern.
c If there is improvement in the presenting signs/symptoms, increase inhaled medications; prescribe oral corticosteroids and antibiotics (if applicable) for 5–7 days and 5 days, respectively. Also schedule short-term medical follow-up (within 2–7 days) for monitoring symptoms, treatment response, individual risk factors, and engagement in self-management. Presentation to an acute-care facility should be considered if there is no improvement or rapid deterioration in symptoms occurs despite initial treatment.

prescription. She used to have a spacer device (but lost it), and her "action plan" when she senses she is starting to have an asthma attack is to take a cold shower, use more salbutamol, and seek out the care of a physician. Although she admitted to occasionally smoking marijuana, she denied cigarette smoking. Her vital signs were as follows: pulse = 100 beats/minute; respirations = 24 breaths/minute; blood pressure = 110/60 mmHg; T = 36.8°C (oral); and SaO$_2$ = 95% on room air. Her PEF was 200 L/min (57% predicted for age, height, and sex). On examination, she was alert and oriented, spoke in full sentences, and was calm. She exhibited expiratory-phase prolongation and musical wheezing throughout the lung fields, and she was not using her accessory muscles of respiration. Her upper respiratory, cardiac, abdominal, and neurological examinations were normal.*

* See discussion of clinical vignettes at the end of section 3.

21.3.2.1 Asthma

Emergency rooms (or equivalent acute-care facilities) are the ideal settings to manage moderate/severe asthma exacerbations that do not improve with self-management and/or the initial management provided in the primary care setting, as well as potentially life-threatening asthma exacerbations.

21.3.2.1.1 ASSESSMENT

A brief medical history, physical examination, and objective measure of lung function (e.g., PEF or FEV$_1$) should precede the prompt initiation of therapy in acute asthma. The patient's clinical condition and response to treatment should be reassessed regularly during their ER stay. Current guidelines recommend lung function to be measured one hour after initial bronchodilator/corticosteroid treatment to document improvement or deterioration. Ordering additional tests (e.g., chest radiographs or laboratory tests) is not routinely recommended in adults, unless other diagnoses need to be ruled out.[1]

21.3.2.1.2 ER TREATMENT

Low-dose oxygen: Significant hypoxemia is common in moderate to severe asthma exacerbations, and therapy should target physiological levels of oxygen. Oxygen therapy either by nasal cannula or mask is recommended to all patients whose saturation is below this parameter (using oximetry when possible).[18] Since hyperoxia has been associated with increased oxidative stress and free radical damage, oxygen saturation above 92% is not recommended.[19]

Inhaled SABA: Inhaled SABA therapy should be administered as early as possible to all patients presenting to the ER with asthma exacerbations in an attempt to reverse airflow obstruction. At comparable doses, nebulizer-delivery products have not been associated with significantly better outcomes than metered-dose inhalers (MDI) delivered by spacer.[20]

Systemic corticosteroids: Systemic corticosteroids (oral or intravenous [IV]) speed the resolution of exacerbations, prevent admission, and relapses, and are recommended to all but the mildest cases of acute asthma.[21] Systemic corticosteroids should be administered within the first hour of presentation when possible. Fifty (50) mg of prednisone for 5–7 days have shown to be effective in the resolution of exacerbations.[22] No benefit has been associated with tapering the dose of oral corticosteroids (OCS) in the short-to-medium term;[23] in adults, very short courses have not replaced standard 7–10–day therapy.

Inhaled corticosteroids (ICS): Although ICS agents are thought to improve asthma control over days to weeks, there is evidence that they are effective in the acute setting. The administration of high doses of ICS within the first hour of ER presentation reduces the need for hospitalization in those patients receiving and not receiving systemic corticosteroids.[24] These observations are likely the result of local vasodilatation, membrane stabilization, and inhibition of the inflammatory cascade.

Short-acting anticholinergics (SAAC): Anticholinergic agents are weak bronchodilator agents, which also decrease mucous production. The combined use of SAAC/SABA has been associated with synergistic effects, especially in severe disease; fewer hospitalizations and greater improvement in pulmonary function, specifically PEF and FEV$_1$, when compared to SABA administration alone.[25]

Aminophylline/theophylline: Methylxanthine agents are weak bronchodilators and respiratory muscle enhancers through their influence on cyclic adenosine monophosphate (cAMP). The IV administration aminophylline is not routinely recommended in the ER management of asthma exacerbations due to lack of effectiveness as a bronchodilator in this setting and increased risk of adverse events when compared to standard inhaled bronchodilators and corticosteroids.[26]

Magnesium sulfate (MgSO$_4$): Intravenous sulfate exhibits its effect on smooth muscles, including those in the respiratory system, and also is a weak anti-inflammatory agent. Administered intravenously (2 g infusion over 20 minutes), MgSO$_4$ is recommended in adults presenting with severe exacerbations who have exhibited blunted response to initial inhaled bronchodilation therapy (e.g., initial FEV$_1$ < 25%–30% predicted, those who fail to respond to initial treatment and have persistent hypoxemia).[27] This agent must be used in combination with systemic corticosteroids and bronchodilators and has a wide margin of safety.

Epinephrine: Epinephrine, a mixed alpha- and beta-receptor agent, is most often used in allergic reactions, such as anaphylaxis. The intramuscular (IM) administration of this agent (adrenaline) is not routinely recommended in the ER management of asthma exacerbations; it is only indicated in acute asthma cases associated with anaphylaxis and allergic angioedema.

Leukotriene receptor antagonists: While these novel and important add-on therapeutic options are commonly recommended and used in chronic asthma, their administration is not routinely recommended in the ER management of asthma exacerbations.[28]

ICS/long-acting β₂-agonist combination agents (LABA): The administration of ICS/LABA agents is not routinely recommended in the ER management of asthma exacerbations.[29]

Antibiotics: Despite the fact that most acute asthma episodes result from exposure to indoor and outdoor environmental triggers and viral upper respiratory tract infections, antibiotics are commonly administered to patients who wheeze, in an attempt to treat any infection (or superinfection). The administration of these agents is only recommended for asthma exacerbations in which there is strong evidence of lung infection or in people who have failed to respond to an initial treatment with aggressive anti-inflammatory agents.

Noninvasive ventilation (NIV): The use of NIV in acute care comes in a variety of forms; however, the general concept is the positive pressure is provided to airways during respiration to maintain airway patency and gas exchange. This airway intervention can be used in patients with severe airflow limitation (usually hypercarbic, hypoxemic, and acidotic) as a strategy to prevent intubation. The use of NIV in the ER for acute asthma is not supported by strong evidence.[30] For example, only one randomized, controlled trial exists, and while positive, the evidence is insufficient for most guidelines to recommend its use in all but the most extreme cases. Nonetheless, given its use in exacerbations for heart failure and COPD in the ER, familiarity, and a desire to avoid intubations in these patients, a trial may be considered. It should be avoided in agitated patients, and concomitant sedation should not be attempted.

Heliox: The administration of heliox (helium/oxygen mixture in a ratio of 80:20 or 70:30) is not recommended for routine ER care of adult asthma. It has been suggested as an alternative for patients not responding to standard therapy.[31]

Intravenous fluids: While many patients with acute asthma have increased insensible losses (e.g., fever, hyperventilation, nausea/vomiting) and decreased fluid intake, most patients are not clinically dehydrated. The administration of IV fluids is therefore not recommended in the routine management of asthma exacerbations; selected patients may need rehydration and correction of electrolyte imbalance.

21.3.2.1.3 DISPOSITION DECISIONS

Most patients with acute asthma respond to therapy and can be safely discharged from the ER with follow-up after several hours of therapy. Patients' clinical condition and lung function one hour after commencement of therapy have shown to predict the need for hospital admissions.[32]

Sociodemographic factors (e.g., female sex, older age, and nonwhite race), asthma history (e.g., previous severe exacerbations), medication factors (e.g., previous use of OCS), and severity at ER presentation have been associated with an increased likelihood of hospitalizations.[33,34]

21.3.2.1.4 POST–ER MANAGEMENT

Management of asthma in the hospital is beyond the scope of this chapter, so emphasis is made on the evidence behind the current recommendations for discharge planning.

21.3.2.1.4.1 Pharmacologic management at ER discharge

Systemic corticosteroids: Systemic corticosteroids (oral or IM) use in the outpatient treatment of exacerbations has been associated with a reduction in relapses and the need for reassessment in the subsequent 7–10 days.[21] Since most patients have preference for oral over IM administration of these agents, short courses of OCS are recommended. Ultrashort doses of agents such as dexamethasone, while used in children,[35] have not proven to be effective in adults and should be avoided.

ICS: Inhaled corticosteroids are widely recommended as first-line agents for mild-to-moderate stable asthma.[36] The addition of ICS agents to OCS has been associated with a significant reduction in relapses, improvement in health-related QoL, and reduction in SABA use, without significant adverse events.[37,38] Given that patients who have an exacerbation of asthma have demonstrated a failure of current management, the addition of ICS agents after an ER visit makes intuitive and guideline-recommended sense. The overall evidence in this field is based on three trials of variable quality and the pooled evidence fails to reach statistical significance (RR = 0.68; 0.46, 1.02); however, it is difficult to ignore a 32% reduction in relapse with a potential of up to a 54% decrease in relapses compared to a possible 2% increase in relapses. Overall, these agents are well tolerated and safe.

ICS/LABA combination agents: Asthma guidelines in adults suggest a step-up to ICS/LABA agents in chronic stable asthma if the regular use of low-to-moderate–dose (moderate in children) agents fails to achieve control.[39] The addition of ICS/LABA agents after an ER discharge for acute asthma has been studied infrequently. There is weak evidence to suggest that patients who experience an exacerbation while already receiving ICS may experience improved QoL and potentially less-frequent relapses if ICS/LABA agents are combined with OCS at discharge.[29] Finally, patients already receiving these agents at ER presentation should continue them at discharge to avoid a step-down in treatment.

Leukotriene receptor antagonists: The use of these agents is not routinely recommended in the post-ER management of acute asthma. Patients already receiving these agents at ER presentation should not have them discontinued if discharged, since this represents a step-down in treatment. Primary care clinicians should reassess the effectiveness of these agents and, if not effective, discontinue to reduce polypharmacy.

21.3.2.1.4.2 Nonpharmacological management at ER discharge

ER visits due to asthma exacerbations have been recognized as ideal scenarios for the identification of gaps in asthma care.[40] Recent asthma guidelines have added content dedicated to the management of asthma exacerbations and highlighted the essential role of the discharge planning.[1] Follow-up 2–7 days after ER presentations for asthma exacerbations and strategies to promote self-management, such as reviewing inhaler techniques, providing written AAPs, and instruction on patient self-monitoring following discharge are recommended.[1,41,42] However, no clear evidence supports the different timing proposed for this visit and the overall effectiveness of this encounter.

A Cochrane systematic review examining the impact of ER-based educational strategies versus standard care showed a statistically significant reduction in hospitalizations but no conclusive reduction in ER visits.[43] A recent systematic review revealed that ER-directed educational interventions targeting either patients or providers increase the chance of having office follow-up visits with PCPs after asthma exacerbations. Their impact on health-related outcomes (e.g., relapse and admissions) remains unclear.[44]

21.3.2.2 Chronic obstructive pulmonary disease

Emergency settings (or equivalent acute-care facilities) are the ideal settings to manage mild ($FEV_1 \geq 80\%$ predicted) or moderate ($50\% \leq FEV_1 < 80\%$ predicted) COPD exacerbations (that don't improve with the initial management provided in the primary care setting), as well as severe ($30\% \leq FEV_1 < 50\%$ predicted) and/or potentially life-threatening exacerbations.[2]

21.3.2.2.1 ASSESSMENT

A focused, brief medical history and physical examination should precede the prompt initiation of therapy in patients presenting with COPD exacerbations. Current guidelines recommend the early provision of respiratory support (supplemental oxygen and ventilation) and pharmacological agents (including bronchodilators, corticosteroids, and antibiotics). The Anthonisen criteria have been used to guide treatment decisions for many years.[45] These criteria require clinicians to evaluate the following symptoms: increased sputum volume, increased sputum purulence, and dyspnea. The presence of three symptoms classifies patients as type I, two symptoms as type II, and one symptom as type III. Additional investigations are helpful in clarifying complications (e.g., complete blood count, venous or arterial blood gases, chest radiographs, serum electrolytes, and sputum collection) and ruling out other diagnoses (e.g., electrocardiogram [ECG], D-dimer to rule out thromboembolic

---

CLINICAL VIGNETTE 21.2

A 65-year-old, retired married male presented to the ER with a seven-day history of progressive shortness of breath, increased sputum volume, and increased sputum purulence. The patient reported a long-standing history of hypothyroidism, hypertension, and type 2 diabetes mellitus; he was diagnosed by a doctor at a clinic as having asthma two years previously. He denied fever or chest pain, and he had been using his "blue puffer" more frequently than in the past. His medications included inhaled salbutamol (1–2 puffs as needed), inhaled tiotropium (e.g., 18 µg, once daily), and inhaled fluticasone (250 mg inhalations, twice daily). He stated he had been immunized against pneumococcal infections; however, not influenza. Despite quitting smoking two years ago, he had a 40 pack-year history of smoking. His vital signs were as follows: pulse = 86 beats/minute; respirations = 20 breaths/minute; blood pressure = 155/95 mmHg; T = 37.4°C (oral); and SaO_2 = 92% on room air. On examination, he was alert and oriented, spoke in short sentences, and did not appear anxious. He exhibited decreased air entry, expiratory prolongation, and wheezing, and he was using his accessory muscles of respiration (e.g., scalene and intercostal muscles). While his throat was clear and trachea was midline, there was a tracheal tug. His heart sounds were normal, there was no peripheral edema, and his jugular veins were not distended. There was no evidence of swollen turbinates or cobblestoning suggestive of postnasal drainage.

---

disease, brain-natriuretic peptide [BNP] to rule out congestive heart failure, advanced imaging, etc.).[2]

21.3.2.2.2 ER TREATMENT

21.3.2.2.2.1 Respiratory support

Oxygen: Early low-dose oxygen therapy is one of the key management components for all patients with COPD presenting to ERs with exacerbations (unless they have indications for ventilatory support).[46] Some medical centers now have capnography monitoring of partial pressure of carbon dioxide (pCO_2); however, limited evidence has been collected to date on the utility of this monitoring in the ER setting.[47] The optimal amount of oxygen needs to be individualized, and it depends on the chronic needs and the severity of the COPD exacerbation. While oxygen saturation above 92% is the goal for most patients with COPD presenting to ERs with exacerbations, saturations between 88%–92% may be acceptable for chronic carbon dioxide (CO_2) retainers.

Ventilator Support: The use of NIV is indicated in patients with respiratory acidosis (arterial pH $\leq$ 7.35 and/or $PaCO_2 \geq$

6.0 kPa, 45 mmHg) and severe dyspnea with increased work of breathing, and/or clinical signs of respiratory muscle fatigue.[2] The high success rate (80%–85%), the reduced number of complications, and the improved outcomes related to intubation and mortality are some of the reasons behind the increased use over time.[48] The use of invasive mechanical ventilation is currently indicated for patients in respiratory or cardiac arrest, hemodynamic instability, massive aspiration, or psychomotor agitation not controlled by sedation; also in those with severe ventricular arrhythmias, diminished alertness (heart rate < 50 beats/minute) and consciousness, NIV failure/intolerability, and inability to mobilize respiratory secretions. Some patients do not tolerate NIV; others arrive at the ER with severe exacerbations or develop respiratory failure while there. Those patients need endotracheal intubation and admission to the intensive care unit.

21.3.2.2.2.2 Pharmacological agents

Bronchodilators: Inhaled SABA or SAAC therapy is recommended for the management of patients presenting to the ER with COPD exacerbations, and the route of delivery can be chosen based on patients' tolerability. Minimal additional benefit has been demonstrated by the use of SABA/SAAC combination therapy in COPD exacerbations.[49] In addition, given the advanced age of many patients with COPD exacerbations and their preexisting cardiac comorbidities, SABA toxicity is a concern, which suggests initiating treatment with SAAC agents. Finally, while the evidence is not as strong in COPD as in asthma, the use of MDI and a spacer device is preferred to nebulization except in the most extreme cases.[50]

Systemic corticosteroids: Systemic corticosteroids (oral or IV) speed the resolution of exacerbations and improve lung function; they also reduce hospital admissions and prevent relapses.[51] In most cases, patients with COPD exacerbations are capable of tolerating oral OCS agents; however, in some cases (e.g., severe dyspnea, vomiting, obtundation/intubation), the use of IV delivery is required.

Antibiotics: The administration of these agents is recommended in patients with COPD presenting to the ER with increasing dyspnea, sputum volume, sputum purulence, and/or requiring mechanical ventilation.[52] Antibiotics reduce sputum purulence, hospital admissions, relapses, and short-term mortality. Although local bacterial resistance patterns should guide clinicians' choice of antibiotics, guidelines recommend an evaluation of the sensitivity to the three most common pathogens (*Streptococcus pneumonie, Haemophilus influenzae, and Moraxella catarrhalis*). Cultures are recommended for patients with frequent exacerbations and severe airflow limitation, as well as those requiring mechanical ventilation, since resistance is common in such cases.

Aminophylline/theophylline: The IV administration of aminophylline/theophylline is not routinely recommended as a first-line therapy in the ER management and should be considered only when there is insufficient response to inhaled SABA/SAAC.[53]

21.3.2.2.3 DISPOSITION

Decisions to admit patients with COPD exacerbations to the hospital are complex. Several factors related to medical history (≥ 2 COPD admissions in the past two years), treatment (receiving OCS for COPD and adjunct ER treatments), and severity at ER presentation (triage score) have shown to predict hospital admissions during COPD exacerbations in Canada.[54] In the United States, sociodemographics (older age, female sex), smoking history, recent use of ICS, activity limitation, higher respiratory rate at ER presentation, and having a concomitant diagnosis of pneumonia have been associated with hospital admissions after visiting the ER for COPD exacerbations.[55] In Nordic countries, anxiety disorders have been associated with an increased risk of rehospitalizations.[56]

21.3.2.2.4 POST–ER MANAGEMENT

Approximately 20%–30% of the patients who are discharged from the ER after being treated for COPD exacerbations will relapse within the next 4 weeks.[10] This chapter makes emphasis on the evidence behind management choices that may influence recovery and relapses.

21.3.2.2.4.1 Pharmacologic management at ER discharge

Oxygen: While all patients should be assessed for the need of supplemental home oxygen before ER discharge, most can be discharged without it.[2] Guidelines for accessing home oxygen therapy vary across jurisdictions, and clinicians are advised to seek local guidance on the requirements.

Systemic corticosteroids: Systemic corticosteroids (oral) prevent relapses, hospital admissions, and reduce the average hospital length of stay.[51] Forty to sixty (40–60) mg of prednisone for 7–10 days have shown to be effective in the resolution of exacerbations. Shorter courses may be recommended for older patients with comorbidities that are potentially exacerbated by systemic corticosteroids (e.g., type 2 diabetes mellitus, heart failure, hypertension).

Antibiotics: Guidelines recommend to discharge patients on antibiotics who exhibit a combination of at least two or more of the following features: increased dyspnea, increased sputum volume, and increased sputum purulence.[57] Considerations regarding antibiotic choice are the same that were mentioned for the ER treatment and short courses (7–10 days or even less) are recommended for the elderly as opposed to longer courses.

21.3.2.2.4.2 Nonpharmacological management at ER discharge

Similar to ER visits due to asthma, visits due to COPD exacerbations represent an excellent opportunity for the assessment of gaps in care. Both, historical (previous urgent care/ER visits) and acute factors (activity limitation and respiratory rate at ER presentation) have been associated with relapse occurrence, and emergency physicians should take them into consideration while making ER decisions.[58]

Medical follow-up after ER presentations for COPD exacerbations is always recommended.[57] A preventive strategy following discharge, such as the use of influenza vaccination, has been associated with reduced rates of influenza-related acute respiratory illness and of COPD exacerbations;[59] the evidence for pneumococcal vaccinations is less robust but sufficient to recommend its use in patients at risk for pneumonia, including patients with COPD.[59] Strategies targeting smoking cessation are recommended due to their decline in the rate of lung function loss and of all-cause mortality.[15] Finally, the benefits derived from an early referral to pulmonary rehabilitation include improvement in functional exercise capacity and QoL, and the reduction of COPD exacerbations, hospitalizations, and health-care costs.[15]

CLINICAL VIGNETTE 21.3

A 59-year-old single male presented to the ER with a three-day history of progressive shortness of breath, without increased sputum volume or purulence. The patient reported a recent history of coronary artery disease, "asthma" since childhood (e.g., atopic disease), and osteoarthritis. He denied fever or chest pain, and he had been using his "green puffer" more frequently than in the past. His medications included inhaled salbutamol (1–2 puffs, four times daily, as needed), inhaled ipratropium bromide (1–2 puffs, four times daily, as needed), and an inhaled combination agent (budesonide/formoterol; 200/6 µg/activation) through a Turbuhaler (one inhalation, twice daily). He stated he had received pneumococcal and influenza vaccinations within the last year. He had a 30 pack-year history of smoking and was "trying to quit." His vital signs were as follows: pulse = 70 beats/minute; respirations = 24 breaths/minute; blood pressure = 128/72 mmHg; T = 36.8°C (oral); and SaO$_2$ = 94% on room air. On examination, he was alert and oriented, spoke in sentences, and did not seem anxious. He exhibited decreased air entry, expiratory prolongation, and wheezing; however, he was not using his accessory muscles of respiration. His throat was clear, trachea was midline, and there was no tracheal tug. His heart sounds were normal, there was no peripheral edema, and his jugular veins were not distended. Breathing through nose was not obstructed, and there was no evidence of postnasal drainage.

21.3.2.3 Asthma-chronic obstructive pulmonary disease overlap

Since the role that patients and PCPs could play in the management of ACO exacerbations has not yet been identified, ERs (or equivalent acute-care facilities) may be the ideal settings to manage patients with combined features of asthma and COPD

who experience rapid and progressive increase in respiratory symptoms or demands in their maintenance medication.

21.3.2.3.1 ASSESSMENT

Similar to asthma and COPD, a focused and brief medical history, physical examination, and objective measure of lung function (e.g., PEF or full spirometry, when possible) should precede the prompt initiation of therapy. Patients' clinical condition and response to treatment should be reassessed regularly during their ER stay if there is an *asthma dominant* clinical profile. If there is a COPD *dominant* clinical profile, additional tests are helpful in clarifying complications (e.g., complete blood count, venous or arterial blood gases, chest X-rays, serum electrolytes, and sputum collection) and ruling out other diagnoses (e.g., ECG, D-dimer, BNP, advanced imaging).

21.3.2.3.2 ER TREATMENT AND POST-ER MANAGEMENT

Most of the patients with ACO have been excluded from both asthma and COPD pharmacological trials. Therefore, the evidence supporting the current pharmacological recommendations for the treatment of this syndrome is limited and mostly extrapolated from the published literature in asthma and COPD.[60] To date, no recommendations have been provided for the ER and post-ER management of ACO exacerbations, and emergency physicians should focus on the stabilization of the dominant clinical profile until there is more conclusive evidence for its specific phenotypes.

CLINICAL VIGNETTE SUMMARIES

In Clinical vignette 21.1, the 25-year-old nursing student with acute asthma responded to three doses of six puffs of inhaled salbutamol and 50 mg of oral prednisone in the ER. Her PEF increased from 57% predicted to 75% predicted during 2 hours of treatment, and she was discharged on oral prednisone for 5 days and encouraged to adhere to her moderate-dose fluticasone. In fact, the social worker was able to apply for assistance with drug coverage. A spacer device was provided, and inhaler techniques were reviewed before ER discharge. An appointment was made with her PCP to review a written AAP, obtain influenza immunization, and reassess her symptoms in 7 days.

In Clinical vignette 21.2, the 65-year-old patient with wheezing, his FEV$_1$/forced vital capacity (FVC) ratio was 62%, and his FEV$_1$ = 1.35 L, confirming the diagnosis of severe COPD. His chest radiograph failed to reveal pneumonia or pneumothorax; however, he was slow to respond to the care provided in the ER (including ipratropium bromide, 6 puffs every 20 minutes × 3, oral prednisone, and oral doxycycline). His arterial blood gas revealed mild respiratory acidosis: pH = 7.30; pCO$_2$ = 55 mmHg; pO$_2$ = 50 mmHg; and

HCO$_3$ = 15 mmol/L. Given his deterioration, he was started on a trial of NIV and admitted to the hospital.

In Clinical vignette 21.3, the 59-year-old patient with wheezing, his prebronchodilator FEV$_1$/FVC ratio was 65%, and his FEV$_1$ = 2.35 L, and he responded to bronchodilators in the ER (> 12% predicted), confirming the diagnosis of ACO. His chest radiograph failed to reveal pneumonia or pneumothorax; and he improved considerably following the care provided in the ER (including ipratropium bromide/salbutamol, six puffs every 20 minutes for an hour, 50 mg of oral prednisone). Given his improvement, he was discharged from the hospital on oral prednisone (50 mg for 7 days); increased combination agent to two activations, twice daily, and instructions to follow-up with his PCP within a week to reassess his symptoms and deal with the other care issues (e.g., need for written ACO action plan, smoking-cessation counseling, immunization, and referral for respiratory education). He did not qualify for antibiotics (ACO with asthma dominant clinical profile) because he only had one of the Anthonisen criteria.

21.4 GAPS IN ACUTE CARE AND RESEARCH OPPORTUNITIES

Despite the dissemination of effective interventions for the management of asthma and COPD exacerbations, variation still exists and undesired outcomes like relapses occur. These outcomes affect the QoL of patients with asthma and COPD, and represent significant costs to the health-care system. Epidemiological and health services research may help identifying relevant factors (e.g., admission/discharge decision tools, unnecessary procedures) and effective strategies (e.g., care bundles) to be considered while making clinical decisions. Methods to standardize patient self-management and medical practice (in and outside the ER), as well as, to facilitate the transitions in care (e.g., hospital and PCP linkages) are needed. The engagement of patients and other knowledge users in research initiatives is a promising approach for the identification of facilitators and barriers for the implementation of research results into day-to-day clinical management. Finally, comparative effectiveness research should be incentivized so there is a rigorous comparison of the different alternatives for the management of these entities.

While initial attempts to define ACO and to measure its human and economic burden have been made, no high-quality data exist upon which to base management recommendations. There is an urgent need to identify ACO phenotypes and their clinical progression so that targeted treatments can be assessed. In addition, nonpharmacological strategies, such as self-management programs, should be adapted to the needs of this specific population and tested using high-quality research methods.

REFERENCES

1. Global Initiative for Asthma. Global Strategy for Asthma Management and Prevention; 2015. Available at www.ginasthma.org.
2. Global Initiative for Chronic Obstructive Lung Disease (GOLD). Global strategy for diagnosis, management and prevention of COPD; 2016. Available at http://www.goldcopd.org/.
3. Gibson PG and Simpson JL. The overlap syndrome of asthma and COPD: What are its features and how important is it?. Thorax. 2009;64:728–735.
4. Ivanova JI, Bergman R, Birnbaum HG et al. Effect of asthma exacerbations on health care costs among asthmatic patients with moderate and severe persistent asthma. J Allergy Clin Immunol. 2012;129:1229–1235.
5. FitzGerald JM, Haddon JM, Bradly-Kennedy C et al. Resource use study in COPD (RUSIC): A prospective study to quantify the effects of COPD exacerbations on health care resource use among COPD patients. Can Respir J. 2007;14:145–152.
6. Kauppi P, Kupiainen H, Lindqvist A et al. Overlap syndrome of asthma and COPD predicts low quality of life. J Asthma. 2011;48:279–285.
7. Akinbami LJ, Moorman JE, Zahran HS et al. Trends in asthma prevalence, health care use, and mortality in the United States, 2001–2010. NCHS Data Brief. 2012;94:1–8. Available at http://www.lung.org/assets/documents/research/asthma-trend-report.pdf.
8. Trends in COPD (Chronic Bronchitis and Emphysema): Morbidity and Mortality. 2013. Available at http://www.lung.org/assets/documents/research/COPD-trend-report.pdf.
9. Rowe BH, Bota GW, Clark S et al. For the MARC Investigators. Comparison of Canadian versus US emergency department visits for acute asthma. Can Respir J. 2007;14:331–337.
10. Cydulka RK, Rowe BH, Clark S et al. Emergency department management of acute exacerbations of chronic obstructive pulmonary disease in the elderly: The Multicenter Airway Research Collaboration. J Am Geriatr Soc. 2003;51:908–916.
11. Shaya FT, Dongyi D, Akazawa MO et al. Burden of concomitant asthma and COPD in a Medicaid population. Chest. 2008;134:14–19.
12. Krahn MD, Berka C, Langlois P et al. Direct and indirect costs of asthma in Canada. Can Med Assoc J. 1996;154:821–831.
13. Mannino DM, Homa DM, Akinbami LJ et al. Chronic obstructive pulmonary disease surveillance—United States, 1971–2000. CDC Surveill Summ MMWR. 2002;51:1–16.
14. Zwerink M, Brusse-Keizer M, van der Valk PD et al. Self management for patients with chronic obstructive pulmonary disease. Cochrane Database Syst Rev. 2014;3:CD002990.

15. Rowe BH, Bhutani M, Stickland MK et al. Assessment and management of chronic obstructive pulmonary disease in the emergency department and beyond. *Expert Rev Respir Med.* 2011;5:549–559.

16. Menezes AM, Montes de Oca M, Perez-Padilla R et al. Increased risk of exacerbation and hospitalization in subjects with an overlap phenotype: COPD-asthma. *Chest.* 2014;145:297–304.

17. Ding B and Enstone A. Asthma and chronic obstructive pulmonary disease overlap syndrome (ACOS): Structured literature review and physician insights. *Expert Rev Respir Med.* 2016;10:363–371.

18. Perrin K, Wijesinghe M, Healy B et al. Randomised controlled trial of high concentration versus titrated oxygen therapy in severe exacerbations of asthma. *Thorax.* 2011;66:937–941.

19. Bryan CL and Jenkinson SG. Oxygen toxicity. *Clin Chest Med.* 1988;9(1):141–152.

20. Cates CJ, Welsh EJ, and Rowe BH. Holding chambers (spacers) versus nebulisers for beta-agonist treatment of acute asthma. *Cochrane Database Syst Rev.* 2013;9:CD000052.

21. Rowe BH, Spooner CH, Ducharme FM et al. Corticosteroids for preventing relapse following acute exacerbations of asthma. *Cochrane Database Syst Rev.* 2007;18:CD000195.

22. Jones AM, Munavvar M, Vail A et al. Prospective, placebo-controlled trial of 5 vs 10 days of oral prednisolone in acute adult asthma. *Respir Med.* 2002;96:950–954.

23. Lederle FA, Pluhar RE, Joseph AM et al. Tapering of corticosteroid therapy following exacerbation of asthma. A randomized, double-blind, placebo-controlled trial. *Arch Intern Med.* 1987;147:2201–2203.

24. Edmonds ML, Milan SJ, Camargo CA et al. Early use of inhaled corticosteroids in the emergency department treatment of acute asthma. *Cochrane Database Syst Rev.* 2012;12:CD002308.

25. Stoodley RG, Aaron SD, and Dales RE. The role of ipratropium bromide in the emergency management of acute asthma exacerbation: A meta-analysis of randomized clinical trials. *Ann Emerg Med.* 1999;34:8–18.

26. Nair P, Milan SJ, and Rowe BH. Addition of intravenous aminophylline to inhaled beta(2)-agonists in adults with acute asthma. *Cochrane Database Syst Rev.* 2012;12:CD002742.

27. Rowe BH, Bretzlaff JA, Bourdon C et al. Magnesium sulfate for treating exacerbations of acute asthma in the emergency department. *Cochrane Database Syst Rev.* 2000;2:CD001490.

28. Ramsay CF, Pearson D, Mildenhall S et al. Oral montelukast in acute asthma exacerbations: A randomised, double-blind, placebo-controlled trial. *Thorax.* 2011;66:7–11.

29. Rowe BH, Wong E, Blitz S et al. Adding long-acting beta-agonists to inhaled corticosteroids after discharge from the emergency department for acute asthma: A randomized controlled trial. *Acad Emerg Med.* 2007;14:833–840.

30. Lim WJ, Mohammed Akram R, Carson KV et al. Non-invasive positive pressure ventilation for treatment of respiratory failure due to severe acute exacerbations of asthma. *Cochrane Database Syst Rev.* 2012;12:CD004360.

31. Rodrigo GJ and Castro-Rodriguez JA. Heliox-driven beta2-agonists nebulization for children and adults with acute asthma: A systematic review with meta-analysis. *Ann Allergy Asthma Immunol.* 2014;112:29–34.

32. Kelly AM, Kerr D, and Powell C. Is severity assessment after one hour of treatment better for predicting the need for admission in acute asthma?. *Respir Med.* 2004;98:777–781.

33. Rowe BH, Villa Roel C, Abu-Laban RB et al. Admissions to Canadian hospitals for acute asthma: A prospective, multicentre study. *Can Respir J.* 2010;17:25–30.

34. Weber EJ, Silverman RA, Callaham ML et al. A prospective multicenter study of factors associated with hospital admission among adults with acute asthma. *Am J Med.* 2002;113:371–378.

35. Altamimi S, Robertson G, Jastaniah W et al. Single-dose oral dexamethasone in the emergency management of children with exacerbations of mild to moderate asthma. *Pediatr Emerg Care.* 2006;22:786–793.

36. Balter MS, Bell AD, Kaplan AG et al. Management of asthma in adults. *CMAJ.* 2009;181:915–922.

37. Rowe BH, Bota GW, Fabris L et al. Inhaled budesonide in addition to oral corticosteroids to prevent relapse following discharge from the emergency department: A randomized controlled trial. *JAMA.* 1999;281:2119–2126.

38. Edmonds ML, Milan SJ, Brenner BE et al. Inhaled steroids for acute asthma following emergency department discharge. *Cochrane Database Syst Rev.* 2012;12:CD002316.

39. Lougheed MD, Lemiere C, Ducharme FM et al. Canadian thoracic society 2012 guideline update: Diagnosis and management of asthma in preschoolers, children and adults. *Can Respir J.* 2012;19:127–164.

40. Lazarus S. Emergency treatment of asthma. *N Engl J Med.* 2010;363:755–764.

41. National Asthma Education and Prevention Program. Expert Panel Report 3 (EPR-3): Guidelines for the diagnosis and management of asthma-summary report 2007. *J Allergy Clin Immunol.* 2007;120:S94–S138.

42. British Thoracic Society Scottish Intercollegiate Guidelines Network. British guideline on the management of asthma. *Thorax.* 2008;63:iv1–iv121.

43. Tapp S, Lasserson TJ, and Rowe BH. Education interventions for adults who attend the emergency room for acute asthma. *Cochrane Database Syst Rev.* 2007;18(3):CD003000.

44. Villa-Roel C, Nikel T, Ospina M et al. Effectiveness of educational interventions to increase primary care follow-up for adults seen in the emergency department for acute asthma: A Systematic Review and Meta-analysis. *Acad Emerg Med.* 2016;23:5–13.

45. Anthonisen N, Manfreda J, Warren P et al. Antibiotic therapy in exacerbation of chronic obstructive pulmonary disease. *Ann Intern Med.* 1987;106:196–204.

46. Celli BR, MacNee W, and Force AET. Standards for the diagnosis and treatment of patients with COPD: A summary of the ATS/ERS position paper. *Eur Respir J.* 2004;23:932–946.

47. Manifold CA, Davids N, Villers LC et al. Capnography for the nonintubated patient in the emergency setting. *J Emerg Med.* 2013;45(4):626–632.

48. Ram FS, Picot J, Lightowler J et al. Non-invasive positive pressure ventilation for treatment of respiratory failure due to exacerbations of chronic obstructive pulmonary disease. *Cochrane Database Syst Rev.* 2004:CD004104.

49. McCrory DC and Brown CD. Anti-cholinergic bronchodilators versus beta2-sympathomimetic agents for acute exacerbations of chronic obstructive pulmonary disease. *Cochrane Database Syst Rev.* 2002;4: CD003900.

50. Woods JA, Usery JB, Self TH et al. An evaluation of inhaled bronchodilator therapy in patients hospitalized for non-life-threatening COPD exacerbations. *South Med J.* 2011;104:742–745.

51. Wood-Baker RR, Gibson PG, Hannay M et al. Systemic corticosteroids for acute exacerbations of chronic obstructive pulmonary disease. *Cochrane Database Syst Rev.* 2005;1:CD0011288.

52. Vollenweider DJ, Jarrett H, Steurer-Stey CA et al. Antibiotics for exacerbations of chronic obstructive pulmonary disease. *Cochrane Database Syst Rev.* 2012;12:CD010257.

53. Barr RG, Rowe BH, and Camargo CA, Jr. Methylxanthines for exacerbations of chronic obstructive pulmonary disease. *Cochrane Database of Sys Rev.* 2003;2:CD002168.

54. Rowe BH, Villa-Roel C, Guttman A et al. Predictors of hospital admission for chronic pulmonary disease exacerbations in canadian emergency departments. *Acad Emerg Med.* 2009;16:316–324.

55. Tsai C-L, Clark S, Cydulka RK et al. Factors associated with hospital admission among emergency department patients with chronic obstructive pulmonary disease exacerbation. *Acad Emerg Med.* 2007;14:6–15.

56. Gudmundsson G, Gislason T, Janson C et al. Risk factors for rehospitalisation in COPD: Role of health status, anxiety and depression. *Eur Respir J.* 2005;26:414–419.

57. O'Donnell DE, Aaron S, Bourbeau J et al. Canadian thoracic society recommendations for management of chronic obstructive pulmonary disease - 2007 update. *Can Respir J.* 2007;14(Suppl. B):5B–32B.

58. Kim S, Emerman CL, Cydulka RK et al. Prospective multicenter study of relapse following emergency department treatment of COPD exacerbation. *Chest.* 2004;125:473–481.

59. Poole PJ, Chacko E, Wood-Baker RW et al. Influenza vaccine for patients with chronic obstructive pulmonary disease. *Cochrane Database Syst Rev.* 2006;25(1):CD002733.

60. Global Initiative for Asthma and Global Initiative for Chronic Obstructive Pulmonary Disease. Diagnosis of Diseases of Chronic Airflow Limitation: Asthma, COPD and Asthma-COPD Overlap Syndrome (ACOS); 2015. Available at www.ginasthma.org and www.goldcopd.org.

Quality of life and health outcomes in asthma, COPD, and asthma-COPD overlap

CHRISTINE F. MCDONALD AND DON D. SIN

22.1 INTRODUCTION

Asthma and chronic obstructive pulmonary disease (COPD) are a huge medical burden worldwide. There are 330 million people globally with asthma and another 384 million individuals with COPD. COPD accounts for 5% of all deaths globally (3 million per year).[1] The most recent estimates suggest that 1 in 12 people have one or both of these disorders.[2,3] Asthma and COPD are distinct disorders, which share some similar clinical features including symptoms (e.g. dyspnea, wheezing, and cough) and airflow limitation. In asthma, however, the airflow limitation tends to be episodic with complete or near complete reversibility during periods of stability or with treatment.[2] The airflow limitation associated with COPD, on the other hand, tends to be persistent, non-reversible, or incompletely reversible, and is often progressive.[3] Some individuals demonstrate clinical features of both asthma and COPD and thus have been recently labeled as patients with asthma-COPD overlap (ACO). The details on ACO epidemiology, definition, and pathophysiology have been discussed in previous chapters. Here, we will focus largely on clinical presentations, health-related quality of life (HRQL) and prognosis of patients with ACO in the context of asthma and COPD, including discussion of a case study that will illustrate the most salient features of ACO on these domains.

CLINICAL VIGNETTE 22.1

Mr I.B. is a single semiretired, 69-year-old magician and television producer living alone. He suffered from childhood asthma and was exposed to environmental tobacco smoke as his father worked for a tobacco company and was a heavy smoker. His mother was a nonsmoker. Hospital emergency room attendance occurred several times with exacerbations of his asthma, but he never required hospital admission. A major improvement in his asthma symptoms came with the introduction of the short-acting β_2-agonist (SABA), and by his early teens he grew out of the condition. In his 20's, Mr. I.B. started smoking, continuing this habit on and off until his early 60s, with a total exposure of 30 pack years. His asthma was largely quiescent during middle age, and he perceived that smoking appeared to help his asthma. In the early 2000s, his asthma recrudesced, and he had several exacerbations of his condition treated with oral corticosteroids by his primary care physician. In 2005, lung function tests showed mild poorly reversible airflow obstruction with post-bronchodilator forced expiratory volume in 1 second (FEV_1)/forced vital capacity (FVC) of 61%, and FEV_1 of 2.36L (73% of predicted), with an increase in the FEV_1 of only 4% from baseline values. The pre- and postbronchodilator FVC was

3.9L (90% of predicted) and 4.10L respectively. Carbon monoxide transfer factor (corrected for hemoglobin) was 72% of predicted. During the next few years, he used inhaled corticosteroid (ICS)/long-acting β_2-agonist (LABA) medications intermittently, tending to cease these after acute attacks had subsided, because of poorly tolerated ICS side effects and resolution of symptoms. He continued to smoke lightly. In 2010 he was hospitalized briefly during an episode of thunderstorm asthma. This author saw him in 2011 after referral with persistent breathlessness and recurrent exacerbations requiring frequent courses of oral corticosteroids. He was still smoking intermittently, described symptoms of mild anxiety and depression, and was minimally physically active. Spirometry revealed a severe obstructive defect with postbronchodilator FEV_1 = 1.77L, VC = 4.2 L, and FEV_1/FVC 43%; demonstrating a dramatic fall in FEV_1 of 116 mLs/year over 6 years, twice the average annual fall in FEV_1 seen in heavy-smoking asthmatics.[40] Spirometry remained stable over months despite ICS/LABA and long-acting muscarinic antagonist (LAMA) therapy and a diagnosis of ACO was made. Despite no personal history of atopy, skin-prick tests (performed during work-up for consideration of anti-Immunoglobulin E [IgE] therapy to better control his asthma) were positive for house dust mite (D. pteronyssinus), grass, and English plantain weed. Treatment included education about his disease, including the importance of maintenance of quit status, pulmonary rehabilitation, continued LAMA/LABA/ICS, psychologist input, and encouragement of regular physical activity. Five years later (2016), lung function was not altered substantially, and his symptoms improved.

22.1.1 DISCUSSION OF CLINICAL VIGNETTE

This patient has features of ACO, with a history of childhood asthma, a significant active and passive smoking history, and persistent chronic airflow limitation. FEV_1 declined acutely and rapidly during continued active smoking and has stabilized now with no decline over the past 5 years. Cessation of smoking, continued physical activity, and regular medication use have seen stabilization of his symptoms. Important elements in this man's treatment were eventual cessation of smoking, constancy of medical review, and psychological support.

22.2 QUALITY OF LIFE IN ASTHMA AND COPD

Both asthma and COPD are associated with impaired HRQL. In an Australian survey of adults aged 15+ years, 39% of those with current asthma rated their health as excellent or very good compared with 58% of those without asthma,[4] while 25% of people with current asthma rated their health as "fair or poor" compared with only 14% of people without the condition. Asthma also impacts psychological health, with the prevalence of one or more anxiety or depressive disorders being at least double than that in the general population.[5] Quality of life in asthma can be measured using a number of measurement tools which have been shown to correlate with symptoms and exacerbations.

The asthma quality of life questionnaire (AQLQ) and its shorter version, the mini-AQLQ, measure the impact of asthma across four domains including symptoms, activity limitation, emotional function, and environmental stimuli.[6,7] Although one would postulate that better asthma control would be associated with better HRQL, few studies have examined this using validated tools. In the Gaining Optimal Asthma Control (GOAL) study of more than 3000 patients,

mean AQLQ score was significantly higher in those who achieved good asthma control than in those who did not.[8] Similarly, in a recent study of asthma in primary care in Portugal, better control of asthma correlated strongly with quality of life as measured with the mini-AQLQ.[9] Supported self-management in patients with asthma including the use of a written action plan, together with self-monitoring and regular review has been shown to reduce emergency room presentations, hospitalizations, and unscheduled consultations, as well as improving HRQL.[10]

Smoking is associated with more asthma symptoms and emergency room visits,[11,12] worse asthma control, and, consequently, worse quality of life, as well as a reduced response to both inhaled and oral corticosteroids. Fortunately, smoking cessation is associated with significant improvements in symptoms, lung function, and quality of life in most, although not all, asthmatics.[13]

Patients with COPD also have impaired health status compared to those without the condition, with determinants of health status impairment including the severity of airflow limitation, level of dyspnea and frequency of exacerbations.[14,15] In the Burden of Obstructive Lung Disease (BOLD) study, a general population–based cross-sectional survey in 17 countries, COPD significantly impacted physical and, to a lesser extent, psychological health status; the impact worsening with increasing COPD severity.[16] The "COPD uncovered" survey, which determined the impact of COPD on a working population, found that 40% of people had been forced to stop working due to their COPD,[17] and other studies have suggested that approximately one in five people is likely to retire prematurely due to their COPD.[18,19] The majority of patients with COPD also have at least one chronic comorbidity. Comorbidity burden presents a significant challenge in the management of patients with COPD. It is associated with increased risk of mortality, longer lengths of hospital stay, and higher readmission rates.[20] A relationship between increasing number of comorbidities and worse quality of life in patients with COPD has also been demonstrated. Although supported self-management is demonstrably beneficial in patients with asthma, its role in patients with COPD is less clear, and further studies are needed to determine which patients or patient groups will be best served by such interventions.[21] Smoking cessation slows lung function decline and improves survival in COPD compared with continued smoking;[22] however data regarding the impact of smoking cessation on quality of life in COPD are limited. In patients with mild COPD enrolled in the Lung Health Study (LHS), a longitudinal study assessing the impact of smoking cessation on FEV_1 decline, the prevalence of symptoms of chronic cough and phlegm, chronic wheeze and breathlessness decreased by more than 80% after 5 years of smoking cessation.[23] Nonetheless, even smokers and former smokers without COPD may have worse quality of life than nonsmokers. In a study of 2,736 current or former smokers and control subjects enrolled in the Subpopulation and Intermediate Outcomes in COPD Study (SPIROMICS), symptomatic current or former smokers with preserved pulmonary function had exacerbations and activity limitation. Quality of life, as measured by the COPD Assessment Test (CAT) score, was significantly worse in current smokers compared with never-smokers.[24]

22.3 CLINICAL PRESENTATION OF ACO

Asthma and COPD often coexist in the same individual. Recognizing this reality, the Global Initiative for Chronic Obstructive Lung Disease (GOLD) and Global Initiative for Asthma (GINA) jointly coined the term "asthma-COPD overlap" (ACO) to describe those individuals who demonstrate clinical features of both asthma and COPD.[25]

In the largest study of its kind, Brzostek and Kokot evaluated 12,103 smokers, who were older than 45 years of age and with a diagnosis of ACO (i.e., having features of both asthma and COPD) by respiratory specialists in Poland (Table 22.1).[26] They found that the most common patient symptom among those with a diagnostic label of asthma was the presence of paroxysmal dyspnea and wheezing, which was noted in 63% of asthmatics. Other common symptoms or signs of asthma were a good therapeutic response to ICSs (which was noted in 53% of asthmatics), a positive skin test to aeroallergens (which was noted in 53% of asthmatics), a family history of atopy (47%), the presence of other allergic symptoms (45%), early onset of bronchial disease (45%), and variability of airflow limitation (42%). Blood eosinophilia was demonstrated in only 24% of the asthmatic patients and elevated serum IgE, defined as blood concentration of > 100 IU occurred in only 8% of asthmatics. In contrast, among those who had a COPD diagnosis by respiratory specialists in Poland, the most common symptoms or signs were persistent airflow limitation defined as postbronchodilator FEV_1 of less than 80% (79%), chronic productive cough (72%), progressive exertional dyspnea (68%), and physical

Table 22.1 What are the common symptoms and signs that persuade clinicians to diagnose asthma and COPD in current or exsmokers presenting to their clinic with respiratory complaints?

Asthma
1. Paroxysmal dyspnea with wheezing (63%)
2. Good therapeutic response to inhaled corticosteroids (53%)
3. Positive skin tests to common aeroallergens (47%)
4. Family history of atopy (46%)
5. Other allergic symptoms (45%)
6. Early onset bronchial disease (45%)
7. Variability of airflow limitation (42%)

COPD
1. Persistent airflow limitation (postbronchodilator FEV_1 less than 80%) (79%)
2. Chronic productive cough (72%)
3. Progressive exertional dyspnea (68%)
4. Clinical signs of emphysema (48%)

Source: Brzostek D. and Kokot M., *Postepy Dermatol Alergol.,* 31, 372–379, 2014.
Note: Listed only those presentations that were endorsed in more than 40% of the cases.

signs of emphysema (48%). Interestingly, poor response to ICSs was reported in only 8% of COPD patients despite the widespread promulgation by experts that COPD is insensitive to these drugs and is a distinguishing feature of COPD (versus asthma). Thus, in the real world, clinicians rarely use poor responsiveness to ICSs to distinguish COPD from asthma.[3]

22.4 SYMPTOM BURDEN AND HEALTH STATUS OF ACO PATIENTS (VERSUS THOSE WITH COPD AND THOSE WITH ASTHMA)

In general, patients with ACO appear to be more symptomatic and have worse health status compared with patients with asthma or COPD alone, although there is considerable heterogeneity of data across studies. The two large systematic reviews and meta-analyses conducted on ACO have affirmed these findings by demonstrating that patients with ACO have greater symptomatic burden and require greater health-care utilization, including emergency room visits and hospitalizations, than individuals with COPD or asthma alone.[27,28]

In a large study of South Korean men and women, who participated in the Fourth Korea National Health and Nutrition Examination Survey of 2007–2009, Chung and colleagues found that individuals with ACO (defined by $FEV_1/FVC < 0.7$ prebronchodilator plus a history of wheezing) were 2.5 times more likely to rate their self-health as "fair" or "poor" compared with control subjects who did not have any airflow limitation or wheezing (Figure 22.1). In contrast, in this study, the prevalence of those who rated their health as "fair" or "poor" was no different between those with asthma and control subjects, and was only very modestly increased in those with COPD only compared with control subjects.[29] Interestingly, ACO patients were more likely to demonstrate moderate to severe airflow limitation compared with all the other groups, including those with only asthma or COPD despite comparable smoking histories (Figure 22.1).

In the COPDGene study, Hardin et al. defined ACO on the basis of self-report of physician diagnosis of asthma before 40 years of age in addition to persistent airflow limitation defined by postbronchodilator FEV_1/FVC < 0.7 in current or former smokers.[30] Among the first 3,570 COPD patients they evaluated, 13% (n = 450) of the subjects met the case definition of ACO. Compared with patients with COPD only, those with ACO were younger (60 years vs. 64 years; p < .001), had lower exposure to cigarettes over their lifetimes (46 pack years vs. 54 pack years; p < .001), were more likely to be females (56% vs. 43%; p < .001), and had less emphysema on thoracic computed tomography (CT) scans. Most importantly, patients with ACO compared with those with COPD only had worse health status as measured by Saint George's Respiratory Questionnaire (SGRQ; 47 points vs. 40 points; p < .001), had more exacerbations (120 per 100 person years vs. 70 per 100 person years; p < .001) and severe exacerbations (34% vs. 21%; p < .001). Symptomatically,

patients with ACO were three times more likely to report having hay fever than patients with COPD (50% vs. 18%; p < .001) (Figure 22.2). One interesting and perhaps unique phenotype associated with ACO (and not frequently found in patients with COPD alone) is atopy and allergic rhinitis. De Marco and colleagues examined this relationship using data from the Gene Environment Interaction in Respiratory Disease (GERD) study, which evaluated approximately 3,000 Italians aged 20–40 years. They found that individuals who had ACO (defined by self-report of asthma and COPD) were two times more likely to report allergic rhinitis compared with individuals who had COPD only.[31] However, because most patients with allergic rhinitis or atopy do not develop airflow limitation, the presence of these conditions is not very useful in defining ACO in clinical practice.

ACO is associated with reduced health status. In the EPI-SCAN Study, for instance, which was a population-based Spanish cohort, examined 3,885 individuals 40–80 years of age and defined COPD by postbronchodilator FEV_1/FVC < 0.7 and ACO by the presence of COPD and self-report of a physician diagnosis of asthma. Miravitlles and colleagues showed that compared with individuals with COPD alone, those who had both COPD (based on spirometry) and asthma (based on self-report) had more dyspnea (modified Medical Research Council Dyspnea score of 1.9 vs. 1.59; p = 0.008) and worse health status (as measured on SGRQ).[32] In terms of SGRQ, the patients with ACO had worse global scores (37 points vs. 25 points; p < .001), which was driven by reduced scores in activity (41 vs. 28; p < .001) and impact domains (23 vs. 12; p < .001).

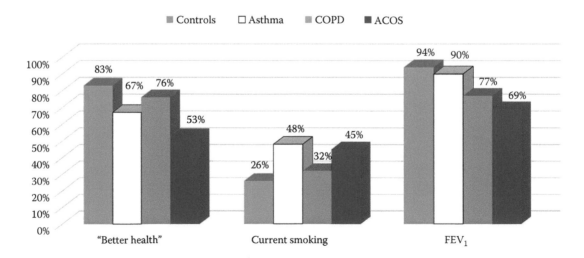

Figure 22.1 General health rating and clinical characteristics of South Korean men and women with asthma, COPD, or ACO. (From Chung JW et al., *Int J Chron Obstruct Pulmon Dis.*, 9, 795–804, 2014.)

"Better Health" is defined by self-rated health status of "excellent," "very good," or "good."
N = 9,104 (overall); 7,634 (controls); 560 (asthma); 700 (COPD); 201 (ACO)
Abbreviations: ACO: asthma-COPD overlap; COPD: chronic obstructive pulmonary disease
All comparisons p < .001

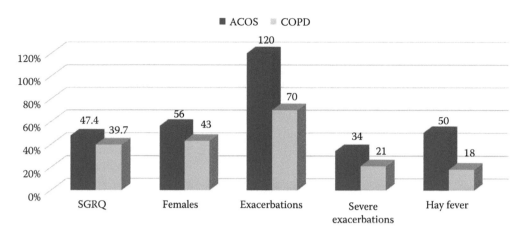

Figure 22.2 Clinical characteristics, health status, and risk of exacerbations in ACO versus COPD in the COPDGene study. (From Hardin M et al., *Eur Respir J.*, 44, 341–350, 2014.)

Exacerbations were defined as events associated with increased symptoms one year prior to study enrollment.
Severe exacerbations were defined as exacerbations requiring emergency room or hospitalization one year prior to study enrollment.
"Better Health" is defined by self-rated health status of "excellent," "very good," or "good."
N = 3,120 (COPD); 450 (ACO)
All comparisons p < .001

22.5 EXACERBATIONS IN ACO PATIENTS

In the PLATINO Study, which was a population-based study in five Latin American countries, individuals with ACO, which was defined by the presence of COPD on the basis of spirometry (i.e., persistent airflow limitation defined as postbronchodilator FEV_1/FVC below 0.7) and asthma (based on self-report of wheezing in the previous 12 months and a bronchodilator response in FEV_1 or FVC of ≥ 200 mL and ≥ 12%) had more respiratory symptoms, worse lung function, and were 2.1 times more likely to experience an exacerbation and four times more likely to become hospitalized than those with COPD alone.[33] Interestingly, unlike another previous study,[34] this study did not show any significant difference in the number of comorbidities between those with ACO and COPD only, or a gender difference between ACO and COPD groups (~53% prevalence of females for each group). However, the PLATINO Study did find that the asthma-only group had significantly greater numbers of female patients than those in the ACO group (75% vs. 54%).

In the COPDgene Study, individuals with ACO were 3.6 times more likely to be a frequent exacerbator (defined as having two or more exacerbations per year), and to experience severe exacerbations requiring hospitalization or ventilatory support in the intensive care unit.[30] These findings have been largely recapitulated in other parts of the world, including in Asia. Rhee and colleagues in South Korea have shown that individuals with ACO were more likely to use emergency rooms and be hospitalized for their respiratory condition compared with individuals with COPD alone.[35]

The totality of data to date suggests that ACO elevates the risk of exacerbations and hospitalizations by 2–3-fold compared with COPD or asthma alone. Moreover, patients with ACO have greater symptom burden and reduced health status compared with those with asthma or COPD alone. Whether ACO increases the risk of respiratory tract infections, thromboembolic disease, or cardiac comorbidities, which are the leading triggers for COPD exacerbations, is not known.

22.6 PROGNOSIS OF ASTHMA, COPD, AND ACO PATIENTS: TRAJECTORY OF LUNG FUNCTION DECLINE FOR PATIENTS WITH ASTHMA, COPD, AND ACO

It is well known that COPD is a risk factor for accelerated decline in lung function over time, though there is tremendous heterogeneity across patients.[36,37] What is more controversial is whether asthma by itself induces accelerated decline in lung function over time. It is notable and interesting that population based studies indicate that approximately 25%–30% of individuals with COPD (defined based on postbronchodilator FEV_1/FVC falling below the lower limit of normal values) are lifetime never-smokers, representing approximately 7% of the general population.[38,39] The main risk factors for COPD among never-smokers are history of asthma and increasing age. Indeed, self-reported history of asthma (which is present in 5%–10% of the general population aged 40 years and older) increases the risk of COPD by ~4–5 fold.[39]

Parental-smoking exposure is also an important but often overlooked risk factor for the development of airflow obstruction in middle age. In the Tasmanian Longitudinal Health Study cohort heavy maternal smoking (>20 cigarettes/day) during childhood was associated with a 2.7-fold higher incidence of airflow obstruction than in those without such exposure.[40] Presence of airway hyper-responsiveness (AHR), which is a cardinal (objective) finding in asthma, also increases the risk of incident COPD by fourfold, independent of other factors including smoking and aging.[41] In the general population, the population risk factor of asthma (defined either by AHR or self-report of a physician diagnosis of asthma) for incident COPD is approximately 20%–25%. To put this in perspective, cigarette smoking, which is an undisputed risk factor for COPD, imposes a population attributable risk of 38% for incident COPD.[41] Moreover, independent of smoking and baseline lung function, AHR as measured by histamine or methacholine, is a strong predictor of COPD mortality in the general population, increasing the risk by 4–15 fold beyond that experienced by those who do not demonstrate AHR[42] (Figure 22.3).

Even in individuals with COPD, AHR is an independent predictor of rapid decline in lung function. Tkacova and colleagues used AHR to define the asthmatic phenotype in patients with COPD.[43] Using the LHS data, which measured AHR to methacholine in patients with mild to moderate COPD (FEV_1 between 70% and 90% of predicted), they found that 24% of these patients demonstrated AHR as defined by a provocation concentration (PC20) of 4 mg/mL or less (to induce a 20% fall in FEV_1). Use of a higher PC20 threshold such as 8 mg/mL increased the prevalence of ACO to 1 in 3 patients with COPD. Importantly, ACO defined by AHR in COPD patients was associated with a faster decline in FEV_1 and increased risk of respiratory but not all-cause mortality over 11 years of follow-up. It should be noted, however, that although AHR is one of the hallmarks

(and defining features) of asthma, its pathophysiology may be quite different in COPD than in asthma. In asthma, for instance, AHR appears to be driven by underlying eosinophilic airway inflammation and disturbances in airway smooth muscle; whereas in COPD, the main risk factors of AHR are altered baseline geometry of the airways and smoking.[44]

What is less known is the impact of lifetime cigarette smoking on the incidence of COPD among asthmatics. In one of the most important studies on this topic, James and colleagues used longitudinal spirometric data from the Busselton Health Study to map out the trajectory of lung function in the population stratified by asthma and smoking status.[45] In terms of FEV_1 decline, the population average for 60 year olds was 36 mL/year in men and 25 mL/year in women. Smoking was the most important risk factor for accelerated decline for both men and women, such that heavy smokers experienced a 50 mL/year decline in FEV_1 in men and a 32 mL/year decline in women (Figure 22.4). Asthma by itself imposed a slightly increased risk of accelerate decline. Male asthmatics experienced on average 40 mL/year FEV_1 decline and female asthmatics experienced a 28 mL/year decline. There was an additive effect of smoking and asthma such that male asthmatics who smoked experienced a 54 mL/year decline and female asthmatics who smoked experienced a 36 mL/year decline (Figure 22.4).

Despite this relatively modest excess risk of FEV_1 decline imposed by asthma or the asthma phenotype, asthmatics are grossly overrepresented in the COPD population by age 60 years, because asthmatics, in general, have smaller lungs at full lung maturity (which occurs between 18 and 25 years of age), and the small excess risk in FEV_1 decline leads to poor lung function with aging. Thus, James and colleagues found that at age 60, an average white, nonsmoking male with asthma in Busselton had FEV_1 that was

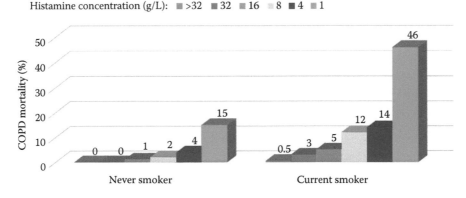

Figure 22.3 COPD Mortality over 30 years in a population according to baseline responsiveness to histamine challenge. (From Hospers JJ et al., *Lancet*, 356, 1313–1317, 2000.)

All comparisons $p < .001$

N = 2,008 (overall); 1,389 (no AHR; 619 (AHR)

AHR is defined as 10% or more decline in the baseline FEV_1 value at histamine concentrations of 16 g/L or less.

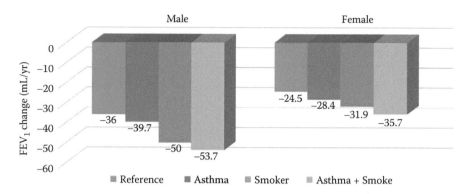

Figure 22.4 Expected FEV$_1$ decline in a 60-year-old white man or woman according to smoking and asthma status. (From James AL et al., *Am J Respir Crit Care Med.*, 171, 109–114, 2005.)

The reference indicates a 60-year-old, white never-smoking man or woman without asthma or COPD.

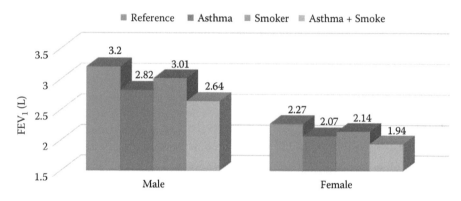

Figure 22.5 Expected FEV$_1$ in a 60-year-old white man or woman according to smoking and asthma status. (From James AL et al., *Am J Respir Crit Care Med.*, 171, 109–114, 2005.)

The reference indicates a 60-year-old, white never-smoking man or woman without asthma or COPD·

approximately 380 mL lower than that observed in a similar nonasthmatic male (we will call the latter individual the "reference male").[40] Interestingly, a similar (heavy) smoking (nonasthmatic) male had FEV$_1$ that was 190 mL lower than the reference male. If the heavy smoker was also an asthmatic, his FEV$_1$ was 560 mL lower than of the reference male (Figure 22.5).

The complex interaction of reduced lung growth and accelerated decline in FEV$_1$ in asthmatics was well described in the Childhood Asthma Management Program (CAMP) study, which followed children aged 5–12 years with annual spirometry until their third decade of life.[46] The CAMP study originally enrolled 1,041 children with a history of chronic asthma and demonstration of AHR based on a methacholine challenge test that resulted in a 20% reduction in FEV$_1$ at a methacholine concentration of 12.5 mg/mL or less. The randomized controlled trial component that evaluated the effects of nedocromil lasted 4.5 years, after which the CAMP cohort was converted to an observational study, which lasted 13 years. Of the CAMP participants, 25% followed a normal lung function trajectory, which was defined as a FEV$_1$ growth curve that was almost always at or above the 25th

percentile of age-, sex-, and height-adjusted normative values in the U.S. general population. Another 25% demonstrated normal growth during childhood and adolescence, but then experienced accelerated (or early) decline in FEV$_1$ during early adulthood. Another 25% demonstrated reduced lung growth during childhood with relatively normal lung decline in adulthood. Finally, the remaining 25% experienced both reduced lung growth during childhood and accelerated (or early) decline in lung function in adulthood. Thus, 2/3 of asthmatic children in the CAMP study demonstrated reduced lung function at age 30. The risk factors for reduced lung function at age 30 were (1) low lung function at age 9, (2) increased bronchodilator response at age 9, (3) AHR at age 9, and (4) reduced body mass index at age 9.[46] Because smoking was infrequent among study participants, the effects of smoking on lung function growth and decline could not be evaluated in the CAMP study.

The additive effects of smoking on asthmatics were well described in the Busselton Health Study, which was discussed earlier, and in the Copenhagen City Heart Study (CCHS). CCHS was a prospective population-based study, which began in 1976 and in which 50% of the study subjects were smokers at enrollment and ~3% were asthmatics. The average FEV_1 decline in those with asthma was 38 mL/year versus 22 mL/year in those without asthma. As with the Busselton Health Study, smoking had an additive effect in accelerating the decline in FEV_1 over 15 years by increasing the rate of FEV_1 decline by 10–20 mL/year.[47] Together, these data suggest that asthmatics have increased risk of COPD (defined by postbronchodilator FEV_1/FVC below 70% or the lower limit of normal on spirometry) between 40 and 80 years of age through two independent mechanisms: (1) reduced lung growth in childhood and (2) accelerated decline in FEV_1 during adulthood. Smoking amplifies this risk (in an additive fashion) by accelerating FEV_1 decline. While there is tremendous variation, on average, asthmatics experience 10 mL/year excess decline in FEV_1 versus nonasthmatics, and smoking adds another 10–20 mL/year decline in FEV_1. Thus, by age 60, 1 in 3 to 1 in 2 asthmatics who smoke throughout their lifetimes will develop COPD (vs. 15%–20% of nonasthmatics who smoke).

22.7 PROPOSED MANAGEMENT OF ACO

Most clinical-trial evidence for asthma or COPD excludes patients with a diagnosis of both conditions; a median of only 5%–7% of patients with airways obstruction would have satisfied inclusion criteria for large, randomized, controlled trials in asthma or COPD, limiting the clinical relevance of such evidence in patients with either asthma or COPD.[48,49] Patients with ACO were excluded from such trials, and thus, treatment for ACO is at this time based on first principles. Treatment goals are similar in asthma, COPD, and ACO, and they include controlling symptoms, improving quality of life, preventing exacerbations and hospitalizations, improving functional outcomes, and, ideally, reducing long-term decline in lung function. GINA/GOLD recommend nonpharmacological strategies, including smoking cessation, physical activity, pulmonary rehabilitation, treatment of comorbidities, and appropriate self-management strategies.[25]

Although asthma is classically associated with eosinophilic inflammation, patients with asthma and persistent airflow obstruction may show a predominant airway neutrophilia and a relative resistance to ICS therapy, the latter the cornerstone of asthma management. Similarly, asthmatic patients who smoke, as well as patients with COPD and neutrophil-predominant inflammation, have disease that is relatively corticosteroid resistant.[50] GINA/GOLD Joint Guidelines on ACO[20] recommend treating patients with ACO initially as for asthma, given the key role of ICS in impacting morbidity and mortality in this condition. Depending on the clinical presentation of a patient with ACO, the patient (if previously treated for asthma) may have already received inhaled combination therapy with ICS/LABA. If not, appropriate treatment is with ICS first,

progressing to combination therapy if the clinical response is inadequate, and subsequently adding treatment with LAMA if needed. If the individual with ACO is a current smoker, as with all patients with airways disease, major efforts should be made to encourage quitting through both psychosocial and pharmacological support, given the known reduction in long-term decline in lung function induced by smoking cessation in COPD. Individuals with asthma who smoke require higher doses of ICSs to induce the same anti-inflammatory effect. As with asthma, there are at present strong recommendations in ACO against use of LABA monotherapy (i.e., without ICS) because of the risk of severe exacerbations and asthma-related death. By contrast, for COPD, LABA monotherapy is actively recommended for milder disease, and use of ICS-only medications is discouraged because of their lower benefit/risk ratio.

22.8 MORBIDITY AND MORTALITY IN ACO

Sorino and colleagues followed patients with ACO, COPD, and asthma for 15 years, and the researchers found that, compared with individuals in the community without any of these airway disorders, those with ACO had a 1.83-fold increase in mortality ($p < .0001$), those with COPD only had a 2.31-fold increase ($p < .0001$), and those with asthma only had a 1.19-fold increase in risk of total mortality ($p = 0.085$).[51]

In the CCHS, ACO was subdivided into two groups: ACO with early onset asthma (asthma onset before 40 years of age) and ACO with late onset asthma (asthma onset $\geq$ 40 years of age). They found that 36% of study participants with any airway disease had ACO. Individuals with late-onset asthma ACO had the highest rate of decline in FEV_1 at 49.6 mL/year, followed by those with COPD only at 39.5 mL/year, early onset asthma ACO at 27.3 mL/year, and healthy former or never-smokers at 21 mL/year.[52] Most importantly, compared with never-smokers without asthma or COPD, total mortality was increased by 1.81-fold in late-onset asthma ACO ($p < .0001$); by 1.44 in early onset asthma ACO ($p = 0.03$); by 1.73 in COPD alone ($p < .0001$); and by 1.05 in asthma alone ($p = 0.73$). For respiratory mortality, the corresponding hazard ratios are 6.36 in late-onset asthma ACO ($p < .0001$); 2.30 in early onset ACO ($p = 0.06$); 3.69 in COPD alone ($p < .0001$); and 2.58 in asthma alone ($p = 0.01$).[47] Compared with COPD only, late-onset asthma ACO is associated with greater risk of total mortality (HR, 1.39; $p = 0.001$) and respiratory mortality (HR, 3.51; $p < .0001$). In contrast, there was no significant mortality difference between COPD alone and early onset asthma ACO.

One major limitation of these studies is the case definition of ACO, which is variable across studies, lacking consistency. Recently, the Spanish Society of Pneumology and Thoracic Surgery (SEPAR) endorsed a case definition based on major and minor criteria. SEPAR recommends the presence of at least one major criterion (history of asthma or bronchodilator response of $\geq$ 400 mL) *or* two minor criteria (IgE > 100 IU or a history of atopy, or bronchodilator response of $\geq$ 200 mL on two different occasions or blood eosinophilia of > 5%) in the presence of fixed airflow limitation. Using this case definition, Cosio and colleagues examined the prevalence of ACO in the COPD History Assessment in Spain (CHAIN) cohort. Of the 831 patients who were diagnosed with COPD on the basis of fixed airflow limitation (FEV_1/FVC < 70% postbronchodilator) and $\geq$ 10 pack years of smoking, 125 patients (15%) met the criteria for ACO.[53] Importantly, 98% of the patients diagnosed with ACO on the basis of the SEPAR criteria maintained their ACO status at a one-year follow-up, suggesting that ACO is a stable phenotype. In this cohort, the use of ICSs was similar between ACO and non-ACO COPD patients; however, the use of LAMA was significantly lower in the ACO than non-ACO COPD patients (62% vs. 72%). Interestingly, patients with ACO had significantly higher one-year mortality than patients with COPD alone, with ACO patients experiencing a mortality that was twofold higher.[53]

Collectively, these data suggest that ACO has a worse prognosis than asthma or COPD alone with more rapid decline in lung function, increased risk of hospitalization, and increased risk of COPD or respiratory mortality. Paradoxically, patients with ACO have been largely excluded from therapeutic trials in asthma and COPD.[54] Thus, there is little evidence-based therapy available for these patients. There is a pressing need to conduct large Phase III trials of therapeutics in patients with ACO.

REFERENCES

1. World Health Organization. Chronic diseases: Burden of COPD; 2016. Available at http://www.who.int/respiratory/copd/burden/en/. Accessed August 21, 2016.
2. Reddel HK, Bateman ED, Becker A et al. A summary of the new GINA strategy: A roadmap to asthma control. *Eur Respir J.* 2015;46(3):622–639.
3. Vestbo J, Hurd SS, Agusti AG et al. Global strategy for the diagnosis, management, and prevention of chronic obstructive pulmonary disease: GOLD executive summary. *Am J Respir Crit Care Med.* 2013;187(4):347–365.
4. Australian Centre for Asthma Monitoring. Asthma in Australia 2011. AIHW Asthma Series no. 4. Cat.no. ACM 22. Canberra: AIHW; 2011.
5. Kuehn BM. Asthma linked to psychiatric disorders. *JAMA.* 2008;299(2):158–160.
6. Juniper EF, Guyatt GH, Epstein RS et al. Evaluation of impairment of health related quality of life in asthma: Development of a questionnaire for use in clinical trials. *Thorax.* 1992;47(2):76–83.
7. Juniper EF, Guyatt GH, Cox FM et al. Development and validation of the mini asthma quality of life questionnaire. *Eur Respir J.* 1999;14(1):32–38.
8. Bateman ED, Bousquet J, Keech ML et al. The correlation between asthma control and health status: The GOAL study. *Eur Respir J.* 2007;29(1):56–62.
9. Correia de Sousa J, Pina A, Cruz AM et al. Asthma control, quality of life, and the role of patient enablement: A cross-sectional observational study. *Prim Care Respir J.* 2013;22(2):181–187.
10. Pinnock H. Supported self-management for asthma. *Breathe.* 2015;11:98–109.
11. Althuis MD, Sexton M and Prybylski D. Cigarette smoking and asthma symptom severity among adult asthmatics. *J Asthma.* 1999;36(3):257–264.
12. Silverman RA, Boudreaux ED, Woodruff PG et al. Cigarette smoking among asthmatic adults presenting to 64 emergency departments. *Chest.* 2003;123(5):1472–1479.
13. Chaudhuri R, Livingston E, McMahon AD et al. Effects of smoking cessation on lung function and airway inflammation in smokers with asthma. *Am J Respi Crit Care Med.* 2006;174(2):127–133.
14. Ståhl E, Lindberg A, Jansson SA et al. Health-related quality of life is related to COPD disease severity. *Health Qual Life Outcomes.* 2005;3:56.
15. Seemungal TA, Donaldson GC, Paul EA et al. Effect of exacerbation on quality of life in patients with chronic obstructive pulmonary disease *Am J Respir Crit Care Med.* 1998;157:1418–1422.
16. Janson C, Marks G, Buist S et al. The impact of COPD on health status: Findings from the BOLD study. *Eur Respir J.* 2013;42(6):1472–1483.
17. Fletcher MJ, Upton J, Taylor-Fishwick J et al. COPD uncovered: An international survey on the impact of chronic obstructive pulmonary disease [COPD] on a working age population. *BMC Public Health.* 2011;11:612.
18. Britton M. The burden of COPD in the U.K.: Results from the Confronting COPD survey. *Respir Med.* 2003;97(Suppl. C):S71–S79.
19. Chapman KR, Bourbeau J and Rance L. The burden of COPD in Canada: Results from the Confronting COPD survey. *Respir Med.* 2003;97(Suppl. C):S23–S31.
20. Almagro P, Cabrera FJ, Diez J et al. Working group on COPD spanish society of internal medicine. Comorbidities and short-term prognosis in patients hospitalized for acute exacerbation of COPD: The EPOC in Servicios de Medicina Interna (ESMI) study. *Chest.* 2012;142(5):1126–1133.
21. Nici L, Bontly TD, ZuWallack R et al. Self management in chronic obstructive pulmonary disease. Time for a paradigm shift? *Ann Am Thorac Soc.* 2014;11(1):101–107.

22. Godtfredsen NS, Lam TH, Hansel TT et al. COPD-related morbidity and mortality after soking cessation: Status of the evidence. *Eur Respir J.* 2008;32(4):844–853.

23. Kanner RE, Connett JE, Williams DE et al. Effects of randomized assignment to a smoking cessation intervention and changes in smoking habits on respiratory symptoms in smokers with early chronic obstructive pulmonary disease: The lung health study. *Am J Med.* 1999;106(4):410–416.

24. Woodruff PG, Barr RG, Bleecker E et al. Clinical significance of symptoms in smokers with preserved pulmonary function. *N Engl J Med.* 2016;374(19):1811–1821.

25. GINA/GOLD Joint Report. Asthma, COPD and asthma-COPD overlap syndrome (ACOS); 2015. Available at http://ginasthma.org/asthma-copd-and-asthma-copd-overlap-syndrome-acos/. Accessed August 1, 2016.

26. Brzostek D and Kokot M. Asthma-chronic obstructive pulmonary disease overlap syndrome in Poland. Findings of an epidemiological study. *Postepy Dermatol Alergol.* 2014;31(6):372–379.

27. Nielsen M, Barnes CB, and Ulrik CS. Clinical characteristics of the asthma-COPD overlap syndrome—A systematic review. *Int J Chron Obstruct Pulmon Dis.* 2015;10:1443–1454.

28. Alshabanat A, Zafari Z, Albanyan O et al. Asthma and COPD overlap syndrome (ACOS): A systematic review and meta analysis. *PlOS ONE.* 2015;10(9):e0136065.

29. Chung JW, Kong KA, Lee JH et al. Characteristics and self-rated health of overlap syndrome. *Int J Chron Obstruct Pulmon Dis.* 2014;9:795–804.

30. Hardin M, Cho M, McDonald ML et al. The clinical and genetic features of COPD-asthma overlap syndrome. *Eur Respir J.* 2014;44(2):341–350.

31. de Marco R, Pesce G, Marcon A et al. The coexistence of asthma and chronic obstructive pulmonary disease (COPD): Prevalence and risk factors in young, middle-aged and elderly people from the general population. *PloS one.* 2013;8(5):e62985.

32. Miravitlles M, Soriano JB, Ancochea J et al. Characterisation of the overlap COPD-asthma phenotype. Focus on physical activity and health status. *Respir Med.* 2013;107(7):1053–1060.

33. Menezes AM, Montes de Oca M, Perez-Padilla R et al. Increased risk of exacerbation and hospitalization in subjects with an overlap phenotype: COPD-asthma. *Chest.* 2014;145(2):297–304.

34. Hardin M, Silverman EK, Barr RG et al. The clinical features of the overlap between COPD and asthma. *Respir Res.* 2011;12:127.

35. Rhee CK, Yoon HK, Yoo KH et al. Medical utilization and cost in patients with overlap syndrome of chronic obstructive pulmonary disease and asthma. *COPD.* 2014;11(2):163–170.

36. Lange P, Celli B, Agusti A et al. Lung-Function trajectories leading to chronic obstructive pulmonary disease. *N Engl J Med.* 2015;373(2):111–122.

37. Zafari Z, Sin DD, Postma DS et al. Individualized prediction of lung-function decline in chronic obstructive pulmonary disease. *CMAJ.* 2016;188:1004–1011.

38. Tan WC, Sin DD, Bourbeau J et al. Characteristics of COPD in never-smokers and ever-smokers in the general population: Results from the canCOLD study. *Thorax.* 2015;70(9):822–829.

39. Thomsen M, Nordestgaard BG, Vestbo J et al. Characteristics and outcomes of chronic obstructive pulmonary disease in never smokers in Denmark: A prospective population study. *Lancet Respir Med.* 2013;1(7):543–550.

40. Perret JL, Walters H, Johns D et al. Mother's smoking and complex lung function of offspring in middle age: A cohort study from childhood. *Respirol.* 2016;21(5):911–919.

41. de Marco R, Accordini S, Marcon A et al. Risk factors for chronic obstructive pulmonary disease in a European cohort of young adults. *Am J Respir Crit Care Med.* 2011;183(7):891–897.

42. Hospers JJ, Postma DS, Rijcken B et al. Histamine airway hyper-responsiveness and mortality from chronic obstructive pulmonary disease: A cohort study. *Lancet.* 2000;356(9238):1313–1317.

43. Tkacova R, Dai DL, Vonk JM et al. Airway hyper-responsiveness in chronic obstructive pulmonary disease: A marker of asthma-chronic obstructive pulmonary disease overlap syndrome? *J Allergy Clin Immunol.* 2016;138:1571–1579.

44. Jones RL, Noble PB, Elliot JG et al. Airway remodelling in COPD: It's not asthma! *Respirol.* 2016;21:1347–1356.

45. James AL, Palmer LJ, Kicic E et al. Decline in lung function in the busselton health study: The effects of asthma and cigarette smoking. *Am J Respir Crit CareMmed.* 2005;171(2):109–114.

46. McGeachie MJ, Yates KP, Zhou X et al. Patterns of growth and decline in lung function in persistent childhood asthma. *N Engl J Med.* 2016;374(19):1842–1852.

47. Lange P, Parner J, Vestbo J et al. A 15-year follow-up study of ventilatory function in adults with asthma. *N Engl J Med.* 1998;339(17):1194–1200.

48. Travers J, Marsh S, Caldwell B et al. External validity of randomized controlled trials in COPD. *Respir Med.* 2007;101(6):1313–1320.

49. Travers J, Marsh S, Williams M et al. External validity of randomised controlled trials in asthma: To whom do the results of the trials apply? *Thorax.* 2007;62(3):219–223.

50. Barnes PJ. Therapeutic approaches to asthma-chronic obstructive pulmonary disease overlap syndromes. *J Allergy Clin Immunol.* 2015;136(3):531–545.

51. Sorino C, Pedone C and Scichilone N. Fifteen-year mortality of patients with asthma-COPD overlap syndrome. *Eur J Intern Med.* 2016;34:72–77.

52. Lange P, Colak Y, Ingebrigtsen TS et al. Long-term prognosis of asthma, chronic obstructive pulmonary disease, and asthma-chronic obstructive pulmonary disease overlap in the copenhagen city heart study: A prospective population-based analysis. *Lancet Respir Med.* 2016;4(6):454–462.

53. Cosio BG, Soriano JB, Lopez-Campos JL et al. Defining the asthma-COPD overlap syndrome in a COPD cohort. *Chest.* 2016;149(1):45–52.

54. Sin DD, Miravitlles M, Mannino DM et al. What is asthma-COPD overlap syndrome? Towards a consensus definition from a round table discussion. *Eur Respir J.* 2016;48:664–673.

Asthma, COPD, and asthma-COPD overlap from the primary care physician perspective

MARK L. LEVY

This chapter discusses the particular challenges faced by doctors and nurses working in primary care management of patients with asthma and chronic obstructive pulmonary disease (COPD). The focus is directed at issues related to diagnosis, differential diagnosis, and ongoing management challenges, as well as identifying when to refer to a specialist. As therapy is dealt with in more detail elsewhere in this book, the reader is directed to those chapters, bearing in mind that patients with features of combined asthma and COPD are generally more at risk than in cases where they suffer from only one of these diseases.[1–3] The reader is also directed to the relevant chapters in the Global Initiative for Asthma (GINA) and the Global Initiative for Chronic Obstructive Lung Disease (GOLD) strategy documents for more information on management of these conditions.[1,2]

CLINICAL VIGNETTE 23.1

G.S. is a 45-year-old man, who consulted his general practitioner in the summer with difficulty sleeping due to coughing. He had been getting short of breath on exertion and suffering from intermittent, nonproductive coughing for the last few weeks; this got worse after he mowed his lawn.

According to his medical notes, he had suffered from episodic cough and wheeze in childhood, but this seemed to resolve in his teenage years although on questioning, he said these symptoms had occurred during the few years he worked as a spray painter in his 20s. He currently worked as a manual laborer, sometimes in a very dusty environment. He had been smoking 20 cigarettes a day from the age of 19 and was living with his wife, also a smoker.

On examination, his fingers were heavily stained with nicotine, his chest was moderately hyperinflated and wheezy with scattered crackles throughout on auscultation. His oxygen saturation was 96% while breathing room air, his peak expiratory flow (PEF) was 70% predicted for his height and age, and his spirogram demonstrated a reversible obstructive airflow pattern with increased predicted FEV_1 percentage after bronchodilation.

Comment: This is a common clinical scenario in primary care where the dilemma for the doctor relates to the diagnosis and which treatment would be appropriate. This man's history strongly suggests undiagnosed childhood asthma, which seems to have an allergic component; he also possibly had occupational asthma during the time he worked as a spray painter. His personal smoking history coupled with passive exposure at home, his dusty work environment, his clinical findings together with evidence of further reaction to triggers (i.e., grass pollen) complicates the diagnostic process—he may have asthma with limited airflow reversibility; however, he may also have mild to moderate COPD or a combination of both diseases (i.e., ACO).

23.1 NATURE OF PRIMARY CARE (GENERAL PRACTICE)

The extensive role of doctors in primary care generally encompasses caring for both the medical and social care aspects of their patient's lives, and more specifically both acute as well as ongoing management of chronic diseases. In most countries, patients' first point of contact when ill is with a primary care physician or nurse. They present with symptoms that may be specific or vague; nonetheless, the clinician has to make a working diagnosis and initiate treatment.

Primary care clinicians are generalists; they have to know about and deal with, on average, more than 400 different types of clinical problems in any one year, in most cases without access to investigations or secondary care opinion. In contrast, the average specialist will only deal with about 20–30 different medical conditions. In contrast with specialist physician practice where patient referrals are usually accompanied by clinical findings and a suggested diagnosis, those presenting to a general practitioner may have a disease affecting any system. The average duration of primary care consultations worldwide varies between five and (unusually) 30 minutes; during this time, the doctor has to establish the presenting complaint, generate a working diagnosis or hypothesis, educate and inform the patient, prescribe appropriately, arrange further investigations and follow-up, and attend to any other ongoing medical issues for the patient.

General practitioners have a few major advantages over their secondary care colleagues; these include time and continuity of care. They usually have access to patient's medical records, coupled with the fact that diagnosis and treatment is not generally limited to a single consultation or event. Once a working diagnosis has been established, and treatment initiated, the diagnosis can be refined with follow-up review, and decisions can be made on the need for a specialist opinion.

In some countries, such as currently in the United Kingdom, patients are registered with a single general practice/primary care provider, and their medical records (from birth onward) are available to all clinicians consulted by these patients. Therefore, provided the medical records are up-to-date, sufficiently detailed, and describe the clinical findings, and underlying rationale for working diagnoses, clinicians can subsequently refine or revise their diagnoses.

Hospital colleagues have the advantage of being provided with a targeted referral letter from primary care, as well as having access to specialist colleagues and investigations, which helps guide the clinician in the direction of the correct diagnosis and subsequent therapy. Together with access to further investigations, such as computed tomography (CT) scans, high-definition ultrasonography, lung biopsy, and more detailed lung function tests, such as the ability to assess diffusion capacity (diffusion capacity of the lungs for carbon monoxide [DLCO] and transfer coefficient [KCO]), clinicians in secondary care are ideally placed to provide primary care clinicians with an accurate diagnosis on patients discharged from the hospital. Unfortunately, many secondary care clinicians are becoming more specialized, which results in at least two possible consequences. First, it is the "luck of the draw" (depending on the health system and country) as to which type of specialist cares for a patient attending a hospital in an emergency; this depends on the duty roster, and a patient with respiratory problems may be attended to by a cardiologist, for example. Secondly, patients may need multiple referrals from general practitioners in primary care until a specialist with appropriate expertise is able to provide a correct diagnosis.

23.2 ACCURATE DIAGNOSIS IS IMPORTANT

Securing an accurate diagnosis is a fundamental aspect of medical care. In the extremely short consultation time available for most general practitioners, it is not often possible to quickly come to a firm diagnosis in patients presenting with respiratory symptoms. Due to time constraints and lack of access to investigations, the initial diagnosis needs to be made based on the clinical history and findings, to be confirmed later.

Respiratory symptoms (cough, wheeze, or shortness of breath), may be due to a number of conditions, for example, and not exclusively, an upper or lower respiratory tract infection, one of the chronic obstructive lung conditions or cardiac disease.[4] Furthermore, in her excellent paper, Reddel describes the complex nature of COPD.[3] She refers to guidelines on asthma and COPD, which are based on evidence derived from studies in which subjects, who are highly selected, are not very representative of the population managed in primary care. For example, patients with asthma have been excluded from COPD studies and vice versa, despite evidence that at least 20% of patients with obstructive lung disease have features of both diseases. How then does a primary care physician decide to treat patients with features of both? It is clear that asthma and COPD are not "clear cut," separate entities, rather that these are heterogeneous conditions comprising many phenotypes.[1–3,5,6]

For primary care physicians, and generalists in secondary care, diagnosis of obstructive lung disease is not a straightforward process. This is even more complex when a patient falls between the care provided by both primary and secondary care clinicians; as illustrated by the following clinical vignette.

CLINICAL VIGNETTE 23.2

M.J. was a 76-year-old man who was admitted to the hospital with fever and severe breathlessness. His current medication, prescribed by his primary care physician, included high-dose inhaled corticosteroids (ICSs) in combination with a long-acting β_2-agonist bronchodilator (LABA). The patient had not been informed of his diagnosis by his primary care doctor. On admission, he had obstructive airflow on spirometry testing, an FEV_1/FVC ratio of 62%, FEV_1 of 68% predicted, and peripheral oxygen saturation of 92%. A chest radiogram suggested lung hyperinflation. An acute asthma attack was diagnosed, and he was treated with 5 mg of nebulized salbutamol, a short-acting β_2-agonist bronchodilator (SABA), oral corticosteroids, broad-spectrum antibiotics, and oxygen. His FEV_1 was 70% predicted posttreatment. After 4 days in the hospital, he was discharged back to the care of his primary care doctor, with a diagnosis of probable COPD based on his predischarge spirometry showing little reversibility of his airflow obstruction.

However, the discharge note advised the primary care physician to repeat the spirometry after a period of 6 weeks following the acute episode. Subsequent repeat spirometry by the primary care nurse found that the FEV_1 had remained at 70% predicted; so, the doctor amended his records, which had previously stated the man had asthma, to a new diagnosis of COPD. Then, in keeping with the national guidance against use of ICSs in mild-to-moderate COPD, he advised the patient to discontinue his ICS treatment. Sadly, this man died mowing his lawn a few months later, and the postmortem found severe macroscopic bronchiolar mucous plugging and thickened basement membrane on histology of the lungs. The man's wife reported at the coroner's inquest, that he had a past history of allergy, and had been treated with inhaled medication in childhood.

Comment: Fixed airflow (irreversible) obstruction may occur in people with longstanding or severe asthma, and it is important to establish from the medical history whether older people with respiratory problems had symptoms in their youth. Someone with childhood asthma can exhibit ongoing respiratory symptoms without reporting these to the doctor. As a result, chronic asthma with fixed airflow obstruction can persist, and patients may tolerate the symptoms without complaining to their doctor. In this clinical vignette, the hospital treated the man's acute problem, and although the primary care clinician was advised to repeat the lung function, the doctor misinterpreted the results in isolation without taking the past medical history into account.

In the case of chronic obstructive lung diseases, the respiratory literature is peppered with studies demonstrating that many patients are treated on the basis of an uncorroborated clinical diagnosis.[7–9] Furthermore, many of the clinical drug trials include patients with so-called "physician-diagnosed asthma or COPD" without corroboratory evidence of an accurate diagnosis. From personal experience, up to 25% of people diagnosed with and on treatment for COPD in North London general practices in the United Kingdom, do not have evidence supporting the diagnosis of this disease. Furthermore, one large Italian study found that 33% of 2,090 patients managed by 540 general practitioners, diagnosed with chronic lung disease (such as COPD and chronic upper-airway disease) had undiagnosed asthma.[7]

Differentiating asthma from COPD in older patients can be challenging. The U.K. National Review of Asthma Deaths (NRAD)[10] investigated 900 asthma deaths during the 12 months from February 2012. Asthma was classified as the underlying cause of these deaths (i.e., ICD-10 code J459) according to the national statistics offices of the four U.K. countries by implementing the algorithm of the World Health Organization (WHO) International Classification of Diseases (ICD).[11] However, following detailed analysis of the clinical records, provided by doctors who had previously cared for them, 39% of these deaths were not due to asthma. Furthermore, a proportion of the doctors believed their patients had suffered from COPD rather than asthma, despite the fact that asthma was recorded on the death certificates; experts concluded that many of these "COPD" patients had suffered from "chronic asthma with fixed airflow obstruction," which resulted in the rapid creation of a new READ code for use in U.K. primary care computerized records.

As the treatment of asthma and COPD differs, and the outcomes are worse when features of both diseases overlap,[1,2] it is very important for these diseases to be accurately differentiated and correctly diagnosed, particularly as the ongoing management often occurs in the primary care sector. Furthermore, detailed research is needed to establish the most-effective therapy based on the phenotypic nature of the patient's obstructive lung disease.[3,6,12]

23.3 THE ASTHMA-COPD OVERLAP (ACO)

The GINA and GOLD strategy documents titled "Diagnosis of asthma, COPD and asthma-COPD overlap (ACO)"[1,2] were simultaneously published in 2015. They define and describe three conditions: asthma, COPD, and ACO, with the aim of assisting nonspecialists (both in primary and secondary care) in differentiating the three conditions. This idea, while welcomed by primary care colleagues (personal communications), has generated widespread debate among specialists.[5,13] The authors argue that the terms asthma and COPD have perhaps outlived their usefulness and do not accurately describe the number of phenotypic manifestations of chronic obstructive respiratory disease encountered in clinical practice. Nonetheless, until there is clear agreement on the use of different descriptive terms for classifying the various phenotypes of these diseases, it seems sensible that the GINA and GOLD recommendations on ACO should be used in primary care (and specifically by general physicians) for diagnosing and deciding on management of these three conditions.

23.3.1 DEFINITIONS

Asthma is a heterogeneous disease, usually characterized by chronic airway inflammation. It is defined by the history of respiratory symptoms such as wheeze, shortness of breath, chest tightness, and cough that vary over time and in intensity, together with variable expiratory airflow limitation.[1]

COPD is a common, preventable, and treatable disease, characterized by persistent airflow limitation that is usually progressive and associated with enhanced chronic inflammatory responses in the airways and the lungs to noxious particles or gases. Exacerbations and comorbidities contribute to the overall severity in individual patients.[1]

Asthma-COPD overlap (ACO) is characterized by persistent airflow limitation with several features usually associated with asthma and several features usually associated with COPD. ACO is therefore identified in clinical practice by the features that it shares with both asthma and COPD.

It is important to note that a specific definition for ACO cannot be developed until more evidence is available about its clinical phenotypes and underlying mechanisms.[1]

23.3.2 DIFFERENTIATING ASTHMA, COPD, AND ACO IN PRIMARY CARE

Ideally, a clear diagnosis should be confirmed before initiating treatment for a patient. However, in primary care the doctor often has to make a preliminary diagnosis, based on a hypothesis using the clinical symptoms and signs, followed by initiation of a trial of therapy.

Someone with obstructive airflow, without a past personal or family history suggestive of asthma, who has been exposed to noxious particles or gasses, particularly with a significant smoking history, and with evidence of obstructive airflow limitation, has probably got COPD. Alternatively, someone with a history of atopy or allergy, a family history of asthma and allergy, and whose chronic intermittent respiratory symptoms started before the age of 30, probably has asthma.

Some patients may have both diseases, some may have asthma with fixed (or at least partly irreversible) airway obstruction,[14] some may have COPD with eosinophilia and/or reversible airflow obstruction; others may have been incorrectly diagnosed with asthma or COPD; whereas some, particularly older patients, may have other comorbid conditions all contributing to the difficulty in making a correct diagnosis.

While there are well-developed research questionnaires available for differentiating asthma from COPD,[15] GINA and GOLD have devised two practical tables, which are helpful in making an initial working diagnosis in primary care. Table 23.1 lists the key features of asthma, COPD, and ACO, while Table 23.2 provides a checklist of features suggestive of asthma or COPD.

A practical approach suggested by GINA and GOLD for primary care and general physicians is to start by determining from Table 23.2, which features apply to a patient and then assigning an initial diagnosis accordingly. Someone with at least three features of asthma or COPD is diagnosed and treated with that disease, and if there are similar numbers of features of both diseases, then ACO should be diagnosed.[1,2] If ACO is diagnosed, then it would be advisable to consult a specialist colleague for assistance with diagnosis; however, treatment for both conditions could be initiated in people with troublesome symptoms while awaiting this opinion.

The challenge then is first to try to confirm the diagnosis in those people assumed to have asthma or COPD by assessing past medical history, family history of asthma, smoking habits and environmental exposures, lung function, and the patient's response to treatment.

23.4 CHRONIC MANAGEMENT IN PRIMARY CARE

Having made an initial diagnosis of asthma, COPD, or ACO, primary care physicians are responsible for ongoing care, including education, monitoring, treatment of exacerbations with subsequent review, and identifying those patients that may need referral for specialist advice.

Table 23.1 Usual features of asthma, COPD, and ACO

Feature	Asthma	COPD	ACO
Age of onset	Usually childhood onset but can commence at any age	Usually > 40 years of age	Usually age ≥ 40 years, but may have had symptoms in childhood or early adulthood
Pattern of respiratory symptoms	Symptoms may vary over time (day-to-day, or ever longer periods), often limiting activity. Often triggered by exercise, emotions (including laughter), dust, or exposure to allergens	Chronic usually continuous symptoms, particularly during exercise, with "better" and "worse" days	Respiratory symptoms including exertional dyspnea are persistent but variability may be prominent
Lung function	Current and/or historical variable airflow limitation (e.g., bronchodilator [BD] reversibility, airway hyperresponsiveness [AHR])	FEV_1 may be improved by therapy, but post-BD $FEV_1/FVC < 0.7$ persists	Airflow limitation not fully reversible, but often with current or historical variability
Lung function between symptoms	May be normal between symptoms	Persistent airflow limitation	Persistent airflow limitation
Past history or family history	Many patients have allergies and a personal history of asthma in childhood, and/or family history of asthma	History of exposure to noxious particles and gases (mainly tobacco smoking and biomass fuels)	Frequently a history of doctor-diagnosed asthma (current or previous), allergies, a family history of asthma, and/or a history of noxious exposures
Time course	Often improves spontaneously or with treatment, but may result in fixed airflow limitation	Generally, slowly progressive over years despite treatment	Symptoms are partly but significantly reduced by treatment. Progression is usual and treatment needs are high
Chest X-ray	Usually normal	Severe hyperinflation and other changes of COPD	Similar to COPD
Exacerbations	Exacerbations occur, but the risk of exacerbations can be considerably reduced by treatment	Exacerbations can be reduced by treatment. If present, comorbidities contribute to impairment.	Exacerbations may be more common than in COPD but are reduced by treatment. Comorbidities can contribute to impairment.
Airway inflammation	Eosinophils and/or neutrophils	Neutrophils ± eosinophils in sputum, lymphocytes in airways, may have systemic inflammation	Eosinophils and/or neutrophils in sputum

Source: The Global Strategy for Asthma Management and Prevention, Global Initiative for Asthma (GINA); 2016. Available at http://www .ginasthma.org. Reprinted with Permission; The Global Initiative for Chronic Obstructive Lung Disease (GOLD); 2016. Available at http://www.goldcopd.org. © Reprinted with Permission.

23.4.1 EDUCATION

Patients with asthma and COPD should be provided with clear information on their medication, how to recognize and what to do in the event of exacerbations and flare-ups, and when to seek medical attention. Patients can benefit from reference to an experienced asthma educator to obtain essential information and teach self-management skills, if available. Education takes time, and the busy clinicians are not always able to provide this type of intervention.

Asthma[16,17] and COPD[18,19] self-management plans (SMPs) are a good method for achieving this intervention and have been demonstrated to improve health status, and to reduce hospitalizations and physician visits. In asthma, the inclusion of PEF measurements (based on personal best) in SMPs is more effective in reducing health-care utilization and improving patient's quality of life.[17]

It is logical that poor inhaler technique renders inhaled medication ineffective,[20–22] and therefore patients must be taught, and be able to demonstrate proper use of their devices.[23] Furthermore, it is essential that medical students, primary- and secondary-care health professionals, and dispensing pharmacists are aware of the common usage errors,[24] and they learn how to select,[25] demonstrate,[26] and assess the use of the increasing numbers of different devices.[27–29]

Table 23.2 List of features suggestive of asthma or COPD

More likely to be asthma if several of ...[a]	More likely to be COPD if several of ...[a]
☐ Onset before age 20 years	☐ Onset after age 40 years
☐ Variation in symptoms over minutes, hours, or days	☐ Persistence of symptoms despite treatment
☐ Symptoms worse during the night or early morning	☐ Good and bad days but always daily symptoms and exertional dyspnea
☐ Symptoms triggered by exercise, emotions (including laughter), dust, or exposure to allergens	☐ Chronic cough and sputum preceded onset of dyspnea, unrelated to triggers
☐ Record of variable airflow limitation (spirometry, peak flow)	☐ Record of persistent airflow limitation (postbronchodilator $FEV_1/FVC < 0.7$)
☐ Lung function normal between symptoms	☐ Lung function abnormal between symptoms
☐ Previous doctor diagnosis of asthma	☐ Previous doctor diagnosis of COPD, chronic bronchitis, or emphysema
☐ Family history of asthma, and other allergic conditions (allergic rhinitis or eczema)	☐ Heavy exposure to a risk factor: tobacco smoke, biomass fuels
☐ No worsening of symptoms over time. Symptoms vary either seasonally, or from year to year	☐ Symptoms slowly worsening over time (progressive course over years)
☐ May improve spontaneously or have an immediate response to BD or to ICS over weeks	☐ Rapid-acting bronchodilator treatment provides only limited relief.
☐ Normal	☐ Severe hyperinflation

Source: The Global Strategy for Asthma Management and Prevention, Global Initiative for Asthma (GINA); 2016. Available at http://www.ginasthma.org. © Reprinted with Permission; The Global Initiative for Chronic Obstructive Lung Disease (GOLD); 2016. Available at http://www.goldcopd.org. © Reprinted with Permission.

[a] Syndromic diagnosis of airways disease, how to use table: Columns list features that, when present, best identify patients with typical asthma and COPD. For a patient, count the number of check boxes in each column. If three or more boxes are checked for either asthma or COPD, the patient is likely to have that disease. If there are similar numbers of checked boxes in each column, the diagnosis of ACO should be considered.

Enabling patients with knowledge and emergency supplies of medication for initiating treatment for exacerbations is important, not only because they may have difficulty accessing medical care early enough, but also to try and abort the attacks and prevent hospitalization. A typical self-management emergency pack for asthma usually includes oral corticosteroid tablets, an extra short-acting bronchodilator inhaler, and a peak-flow meter to monitor progress. In COPD, this would also include corticosteroid tablets and a course of broad-spectrum antibiotics. These SMPs should be agreed upon and adjusted according to the patient's understanding of their disease, and will differ according to a physician's personal approach and the regulations specific to different countries.

In all cases, patients should be taught to seek medical assistance soon after initiating these medications, mainly so the clinician can assess the severity and progress of the attack, to establish whether there were any preventable factors preceding the attack, and so that treatment and preventative measures can be optimized according to local guidelines.

23.5 MONITORING AND FOLLOW-UP

Key issues in managing chronic obstructive airflow diseases is first to acknowledge these are chronic conditions requiring ongoing attention, and also to recognize when a patient is not responding to treatment. The diagnosis may be wrong, comorbid conditions may be adversely affecting disease control, the patient may not have been prescribed or may not be taking appropriate medication, or the patient may not be administering their drugs correctly. Simply treating patients for acute flare-ups or exacerbations without recognizing these issues signify failure of treatment, is insufficient.

Following initial diagnosis and treatment, and after approximately 6 to 8 weeks or sooner following treatment for an acute attack (i.e., within a few days), a follow-up evaluation should then be arranged, to assess progress and either amend the treatment or referral to a specialist if the patient has not responded as expected.

After the initial diagnosis, further testing that could be arranged should include the following:

- Quality-assured spirometry with reversibility testing following administration of inhaled short-acting β_2-agonist bronchodilator helps both in diagnosis and in establishing severity plus risk of the disease.
- Serial PEF charts and allergy tests where indicated (skin-prick tests and specific IgE) in those patients suspected with asthma
- Blood counts and chemistry are important to identify risk factors (e.g., high eosinophil counts in asthma) and comorbid conditions (like metabolic syndrome) in asthma and COPD
  - Chest X-ray in patients with newly diagnosed COPD or ACO, because of the relatively high incidence of lung cancer and other cardiorespiratory conditions in these patients.

23.6 LUNG FUNCTION TESTS

Spirometry is regarded as the gold standard test for diagnosing obstructive airflow and reversibility. As the test results are used as a basis for diagnosis and selection of therapy options, it is essential these are performed by trained individuals, and must be of a high standard for quality assurance.[30] The spirometric features of asthma, COPD, and ACO are detailed in Table 23.3. While the absolute cutoff of 70% for FEV_1/FVC is advocated for diagnosing obstructive airflow,[2] there is some controversy as this system, compared with utilizing the Lower Limit of Normal (LLN) results in underdiagnosis of younger females and overdiagnosis of older patients.[31]

While spirometry may be the ideal test for lung function, this is not always available or practical in the primary care setting.

As normal lung function may be present at times, by definition, in the people with asthma, it is not practical in primary or specialist practice, to perform serial spirometry investigations in those with a suggestive clinical history. Therefore, apart the from usual bronchoprovocation tests (e.g., with methacholine) whenever available, serial PEF testing can be included in the investigation of people with suspected asthma with normal spirometry on initial investigation. This is a simple test, utilizing a cheap, portable instrument, which can provide serial readings taken by the patient. As it is effort-dependent, proper technique should be taught and demonstrated. These readings can be done when at and away from work to identify an occupational component,[32] before and after bronchodilator treatment to identify reversible airflow obstruction, and at different times of the day to identify diurnal patterns.[1] PEF variability of > 10% in adults supports a diagnosis of asthma, using the following formula for analyzing a twice-daily PEF chart: [(day's highest minus day's lowest)/mean of day's highest]. Physicians do need to be aware that readings may vary between individual peak-flow meters,[33] and, therefore, patients should ideally use the same PEF meter to monitor their asthma.

Table 23.3 Spirometry: Differentiating asthma, COPD, and ACO

Spirometric variable	Asthma	COPD	ACO
Normal FEV_1/FVC pre- or post-BD	Compatible with diagnosis	Not compatible with diagnosis	Not compatible unless other evidence of chronic airflow limitation
Post-BD FEV_1/FVC < 0.7	Indicates airflow limitation but may improve spontaneously or on treatment	Required for diagnosis (GOLD)	Usually present
FEV_1 ≥ 80% predicted	Compatible with diagnosis (good asthma control or interval between symptoms)	Compatible with GOLD classification of mild airflow limitation (categories A or B) if post-BD FEV_1/FVC < 0.7	Compatible with diagnosis of mild ACO
FEV_1 < 80% predicted	Compatible with diagnosis, risk factor for asthma exacerbations	An indicator of severity of airflow limitation and risk of future events (e.g., mortality and COPD exacerbations)	An indicator of severity of airflow limitation and risk of future events (e.g., mortality and exacerbations)
Post-BD increase in FEV_1 ≥ 12% and 200 ml from baseline (reversible airflow limitation)	Usual at some time in course of asthma, but may not be present when well-controlled or on controllers.	Common and more likely when FEV_1 is low	Common and more likely when FEV_1 is low
Post-BD increase in FEV_1 > 12% and 400 ml from baseline (marked reversibility)	High probability of asthma	Unusual in COPD. Consider ACO	Compatible with diagnosis of ACO

23.7 ROUTINE REVIEW

The traditional model for managing obstructive lung disease separates primary from secondary care. Patients are managed predominantly in primary care, and specialist assistance is sought for diagnosis and intermittently for emergency management. Given recent reports of poor outcomes, and marked variability in standards of care and outcomes,[34] perhaps it is time to rethink the way chronic respiratory disease is managed.

One suggestion pertaining to asthma includes[35] specialists providing outreach community clinics. There are models for providing COPD care involving an integrated approach. For example, a scheme in the northern Netherlands where patients with suspected obstructive lung disease are referred from primary to secondary care specialists, who then provide a remote-access advisory service on diagnosis and management.[36] This latter system has successfully demonstrated improved outcomes in terms of quality of life and control of patients with asthma and COPD, and may be even more feasible with the advent of telemedicine technology.

In some countries, such as the United Kingdom, chronic disease review is delegated to nurses or health-care assistants, who utilize a pro-forma checklist for doing the review. A routine review is aimed at confirming the diagnosis, assessing current control of the disease and its impact on the person's life, assessing adherence to medication, appropriateness of drugs and dosages, identifying risk factors (modifiable and otherwise), and optimizing care to reduce risk and achieve best-possible control of the disease. Therefore, patients with asthma or COPD should be reviewed in primary care by someone trained in managing these diseases. Timing of reviews will vary depending on the patient's circumstances, the severity of disease (i.e., ideally once or twice a year or more for patients with severe, difficult-to-control asthma), and soon after each exacerbation.

Objective validated questionnaires are used in research studies and could be incorporated in the routine primary care assessment of control and disease impact of asthma and COPD. Examples of these are, for asthma, the Asthma Control Questionnaire (ACQ),[37] Asthma Quality of Life Questionnaire (AQLQ),[38] and in COPD, the Clinical COPD Questionnaire (CCQ),[39] Medical Research Committee (MRC) dyspnea score or mMRC (modified MRC), Saint Georges Respiratory Questionnaire (SGRQ),[40] or COPD Assessment Test (CAT)[41] questionnaires.[1,2]

23.7.1 RECOGNIZING RISK

Assessment of asthma control is clearly demonstrated in Table 23.4. Current asthma control is assessed using four questions. Clearly, if someone has poor current symptom control, the patient's therapy needs to be optimized. However, if their disease is well controlled, a further assessment is needed to identify any risk factors for future attacks

or asthma death. These are listed for asthma in Table 23.4 and COPD in Figure 23.1.

Asthma control assessment includes two main components: current symptom control, which is assessed using presence of symptoms plus the patients need for reliever medication, and risk factors for future attacks.

Unfortunately, many clinicians only assess current symptoms, which simply provide information on the patient's status at the time of the assessment. Through education and optimization of care to reduce modifiable risk factors and noting the presence on nonmodifiable factors, future asthma attacks and deaths may be prevented. Section A in Table 23.4 lists four questions related to current symptoms. If the patient has poor current control, medication or the device may need changing. However, if the patient is well controlled currently, an assessment of risk is still indicated.

Section B of Table 23.4 summarizes the risk factors that, if present, should be addressed at the time of assessment. For example, someone using excess relievers or insufficient preventer medication, or with poor inhaler technique, may need advice and optimization of treatment. Furthermore, someone who has had a recent attack could be recalled for an earlier review, and patients who are at heightened risk, for example with a history of reduced FEV_1 percentage predicted below 60% and/or a previous life-threatening attack could be referred to a severe asthma service for advice.

A common misconception among clinicians is that asthma severity is determined by the amount of drug(s) prescribed, which is an incorrect assertion. Severity of asthma is defined as *the amount of treatment needed to control asthma*, not the amount of treatment prescribed.[42,43] Therefore, an assessment of asthma control and risk, together with the guideline treatment step is used to classify severity. Most of the patients in the U.K. NRAD[10] were misclassified with mild or moderately severe asthma; only 19% of those who died had a record of an assessment of asthma control.

In the case of COPD, GOLD has developed a system for assessing risk (see Figure 23.1). This is based on symptoms, impact on health, quality of life, spirometric classification of severity, and risk of exacerbations. Symptoms and health-related quality of life (HRQL), and the impact of HRQL, is assessed through questionnaires; i.e., the CAT and the MRC COPD symptom scores. Risk of exacerbations is determined by the patient's history of exacerbations.

Finally, the GOLD classification of severity according to spirometry ranging from mild to severe in patients with $FEV_1/FVC < 0.70$, (i.e., defined as having obstructive airflow limitation) is as follows[2]:

- GOLD 1: Mild = $FEV_1 \geq \_80\%$ predicted
- GOLD 2: Moderate = $50\% \leq FEV_1 < 80\%$ predicted
- GOLD 3: Severe = $30\% \leq FEV_1 < 50\%$ predicted
- GOLD 4: Very Severe = $FEV_1 < 30\%$ predicted

Through the use of Figure 23.1, clinicians can allocate patients to one of four categories of risk to help guide treatment decisions (such as referral for pulmonary rehabilitation

Table 23.4 GINA Assessment of asthma control

A. Asthma symptom control			Level of asthma symptom control		
			Well controlled	Partly controlled	Uncontrolled
In the past 4 weeks, has the patient had:					
• Daytime asthma symptoms more than twice per week?	Yes ☐ No ☐		None of these	1–2 of these	3–4 of these
• Any night waking due to asthma?	Yes ☐ No ☐				
• Reliever needed for symptoms* more than twice per week?	Yes ☐ No ☐				
• Any activity limitation due to asthma?	Yes ☐ No ☐				

B. Risk factors for poor asthma outcomes

Assess risk factors at diagnosis and periodically, particularly for patients experiencing exacerbations. Measure FEV_1 at start of treatment, after 3–6 months of controller treatment to record the patient's personal-best lung function, then periodically for ongoing risk assessment.

Potentially modifiable independent risk factors for flare-ups (exacerbations)
- Uncontrolled asthma symptoms
- High SABA use (with increased mortality if > 1 × 200-dose canister per month)
- Inadequate ICS: not prescribed ICS, poor adherence, incorrect inhaler technique
- Low FEV_1, especially if <60% predicted
- Major psychological or socioeconomic problems
- Exposures: smoking, allergen exposure if sensitized
- Comorbidities: obesity, rhinosinusitis, confirmed food allergy
- Sputum or blood eosinophilia
- Pregnancy

Other major independent risk factors for flare-ups (exacerbations)
- Ever intubated or in intensive care unit for asthma
- ≥ 1 severe exacerbation in last 12 months

> Having one or more of these risk factors increases the risk of exacerbations even if symptoms are well controlled.

Risk factors for developing fixed airflow limitation
- Lack of ICS treatment
- Exposures: tobacco smoke, noxious chemicals, occupational exposures
- Low initial FEV_1, chronic mucus hypersecretion, sputum or blood eosinophilia

Risk factors for medication side effects
- *Systemic:* frequent OCS; long-term, high-dose, and/or potent ICS; also lacking P450 inhibilors
- *Local:* high-dose or potent ICS, poor inhaler technique

Source: The Global Strategy for Asthma Management and Prevention, Global Initiative for Asthma (GINA); 2016. Available at http://www.ginasthma.org. © Reprinted with Permission; The Global Initiative for Chronic Obstructive Lung Disease (GOLD); 2016. Available at http://www.goldcopd.org. © Reprinted with Permission.

or prescription of ambulatory oxygen) and the need for specialist referral.

In the management of COPD and asthma in primary care, failure to classify severity of disease and risk of future attacks may result in inadequate or inappropriate treatment, or a referral for specialist advice when needed.

23.7.2 NONPHARMACOLOGICAL TREATMENT

Chronic exposure to environmental pollution (either inside or outside the home) should be reduced or eliminated, and regular exercise should be encouraged (with pulmonary rehabilitation in COPD). Weight reduction, healthy diet, and breathing exercises are of benefit.[1,2]

23.7.3 DRUG TREATMENT

Treatment of asthma and COPD in primary care varies from one country to another. Often this relates to the funding system, where in some countries, specialist initiation of treatments is required. Overall, the treatment of these two diseases follows a stepwise progression, which is described in detail in the GINA[1] and GOLD[2] strategy documents, as well as in local country-based systems.

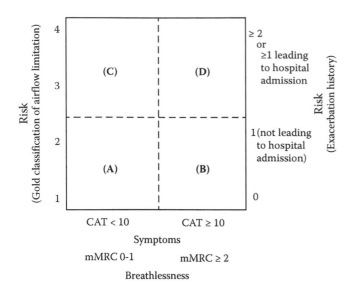

Figure 23.1 GOLD assessment using symptoms, breathlessness, spirometric classification, and risk of exacerbations. (From The Global Strategy for Asthma Management and Prevention, Global Initiative for Asthma (GINA); 2016. Available at http://www.ginasthma.org. © Reprinted with Permission; The Global Initiative for Chronic Obstructive Lung Disease (GOLD); 2016. Available at http://www.gold-copd.org. © Reprinted with Permission.)

In asthma, treatment includes low- to high-dose ICSs, with the addition of long-acting β_2-agonist bronchodilators (LABAs), and additional drugs depending on severity. In addition, short-acting bronchodilators (SABAs) are used for relief treatment and when there is increased need for these drugs, which serve as an early warning system of impending attacks. Newer combination therapies with three drugs are available in some countries; their role in asthma care is currently being investigated.

In COPD, treatment begins with bronchodilators in mild to moderate cases, with the addition of ICSs as the disease severity progresses. As in the case of asthma, newer triple combinations of drugs are licensed in some countries, with ongoing studies.

In those patients with mixed asthma and COPD, care needs to be taken to ensure that both diseases are treated appropriately, in particular, starting ICSs in patients with mild, persistent asthma. Medications for treatment of asthma and COPD are discussed more extensively in Chapter 17.

23.7.4 COMORBIDITIES

Patients health status and symptoms may be adversely affected due to comorbid conditions associated with asthma and COPD. Given the generalist nature of expertise of primary care physicians, they are often well placed to identify and treat these conditions. In asthma, conditions such as chronic rhinitis, gastroesophageal reflux, dysfunctional breathing, obstructive sleep apnea, and psychological problems should be diagnosed and treated. Weight loss should be advised in the obese patient. Similarly, patients with COPD are also prone to a number of comorbidities, such as metabolic syndrome, osteoporosis, and cor-pulmonale, which need to be identified and managed either by the primary care physician or in conjunction with an appropriate specialist.

Finally, some of the barriers and facilitators in optimizing respiratory care in primary care form the perspective of health-care professionals, as well as patients, are summarized in Table 23.5. (The Global Strategy for Asthma Management and Prevention, Global Initiative for Asthma (GINA); 2016. Available at http://www.ginasthma.org. Reprinted with permission.)

23.8 CONCLUSIONS

Health professionals working in primary care are faced with considerable challenges in managing patients with chronic obstructive lung diseases such as asthma and COPD. The key to this role is the recognition that these are chronic, relapsing conditions that must not be treated as if they are acute diseases. The primary care physician has a critical role in the diagnosis, identification of risk,

Table 23.5 Barriers and facilitators to optimal respiratory care in primary care practice

Primary health-care providers	Patients and their families
Insufficient knowledge of guideline recommendations	Low health literacy
Lack of agreement with recommendations or expectation that they will be effective	Insufficient understanding of their disease, its management, and failure to adhere to medical advice
Resistance to change; ingrained habits	Lack of agreement with doctor's recommendations
Inadequate skill in lung function testing and interpretation	Cultural and economic barriers
External barriers (organizational, health policies, financial constraints)	Peer influence and advice on medication and behavior
Lack of time and resources	Attitudes, beliefs, preferences, fears, and misconceptions
Lack of provision of patient education resulting in preventable acute exacerbations	
Lack of support from secondary care colleagues	

initiation of treatment, ongoing monitoring, and patient education. For difficult-to-control symptoms, the primary care physician should seek further advice from a respiratory therapist who can help address environmental issues and other comorbidities that are obfuscating improved outcomes. Guidelines have provided consensus evidence-based practical approaches that have carefully considered global differences in health care. However, access to health care and more advanced therapies due to economics no doubt continues to remain a problem for many countries.

REFERENCES

1. The Global Strategy for Asthma Management and Prevention, Global Initiative for Asthma (GINA); 2016. Available at http://www.ginasthma.org.
2. The Global Initiative for Chronic Obstructive Lung Disease (GOLD); 2016. Available at http://www.goldcopd.org.
3. Reddel HK. Treatment of overlapping asthma-chronic obstructive pulmonary disease: Can guidelines contribute in an evidence-free zone? *J Allergy Clinical Immunol.* 2015;136(3):546–552.
4. Levy ML, Fletcher M, Price DB et al. International primary care respiratory group (IPCRG) guidelines: Diagnosis of respiratory diseases in primary care. *Prim Care Resp J.* 2006;15(1):20–34.
5. Pavord I, Bush A. Two lovely black eyes; oh, what a surprise! *Thorax.* 2015;70(7):609–610.
6. Gibson PG and McDonald VM. Asthma-COPD overlap 2015: Now we are six. *Thorax.* 2015;70(7):683–691.
7. Magnoni MS, Caminati M, Senna G et al. Asthma under/misdiagnosis in primary care setting: An observational community-based study in Italy. *Clin Mol Allergy.* 2015;13:26.
8. Martinez CH, Mannino DM, Jaimes FA et al. Undiagnosed obstructive lung disease in the United States associated factors and long-term mortality. *Ann Am Thorac Soc.* 2015;12(12):1788–1795.
9. Tinkelman D, Price D, Nordyke R et al. Misdiagnosis of COPD and asthma in primary care patients 40 years of age and over. *J Asthma.* 2006;43(1):75–80.
10. Why asthma still kills: The National Review of Asthma Deaths (NRAD) Confidential Enquiry report Royal College of Physicians. London; 2014. Available at http://www.rcplondon.ac.uk/sites/default/files/why -asthma-still-kills-full-report.pdf.
11. The International Classification of Diseases (ICD): World Health Organisation; 2013. Available at http://www.who.int/classifications/icd/en/.
12. Bateman ED, Reddel HK, van Zyl-Smit RN et al. The asthma-COPD overlap syndrome: Towards a revised taxonomy of chronic airways diseases? *Lancet Resp Med.* 2015;3(9):719–728.
13. Gibson PG and Simpson JL. The overlap syndrome of asthma and COPD: What are its features and how important is it? *Thorax.* 2009;64(8):728–735.
14. Vonk JM, Jongepier H, Panhuysen CIM et al. Risk factors associated with the presence of irreversible airflow limitation and reduced transfer coefficient in patients with asthma after 26 years of follow up. *Thorax.* 2003;58(4):322–327.
15. Tinkelman DG, Price DB, Nordyke RJ et al. Symptom-based questionnaire for differentiating COPD and asthma. *Respiration.* 2006;73(3):296–305.
16. McDonald VM and Gibson PG. Asthma education. In JA Bernstein, ML Levy eds., *Clinical Asthma:Theory and Practice.* London: CRC Press, 2014; 127–137.
17. Gibson PG and Powell H. Written action plans for asthma: An evidence-based review of the key components. *Thorax.* 2004;59(2):94–99.
18. Gadoury MA, Schwartzman K, Rouleau M et al. Self-management reduces both short- and long-term hospitalisation in COPD. *Europ Resp J.* 2005;26(5):853–857.
19. Bourbeau J. Disease-specific self-management programs in patients with advanced chronic obstructive pulmonary disease: A comprehensive and critical evaluation. *Dis Manage Health Outcomes.* 2003;11(5):311–319.
20. Melani AS. Inhalatory therapy training: A priority challenge for the physician. *Acta Biomed Ateneo Parm.* 2007;78(3):233–245.
21. Molimard M and Gros VL. Impact of patient-related factors on asthma control. *J Asthma.* 2008;45(2):109–113.
22. Levy ML, Hardwell A, McKnight E et al. Asthma patients' inability to use a pressurised metered-dose inhaler (pMDI) correctly correlates with poor asthma control as defined by the Global Initiative for Asthma (GINA) strategy: A retrospective analysis. *Prim Care Resp J.* 2013;22(4):406–411.
23. Asthma. NICE quality standard 25 (2013): National Institute for Health and Clinical Excellence 2013; Available at http://publications.nice.org.uk/quality -standard-for-asthma-qs25. Accessed March 6, 2013
24. Sanchis J, Corrigan C, Levy ML et al. Inhaler devices—From theory to practice. *Respir Med.* 2013;107(4):495–502.
25. Vincken W, Dekhuijzen PNR, Barnes P et al. The ADMIT series—Issues in inhalation therapy. 4) How to choose inhaler devices for the treatment of COPD. *Prim Care Resp J.* 2010;19(1):10–20.
26. Lavorini F, Levy ML, Corrigan C et al. The ADMIT series—Issues in inhalation therapy. 6) training tools for inhalation devices. *Prim Care Resp J.* 2010;19(4):335–341.
27. Press VG, Arora VM, Shah LM et al. Teaching the use of respiratory inhalers to hospitalized patients with asthma or COPD: A randomized trial. *J Gen Intern Med.* 2012;27(10):1317–1325.

28. Takemura M, Kobayashi M, Kimura K et al. Repeated instruction on inhalation technique improves adherence to the therapeutic regimen in asthma. *J Asthma.* 2010;47(2):202–208.

29. Takemura M, Mitsui K, Itotani R et al. Relationships between repeated instruction on inhalation therapy, medication adherence, and health status in chronic obstructive pulmonary disease. *Int J COPD.* 2011;6(1):97–104.

30. Levy ML, Quanjer PH, Booker R et al. Standards for diagnostic spirometry within session repeatability in primary care. *Prim Care Resp J.* 2012;21:252–253.

31. Miller MR and Levy ML. Chronic obstructive pulmonary disease: Missed diagnosis versus misdiagnosis. *BMJ (Online).* 2015;351.

32. Huggins V, Anees W, Pantin C et al. Improving the quality of peak flow measurements for the diagnosis of occupational asthma. *Occup Med.* 2005;55(5):385–388.

33. Miller MR, Hankinson J, Brusasco V et al. Standardisation of spirometry. *Euro Resp J.* 2005;26(2):319–338.

34. European Respiratory Society. European lung white book; 2013. Available at http://www.erswhitebook.org/.

35. Levy ML and Winter R. Asthma deaths: What now? *Thorax.* 2015;70(3):209–210.

36. Metting EI, Riemersma RA, Kocks JH et al. Feasibility and effectiveness of an Asthma/COPD service for primary care: A cross-sectional baseline description and longitudinal results. *NPJ Primary Care Resp Med.* 2015;25:14101. doi: 10.1038/npjpcrm.2014.101.

37. Juniper EF, O'Byrne PM, Guyatt GH et al. Development and validation of a questionnaire to measure asthma control. *Eur Respir J.* 1999;14(4):902–907.

38. Juniper EF, Guyatt GH, Ferrie PJ et al. Measuring quality of life in asthma. *AM Rev Resp Dis.* 1993;147(4):832–838.

39. van Der Molen T. Clinical COPD questionnaire. Biomed central [Internet]. 1999. Available at http://www.biomedcentral.com/content/supplementary/1465-9921-7-62-S1.PDF.

40. Jones PW, Quirk FH, and Baveystock CM. The St George's respiratory questionnaire. *Respi Med.* 1991;85(Suppl. B):25–31.

41. Jones PW, Brusselle G, Dal Negro RW et al. Health-related quality of life in patients by COPD severity within primary care in Europe. *Resp Med.* 2011;105(1):57–66.

42. Reddel HK, Taylor DR, Bateman ED et al. An official American thoracic society/European respiratory society statement: Asthma control and exacerbations - standardizing endpoints for clinical asthma trials and clinical practice. *American J R Critical Care Med.* 2009;180(1):59–99.

43. Taylor DR, Bateman ED, Boulet LP et al. A new perspective on concepts of asthma severity and control. *Eur resp J.* 2008;32(3):545–554.

Index